A–Z of

Plastic Surgery

Matthew Fell is the nationally appointed Cleft Lip and Palate Training Interface Group (TIG) Fellow at the Spires Cleft Centre in Oxford and Salisbury for 2023/2024. Matthew qualified from Manchester University Medical School in 2011 and completed his Plastic Surgery training in Exeter and Bristol within the South West Deanery, and undertook specialist Cleft and Craniofacial training at the Royal Children's Hospital in Melbourne, Australia in 2022. He is an Honorary research fellow with the Cleft Collective at the University of Bristol, a Trustee for the CLEFT charity (www.cleft.org.uk) and holds an advisory role for Transforming Faces (www.transformingfaces.org).

Susan Hendrickson studied at Oxford University and University College London and undertook Foundation and Core Surgical Training in London before embarking on her plastic surgical training in Bristol and the Southwest. She undertook specialist fellowships in extremity trauma reconstruction and breast microsurgical reconstruction in London, Bristol and Sydney, Australia. She has a passion for microsurgery and extremity trauma reconstruction and enjoyed working on this book while revising for her FRCS(Plast) with Matt, her co-author, colleague, and friend.

Andrew Hodges is a plastic surgeon currently working for CURE International in Zimbabwe and wrote the first edition of the A-Z during his plastic surgery training in Exeter and Plymouth, UK. After his training he spent 15 years as a plastic surgeon in Uganda and 3 years in the Philippines.

For recommended web links for this title, visit www.oxfordreference.com/page/geog when you see this sign.

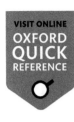

The most authoritative and up-to-date reference books for both students and the general reader.

Many of these titles are also available online at www.oxfordreference.com

A–Z of
Plastic Surgery

SECOND EDITION

MATTHEW FELL
SUSAN HENDRICKSON
ANDREW HODGES

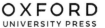

OXFORD
UNIVERSITY PRESS

OXFORD
UNIVERSITY PRESS

Great Clarendon Street, Oxford, OX2 6DP,
United Kingdom

Oxford University Press is a department of the University of Oxford.
It furthers the University's objective of excellence in research, scholarship,
and education by publishing worldwide. Oxford is a registered trade mark of
Oxford University Press in the UK and in certain other countries

© Oxford University Press 2024

The moral rights of the authors have been asserted

Published in the United States of America by Oxford University Press
198 Madison Avenue, New York, NY 10016, United States of America

British Library Cataloguing in Publication Data

Data available

Library of Congress Control Number: 2024934064

ISBN 978-0-19-285895-5

Printed and bound by
CPI Group (UK) Ltd, Croydon, CR0 4YY

Links to third party websites are provided by Oxford in good faith and
for information only. Oxford disclaims any responsibility for the materials
contained in any third party website referenced in this work.

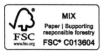

Contents

Preface to the 1st Edition

Plastic surgery is an extremely broad subject and the trainee in this specialty is required to assimilate a large amount of information. The *A–Z of Plastic Surgery* has been written as an aid to learning and revising this material and as a reference book. Although it is written in an encyclopaedic format, it does not claim to be a complete text. The concise style should enable subjects to be grasped rapidly. However, this book does not replace, but rather complements fuller chapter-based texts. The primary focus is for plastic surgery trainees, but it will also be of value to the specialist as a reference text and to medical workers in allied specialties. In a book of this scope and size there will inevitably be controversy as to what should be included or omitted, and under which heading. In this rapidly changing and expanding specialty, the author would welcome contributions and comments from readers—particularly to augment existing entries or to suggest new entries. These will be incorporated into the second edition.

Andrew Hodges
Consultant Plastic Surgeon
Mengo Hospital, Kampala, Uganda

Preface to the 2nd Edition

We were honoured to take this opportunity with Andrew to update the *A–Z of Plastic Surgery*. We trained together in London and the Southwest of England and share a passion for developing plastic surgery services in low- and middle-income countries. Andrew Hodges and his wife Sarah have been an inspiration for many years due to their never-ending energy, natural inquisitiveness and commitment to populations in less resourced settings around the globe. The Hodges returned to the United Kingdom briefly in 2017 to work in Exeter, which coincided with our higher surgical training and led to this team effort for the updated second edition.

We combined our subspecialty interests of limb reconstruction/trauma and cleft/craniofacial respectively with our coordinated campaign to prepare for the FRCS Plast examination to update this edition with oversight from Andrew. We wanted to retain the concise and compact nature of the first edition whilst modernizing the content. Plastic surgery continues to evolve at a rapid pace and the innovations are extraordinarily exciting for patients and clinicians alike. We look forward to being a part of this specialty and to bearing witness to further improvements that future editions of the *A–Z* will document.

Matthew Fell and Susan Hendrickson

This book is dedicated to Matthew's wife Tessa and his children Poppy and Florence, Susan's husband James and her children Annabel and Eliza and Andrew's wife Sarah and his children Naomi, Sam and Rachel.

Acknowledgements

We are grateful to the plastic surgeons and wider interdisciplinary team who have inspired and taught us around the world.

Both Matthew and Susan are grateful to their trainers and mentors in the South West, including Umraz Khan, Thomas Chapman, Emily West, Sankhya Sen, Thomas Wright, George Wheble, James Henderson, Chris Wallace, Sherif Wilson, Rachel Tillett, Philippa Jackson and Rachel Clancy. Matthew would also like to thank Gus McGrouther, Mark McGurk, Per Hall and Marc Swan, and Susan would like to thank Shehan Hettiaratchy, Joe Dusseldorp and David Kulber.

Andrew would like to acknowledge Tim Goodacre, who first introduced him to this exciting specialty, and plastic surgeons in Exeter, Peter Saxby, John Palmer, Vik Devaraj and Chris Stone, who helped him throughout his training and particularly in preparation for the final plastic surgery examinations.

We thank James Henderson for his talented cover design. We are grateful to Oxford University Press, James Oates, Caroline Smith and the rest of the team for their assistance in publishing this book, and for their valuable comments and suggestions.

How to use this book

- Entries are arranged in alphabetical order. Some subjects are grouped under one main heading.
- Words that are *italicized* and <u>underlined</u> are cross references to other entries. Other cross references are shown by small capitals.
- Abbreviations have been used to maintain the concise style. A list of abbreviations is available at the end of the book.

Abbé flap to Axonotmesis

Abbé flap

- A pedicled two-stage lip-switch flap for reconstructing moderate-sized defects of the lip.
- Especially useful to reconstruct a central defect on the upper lip, although can also be used for lower lip defects.
- Blood supply is from the labial artery, which lies deep to the orbicularis oris muscle at approximately the level of the vermilion-cutaneous junction.
- Measure the anticipated defect before excision and plan the flap so that the width of the vermilion is slightly less than the segment being replaced, to allow for stretch and minimize donor morbidity.
- The Abbé flap may be quadrilateral, forked or winged to assist closure of the donor lip defect.
- Make a full thickness incision on one side of the flap and use the identified position of the labial artery to assist with preservation of the blood supply when making an incision through skin and muscle only on the other side of the flap.
- The lower lip can sacrifice 25–35% of its length.
- While pedicle remains attached the patient requires a soft diet.
- Divide the flap in 2–3 weeks.

See LIP RECONSTRUCTION. *See* SECONDARY LIP AND NASAL DEFORMITIES.

Abdominal wall anatomy

Function: abdominal wall muscles important for posture, standing, walking and bending.

Components:
- Soft tissue cover.
- Laterally based musculoaponeurotic system:
  - *External oblique:* from lower 8 ribs, inserts into iliac crest and forms inguinal ligament;
  - *Internal oblique:* from lumbodorsal fascia, iliac crest and inguinal ligament. Lower fibres form conjoint tendon. Superior fibres insert into linea alba and rib cartilages 7–9;
  - *Transversus abdominis:* from lower 6 ribs, lumbodorsal fascia and iliac crest into linea alba and conjoint tendon.
- Central muscles:
  - *Rectus abdominis:* paired longitudinal muscles from symphysis to xiphoid and ribs 5–7 and enclosed in rectus sheath;
  - *Pyramidalis:* small triangular muscle superficial to rectus abdominus. From pubis to linea halfway between symphysis and umbilicus.

The linea semilunaris runs along the lateral edge of the rectus abdominis and is the site of union where tendons of the lateral abdominal muscles meet the rectus sheath. The arcuate line is the inferior margin of the posterior rectus sheath and lies midway between umbilicus and pubis. Above this the internal oblique aponeurosis splits and half passes deep to rectus. Below this the posterior rectus sheath is only composed of transversus abdominis. Neurovascular structures lie between internal oblique and transversus abdominis and this is where a transversus abdominis plane (TAP) block is delivered.

Blood supply can be considered in the zones described by Huger:
- *Zone 1:* lies centrally in the vicinity of the rectus abdominis muscle and is supplied by the superior epigastric artery and deep inferior epigastric artery.
- *Zone 2:* lies across the caudal end of the abdominal wall and is supplied by the superficial inferior epigastric artery, the superficial circumflex iliac artery and the superficial external pudendal artery.
- *Zone 3:* encompasses the two lateral aspects of the abdominal wall and is supplied by the thoracic and lumbar intercostal arteries.

Abdominal wall reconstruction

Indications:
- *Trauma.*
- *Tumour:* Desmoid, Dermatofibrosarcoma protuberans.
- *Radiation.*
- *Infection:* Gas gangrene, Necrotizing fasciitis.

- *Iatrogenic: Incisional hernia.*
- *Congenital: Omphalocoele, Gastroschisis, Prune belly syndrome.*

Pre-operatively:
- Manage risk factors for complications including smoking, obesity, nutritional status, wound healing problems and chronic lung disease.
- CT to provide details of defect, quality of muscles and loss of domain.

Procedures:
- *Skin only defects:* consider direct repair, skin grafts or local flaps based on vessels supplying the abdominal skin.
- *Myofascial defects:* component separation is the mainstay:
  - Anterior component separation via incision through the external oblique aponeurosis at linea semilunaris. Good for superior defects;
  - Posterior component separation and transverse abdominis release (TAR) allows greater medialization and ample space for mesh placement;
  - Possible to do anterior on one side and posterior on the other but not both on one side.
- *Full thickness defects:* if primary repair not feasible consider:
  - Pedicled flaps—rectus abdominis, external oblique, latissimus dorsi, tensor fascia lata or rectus femoris;
  - Free flaps or abdominal wall transplant.
- *Mesh:* the use of mesh has been associated with superior repairs in abdominal hernia repair compared to sutures alone. Mesh can be synthetic, biologic or biosynthetic. Location of the mesh is more important than fixation and options include onlay, inlay or sublay.

Post-op considerations:
- High-care setting and bed rest initially.
- Fluids and nutrition in line with evidence of bowel motility.
- Drains to reduce risk of seroma.
- Abdominal binder.

Abdominoplasty
- A procedure which aims to provide a flatter, narrower abdomen by excising skin and fat excess and addressing rectus divarication, generally by using a lower transverse abdominal scar.

Operation:
- Mark skin incision with a large ellipse. The lower line passes just above the pubic hairs and is flattened centrally. For a full abdominoplasty, the upper line will be around the level of the umbilicus.

- Elevate flap at sub-Scarpa's level, can leave thin layer of tissue intact over the deep muscle fascia (theoretically preserves lymphatics). Proceed up to xiphoid if needed.
- Dissect out umbilicus.
- Limit lateral dissection to preserve lateral skin perforators.
- Consider plication of the rectus sheath.
- Pull the skin flap inferiorly and make the upper incision.
- Suture flap and find new location for the umbilicus.

Variations:
- *Mini abdominoplasty:* superior extent of undermining limited to umbilical level.
- *Lipo-abdominoplasty:* combines liposuction with abdominoplasty.
- *Fleur-de-lis:* inverted T-shaped excision of skin and fat to address central tissue excess.
- *Panniculectomy:* amputation of apron without undermining.
- *Circumferential abdominoplasty:* for circumferential tissue excess.

Complications:
- *Early:* nerve injury, asymmetry.
- *Later:* thromboembolism, respiratory difficulties, skin necrosis, wound dehiscence, wound infections, haematoma, seroma.

Abductor pollicis brevis
APB: most superficial muscle of thenar eminence.

Origin: transverse carpal ligament, palmaris longus and there may also be another slip from abductor pollicis longus.

Insertion: the tendon is adherent to the radial side of the MCP joint capsule. A few fibres join FPB and radial sesamoid. The rest join the extensor expansion.

Nerve supply: median nerve.

Action: abduction of the thumb at the carpometacarpal and MCP joint. This is a forward movement in the anteroposterior plane.
See MUSCLES.

Abductor pollicis longus
Origin: dorsum of radius, ulnar and interosseous membrane. It runs obliquely around the radius coursing over the wrist extensors. It runs in the 1st extensor compartment with extensor pollicis brevis and may have several slips.

Insertion: lateral 1st metacarpal. It gives off a slip to trapezium and another to APB.

Nerve supply: posterior interosseous nerve.

Action: abducts the thumb through slip to APB. Extends the thumb and radially deviates the wrist.

See MUSCLES.

Absorbable polymers
Synthetic:
• Used for sutures and investigated for other devices such as plates and screws (LactoSorb™).
• One class of polymers used is the alpha-hydroxy acids including L-lactic acid, glycolic acid and dioxanone.
• As polymers these are:
  ○ *PLLA:* poly-l-lactic acid;
  ○ *PGA:* polyglycolic acid;
  ○ polydioxanone.
• PLLA and PGA are used together. Breakdown is by hydrolytic scission of the ester bond.
• PGA is degraded more rapidly than PLLA.
• Dexon™ is pure PGA. Vicryl™ is 8% PLA, 92% PGA.

Natural:
• Many materials are produced from *Collagen*.
• Haemostatic properties can be reduced by isolating collagen into fibrils.
• The haemostatic properties can also be utilized.

See ALLOPLASTS.

Acanthosis
Hyperplasia of epithelium. *See* SKIN.

Accutane
Isotretinoin. The synthetic retinoid derivative 13-*cis*-retinoic acid (Accutane™) used for severe *Acne vulgaris*. The dose is 1 mg/kg body weight for an initial 4-5-month course of therapy. It reduces sebum excretion and is anti-inflammatory. Side effects can be limiting, including dry skin, dry eyes, dry mucous membranes, nosebleeds and mood disturbance. Female patients must take contraception during treatment due to risk of severe congenital defects. Acne may worsen initially before improving.

Acne vulgaris
• Acne vulgaris is a common skin disorder seen in adolescents and young adults.
• Seborrhoea, small comedones, and inflammatory papulopustules found.
• Acne conglobata is the severe form with deep cysts and sinuses with extensive scarring of face back and chest.

Management:
• Dietary control does not appear to be beneficial.
• Topical medications with benzoyl peroxide, topical antibiotics or tretinoin (retinoic acid).

• Skin hygiene and long-term administration of antibiotics, such as tetracycline, has been helpful.
• Ultraviolet rays and superficial X-ray therapy are effective, but with unacceptable long-term effects.
• *Accutane* is effective for severe acne.
• Dermabrasion, laser resurfacing and collagen injections may help reduce the scarring. Incision of the cystic lesions reduces the inflammation that produces the scarring.

Acrochordon
• Common papillomatous lesion occurring in middle adult life.
• Multiple, fleshy, skin-coloured tags.
• Occur mainly on neck, upper chest and axilla.
• The only symptoms relate to local irritation.
• Excise with scalpel or scissors.

See MESODERMAL TUMOURS.

Acrosyndactyly
• One of the *Congenital hand anomalies*.
• Fusion of digits distally.
• Mainly sporadic, non-hereditary occurrence.
• Associated with *Constriction ring syndrome*.
• Bilateral in 50%, but asymmetric.
• Also associated with craniofacial syndactyly, such as *Apert's syndrome*, in which it is symmetrical.

Management:
• *Type 1:* conjoined fingertips with normal webspaces—separation and contouring of tips.
• *Type 2:* conjoined fingertips and incomplete webspace formation—separation of tips and deepening of webspace.
• *Type 3:* sinus tracts are the only separation between absent webspaces and joined digits—requires formal syndactyly release.

Actinic keratosis
Also called senile keratosis and solar keratosis.
• Often multiple well-circumscribed, erythematous scaly lesions occurring on sun exposed skin due to the cumulative effect of UV exposure.
• The most frequently occurring premalignant cutaneous condition. More common if genetically predisposed. Over time may progress to *SCC* and 20–25% become invasive. SCCs arising from actinic keratosis rarely metastasize.
• Microscopically get hyperkeratosis with dyskaryosis and acanthosis. In the dermis there is an actinic elastosis with inflammatory infiltrate.

Management:
• Lesions may regress if sun exposure is limited.

- Treat with excision, curettage, liquid nitrogen, 5-fluorouracil (efudex), chemical peel, dermabrasion and photodynamic therapy (*PDT*).

  See CUTANEOUS HORN.

Adductor pollicis
Origin:
- *Oblique head:* transverse carpal ligament, anterior surface base of 2nd and 3rd metacarpal.
- *Transverse head:* from anterior surface of shaft of 3rd metacarpal. Two heads join. The transverse fibres insert mainly into the medial sesamoid and the oblique into the extensor expansion.

Insertion: with the 1st palmar interosseous into medial side of base of proximal phalanx.

Nerve: deep branch of ulnar nerve.

Action: adduction of the thumb at the carpo-metacarpal and metacarpophalangeal joint. This is a backward movement in an anteroposterior plane.

  See MUSCLES.

Adipofascial flaps
A flap comprised of fascia and overlying fat. Essentially, the same as a fasciocutaneous flap with the skin dissected away from the flap.

Anatomy:
- Dermal and fascial plexuses exist in subcutaneous tissues. Both gain their blood supply from perforators.
- In adipofascial flaps the tissues are divided between plexuses leaving the dermal and subdermal plexuses to supply the skin and the fascial plexuses are taken with the flap to supply it.
- Three perifascial plexuses are described—sub-, intra- and prefascial plexuses. All anastomose, but only pre- and subfascial plexuses receive branches from perforators. The prefascial plexus (superficial to fascia) is dominant.

Properties: adipofascial flaps are easy to raise, are more malleable and conform better than fasciocutaneous flaps. They are not so robust and require a skin graft onto the flap.

Indications:
- *Lower limb:* medial flaps use posterior tibial perforators. Usually 2–5 of these, fairly constant. There are usually 4–5 anterior tibial perforators. The perforators to the peroneal artery are less predictable, but usually number 4–5.

- *Upper limb:* small adipofascial flaps can be raised from the dorsum of the finger to cover finger tips or exposed bone.

Adnexal tumours of the skin
- Benign or malignant tumours of the skin appendages and classified by the degree of differentiation to sweat and sebaceous glands, and hair follicles.
- In adnexal tumours, the relationship between stromal and epithelial components is maintained though distorted to varying degrees.
- They are also termed organoid or appendageal tumours or *Hamartomas*.
- A tumour with fully developed appendageal structures is called a *Naevus*.
- A tumour with incomplete development of structures is an *Adenoma*.
- A poorly organized tumour is an *Epithelioma*.

Adrenaline
- Extensively used in plastic surgery to produce vasoconstriction, which reduces blood loss during surgery.
- Adrenaline can cause cardiac arrhythmias especially in conjunction with halothane.
- The maximum recommended dose is 10 ml of 1:100,000 (100 µg) over 10 minutes or 30 ml (300 µg) over 1 hour.
- 1 ml 1:1,000 in 200 ml = 1:200,000.
- Topical soaks for haemostasis can be 1:10,000.
- The total dose of adrenaline should *not* exceed 500 µg and it is essential not to exceed a concentration of 1 in 200,000 (5 µg/ml) if more than 50 ml of the mixture is to be injected.
- Generally avoided in end arteries, such as digital vessels, although several trials have shown no adverse effects in such situations.

Adson's test
A test used in the assessment of *Thoracic outlet syndrome*.
- Patient stands with arm adducted against front of trunk. Feel radial pulse.
- Extend neck and turn chin to affected side. This stretches and tightens the *Scalene* muscles causing neural or arterial compression by scissoring effect.
- Now take a deep breath. This depresses the first rib. Hold breath while traction is applied to arm and feel the pulse. Loss of pulse volume or neurological signs gives a positive result.
- Reverse Adson's test: patient in same position, but patient flexes neck and rotates chin to contralateral side to shorten the scalenes. Push down with chin against chest to contract scalenes. This may reproduce symptoms when there is scalene hypertrophy.

Advancement flaps
A local random pattern flap where tissue is advanced to fill an adjacent defect. Examples include:

- *Single pedicle:* raised as a square or rectangle with two parallel cuts along the sides of the defect. *Burow's triangles* are excised from the base of the flap to help advancement.
- *Bipedicled advancement flap:* useful for long defects in extremities. An incision is made parallel to the defect and the flap attached at either end is advanced. As there is a blood supply from either end a longer length to width ratio is possible. The donor defect can be grafted.
- *V–Y advancement flap*.

Aeromonas hydrophila
- Gram-negative anaerobic rod.
- Aid the nutrition of leeches by producing enzymes to break down red blood cells and haemoglobin.
- Usually sensitive to quinolones such as ciprofloxacin.

Aesthetic unit
Gonzalez-Ulloa in 1956 divided the face into regional aesthetic units, based on the microscopic study of facial skin thickness, to aid in the planning of reconstruction. Some principles of reconstruction by units are:

- Facial aesthetic units are adjacent three-dimensional areas of characteristic skin quality, thickness, surface outline and contour. The wound may need to be enlarged and normal tissue to be discarded to allow a whole aesthetic unit to be reconstructed.
- Scars are best positioned in the borders between units where they will be less apparent.
- Donor material should be chosen for similar quantity and quality.

Ageing face
The face is prone to display signs of ageing due to the highly mobile mimetic muscles in the anterior face, which lack the presence of a deep fascia around the eyes and mouth.

Anatomy and ageing:
Soft tissues of the face are arranged into five layers:

1. *Skin:* areas with thin dermis more susceptible to ageing—becomes thin with loss of elasticity. Loss of fibroblasts and collagen reduces capacity to resist constant force of muscles and deep rhytids are apparent at rest.
2. Subcutaneous fat organized into discrete compartments such as malar fat pad and nasolabial fold. Separation and descent of compartments occurs with ageing.
3. *Musculoaponeurotic layer:* muscles atrophy with age.
4. Areolar tissue containing soft tissue spaces (upper temporal, pre-zygomatic, pre-masseter and buccal) and retaining ligaments (zygomatic osseocutaneous, mandibular osseocutaneous, platysma-auricular and anterior platysma-cutaneous ligaments). Retaining ligaments attenuate with age and become posteriorly displaced due to bony absorption.
5. *Deep fascia:* deep temporal above the zygomatic arch and masseteric below.

Chronology:
- *30s:* redundant eyelid skin, crow's feet.
- *40s:* prominent nasolabial folds, forehead furrows.
- *50s:* neck rhytids, jowls.
- *60s+:* skin atrophy with increasing wrinkles.

Air embolus
Air entering the circulation, usually through the veins. Complication seen in *Neck dissection* and neurosurgery from air entering the internal jugular vein. Air enters the heart and is compressed, rather than expelled. Air froths in the chamber and reduces cardiac output.

Treatment:
- Fill the wound with fluid to reduce further embolisms.
- Lie the patient on the side with head down and aspirate the heart directly or aspirate through a central line.

Albinism
- The absence of melanin in ectoderm-derived tissues, leading to characteristic hypopigmentation.
- Number and distribution of melanocytes are maintained (unlike piebaldism and vitiligo), therefore melanoma can occur.
- Due to mutation of genes, which regulate melanin synthesis.
- Equal incidence in sex and race.
- Most are autosomal recessive traits.
- The skin is very sensitive to the carcinogenic action of UVB radiation.

Albright syndrome
See MCCUNE-ALBRIGHT SYNDROME.

Alginates
- Derived from seaweed.
- They contain calcium, which activates the clotting cascade when exchanged with sodium in the wound.

- They are very absorbent and become gelatinous upon absorbing moisture.
- They are used clinically for both their haemostatic and absorbent properties.
- Examples include Sorbsan™ and Kaltostat™.

See DRESSINGS.

Allen's test
- To test the integrity of arterial anastomosis between the radial and ulnar side of the hand.
- Empty hand by making a fist and occlude radial and ulnar artery.
- Release one artery, the hand should fill with blood immediately.
- A similar test can be applied to the finger to confirm the presence of two digital arteries.

Alloderm™
An immunologically inert dermis derived from human cadaver.

Allodynia
Marked pain from a usually non-noxious stimulation. *See* CRPS.

Alloplasts
An alloplast is a relatively inert foreign body implanted into tissue.

Advantages: no donor site morbidity, quick, unlimited supply, can be prefabricated, selected resorption.

Classification:
- Liquid or solid. The physical form determines whether it will be encapsulated or whether fibrous tissue will penetrate the implant.
- Biological or synthetic.
- Permanent or absorbable.

Properties: ideal properties of an alloplast are:
- Inert.
- Strong.
- Ability to shape.
- Non-toxic, non-carcinogenic, non-allogenic.
- Sterile.
- Withstands stress.

Liquids:
- *Injectable collagens.*
- *Hyaluronic acid preparations.*
- *Silicone.*

Metals:
- *Stainless steel.*
- *Vitallium.*
- *Titanium.*
- *Gold.*

Polymers:
- *Polyethylene.*
- *Polypropylene.*
- *Methylmethacrylate.*

- *Cyanoacrylates.*
- *Fluorocarbons.*

Ceramics:
- *Hydroxyapatite.*
- *Others:* calcium sulphate and calcium phosphate. *Absorbable polymers*, *sutures*.

Fibrous tissue interface: around an implant there is a dead space into which fibroblasts and macrophages migrate. As a result of this chronic inflammatory response, fibrous encapsulation occurs. This is termed implant bursitis.

Bonding and Osseointegration: bonding can be mechanical or chemical. Mechanical bonding occurs when there is in-growth into a porous substance. Chemical bonding occurs by molecular adsorption and is poorly understood. Osseointegration refers to bone on an implant surface with no intervening fibrous tissue.

Carcinogenicity: chromium and nickel are known carcinogens. There are few reports of tumours around implants. Some studies following hip implants have suggested an increase in lymphatic and haemopoietic cancers, but a decrease in breast and colon cancer.

Biomaterial failure: due to wear, e.g. by abrasion and fatigue, or corrosion, where the implant is lost by chemical reaction.

Alopecia
Androgenic alopecia accounts for 95%—due to action of testosterone and dihydrotestosterone leading to miniaturization of the hair follicle and shortened anagen phase:

- Non-androgenic alopecia (rarer causes):
  - Metabolic—iron deficiency anaemia, thyroid disease, polycystic ovaries;
  - Telogen effluvium—prolonged high fever, acute psychiatric illness;
  - Infectious disease—herpes simplex, herpes zoster;
  - Autoimmune—alopecia areata;
  - Trauma—traction alopecia and burns;
  - Medications—beta blockers, ACE inhibitors and birth control pills.

Management options:
- Wigs.
- Medical with anti-androgens: topical Minoxidil or oral Finasteride.
- Laser to promote thickening and growth induction of existing follicles.
- Surgical:
  - Tissue expansion;
  - *Hair restoration with local flaps*;
  - *Hair transplantation.*

See BURNS RECONSTRUCTION.

Alveolar carcinoma
See HEAD AND NECK CANCER.
- Third most common site.
- Usually over 50 years.
- Lower jaw is more common than upper jaw, particularly behind the bicuspid teeth.
- Less directly related to tobacco and ethanol.
- Sometimes linked to poor dental hygiene and dentures.
- Commonly present with ulcers without pain.
- Spread is initially lateral. Dental caries can be a site of invasion. If bone is invaded the neurovascular bundle (NVB) is at risk. Direct mandibular invasion is common.
- Regional node metastasis is more common with carcinoma of the lower alveolus than of the upper alveolus mainly to levels I–III.

Treatment:
- For T1N0 lesions, a localized excision with marginal mandibular resection can be accomplished through the mouth.
- More extensive lesions with more significant mandibular involvement require a lip split, cheek flap and mandibular resection.
- In the upper jaw, a partial maxillectomy is performed through a modified Weber-Fergusson incision. With more invasive lesions that have broken into the maxillary antrum, total maxillectomy is indicated. More extensive involvement (e.g. ethmoid sinus) will require an anterior cranial fossa approach.
- If access to the neck is required for reconstruction, perform a selective neck dissection for an N0 neck. Palpable nodes make this procedure mandatory.
- Small tumours may be treated with external beam irradiation. Osteoradionecrosis may occur if larger tumours are irradiated.
- Large tumours or node positive tumours are irradiated after resection.

Ambiguous genitalia
See EMBRYOLOGY. In cases of ambiguous genitalia, assign patients sex before the age of 2. Assess by a geneticist and paediatrician. The most common cause is congenital adrenal hyperplasia.

Female pseudohermaphroditism:
- 46XX usually with congenital adrenal hyperplasia.
- Increased androgen production due to a deficiency of the enzyme 21-hydroxylase.
- The appearance of the external genitalia varies from a mildly enlarged clitoris to a normal penis with terminal meatus.
- These children should be raised as female and can be fertile.

- Surgical correction may be necessary. Perform at 3–6 months, clitoral recession and vaginoplasty.

Male pseudohermaphroditism:
- 46XY.
- Have defects in androgen synthesis and other causes of incomplete virilization.
- It may be advisable to raise as a female as there will always be an inadequate phallus. Orchidectomy and vaginal reconstruction will be required. May be due to:
  - Enzyme 5-α reductase resulting in decreased testosterone production;
  - Testicular feminization syndrome, with absence of androgen receptors.

True hermaphrodite:
- 46XX or 46XY or mosaic karyotype with both testicular and ovarian tissue.
- Very rare.
- Patients have an ovary one side and a testis on the other or bilateral ovotestes.
- Raise as female as they will have an inadequate phallus. Remove the testes.

Mixed gonadal dysgenesis:
- Most have 46XY/46XO karyotype with testis on one side and streak gonad on the other.
- The normal testis has a high risk of developing gonadoblastoma.
- These patients should be raised as female. Perform gonadectomy, clitoral recession and vaginoplasty.

Pure gonadal dysgenesis:
- 45X0, 46XX or 46XY karyotype.
- Usually present with delayed adolescence.
- Bilateral streak gonads. High malignant potential and gonadectomy is recommended.

Ameloblastoma
- Benign odontogenic tumour deriving from ameloblasts that do not differentiate to the stage of enamel formation.
- More commonly located on mandible than maxilla.
- Can be locally aggressive.
- Treatment via surgical excision or enucleation.

Amplitude: of tendon excursion
See TENDON TRANSFERS. Donor muscles should have similar excursion to that which is replaced.
- Excursion of wrist flexors and extensors is 3 cm, finger extensors is 5 cm, finger flexors is 7 cm.
- Increase amplitude of donors by tenodesis effect and by freeing fascial attachments.

Amyotrophic lateral sclerosis (ALS)

- A type of motor neuron disease with atrophy of skeletal muscles of the body.
- Causes degeneration of motor neurons.
- Patients with ALS have weakness, atrophy and fasciculations.
- Often asymmetric.
- No loss of sensation.
- One-third of patients present with upper limb symptoms.

Anaesthesia

See ASA CLASSIFICATION. *See* LOCAL ANAESTHETICS. *See* TUMESCENT ANAESTHESIA.

Anaplastic Large Cell Lymphoma (Breast Implant Associated)

See BREAST IMPLANT-ASSOCIATED ANAPLASTIC LARGE T-CELL LYMPHOMA (BIA-ALCL).

Andre-Thomas sign

- In *Ulnar nerve palsy*.
- The deformity of clawing is made worse by an unconscious effort to extend the fingers by tenodesing the extensor tendons with palmar flexion of the wrist.

Aneurysmal bone cyst

- Blood-filled cysts lined with fleshy membrane.
- 50% occur secondary to other tumours.
- 20s–30s.
- Tendency to recur, can be aggressive.

XR: metaphyseal expansile lesion with a thin rim of reactive bone.

Treatment: en bloc bone excision and strut graft.

See BONE TUMOURS.

Aneurysms—upper limb

See VASCULAR INJURIES.

- Most are due to trauma and infection.
- Traumatic aneurysms are most commonly found in the thenar and hypothenar eminence, and the superficial arch.
- True aneurysms contain all layers of the vessel wall. False aneurysms are pulsating haematomas and occur after penetrating injury.
- Most patients complain of a pulsatile mass. It may be difficult to distinguish from a ganglion.
- Arteriography may be useful.

Treatment: resect and repair pseudoaneurysms. Ligation may be adequate if there is no vascular compromise.

Angel kiss

See NAEVUS FLAMMEUS NEONATORUM. A macular vascular birthmark seen on the upper lip, which fades spontaneously.

Angioblastoma of Nakagawa

See TUFTED ANGIOMA.

Angiofibroma

- Skin lesions usually found on the lower central face.
- Fibrous, erythematous papule 1–3 mm in size.
- When multiple they are associated with the *Tuberous sclerosis* complex (Bourneville's disease) and occur on the cheeks and chin.
- Treatment is by dermabrasion, laser or excision.
- Peri-ungual angiofibromas (Koenen's peri-ungual tumours) also are often present in this syndrome.

Angiogenesis

- Angiogenesis is the process of forming new blood vessels.
- Platelets secrete PDGF, which attracts macrophages and granulocytes and promotes angiogenesis.
- The macrophage plays a key role in angiogenesis by releasing angiogenic substances, including tumour necrosis factor-alpha (TNF-α) and basic fibroblast growth factor (bFGF).
- *VEGF*, released by keratinocytes is also a potent stimulator of angiogenesis.

See WOUND HEALING. *See* CYTOKINES AND GROWTH FACTORS.

Angiosarcoma

See SARCOMA.

- Rare vascular neoplasm.
- Aggressive, recurs locally, spreads widely and has a high rate of vascular and lymphatic metastasis.
- 50% occur in the head and neck.
- M:F 8:1.
- Associated with irradiation and some environmental carcinogens.
- Soft violaceous painless compressible mass.
- Treat with wide excision and radiotherapy.

Angiosome

- Manchot studied skin territories in 1889. Salmon expanded this in 1930s, and Taylor and Palmer developed the angiosome concept in 1987.
- An angiosome is a three-dimensional composite block of skin, soft tissues and bone supplied by branches of a single source artery.
- Choke vessels link adjoining angiosomes and may regulate flow between them. The veins do not contain valves and are called oscillating veins as blood may flow in either direction.

- The *anatomic* territory is the area of tissue supplied by an artery before anastomosing with adjacent vessels.
- The *dynamic* territory of an artery is that which stains with fluoroscein.
- The *potential* territory is that which can be included if the flap is delayed.
- Flap principles are that a random flap can support one angiosome. An axial pattern flap can support another angiosome perfused via a choke vessel in a random cutaneous fashion.

Anatomic concepts of blood supply developed by Taylor and Palmer:
- Blood supply detours through muscles.
- Arteries link to form continuous unbroken network.
- The intramuscular territories of arteries and veins match.
- The viability of a muscle flap is dependent on the size and number of its vascular territories.
- The vessels hitchhike with nerves.
- The vessels follow connective tissue framework.
- Vessels radiate from fixed to mobile areas.
- There is a direct relationship between muscle mobility, and the size and density of the supplying vessels.
- Vessels tend to have a constant destination, but a variable origin.
- The territory of the intramuscular arteries obeys the law of equilibrium.
- Vessel size and orientation are the product of tissue differentiation in the area.
- The muscles are the prime movers of venous return.
- As arterial territories are linked by choke vessels, so the venous territories are linked by oscillating veins, which are devoid of valves.

Angle classification of occlusion
- System for describing dental occlusion in the anteroposterior plane developed by Edward Angle.
- The upper first molar is the point of reference in describing the anteroposterior relationship of the mandible and maxilla.
- This classification only tells of the relationship of mandible to maxilla. It doesn't say which is malpositioned or what the cause is.
- *Class I occlusion:* the mesiobuccal cusp of the maxillary first molar articulates within the mesiobuccal groove of the lower first molar.
- *Class II malocclusion:* the lower first molar is distal to the upper first usually 1/2 to a full cusp. In Division 1 the upper anterior teeth

are flared forward, in Division 2 the anterior upper and lower teeth are retruded with overbite.
- *Class III malocclusion:* the mandibular dentition is positioned mesial to maxillary dentition. (NB Mesial means situated toward the middle of the front of the jaw along the curve of the dental arch.)

  See ORTHOGNATHIC SURGERY. *See* TEETH.

Anterior interosseous syndrome
- Anterior interosseous nerve is a branch of the median nerve supplying FPL, FDP (index and middle) and pronator quadratus.
- Compression produces pain in the forearm and a weak pinch grip (O sign).
- Test pronator quadratus by strength of resisted forced supination with elbow flexed to eliminate humeral head of pronator teres.
- EMG may be helpful.
- Incomplete syndromes can occur.
- Distinguish from *Parsonage–Turner syndrome*.

Compression points:
- Fibrous bands of pronator teres muscle between the superficial and deep heads.
- FDS bands.
- Gantzer's muscle, an accessory head of FPL.
- Aberrant radial artery.
- Thrombosis of the ulnar collateral vessel.
- As a complication of forearm fracture.
- Accessory bicipital aponeurosis.
- Enlarged communicating veins.

Treatment:
- Majority will resolve spontaneously.
- Plan to explore if there is confirmation on nerve conduction studies and if there is no improvement after 2–3 months. Surgical exposure as for *Pronator syndrome*. Release the deep head of pronator teres and suture the deep head to the superficial head.
- Interfascicular neurolysis of the anterior interosseus nerve 2–7.5 cm below the elbow is probably warranted if no obvious compression identified.

Anterolateral thigh flap
- A workhorse fasciocutaneous flap raised from the anterolateral aspect of the thigh.
- Described by Song 1984 with a septocutaneous perforator, but often only musculocutaneous perforators are present.
- *Arterial supply:* perforators from descending branch of the lateral circumflex femoral system. Perforators reach the skin either via inter-muscular septum between vastus

lateralis and rectus femoris (20%) or traverse through the vastus lateralis muscle (80%). The largest perforator usually reaches the deep fascia 2 cm inferolateral to the midpoint of a line between the ASIS and the superolateral corner of the patella.

- *Venous drainage:* usually two venae commitantes accompany the descending branch of the lateral circumflex femoral artery.
- This flap can be raised as a proximally or distally based pedicled flap or more commonly as a free flap. It can be raised below the fascia or suprafascially if a thin flap is required.

Operative technique:
- Supine position.
- Landmarks—flap is designed over a line drawn from ASIS to lateral edge of patella:
  ○ 4 cm circle at midpoint of line is highest density of perforators—can be identified with ultrasound doppler;
  ○ Junction proximal and middle third of line locates TFL perforator lifeboat (ascending branch from the lateral femoral circumflex).
- Anterior incision first—incise through deep fascia onto rectus and dissect to septum to identify perforators. Can perform posterior incision first to protect TFL perforator.
- Open septum between rectus and vastus lateralis to identify main arterial vessel and locate perforators.
- Then incise posterior border of skin flap.
- Can close donor site primarily if 8–12 cm wide.

Antia-Buch Flap
- A one-stage reconstruction for helical defects with condrocutaneous flaps.
- A superior and inferior flap are mobilized and advanced.

Apert's hand *See* APERT'S SYNDROME.
- All involved portions of upper limb have skeletal unions, incomplete joint segmentation and incomplete separation of rays.
- All hands have skeletal coalitions, distal bifurcation of tendons, nerves and vessels, distal intrinsic insertions and complex syndactylies.
- Shoulder and elbow synostosis may occur especially with type 1 and 2 hands. A discrepancy in size in shoulder may cause reduced ROM with growth. Most have normal elbow motion.
- Hand features are short, radially-deviated thumb, osseous syndactyly and symbrachydactyly of central 3 rays, simple

syndactyly of 4th web and variable syndactyly of 1st web. Carpal coalitions occur, particularly between capitate and hamate, and 4th and 5th metacarpal.
- Ideally treatment is performed bilaterally between 4–12 months of age. Earlier treatment leads to relapse.
- Ideally perform two bilateral releases before the age of 2, mobilize 5th ray, and lengthen and realign thumb when 4–6 years.

Classification: Upton.
- *Type I:* spade hand. Complex syndactyly of digits 2–5 with the thumb and little fingers free.
- *Type II:* spoon or mitten hand. Complex syndactyly of digits 2–5 with simple syndactyly of thumbs or thumbs free.
- *Type III:* rosebud hand. All 5 digits involved in complex syndactyly.

See APERT'S SYNDROME.

Type I:
- Least severe and most common.
- Thumb radial clinodactyly and shallow web.
- Side to side fusion of fingers 2–4 with phalangeal fusion at DIPJ, spade hand.
- Simple syndactyly of 4th and 5th finger.
- Mobile MCPJs, stiff IPJs.

Treatment:
- 4–12 months separate 2nd and 4th web, after 6/12 separate 3rd web. Division of transverse metacarpal ligaments will increase mobility.
- Get frequent tendon, nerve and vessel anomalies.
- Perform osteotomies, which may be through cartilaginous bars of IPJs at time of releases.
- Age 3–5, correct thumb clinodactyly with opening-wedge osteotomy through middle of proximal phalanx. Use bone from iliac crest. Release 4–5th metacarpal synostosis with interposition of dermal graft.

Type II:
- Thumb joined to index in complete simple syndactyly, but have separate nails.
- Central fusion gives concave palm, mitten or spoon hand. Conjoined nail. Abnormalities of index proximal phalanx.
- Complete syndactyly between 4th and 5th fingers.

Treatment:
- Release 2nd and 4th web at the same time as 1st web. Need to excise fascial bands between thumb and index.
- If not too tight use 4-flap Z-plasty, otherwise use Y-V. Perform capsulotomy of CMCJ.

- If index finger proximal phalanx is abnormal and radially deviated it may be better to ablate early.
- Later correction of thumb clinodactyly as for type I.

Type III:
- Most severe, least common.
- Tight osseous and cartilaginous union between fingers 1–4 with single conjoined nail with index and thumb being indistinguishable, hoof or rosebud hand.
- Thumb radial clinodactyly less severe, but thumb is smaller.

Treatment:
- Perform index ray resection at time of 1st web release. Use dorsal advancement flap, and re-advance with subsequent procedures. Release 4th web at the same time.
- At time of 1st web release perform osteotomy across DIPJs with a transverse K-wire, which converts this to a type I hand.

Apert's syndrome
Acrocephalosyndactyly characterized by bicoronal synostosis, midface hypoplasia, cleft palate, and complex syndactyly.
- Most are sporadic, but also autosomal dominant inheritance.
- Mutation in *Fibroblast growth factor receptor* 2 (FGFR2).
- Incidence is 1/160,000 live births.
- Craniosynostosis most commonly affects the two coronal sutures but also potential cranial base synostosis.
- The face has a steep forehead and a groove above the supra-orbital ridge. Orbits are shallow with hypertelorism and down slanting of palpebral fissures.
- The mid-third of the face is hypoplastic with a normal mandible.
- The nose is beaked.
- Decreased patency of posterior nasal choanae may result in obstructive apnoea.
- 30% have a cleft palate.
- Mirror image abnormalities of hands and feet with an inverse relationship between the severity of craniofacial abnormality and the severity of hand anomalies.
- Syndactyly of fingers 2, 3 and 4 is present and the whole hand may be fused. If the thumb is free, it is broad and radially deviated. The feet are similarly involved. Acrosyndactyly of hands graded from I–III with increasing severity:
  - *Class 1:* the little finger and thumb are separate;

  - *Class 2:* only the thumb is free;
  - *Class 3:* the whole hand is involved.
  See CRANIOSYNOSTOSIS. *See* APERT'S HAND.

Aplasia cutis congenita
- Rare, sporadic congenital deformity most often in first-born females.
- Get failure of differentiation of skin ranging from total absence of skin, fat, skull, dura and occasionally underlying brain. Scalp is involved in 60% of cases and ulcers may be multiple.
- Mostly occurs in the midline in the area of the posterior fontanelle.
- Ulcers are sharply marginated with a red base and usually heal rapidly by secondary intention.

Aetiology: may be chromosomal, placental infarcts, amniotic adhesions or pressure necrosis. Also associated with hydrocephalus, facial clefts and spina bifida.

Management:
- May heal with dressings, which should be kept moist.
- For large defects with exposed brain, dura or skull, provide soft tissue cover and reconstruct bone later.
- Use local flaps and possibly tissue expansion.
  See SCALP RECONSTRUCTION.

Apocrine cystadenoma
- A small, benign, translucent nodule, usually appearing on the face.
- Often pigmented and may contain brownish fluid.
- It may be confused with melanoma or pigmented basal cell naevus.

Apocrine glands
- *Sweat glands* found in axilla and groin.
- They start to function in puberty and give an odour due to bacterial decomposition.
- They have a sympathetic adrenergic nerve supply.

Apocrine tumours
See APOCRINE CYSTADENOMA. *See* SYRINGOCYSTADENOMA PAPILLIFERUM. *See* CHONDROID SYRINGOMA.

Arachnodactyly
Unusually long slender fingers.

Arnez and Tyler classification
Classification for *Degloving injuries*.
- *Type 1:* abrasion, but no degloving. Wound edge excision followed by single stage reconstruction possible.
- *Type 2:* non-circumferential degloving. Single stage debridement and reconstruction

possible. If degloved skin flaps are not devitalized, they may be sutured back in place, but caution is required in this approach.

- *Type 3:* circumferential degloving. Degloved skin usually excised in its entirety. Single stage debridement and reconstruction possible if underlying tissue is carefully assessed and found to be healthy.
- *Type 4:* circumferential degloving plus avulsion between deep tissue planes. Requires serial conservative debridement and delayed reconstruction.

Arteriovenous fistulae

Rare in the upper extremity with the exception of high flow *AV malformations* and surgically made AV fistulae. High output failure rarely occurs distal to the elbow. Most become manifest in the first ten years of life. Most traumatic fistulae are due to penetrating *Vascular injuries*. An arteriogram will help guide treatment. Fistulae with bony involvement are poorly controlled by excision. Diffuse digital masses respond poorly to simple excision. Amputation may be required.

Arteriovenous malformations

- These are the most difficult *Vascular malformations* to treat.
- They can be high flow and haemodynamically active.
- Pure arterial malformations such as aneurysms are rare but they can occur with AVMs.
- The epicentre of an AVM is called the nidus and consists of arterial feeders, micro- and macro-arteriovenous fistulas (AVFs), and enlarged veins.
- AVM is present at birth and can either manifest in infancy, or appear later.
- Intracranial AVM is more common than extracranial AVM, followed in frequency by AVM of the limbs, trunk and viscera.
- Some may be hormonally active. The fast-flow nature may not be recognized until trauma or puberty stimulate expansion.
- AVMs develop ischaemic skin changes, ulceration, intractable pain, and intermittent bleeding. Low-flow lesions may be associated with skeletal hypertrophy, high-flow with destruction. May present as emergency with haemorrhage or cardiac failure.

Staging: clinically by Schobinger.

- *Stage I:* blush/stain, warmth and AV shunting.
- *Stage II:* stage I with enlargement, tortuous veins, pulsations, thrill and bruit.
- *Stage III:* stage II with either dystrophic changes, ulceration, bleeding, persistent pain or destruction.
- *Stage IV:* stage II with cardiac failure.

Treatment: *see* VASCULAR MALFORMATIONS.

Arthrodesis
Wrist:

- For pain, reconstruction following tumour resection, instability.
- Remove all articular surface, maintain carpal alignment and height, use internal fixation, bone graft and splint until radiological union.
- Optimal position is 15° extension 5° ulnar deviation. If both wrists are being fused place dominant hand in extension and non-dominant in flexion for personal hygiene.
- Use bone graft, bone blocks, intramedullary rods, interosseus wires, external fixators and dorsal plates.

See PROXIMAL ROW CARPECTOMY.

Limited fusions:

- *Triscaphe arthrodesis (STT):* for rotary subluxation of the scaphoid, non-union, Kienböck's, triscaphe arthritis, DISI.
- *Lunotriquetral arthrodesis:* for lunotriquetral ligament tears and instability.
- *Capitolunate arthrodesis:* mid-carpal degenerative arthritis.
- *Scaphocapitate arthrodesis:* for rotary subluxation of the scaphoid, *Kienböcks*, mid-carpal instability.
- *Capitate-lunate-hamate-triquetral (four corner):* for ulnar mid-carpal instability, SLAC, scaphoid non-union.

Fusion across radio-carpal joint gives the greatest loss of movement. A single row fusion gives the least loss of motion.

Small joint arthrodesis:

- *Indications:* pain, instability, deformity and loss of neuromuscular control.
- *Position:* individualize to particular patient:
  o MCP joints cascade radial to ulnar, 25° for the index and add 5° for each digit;
  o PIPJ cascade from 40° in index to 55°;
  o DIPJ fuse in 0° flexion, possibly 5–10° supination for index and middle to achieve pinch grip;
  o Thumb, keep length. IPJ fuse in slight flexion (recommended between 0–15°). MCPJ 5–15°. CMC fuse with 40° palmar abduction and 20° of radial abduction.
- *Surface preparation:*
  o Avoid shortening;
  o Cup and cone method enables accurate positioning;
  o Remove all the articular cartilage.

- *Fixation options:*
  - K-wires: crossed;
  - *Interosseous wiring:* stronger than K-wires;
  - *Tension band wiring:* use for MCP joints and pip joints. Compression is produced by the dorsally placed tension band.

DIPJ: approach through <u>H incision</u>. Section extensor tension. Flex joint and excise collateral ligaments to increase exposure. Fix with either Herbert screw or interosseous wire and oblique K-wire. For the IPJ can use 90-90 wires or if bone stock poor use K-wire.

PIPJ dorsal longitudinal incision. Split extensor tendon and elevate to either side. Cut central tendon and collaterals. Use 90-90 wires or tension band wiring.

MCPJ: expose through longitudinal incision in skin and on radial side of finger. Excise collaterals. Fix with mini plate.

Arthrogryposis

- Greek meaning curved joint.
- Many causes but all have in common immobility of the joints *in utero.*
- This may be due to abnormal muscles, abnormal neurology or crowding due to oligohydramnios, bicornuate uterus, etc. *Beal's syndrome* is a contractural arachnodactyly.
- *Findings:* contractures, usually bilateral, adduction and internal rotation of shoulders, fixed flexion or extension of elbows and knees. Club-like hands and wrists, thin waxy skin.
- *Treatment:* dynamic and static splintage, occasionally surgery.

See CONGENITAL HAND ANOMALIES.

Arthroplasty

- **Wrist:** inflammatory, degenerative and post-traumatic arthritis. Arthroplasty most commonly performed in RA. Contraindicated if there are poor wrist motors.
- **PIPJ:** silicone implant arthroplasty may be performed through a palmar, lateral or dorsal approach. For a dorsal approach the extensor mechanism is opened. Collateral ligaments and volar plate are released. The articular surfaces are removed, osteophytes are removed, the medullary canal reamed and the implant inserted. Repair the collateral ligament. Commence active motion immediately. Protect finger from lateral stress.
- **MCPJ:** *Swanson's arthroplasty.*

Arthroscopy—wrist

Indications: diagnose and treat pain, tears of ligaments and TFCC. Remove loose bodies.

Portals:
- Named by the extensor compartments, e.g. 3-4 portal is between 3rd and 4th dorsal compartment.
- The 5 used are 1-2, 3-4, 4-5, 6R and 6U—radial and ulna to FCU.
- 3-4 and 4-5 most commonly used, the former for visualization and the latter for instrumentation.
- With 1-2 the nerve and artery are at risk. With 6U dorsal branch of ulnar nerve at risk.
- Some surgeons pre-inflate the joint. Lunotriquetral ligament is best seen through 6R.
- *Mid-carpal joint:* three mid-carpal portals—mid-carpal radial (MCR), ulnar (MCU) and scaphotrapeziotrapezoid (STT).

ASA classification

Classification adopted by the American Society of Anaesthesiologists for assessing preoperative physical status.
- *I:* healthy.
- *II:* mild systemic disease.
- *III:* moderate systemic disease, some functional limitation.
- *IV:* severe systemic disease, constant threat to life.
- *V:* moribund patient, unlikely to survive 24 hours.

Aspergillosis

- An opportunistic fungal infection seen in immunocompromised patients, e.g. aplastic anaemia, leukaemia and major burns.
- It is not seen in healthy individuals.
- Invasive aspergillosis usually requires surgical debridement in addition to anti-fungal agents to eradicate infection.

See FUNGAL HAND INFECTIONS.

Aspirin

- Has an inhibitory effect on platelet aggregation.
- Irreversible inactivation of cyclo-oxygenase (COX) enzyme, which blocks thromboxane A2 and prostaglandin production.

See MICROSURGERY.

Atasoy volar V–Y flap

- Used in the treatment of *Fingertip injuries.*
- Volar Y-V flap taken from defect down to DIP joint.
- Raise with NVB and free fibrous septa. Tension free closure. 5–10 mm advancement may be possible.
- Also known as Tranquilli–Leali flap.

Ataxia-telangiectasia

See LOUIS–BAR SYNDROME.

ATLS: Advanced Trauma Life Support

A system of trauma care that involves systematic prioritized evaluation and treatment aimed specifically at preventing deaths in the 2nd peak (minutes to hours after trauma) and minimizing morbidity and mortality in the 3rd peak (days–weeks) by optimizing initial trauma care.

- Prehospital management.
- Triage.
- Primary survey:
  - A: airway and cervical spine control;
  - B: breathing and ventilation;
  - C: circulation haemorrhage control;
  - D: disability; AVPU—Alert, Vocal stimulus, Painful stimulus, Unresponsive;
  - E: exposure and environmental control.
- Resuscitation and repeat primary survey until stabilized.
- Secondary survey.
- Post-resuscitation monitoring.
- Definitive care.

Atypical fibroxanthoma

- A small, firm nodule with crusting. Similar in appearance to a BCC.
- Occurs in the elderly on the head and neck.
- Histologically see atypical spindle and giant cells with a lot of mitoses.
- Treat with simple excision and it rarely recurs.
- If it invades deeply it is called a *Malignant fibrous histiocytoma* and can resemble basal cell epithelioma. Appears on chronically sun-exposed parts of the head and neck, particularly in the pre-auricular area in older persons.

  See PSEUDOSARCOMATOUS LESIONS.

Axial flaps

A flap raised with a known vessel that increases the length to width ratio available.

- *Direct:* contain a named artery in the subcutaneous tissues. Examples include the *Groin flap* and *Deltopectoral flap.* They may include a random element in the distal portion.
- *Fasciocutaneous flap:* based on vessels running within or near the fascia.
- *Musculocutaneous flaps.*
- *Venous flaps.*

Axilla

Boundaries:

- *Anterior:* pectoralis major, subclavius, pectoralis minor.
- *Posterior:* subscapularis, latissimus dorsi, teres major.
- *Medial:* ribs 4–5, serratus anterior.
- *Lateral:* coracobrachialis and biceps.

Nerves:

- *Intercostobrachial nerve:* sensory innervation to upper medial arm.
- *Long thoracic nerve:* to serratus anterior. From C5-7. Division cause winging of the scapula.
- *Thoracodorsal nerve:* from posterior cord to latissimus dorsi.
- *Medial pectoral nerve:* pectoralis major and often wraps around the lateral border of pectoralis minor.

Axillary burn contractures
Classification (Kurtzman and Stern):

- *Type 1:* single axillary fold—amenable to local tissue rearrangement.
- *Type 2:* both axillary folds—usually amenable to local tissue rearrangement.
- *Type 3:* Involvement of both axillary folds and axillary dome—requires resurfacing with skin graft or flap.

Axillary dissection

Aims to remove lymph nodes from all three of Berg's levels of axillary nodes:

- *I:* lateral to lateral border of pectoralis minor.
- *II:* under pectoralis minor.
- *III:* medial to pectoralis minor muscle.

Operative steps:

1. Position: supine with arm out on board, draped for mobility.
2. U-incision with skin flap raised deep to clavipectoral fascia.
3. Definition of borders of axilla:
   a. Along pectoralis major anteriorly;
   b. Along latissimus dorsi posteriorly;
   c. Up axillary vein ligating branches going into the axillary contents.
4. Decision on pectoralis minor access level 2 and 3 nodes and intrapectoral nodes of Rotta—controversy about whether to excise pectoralis minor for oncological clearance.
5. Preservation of axillary contents: long thoracic nerve and thoracodorsal bundle.
6. Remove lymph node content, dissecting distally to proximally on a broad front from anterior to posterior to converge on axillary vein.
7. Closure in layers with consideration of suction drain.

Axillary nerve

C5-6 roots from the posterior cord. Supplies deltoid and teres minor.

Axonotmesis

Axonal damage with Wallerian degeneration.

See SEDDON AND SUNDERLAND CLASSIFICATIONS OF NERVE INJURY.

Bactigras

Paraffin gauze impregnated with chlorhexidine. *See* DRESSINGS.

Baker classification

Classification of capsular contracture (1975):

- *I:* breast soft, implant not palpable.
- *II:* minimal: implant palpable not visible.
- *III:* moderate: implant palpable and visible.
- *IV:* severe: hard, painful with distortion of breast.

    See BREAST AUGMENTATION. *See* BREAST IMPLANTS.

Balanitis xerotica obliterans (BXO)

- Male genital form of *lichen sclerosis*, which is a chronic, progressive, sclerosing inflammatory dermatosis of unclear aetiology.
- Chronic BXO predisposes to SCC.
- There may be a viral association and HLA association.
- Increased in obese patients.
- Dyskaryosis and inflammatory changes in the early stages lead to fibrosis and skin atrophy.
- The prepuce becomes adherent to the glans with a white stenosing band at the end of the foreskin and a haemorrhagic response to minor trauma leading to phimosis and stenosis.

Treatment:

- Steroid creams for early disease in children.
- Circumcision, meatoplasty.
- Excise advanced disease and apply a buccal mucosal graft in which BXO does not recur.

Balding

See HAIR RESTORATION.

Banff classification

A system for grading histological rejection in graft skin in human vascularized composite allotransplantation:

- *Grade 0:* no sign of rejection.
- *Grade 1:* mild perivascular infiltration.
- *Grade 2:* advanced infiltrates with or without mild involvement of epidermis.
- *Grade 3:* additional epithelial apoptosis, dyskeratosis and/or keratinolysis.
- *Grade 4:* frank necrosis of epidermis or other skin structures.

Bannayan syndrome

Microcephaly, multiple vascular malformations and multiple lipomas.

Basal cell carcinoma

- 95% of BCCs occur between 40–80 years, 85% in the head and neck.
- It is the most common malignancy in Caucasians.
- BCCs arise from pluripotential cells of the basal layer of the epithelium or pilosebaceous follicles.
- Do not tend to occur on non-hair bearing skin.
- Almost never metastasize.

Carcinogens:

- *Ultraviolet radiation (UV).*
- *Ionizing radiation.*
- *Chemicals:* arsenic, psoralens, nitrogen mustard and atmospheric pollutants have been implicated.

Inherited conditions:

- *Xeroderma pigmentosa.*
- *Gorlin's syndrome.*
- *Albinism* with increased risk of BCC and SCC.
- *Epidermodysplasia verruciformis.*
- *Muir–Torre syndrome.*
- *Porokeratosis.*
- *Bazex–Dupre–Christol syndrome.*

Types:

- *Nodular:* most common. Usually single on face. Translucent papules. Grow slowly and ulcerate.
- *Superficial:* often multiple, usually trunk, erythematous, scaly.
- *Infiltrative:* also morphoeic, yellow-white, morpheaform, and ill-defined borders. More often recur.
- *Pigmented:* like nodular with pigment.
- *Trabecular: see* Merkel cell tumour.

- *Adnexal:* arise from sebaceous sweat glands. Uncommon and appear as solitary tumours in older patients. No particular features, grow slowly, tend to recur locally and metastasize regionally.

Dermoscopy features:
- Absence of pigment network.
- Arborizing vessels.
- Focal ulcerations.
- Blue nests—resulting from the Tyndall effect when BCC is located in the dermis.

Histology:
- Oval cells with deeply staining nuclei and scant cytoplasm.
- Irregular masses of basaloid cells in the dermis, with the outermost cells forming a pallisading layer on the periphery.
- A fibrous reaction in the surrounding stroma.
- 95% are attached to the epidermis, the rest are attached to a hair follicle.
- *Broder's classification*.

Features of high risk:
- Patient factors:
  - Immunosuppression and prior radiation.
- Macroscopic factors:
  - Size above 2 cm;
  - Site—lesions on central face are at higher risk of recurrence;
  - Poor definition of margins.
- Microscopic factors:
  - Histological subtype;
  - Aggressive features—invasion;
  - Recurrent lesion.

Treatment options for isolated BCC:
- Surgical excision with predetermined peripheral margin and deep to superficial fascia:
  - Low-risk lesions can be excised with 4 mm margin for 95% clearance rate;
  - High-risk lesions can be excised by wider margins of 5 mm for 95%.
- Consider Mohs for high risk of incompletely excised or recurrent lesions. If Mohs not available, other margin control approaches such as the *Linguine technique*, intraoperative frozen section and delayed reconstruction can be employed.
- Destructive techniques: non-surgical:
  - Topical *Imiquimod* or *Fluorouracil*—may be effective for low risk superficial BCCs;
  - Photodynamic therapy;
  - *Radiotherapy*.
- Destructive techniques: surgical:
  - Cryosurgery;
  - Curettage;
  - Ablative laser.

- **Incomplete excision and recurrence**:
  - Incomplete or close (<1 mm) margins in 4–7%. Re-excision will include residual tumour in less than 50%. Can also consider Mohs and radiotherapy. Observation may be appropriate if only peripheral margins involved as only 17% recur;
  - 36% of patients with a BCC develop a second primary within 5 years.

Treatment options for multiple BCCs (i.e. Gorlin's):
- Targeted surgical excision for problematic lesions.
- Topical therapies for superficial lesions.
- Electrochemotherapy.
- Vismodegib—hedgehog pathway inhibitor.

See SQUAMOUS CELL CARCINOMA. *See* NAEVUS SEBACEOUS.

Basal osteotomy
For 1st *CMC joint OA*.
- Can provide good stable pain free CMC movement.
- Closing wedge osteotomy.
- 4-cm incision centred on prominence of 1st CMC joint in line with shaft. Retract EPL, expose proximal third of metacarpal.
- Site of osteotomy should be 1 cm from joint. Strip periosteum circumferentially and insert levers. Mark osteotomy—5 mm wide for 20–30° abduction.
- Wide part of wedge is directed so as to cause abduction on closing the wedge, insert interosseous wire.
- Excise bone wedge keeping far cortex intact. Close wedge. Insert wire and plaster in corrected position for 6/52.

Bayne and Klug classification of radial dysplasia
- *I:* short radius.
- *II:* hypoplastic radius.
- *III:* partial absence of radius.
- *IV:* total absence of radius.

See RADIAL CLUB HAND.

Bazex–Dupré–Christol syndrome
- X-linked disorder.

• Follicular atrophoderma, congenital hypotrichiosis, basal cell naevi and _Basal cell carcinomas_.

Beal's syndrome
Contractural arachnodactyly syndrome. Initially thought to be _Marfan's_ with _Arthrgryposis_.

BEAM: Bulbar Elongation and Anastomotic Meatoplasty
• One stage treatment for _Hypospadias_.
• The whole length of urethra is dissected and advanced to lie at the level of the normal meatus.
• Up to 5 cm advancement can be achieved.

Bean syndrome
See BLUE RUBBER BLEB SYNDROME.

Becker's flap
• Fasciocutaneous dorsal ulnar artery flap.
• Based on the dorsal branch of the ulnar artery supplying the dorsal ulnar border of the forearm. Arises 2–4 cm proximal to pisiform and passes between the ulna and flexor carpi ulnaris.
• It pierces the deep fascia a few centimetres proximal to the pisiform so it can be used as a distal island flap without sacrificing the ulnar artery.

Becker's naevi
• Acquired pigmented patches.
• Incidence of 1:200, M:F 5:1.
• Appears in adolescence, exaggerated by sunshine.
• Occurs on the upper trunk and arms.
• It gradually spreads, and becomes darker and hairy with acne lesions within it. The melanocytes are excessively active and the epidermis is thickened with enlarged sebaceous glands.
• Q-switched ruby (694 nm) and pulsed dye _Lasers_ (510 nm) may be effective.

See NAEVUS.

Beds—for pressure sores
• Patients are assessed for the risk of developing a pressure sore by using the _Waterlow score_.
• _10+ risk:_ foam mattress such as soft foam premier which contains a contoured insert pad.
• _15+ risk:_ alpha excel has an overlay pressure-relieving mattress.
• _20+:_
   ○ _Dynamic floatation:_ Nimbus 3™;
   ○ _Alternating pressure system:_ Pegasus™;
   ○ _Air fluidized bead bed:_ Clinitron™;

   ○ _Low air loss:_ Mediscus™, cells inflate and deflate independently.

Belfast regimen
• A regimen of early active mobilization after flexor tendon repair.
• A dorsal splint is worn, which leaves the fingers free to flex.
• The wrist is held between neutral and 30° flexion. MCP extension limited to 70° flexion. Hyperextension of IPJs is prevented beyond neutral.
• Active mobilization consists of:
   ○ Passive flexion;
   ○ Passive flexion and hold, to maintain muscle function;
   ○ Active flexion, to create tendon glide and limit adhesions.

See TENDON. _See_ FLEXOR REPAIR.

Bell's palsy
• Idiopathic paralysis of the facial nerve.
• Described by Charles Bell in 1814.
• Originally referred to facial nerve paralysis from any cause.
• A diagnosis of exclusion.
• It may be a viral infection with swelling of the nerve in the tight intratemporal course.
• 80% recover full function, which begins within 4 weeks.

See FACIAL NERVE.

Bell's phenomenon
• Upward movement of eye with closure of eyelid. A normal defence reflex present in approximately 75% population.
• Bell's phenomenon has protective mechanism on tear film stability and ocular surface. An abnormal Bell's associated with a higher risk of complications following eyelid surgery.
• Test by holding upper lid open, while patient attempts gentle closure of the eye.

See PTOSIS.

Below knee amputation
See SKEW FLAP. _See_ LONG POSTERIOR FLAP.

Benelli mastopexy
Characterized by concentric skin excision around the areola, which moves the nipple superiorly. Useful for mild and moderate ptosis. It may also help in the constricted or tuberous breast with mild to moderate laxity.

• Technique allows for parenchymal repositioning; parenchymal criss-cross flaps can cone the breast tissue and may help increase projection.
• Tendency for the scar to stretch is combated with a non-absorbable purse string suture, as

well as nylon cross sutures to reduce areolar herniation.

- Three problems may occur:
  - ○ The areola may enlarge;
  - ○ The scar may be hypertrophic;
  - ○ Breast contour may be flattened.

See MASTOPEXY.

Bennett's fracture

- Two-part intra-articular fracture-subluxation at base of thumb metacarpal. Oblique fracture through volar beak, which is held by the palmar oblique (beak) ligament.
- Inherently unstable due to APL pulling first metacarpal radially and proximally.
- Reduce by pronation of first metacarpal, abduction, longitudinal traction and counter-pressure at base of thumb.
- Treatment options:
  - ○ Conservative in Bennett's cast (below-elbow thumb spica with thumb held in plane of palm to reduce pull of APL) if fracture non-displaced;
  - ○ Closed reduction and internal fixation with K-wires—most common treatment modality due to instability of the fracture;
  - ○ Open reduction internal fixation—may be indicated in large fragment if closed reduction failed.
- Reverse Bennett's fracture occurs in the base of the 5th metacarpal.

See ROLANDO FRACTURE.

Bernard lip reconstruction

- Used for *Lip reconstruction* with significant-sized defects.
- Advances full thickness flaps with triangular excision to allow proper mobilization.
- May have diminished sensation and mobility which may be lessened in *Webster modification*.

Bier's block

- Intravenous regional anaesthesia which lasts 90 minutes.
- Cannula placed in arm which is exsanguinated and a tourniquet applied.
- 4–6 mg/kg of 0.5% lignocaine without adrenaline (not bupivicaine, which is cardiotoxic) is injected slowly.
- The tourniquet should be on for at least 25 minutes to reduce the risk of generalized spread of lignocaine.
- If tourniquet pain is a problem, inflate a second more distal.

Bilhaut–Cloquet operation

- May be used to correct distal *Thumb duplication* (i.e. Wassel type 1 and 2).
- Both elements of the duplicated thumb are reduced and joined.
- Nail plates are removed, the outer segments approximated and the nail bed repaired.
- It can be modified by taking unequal portions of each finger. This avoids the central longitudinal nail bed repair and reduces the risk of subsequent nail irregularities.

Bilobed flap

- A double transposition flap with 2 lobes.
- Most commonly used for reconstruction of small to median nasal skin defects up to 1.5 cm diameter.
- The initial design by Esser described a 180° rotation over the entire flap whereas the modification by Zitelli described a 90° rotation (approximately 45° per lobe)

Principles:

- 1st lobe adjacent to the defect should be same diameter and thickness as defect. At base of 1st lobe, submuscular undermining onto perichondrium can facilitate flap inset and decrease pin-cushioning.
- 2nd lobe should be placed in area of tissue laxity and can be half the diameter of defect to facilitate direct closure.
- Excise a triangle of dog-ear between defect and flap pivot point before the flap is rotated.

Limitations:

- Associated with pin-cushioning.

See NASAL RECONSTRUCTION.

Binder's syndrome

- A congenital condition, most often occurs sporadically.
- Also known as nasomaxillary hypoplasia.
- Characterized by hypoplasia of central face with the nose appearing pushed in with malocclusion.
- It may be due to an inhibition of the ossification centre that would have formed the lateral and inferior borders of the piriform apertures.

Treatment options:

- *Le Fort osteotomies* with advancement of maxilla until teeth occlude.
- Augmentation rhinoplasty with costal cartilage grafts or synthetic silicone implants can be performed.

Binderoid cleft

- A subset of cleft lip and palate with associated nasolabiomaxillary hypoplasia and orbital hypotelorism.

- Nasal septum tends to be hypoplastic and nasal alar cartilages are small.

Biobrane™
- A dressing used for partial thickness wounds including burns.
- A bilaminate semi-permeable silicone membrane bonded to a thin layer of nylon fabric which is bound to modified porcine dermal collagen.
- It is available as a glove, which allows active movement during healing.
- It cannot be used for deeper or full thickness wounds.

Biological skin substitutes
- *Allograft: Cadaver skin.*
- *Xenograft:* pigskin. Less expensive, doesn't last as long, and doesn't cause wound bed vascularization.
- *Biobrane™.*
- *Human amniotic membrane.*
- *Transcyte™.*
- *Integra™.*

See BURNS. *See* TRANSPLANT IMMUNOLOGY.

Biomaterials
See ALLOPLASTS.

Bites
- *Human:* aerobic pathogens include *Staph. aureus* and *epidermidis*, and *Streptococci*. Anaerobic bacteria include *Peptostrep. peptococci, Eikenella corodens* and *bacteroides*.
- *Animal:* dogs and cats also have *Pasteurella multocida*. Dog bites tend to cause abrasions, tears and avulsions with an infection rate of approximately 20%. Cat bites tend to be deeper puncture wounds due to long slender teeth and can cause infection in 50%.

Bite wound management principles:
- Copious irrigation.
- Debridement if frank infection or devitalized tissue.
- Prophylactic antibiotics as per local guidance.
- Tetanus prophylaxis if indicated.

Blauth and Gekeler classification of symbrachydactyly
- *Short finger:* four short stiff coalesced fingers, normal thumb.
- *Oligodactylic:* central aplasia and cleft.
- *Monodactylic:* aplasia of all fingers, thumb preserved.
- *Peromelic:* transverse absence of all digits at metacarpal level.

See SYMBRACHYDACTYLY.

Blauth classification for thumb hypoplasia
See THUMB HYPOPLASIA.

Blepharochalasis
- A rare inherited condition with recurrent episodes of eyelid oedema.
- This results in ptosis due to an attenuated levator aponeurosis.
- Eyelid skin remains excessive.
- The term *Dermatochalasis* should be used for involutional skin excess.

Blepharomelasma
Dark discolouration of eyelid skin.
See BLEPHAROPLASTY.

Blepharopachynsis
Thickening of eyelid skin.
See BLEPHAROPLASTY.

Blepharophimosis
Congenitally small palpebral fissures caused by a triad of *Ptosis, Epicanthal folds* and *Telecanthus*.
See PTOSIS—EYELID.

Blepharoplasty
A procedure to shape the appearance of the eyelids and create lid creases. Eyelid skin is removed. Orbicularis muscle and excessive orbital fat may also be removed.

Assessment: ask whether the patient wears contact lenses, suffers from dry eyes or diplopia.

Examination: assess position of the eyebrow, eyelid pathology, fat pads, lagophthalmos, position of eyelid in relation to the eye.
- *Compensated brow ptosis:* as the patient opens the eyes the eyebrow moves up.
- *Snap test:* distract eyelid, >1 second to return is abnormal.
- *Distraction test:* lax if the lower lid can be pulled more than 7 mm from the globe.
- *Fat pads:* push on globe and look for herniation.
- *Lateral herniation:* may be lacrimal gland;
- *Bell's phenomenon.*
- *Enophthalmos:* look at position of globe from above.
- *Visual fields.*
- *Visual acuity.*

Operation:
- *Upper blepharoplasty:* while patient is supine design upper eyelid incisions. Elevate the eyebrow manually. Make caudal incision first. In the crease in younger patients, 1 mm above in older patients. Gently stretch the skin. Pinch the skin and mark the upper incision. Extend the upper mark laterally and medially.

Examine and mark the fat pads. Excise skin, with orbicularis if required. Consider incising orbital septum to expose the pre-aponeurotic fat pad and remove with careful haemostasis. If the lacrimal gland is prominent it may need to be elevated and secured. A lateral canthopexy may be required.

- *Lower blepharoplasty:* more complex than upper lid blepharoplasty and associated with higher risk of complications. Choice between subciliary incision (good for dealing with excess skin; a pinch blepharoplasty can be used to remove excess skin without undermining to reduce lid malposition) and transconjunctival incision (good for dealing with prominent fat; a pre-septal approach facilitates the release of the orbital septum at the arcus marginalis and re-draping of post-septal fat; a post-septal approach facilitates excision of excess fat). Glat advocated a 'no touch technique' to maintain the integrity of the tarsal plate and orbicularis muscle to reduce the risk of ectropion.
- *Compensated brow ptosis:* if the resting position of the brow has dropped, frontalis contracts to elevate brow and lid. Lid resection allows relaxation of frontalis and the position of the eyelid remains unchanged. A brow lift may be required prior to performing a blepharoplasty.

Complications:

- Early:
  - Loss of vision;
  - Retrobulbar haematoma—if this occurs decompress surgically via lateral canthotomy as an emergency; acetazolamide and mannitol can also be given;
  - Injury to inferior oblique muscle;
  - Wound dehiscence.
- Later:
  - Ectropion;
  - Over or under correction;
  - Dry eye syndrome;
  - Epiphora.

Blepharoptosis

Drooping of the upper lid.
See PTOSIS—EYELID.

Blood flow

Muscular tone of vessels is controlled by:

- *Sympathetic nerve supply:* these regulate flow by:
  - Increasing arteriolar tone and precapillary sphincter tone which decreases blood flow;
  - Decreasing AVA tone enabling blood to bypass the capillary bed.

- *Pressure:* an increase in intraluminal pressure results in vasoconstriction and a decrease causes vasodilatation. This is the explanation for hyperaemia after releasing the tourniquet.
- *Humeral factors:*
  - Adrenaline and noradrenaline cause vasoconstriction;
  - Histamine and bradykinin cause vasodilatation;
  - Low O_2, high CO_2 and acidosis result in vasodilatation.
- *Temperature:* increase in temperature produces cutaneous vasodilatation and flow, which bypasses the capillary beds.

Blood supply to skin

Six layers of vascular plexuses:

- *Subfascial plexus:* small plexus under the fascia.
- *Prefascial plexus:* larger plexus, prominent on limbs, predominantly supplied by fasciocutaneous vessels.
- *Subcutaneous plexus:* in superficial fascia. Predominant in torso, supplied by musculocutaneous vessels.
- *Subdermal plexus:* main plexus supplying skin.
- *Dermal plexus:* arterioles, important for thermoregulation.
- *Subepidermal plexus:* contains small vessels without muscles. Predominantly nutritive and thermoregulatory.

Blood supply to upper limb

- *Radial artery.*
- *Ulnar artery.*
- *Dorsal carpal arch.*
- *Superficial palmar arch.*
- *Deep palmar arch.*

Blood vessels
Anatomy:

- The inner layer consists of basement membrane with endothelial cells sitting on it.
- The next layer is the intima composed of elastin.
- Next is the media made of collagen and smooth muscles.
- The outer layer is the adventitia with the vasa vasorum.

Injury and repair:

- After injury endothelium is regenerated from endothelial cells from the edge.
- At an anastomosis get healing of all layers.
- Initially platelets aggregate on exposed collagen, but by the end of a week the endothelium proliferates and sutures are covered by 2 weeks.

Blue naevus
- Round, solitary bluish skin lesion.
- Found on dorsum of extremities or buttocks and often present at birth.
- F:M 2:1.
- Very low malignant potential.
- Due to arrested migration of melanocytes bound for the dermo-epidermal junction.
- Naevus of Ota occurs in area of 1st and 2nd trigeminal nerve.
- Naevus of Ito occurs in the dermatome of the upper chest.
- Current treatment is excision though lasers should be effective.

See NAEVUS. *See* OTA, NAEVUS OF. *See* ITO, NAEVUS OF.

Blue rubber bleb naevus
- Congenital condition with sporadic cause.
- Characterized by multifocal *venous malformations* on the skin and in the gastrointestinal tract.
- The skin lesions are soft, blue and nodular; they can occur anywhere, but are typically located on the hands and feet.
- The gastrointestinal lesions can lead to recurrent intestinal bleeding which can be severe, requiring repeated transfusions.

Body dysmorphic disorder (BDD)
- Preoccupation with an imagined defect in one's appearance.
- If a physical anomaly is present, the person's concern is markedly excessive. Patients with BDD have a high risk of committing suicide.
- The most common preoccupation is with the nose.
- Surgery tends to increase the preoccupation and the dissatisfaction.
- Patients turned down for surgery may attempt DIY surgery.
- BDD tends to begin in adolescence.
- Men and women show differing concerns for different body parts.

Body Mass Index (BMI)
Measured by body weight (kg) divided by height^2 (m):

- Normal — 20–25 kg/m^2
- Overweight — 25–30 kg/m^2
- Obese — 30–35 kg/m^2
- Morbidly obese — 35–55 kg/m^2
- Super morbidly obese — >55 kg/m^2

See OBESITY.

Bolam Principle
- A legal test to determine medical negligence using the standard of care expected of a doctor when compared to the standard of a responsible body of medical opinion. Has now been superseded by *Montgomery v. Lanarkshire Health Board (2015)*.
- Based on Bolam versus Friern Hospital Management Committee 1957: electroconvulsive therapy administrated with no restraints or muscle relaxant and the patient fell off the trolley sustaining an acetabular fracture.
- By this ruling, doctors defending *negligence* actions could rely on evidence of opinion from colleagues to justify their actions even if there is a body of opinion that would take the contrary view.

See ETHICS.

Bolitho Principle
- Built upon the *Bolam Principle* by requiring the body of opinion to have a logical basis, and the judge must be satisfied that the experts have considered the question of comparative risks and benefits, and reached a defensible conclusion. It was no longer enough for the defence to put up experts to say they genuinely believe a doctor's actions conformed with accepted practice.
- Based on Bolitho versus City and Hackney Health Authority, 1997: a case of a child admitted for observation with respiratory difficulties. The registrar did not attend when called, the child died and the medical experts were divided on whether it would have made any difference.

See ETHICS.

Bone
To maintain function, bone must regenerate.

Anatomy: bone is generated by osteoblasts. They are surrounded by their matrix and they are trapped. Once trapped they become smaller and become osteocytes.

- *Enchondral:* bones (long bones and iliac crest) start as cartilage precursor, which ossifies.
- *Membranous:* bones (face, calvarium and ribs) lay down bone directly within a vascularized membranous template. Membranous bones are more vascular but less strong.
- *Cortical:* bone has concentric lamellae around Haversian canals containing blood vessels.

- *Cancellous:* bone has large and small units of bone—trabeculae and spicules. Also have osteocytes, though not as compact as cortical bone. Bone is only 8% water. The matrix is 98% collagen (type I).
- *Blood supply:* of long bones from a primary nutrient artery, proximal and distal metaphyseal vessels and the periosteum. Though the endosteal circulation is dominant in undisplaced fractures, in displaced fractures, the main blood supply is derived from the periosteum.

Healing:
- *Primary healing:* if bone is rigidly fixed. Get restoration of normal bone structure without the inflammatory and proliferative phase. Callus is not formed. Osteoclasts first cross the fracture line in a cutting cone, allowing ingrowth of blood vessels and mesenchymal stem cells (MSCs), which differentiate into osteoblasts.
- *Secondary healing:* occurs if fragments are not rigidly fixed or if there is a gap. If the fracture is widely displaced or mobile then scar tissue bridges the gap forming a non-union. In more favourable conditions, new bone formation occurs.

Phases of secondary bone healing:
- *Haematoma and Inflammation:* osteoclasts remove debris. Associated with pain. Platelets release PDGF and TGF which promote MSC proliferation.
- *Cellular proliferation:* periosteal and endosteal.
- *Callus formation:* immature woven bone, osteoid laid down by osteoblasts and mineralized with hydroxyapatite:
  - *Soft callus:* neovascularization mainly from periosteum. Precursor cells differentiate into fibroblasts, chondroblasts and osteoblasts. These produce collagen, cartilage and osteoid that makes up callus. Mainly type II collagen;
  - *Hard callus:* soft callus is mineralized. 3–4 weeks after injury. Osteoclasts remove all dead bone and type II collagen is replaced by type I collagen. Calcium hydroxyapatite is deposited. Initially get woven bone.
- *Remodelling:* cortical structure and medullary cavity are restored. Fibres are reorientated along stress lines (Wolf's law). Woven bone is remodelled into lamellar bone.

Guided bone regeneration: controlled stimulation of new bone into a defect by osteoconduction, osteoinduction or osteogenesis. Periosteum provides a source of osteoprogenitor cells and blood supply. The periosteum may

also provide a barrier to the in-growth of fibrous tissue. Other membranes have been tried in place of periosteum. PTFE sheets have been used. Resorbable barriers are being evaluated.

See ILIZAROV.

Bone graft
Source:
- *Autogenous:* preferred due to improved take. Autogenous grafts contain cells and growth factors. Cancellous bone has these in greater amounts. Cortical bone provides bulk. Grafts can be vascularised or free, inlay or onlay.
- *Allogenic implants:* bone transplanted between individuals. As the cells are killed it is not an allograft, but an implant. Less predictable than autografts. Get delayed vascularization, resorption and poor osteogenic capacity.
- *Xenogenic transplant:* first performed in 1668 when a Dutch surgeon put pig calvarium into a Russian soldier. The Russian church demanded its removal 2 years later during which he died. Xenogenic grafts are presently not performed.

Bone graft mechanisms:
- *Osseointegration:* graft adheres to the host tissue.
- *Osteoconduction:* cells migrate from the bone ends into the graft, which acts as a scaffold.
- *Osteoinduction:* precursor cells within local tissues are stimulated to become osteocytes, which move into the graft. Osseo-induction is controlled by bone morphogenic proteins (BMPs).
- *Osteogenesis:* formation of new bone by surviving cells in the bone graft. This only occurs in vascularized bone grafts.

Graft survival:
- *Systemic factors:* are similar to those affecting *Wound healing*.
- *Intrinsic graft factors:* grafts with intact periosteum and membranous bones undergo less absorption.
- *Graft placement factors:* particularly if in a normal bone site, quality of bed, graft fixation.

Bone substitutes *Polymethylmethacrylate, Polytetrafluoroethylene.*

Bone morphogenetic proteins (BMPs)
- Osteoinductive growth factors. BMPs are responsible for bone regeneration.
- Multiple BMPs exist. 15 have been identified, and all apart from BMP-1 belong to the TGF-β family.
- Bone produced at non-bony sites may be caused by the presence of BMPs.

- BMPs can be used instead of autologous bone grafts for procedures such as alveolar bone grafting but pathological and oncological concerns have limited widespread clinical use.

Bone tumours

Hand bone tumours account for 5% of bone tumours and 2% of malignant bone tumours.

- *Aneurysmal bone cyst.*
- *Chondroblastoma.*
- *Chondromyxoid fibroma.*
- *Chondrosarcoma.*
- *Enchondroma.*
- *Ewing's sarcoma.*
- *Fibrous dysplasia.*
- *Giant cell tumour of bone.*
- *Histiocytosis.*
- *Osteochondroma.*
- *Osteogenic sarcomas.*
- *Osteoid osteoma.*
- *Osteoblastoma.*
- *Unicameral bone cyst.*
- *Metastatic carcinoma.*
- *Myeloma.*
- *Non-ossifying fibroma.*

Classification: *Enneking's system.*

Clinical presentation: pain is a common symptom. Family history is important for some diseases with a high association with tumours.

Investigations:
- Hypercalcaemia is common.
- Alkaline phosphatase is elevated in 50% of patients with osteosarcoma.
- Lactate dehydrogenase is elevated with Ewing's sarcoma.
- Perform plain XRs. Assess the bone, the tumour and the matrix. Bone scans are not very useful.
- MRI is useful to assess intramedullary extent.
- CT is useful to detect matrix calcification. CT of the chest is important.
- USS differentiates cystic from solid masses.
- PET is useful for some carcinomas such as hepatic carcinoma and melanoma.

Principles: without surgery, the tumour will recur. The options for resection are intracapsular, marginal, wide (intracompartmental) and radical (extracompartmental). The aim is to cure the patient of the tumour, preserve the limb and preserve function if possible.

- *Biopsy:* a tissue diagnosis is important. Perform an incision longitudinally over the tumour closest to the skin within one compartment. Frozen section may be used to ensure a good sample of the tumour has been taken. FNA and core biopsies can be used if the pathologist is confident. The incision or core tract will require complete excision at the time of definitive surgery.
- *Curettage:* this is not curative and is reserved for recurrent or stage 3 tumours. The cavity can be filled with bone cement or treated with liquid nitrogen. Bone graft or allograft can be used to fill the defect.
- *Resection/amputation:* most primary tumours are located in the metaphysis and require sacrifice of the joint.

Bonnet–Dechaume–Blanc

Telangiectatic facial birthmark with intracranial AVM.

See VASCULAR MALFORMATIONS.

Boss—carpometacarpal

- Bony prominence usually arising at the base of the second and third metacarpal.
- The joint becomes hypertrophic with an overlying bursa, and tendons may bowstring over the swelling.
- Possibly secondary to trauma.
- *XR:* use a carpal boss view taken in 30–40° supination and 20–30° ulnar deviation.

Treatment:
- *Conservative:* splint, NSAIDS and steroid injection.
- *Surgical:* excise the boss through a longitudinal or transverse incision. Retract extensors. Make a longitudinal incision over the boss. Expose the boss subperiosteally. Elevate part of ECRB from the bone. Excise the boss with an osteotome until normal cartilage is seen. Inadequate excision results in persistent pain and swelling, so the entire boss needs to be excised, exposing the CMC joint. A ganglion at this site will require excision of the ganglion and the boss.

Botulinum toxin

- Seven serologically distinct exotoxins *A-G* produced by strains of *Clostridium botulinum* that prevent the release of acetylcholine at the neuromuscular junction to treat striated muscle spasm, resulting in flaccid paralysis.
- Type A toxin consists of a heavy and light chain that works at the pre-synaptic neuronal cell membrane to cleave SNAP-25. It is used for focal spasticity and blepharospasm and off-licence for cosmetic purposes, most commonly improving rhytids, paralysis of the depressor anguli oris or mentalis and softening of platysmal bands.

- Type B toxin also works at the pre-synaptic terminal but cleaves synaptobrevin and is licenced for use in spasmodic torticollis.
- Botox* is supplied dry in vials containing 100 Mouse Units (MU). It is unstable and must be kept in a freezer. It is reconstituted in 2 ml of saline. Toxic dose in humans is 3,000 MU.
- Paralysis appears within 24–48 hours of injection with peak action at 7–10 days.
- Contraindications include motor neurone disease, myasthenia gravis, Lambert-Eaton myasthenic syndrome, pregnancy and lactation and psychological instability.

Bouchard's node
Osteophyte developing at the PIP joint. Seen in osteoarthritis.

Boutonnière deformity
- Flexion of the PIP joint and extension of the DIP joint.
- Due to a disruption of the extensor mechanism. The central slip is often disrupted and the lateral bands move volarly and become flexors of the PIP joint. The FDS tendon now has nothing to resist it and unopposed flexion occurs. With time the lateral bands contract and their pull on the oblique retinacular ligament (ORL) pulls the DIP joint into hyperextension. The MCP joint also moves into hyperextension.

Assessment:
- Active and passive ROM of DIP joint and PIP joint.
- Check tightness of ORL by extending PIP joint and assessing tension at DIP joint.

Classification by Nalebuff:
- *Stage 1:* dynamic, passively correctable.
- *Stage 2:* established deformity which cannot be passively corrected.
- *Stage 3:* established deformity with secondary PIP joint changes.

Treatment:
- Acute central slip divisions should be repaired.
- Stage 1and 2 problems should be splinted to stretch volar structures, lateral bands and the ORL.
- Stage 3 problems are difficult to correct. Joint release may be performed. Central slip reconstruction, lateral band release, arthrodesis or arthroplasty may be required.

Bouvier's manoeuvre
- A test for integrity of the central slip and lateral bands of the extensor mechanism. Used in the assessment of claw hand in *ulnar nerve palsy*.

- To perform the test, the examiner blocks MCPJ hyperextension and patient is asked to extend the IPJs of digits:
  ○ Normal if IPJs actively extended—suggests static anti-claw procedures to produce MCPJ flexion should improve claw;
  ○ Abnormal if IPJs cannot be extended actively—if the IPJs can be extended passively then the patient may benefit from dynamic anti-claw procedures to provide coordinated MCPJ flexion and PIPJ extension. Fixed deformity of the IPJs suggests an intrinsic joint deformity that would not respond to an anti-claw procedure.

Bowen's disease
- An intra-epithelial *squamous cell carcinoma* (carcinoma-*in-situ*). 10% become invasive after many years with 1/3 of those developing metastatic disease.
- Seen in older patients in sun exposed and covered areas.
- Found on skin or mucous membrane (*Bowen's of mucous membranes*). Most are solitary with a long clinical course.
- More common in men than women.
- Appearance of sharply defined erythematous reddish scaly plaque with pruritus and superficial crusting.
- Histologically see hyperkeratosis and acanthosis with disordered epithelium and frequent mitoses, but no dermal invasion.
- Treat with excision or curettage.
- There is also a relation between Bowen's disease and internal malignancies.

Boyes sublimis tendon transfer
For *Radial nerve palsy*:

• PT	→	ECRB
• FDS middle	→	EDC 2–5
• FDS ring	→	EPL, EIP
• FCR	→	APL, EPB

Bra
See CUP SIZE.

Brachial plexus—anatomy
- 5 nerve roots (C5–T1).
- 3 trunks (upper, middle, lower).
- 6 divisions (3 posterior, 3 anterior).
- 3 cords (lateral, medial and posterior).
- 4 major nerves (median, ulnar, radial and musculocutaneous).
- *Dorsal root:* sensory afferents, cell bodies in the dorsal root ganglion.
- *Ventral root:* motor efferents (relay in anterior horn cells).

- Dorsal and ventral roots combine to form spinal nerves which split into anterior and posterior rami. The major plexuses are formed from the anterior rami. The posterior rami become the posterior intercostal nerves.

Roots: C5–T1, variably C4 and T2. lie behind scalenus anterior.

Trunks: upper, middle, lower between the anterior and middle scalenes. Cross lower part of posterior triangle.

Division: anterior and posterior. Each trunk divides at the lateral edge of first rib. Lie behind clavicle.

Cords: lateral, medial and posterior. Formed by the combinations of divisions and named in relation to the axillary artery. The anterior division of lower trunk continues to become the medial cord, the posterior divisions join to become the posterior cord and the anterior division of lower joins with anterior division of upper to become the lateral cord.

Nerves: commence at the lateral border of pectoralis minor.

Examination based on anatomy:
C5 and C6 roots and upper trunk:

- *Dorsal scapular nerve supplies rhomboids:* squeeze shoulder blades and palpate.
- *Long thoracic nerve supplies serratus anterior:* push wall.
- *Suprascapular nerve supplies supra- and infraspinatus:* look at muscle bulk and test for external rotation of the shoulder.
- *Third branch joins middle trunk to form axillary nerve:* test abduction of shoulder, palpate deltoid.
- *Lateral pectoral nerve:* clavicular head of pectoralis major, don't examine.
- *Musculocutaneous nerve:* biceps and sensation lateral arm.
- *Upper trunk contribution to median nerve:* supplies FCR and pronator teres. Test FCR with wrist flexion and palpation. Test PT with pronation against force at 90°.

C7 root:
This is like examining the radial nerve with subscapularis.

- *Assess internal rotation and latissimus dorsi:* push down on hips and palpate.
- Axillary nerve has already been tested.
- Final branch is radial nerve. Brachioradialis and ECRL/B are supplied by C6, EPL and EDC supplied by C7 and 8. Test sensation.

C8–T1 root:
- *Medial pectoral nerve:* supplies pectoralis major.
- *Medial cutaneous nerve of the arm and forearm:* test sensation.
- Contribution to median nerve supplying FDS, FDP index and middle, FPL, APB.
- Terminates as ulnar nerve.
  Also note pain, fractures, phrenic nerve palsy and *Horner's syndrome*.

Brachial plexus injury—adult
Injury: Most occur following a high energy traction injury during an RTA. The aim of the assessment is to identify the anatomical level of the injury as this will dictate the management options available.

Diagnosis:
- *History:* the nature of the force. The position of head and arm. Shoulder abduction will suggest lower root injury. If the arm is pulled down it is more likely to involve upper roots. Traction will cause a central C7 injury.
- *Examination:* to assess likelihood of pre-ganglionic injury look for Horner's syndrome and test the proximal branches: long thoracic nerve to serratus anterior (winging of the scapula) and dorsal scapula nerve to rhomboids (inability to squeeze shoulders together). Then test sensation in each dermatome and muscles in each myotome and record MRC grade.
- *Electrodiagnostic studies:* need to wait for Wallerian degeneration for it to be effective so can first do neurophysiology at 3 weeks:
  - Low amplitude potentials suggest re-innervation;
  - Diminished fibrillations and sharp waves and activated muscle units suggest re-innervation, but do not correlate with function;
  - Sensory nerve action potential (SNAP)—in a pre-ganglionic root avulsion sensory SNAPs will be intact (due to their location in the dorsal root ganglion) but motor SNAPS will be absent. In a post-ganglionic injury both sensory and motor SNAPs will be absent.
- *Neuroradiology:*
  - MRI is the gold standard and can reveal pseudomeningoceles around the spinal cord to indicate root avulsion;
  - MRA/CTA may be required if suspicion of vascular injury.

Indications for surgical exploration:
- Open injury—mechanism increase risk of non-continuity.

- Concomitant injury requiring exploration, i.e. vascular or orthopaedic.
- Imaging suggested non-continuity.

b

Timing of surgery:
- Open injuries should be explored acutely.
- The timing of operative exploration in closed injuries is controversial because spontaneous recovery is associated with better outcomes yet if surgery is indicated, the sooner the better. Early exploration (within 2 weeks) is associated with improved MRC grades following nerve grafting of ruptures.

Priorities: aim is to restore use and prevent amputation.
- *Shoulder stabilization:* prevents subluxation— by neurotization of the suprascapular nerve with intraplexus nerve donor or accessory nerve.
- *Elbow flexion:* musculocutaneous nerve is restored with intraplexus donors or extraplexus donors such as intercostals.
- *Sensation:* median nerve neurotization from sensory intercostals or cervical plexus.
- *Hand function:* priorities are finger flexion and extension, then intrinsics and thumb opposition and abduction.

Operative procedures: the final diagnosis can only be made at exploration. Use intra-operative neurophysiology (somatosensory evoked potentials SSEPs) to establish continuity between peripheral nerves and central nervous system.
- *Direct nerve repair:* usually only possible for a fresh cut.
- *Nerve grafting:* for bridging post-ganglionic ruptures or neuromas in continuity. Ensure nerve grafts are reversed, splayed (to enhance re-vascularization) and not under tension. Common donor nerves: sural (40 cm), medial/lateral cutaneous nerves of arm and forearm, superficial branch of the radial nerve.
- *Nerve transfer (Neurotization):* for pre-ganglionic injuries (where nerve grafting is not an option) and some post-ganglionic injuries where the regrowth distance is too long. Donor nerves can be:
  - *Intraplexal:* Oberlin 1 (ulnar nerve fascicle to biceps branch of musculocutaneous) and Oberlin 2 (median nerve fascicle to brachialis branch of musculocutaneous) for elbow flexion;
  - *Extraplexal:* spinal accessory nerve, intercostal nerves cervical plexus, phrenic (partial), hypoglossal, contralateral pectoral, contralateral C7.

Secondary reconstruction: these may be necessary if only partial recovery occurs with the above procedures.
- *Shoulder:* aim for abduction and external rotation with tendon transfers such as latissimus dorsi for external rotation and trapezius advancement for abduction. Free muscle transfer can be used, e.g. gracilis and adductor longus on a single pedicle.
- *Elbow:* pedicled latissimus dorsi can restore elbow flexion. Forearm flexors have been moved proximally to act on the elbow. Free transfers used are latissimus dorsi, gracilis (but not very strong), vastus lateralis and rectus femoris for biceps.
- *Wrist:* fuse in global avulsion as restoration of wrist function is not feasible.

Prognosis: determined by the type of lesion, age, denervation time, degree of root involvement, surgical technique and patient compliance.

Brachial plexus injury—obstetric
Incidence 1:1,000. Most recover, 10% are severe.

Aetiology:
- Injury to brachial plexus caused by excess traction of baby's neck during delivery.
- Upper palsy involving C5-6 +-7 (Erb's palsy) is the most common presentations and can be a consequence of shoulder dystocia. See a 'waiter's tip' deformity with internally rotated and adducted shoulder, extended elbow, pronated forearm and flexed wrist. C5 has strong dural attachment so ruptures. C6 and C7 will avulse at the roots.
- C8 and T1 are usually only injured once the other roots are completely avulsed. However, Klumpke's is lower root due to hyperabduction in breech delivery.
- Overall 50% will recover spontaneously, 5% will need nerve surgery in infancy and 30% will need shoulder stabilization at a later stage.

Classification: by *Narakas*.
1. Mild C5-6: neuropraxia and axonotmesis— isolated paralysis of shoulder and biceps— 60% recovery.
2. C5-7: varying from neuropraxia to neurotmesis—paralysis of shoulder, biceps and forearm extensors—30% recovery.
3. C5-T1: complete dense paralysis but without Horner's—10% recovery—more likely to need nerve surgery.
4. C5-T1: with Horner's 5% recovery.

Prognosis:
- Any partial lesion has a better prognosis.
- Good grasp at 8/52 is likely to recover well.

- No recovery by 6/12 is unlikely to improve much.
- Breech delivery gives the most severe injuries.

Indications for operation:
- Assess at 3 months to see if surgery required and use Toronto Prognostic score to help make the decision.
- Indications for operative intervention are poor shoulder flexion and abduction, minimal elbow flexion, wrist drop and Horners syndrome, i.e. Narakas 2–4 with little sign of recovery at 3 months.

Investigation:
- Neurophysiology and MRI at 4 months.

Management:
- Conservative: once the diagnosis is made, assess every 3 months until age 1 year, then 6 monthly until plateau, then annually for life to monitor for shoulder tightness. Assess using the Mallett score of shoulder function and look for the Trumpeting sign. Physio to perform external rotation stretch and maintain supple joints.
- Surgical: timing is controversial and can be early (3 months) or later (9 months). Principles:
  - Supra-clavicular approach—often see neuromas in upper and middle trunks;
  - Exploration with SSEP to confirm pattern of change;
  - Graft any ruptures or neuromas;
  - Spinal Accessory to SSN.

Brachioplasty
- A procedure to re-contour the arm involving an excision of excess skin.
- Excess of fat alone without skin redundancy can be treated with liposuction alone.
- Horizontal redundancy of skin can be managed with a wedge, elliptical or T-incision in the axillary fold.
- Horizontal and vertical redundancy of skin requires an extended brachioplasty with an incision from the axilla to elbow.
- To reduce the risk of damage to sensory nerves and lymphatics (leading to lymphoedema), liposuction is recommended prior to skin excision to deflate the tissues.

Brachioradialis
Origin: proximal 2/3 of lateral supracondylar ridge of humerus and intermuscular septum proximal to ECRL. It lies on the radial aspect of forearm, crossing ECRL and PT.

Insertion: styloid process of radius and ante-brachial fascia. The latter is divided if the tendon is used as a tendon transfer.

Nerve supply: radial nerve.

Action: flexes elbow joint, supinates the pronated forearm, weak pronator of supinated forearm.
See MUSCLES.

Brachydactyly
Unusually short fingers.

Brachytherapy
- Radiotherapy treatment by implantation of radioactive material.
- Originally radium needles were used but now iridium 192 is implanted in wires.
- Plastic tubes are inserted at the time of operation.
- These are then loaded with radioactive seeds. This can be performed manually or it can be automated to reduce radiation exposure to the technicians.
- Useful in tongue and mouth lesions. Also used to treat keloid scars.
- May be preferable for posterior 1/3 of tongue tumours, which cross the midline which would otherwise require a debilitating total glossectomy.
- High risk of osteoradionecrosis.
See RADIATION.

Bracka repair for hypospadias
This is a two-stage reconstruction for hypospadias which is usually indicated in a proximally located ventral meatus or where the urethral plate is insufficient for single stage tabularization. It is a modification of the original Cloutier operation for *Hypospadias* repair.

First stage: aims are to correct chordee, excise the hypoplastic urethral plate and apply a FTSG. FTSG can be harvested from inner surface of prepuce or buccal mucosa. Post-op remove dressing and catheter at 1 week.

Second stage: aims to tubularize the skin graft to form a neo-urethra. Perform when the graft is well healed and softened (usually 3-6 months after the first stage).

Results: fistula rate of 5% reported by Bracka in 1995, but 15% by trainees in the same unit.

Branchial cysts
- Branchial cleft anomalies are the most frequently occurring masses in the lateral neck.
- They occur because of failure of maturation of the first and second branchial arches. The remnant remains trapped in the neck. Most branchial cleft anomalies involve first and second branchial pouch complexes.
- Between the arches are clefts. The 2nd, 3rd, 4th clefts are usually obliterated by the 6th week. If they persist they become a sinus or cyst.

- They occur along the anterior border of the sternocleidomastiod.
- May present at any age, usually present by 8 years of age.
- Cysts are soft non-tender.
- They often become infected which should be treated prior to excision.
- Require imaging prior to surgery to define cleft anatomy.
- Definitive management is complete surgical excision. Incomplete excision has high incidence of recurrence. The tract may be cannulated or dye injected during excision to aid visualization. The tract should ultimately be ligated and divided at its source.

Cysts:
- *First branchial cleft cysts:* very rare. Get dimple or tract close to parotid (between external auditory canal and submandibular area), associated with facial nerve.
- *Second branchial cleft cysts:* most common. Occurs at the junction of middle and lower thirds of sternocleidomastoid in the direction of the tonsillar fossa between internal and external carotid artery. May have intermittent and chronic drainage. Can be intimately associated with glossopharyngeal and hypoglossal nerve.
- *Third branchial cleft cysts:* rare.
- *Fourth branchial cleft cysts:* runs behind the internal carotid artery then beneath the subclavian artery on the right and aortic arch on the left, opening into upper oesophagus.

See HEAD AND NECK EMBRYOLOGY.

Branemark implant
See OSSEOINTEGRATION.

BRCA
- *BRCA1* and *BRCA2* are tumour suppressor genes present in all women.
- Mutations in these genes increase the risk of developing *Breast cancer* and ovarian cancer. There is an 85% lifetime risk of developing breast cancer and 65% risk for ovarian cancer.
- 1:300 women are carriers of mutations of *BRCA1* gene.
- Autosomal dominant inheritance.
- Present in 2% of women with breast cancer.

Breast
Anatomy:
- The breast develops from ectoderm. The milk line forms in the 5th week of gestation. Incomplete involution of the milk ridge produces accessory nipples.
- At adolescence the breast grows and differentiates with ptosis developing after the

age of 16. At menopause glandular involution occurs.
- The breast is mainly fibrous with around 15 main ducts running through to drain at the nipple. Each duct drains a lobe and lobes are separated by fibrous septae. The ligaments of Astley-Cooper attach deep fascia to skin and provide support.

Boundaries: 2nd to 7th rib, sternal edge to anterior axillary line overlying the pectoral fascia and serratus anterior, external oblique and rectus abdominis.

Blood supply:
- *From perforating branches of the internal thoracic artery (60%):* medial portion.
- *The lateral thoracic artery:* lateral portion.
- *Thoracoacromial axis:* pectoral branches.
- *Lateral branches from the 3rd, 4th and 5th posterior intercostal arteries:* lower outer portion.
- Veins follow arteries.

Lymphatics: lymph drains via interlobular vessels to the subareolar plexus and parallels the venous system. 75% drains to the axilla via the pectoral nodes. Medial parasternal lymph nodes carry 3–20% of lymph along the internal thoracic chain.

Nerve supply: sensory innervation from:
- The supraclavicular nerves of the 3rd and 4th branches of the cervical plexus.
- The anterior cutaneous nerves from the 2nd–6th intercostal nerves.
- The anterior branches of the lateral cutaneous nerves from the 3rd–6th intercostal nerves. Sensation to the nipple is primarily from the lateral cutaneous branch of the 4th intercostal nerve.

Shape:
- The shape varies but in the mildly ptotic breast, most of the fullness is in the inferior half.
- The nipple to inframammary fold distance measures 5–6 cm in the 'ideal' breast.
- The nipple-areolar complex is the point of maximum projection and measures 35–45 mm in diameter.

Accessory breast tissue:
- Due to failure of regression of ectoderm or mesoderm along the mammary line. <2% of children.
- M:F 1:2.
- Accessory nipples are confused with pigmented naevi and breast tissue with lipomas.
- May develop the same pathological diseases as breast.

Breast augmentation
A commonly performed cosmetic procedure with multiple options available. Usually involves the insertion of breast implants but augmentation can also be performed with autologous fat grafting. Careful patient selection is imperative and patients should be encouraged to be involved with decision making.

History of breast augmentation:
- Czerny transplanted a lipoma in 1895.
- Cronin and Gerow inserted a silicone prosthesis in 1962.

Assessment:
- Current bra size and desired bra size. Do they want a change in size or shape or both?
- Presence of ptosis, chest wall deformities and tuberous breasts will impact on options.
- 'Pinch test' for skin envelope thickness—<2 cm not appropriate for subglandular pocket.
- Measure:
  - Sternal notch to nipple distance to document asymmetry;
  - Nipple to IMF distance—may indicate if IMF needs to be lowered if <8–9 cm on stretch;
  - Breast base width—informs implant choice.
- Up to date mammography as per local/national guidance.

Implant shape:
- Anatomical—reproduces natural tear drop shape of breast with lower pole fullness but can become malpositioned if it rotates in the pocket. Choice of projection and height of implant.
- Round—provides patients with upper poll fullness which may be cosmetically advantageous and does not malposition with rotation. Choice of projection only.

Implant size:
- Volume measured in cubic centimetres (cc).
- The High Five (Tebbetts and Adams 2006) and ICE principles (Mallucci 2016) have been published to assist in planning.

Implant surface:
- Textured—based on ISO scale can be macro (>50 micrometres) or micro (<50 micrometres) textured. May be associated with lower capsular contracture rate and less migration but have thicker shells so may be more palpable and have been associated with *Breast Implant Associated Anaplastic large cell lymphoma (BIA-ALCL)*.
- Smooth—less palpable so may be beneficial in patients with less parenchymal coverage but prone to migration.

Implant contents:
- Saline.
- Silicone.

Incisions:
- Inframammary with good exposure but more noticeable scar. Most commonly used incision and associated with the lowest risk of infection.
- *Peri-areolar:* with good scar, but possibly nipple paraesthesia.
- Axillary with no scar on the breast but decreased exposure.
- Endoscopic placement through umbilical or axillary route.

Position of implant:
- *Subglandular:* below breast tissue, above fascia. Provides good projection and shape but may be associated with high capsular contraction rates especially in thin parenchymal coverage when upper pole pinch test <2 cm.
- *Subfascial:* beneath pectoral fascia but above the pectoralis major muscle.
- *Submuscular:* below pectoralis and rectus abdominus. Theoretically lower capsular contracture rates and good preservation of nipple sensation. Disadvantage of animation deformity and lateral displacement of implant over time, double bubble deformity, more dissection and increased bleeding risk.
- *Tebbett's dual plane pocket:* the implant is positioned subpectorally, but the parenchymal-muscle interface is altered by varying degrees of subglandular pocket dissection to change the soft tissue relationships and allow the nipple to lie at the most projecting part of the implant. This allows the implant to be placed along the IMF and reduces risk of a 'double bubble' deformity.

Adams 14-point plan to reduce risk of infection in Breast Augmentation:
1. IV antibiotics at induction.
2. Avoid peri areola and transaxillary incisions as shown to be associated with capsular contracture.
3. Use nipple shields to avoid spill of bacteria.
4. Perform careful atraumatic dissection.
5. Careful haemostasis.
6. Avoid dissection into parenchyma.
7. Use a dual-plane pocket.
8. Perform pocket irrigation with betadine.
9. Minimize skin contamination.
10. Minimize implant open time.
11. Change surgical gloves before handling implant.
12. Avoiding drains.

13. Use layered closure.
14. Use antibiotics prophylaxis to cover subsequent procedures.

Complications:
Early:
- Nerve injury to _Nipple_ with decreased sensation in 15%.
- Bleeding.
- Infection incidence is 2.2%, most commonly with _Staph. epidermidis._ Explantation usually required.

Later:
- _Capsular contracture:_ CORE studies suggest 1% annual risk: 1/10 at 10 years.
- Rippling.
- Malposition.
- Scarring.
- _Rupture:_ around 2% per year, but less with newer implants.
- _Breast Implant Associated Anaplastic large cell lymphoma (BIA-ALCL):_ up to date UK incidence reported via MHRA.
- _Breast implant illness._

Breast cancer
- _Incidence:_ 1:8. The most common cancer in women. 25,000–33,000 new cases per year in Britain.
- _Risk factors:_ female sex, age, personal or family history of breast cancer, oestrogen exposure (first pregnancy >30 years, nulliparity, early menarche and late menopause, hormone replacement therapy (HRT) and oral contraceptive pill), reduced risk with breastfeeding, radiation to chest.
- _Inheritance:_ BRCA carriers have 85% lifetime risk.

Presentation:
- Symptomatically with breast lump.
- Identification through screening programme.

Investigation:
- Triple assessment is gold standard, with grades 1–5 allocated in each of the PMB categories:
  - P—clinical examination of breast, axilla and supraclavicular fossa;
  - M—imaging by mammography has a sensitivity of 90% and specificity of 95% +/– USS for dense breasts (especially younger patients);
  - B—histology ideally by image guided core biopsy to facilitate differentiation of subtype and receptor status.

Subtypes:
- Non-invasive:
  - Ductal carcinoma _in situ_ (DCIS):
    - Dysplasia in the epithelial cells of the mammary ducts;
    - 10% bilateral, 20% multicentric, 30% become invasive;
    - Small, local excision; larger, mastectomy;
  - Lobular carcinoma _in situ_ (LCIS):
    - A marker of breast cancer;
    - 40% bilateral, 60% multifocal;
    - 1% chance per year of developing invasive breast cancer;
    - Treat by observation or bilateral mastectomy.
- Invasive:
  - 75% are ductal;
  - 10% are lobular. Often ER positive, more likely to be bilateral and may not be identified on a mammogram;
  - Other subtypes: medullary, tubular, papillary, mucinous, adenoid cystic; inflammatory.

Receptor status:
- Hormone receptors (oestrogen ER and progesterone PR). 70% breast cancers are ER+ve and associated with better prognosis.
- ERBB2-ve associated with better prognosis but better improved outcome now for ERBB2+ve with Herceptin.
- Triple negative (ER/PR/ERBB2-ve) associated with worst prognosis due to limited treatment options and an indication for chemotherapy.

Classification:
- _TNM:_
  - _Tumour:_
    - _T1:_ <2 cm;
    - _T2:_ 2–5 cm;
    - _T3:_ >5 cm;
    - _T4:_ tumour invades skin and chest wall.
  - _Lymph nodes:_
    - _N1:_ ipsilateral mobile axillary lymphadenopathy (levels I, II);
    - _N2a:_ as above but fixed;
    - _N2b:_ ipsilateral internal mammary nodes;
    - _N3a:_ ipsilateral infraclavicular nodes;
    - _N3b:_ ipsilateral internal mammary and axillary nodes (levels I, II);
    - _N3c:_ ipsilateral supraclavicular nodes.
  - _Metastasis:_
    - _M1:_ supraclavicular nodes or distant metastases.

Staging:

Stage	T	N	M
0	Tis	N0	M0
1A	T1	N0	M0
1B	T0-1	N(Micro)	M0
2A	T0-1	N1	M0
	T2	N0	M0
2B	T2	N1	M0
	T3	N0	M0
3A	T0-3	N1-2	M0
3B	T4	N1-2	M0
3C	Any T	N3	M0
4	Any T	Any N	M1

Predicted 5-year survival:

- Stage 1—92%.
- Stage 2—73%.
- Stage 3—50%.
- Stage 4—13%.

There are tools that can be used in clinic to help work decision making and calculation of risk:

- Nottingham Prognostic Index.
- Adjuvant! (online tool).
- PREDICT (online tool).

Oncological treatment:
- *Surgical excision:*
  - Wide local excision (with radiotherapy) can be considered in small unifocal tumours with favourable pathological profiles— NSABP trials demonstrated equivalent overall and disease-free survival following WLE+RT and modified radical mastectomy;
  - Mastectomy—indicated in multifocal breast cancer, widespread DCIS, high risk tumours, large tumours in small breasts and previous breast cancer or radiation. Types of mastectomy:
    - Nipple-sparing—removal of breast parenchyma with preservation of skin envelope and NAC. May be suitable in prophylactic mastectomies and tumours located away from the nipple with favourable pathological features. Many advocate a biopsy from beneath the NAC;
    - Skin-sparing—removal of breast parenchyma but with preservation of the skin envelope;
    - Simple—removal of breast parenchyma and skin envelope. NSABP trials demonstrated equivalent overall and disease-free survival following simple mastectomy or radical mastectomy;

- Modified radical = simple + axillary node clearance;
- Radical = radical + pectoralis major removal.
- *Adjuvant radiotherapy:* usually dose of 40Gy in 15 fractions. Indications:
  - Pre-op factors—nodal burden and tumour size;
  - Post-op factors—lymphovascular invasion and posterior distance to the chest wall.
- *Axillary surgery:* in the absence of clinical axillary lymph node disease, sentinel lymph node biopsy (SLNB) is performed at the time of tumour excision or prior (upfront SLNB). A positive SLNB can be treated with either axillary lymph node dissection (ALND) or radiotherapy (AMAROS Trial demonstrated equivalent 5-year survival rates but less morbidity with RT). Clinical axillary lymph node involvement is managed by axillary lymph node dissection (ALND).
- *Systemic treatment:* treatment regimen is determined by receptor status:
  - ER+ tumours receive either tamoxifen (an anti-oestrogen, especially for pre-menopausal women) or aromatase-inhibitors such as anastrozole (especially for post-menopausal women as acts at periphery). Treatment is for 5–10 years. Stop tamoxifen 4 weeks pre-operatively as increases risk of venous thromboembolism;
  - ERBB2+ tumours receive targeted immune therapy, e.g. trastuzumab (Herceptin) for 1 year. Trastuzumab works synergistically with chemotherapy;
  - Triple-negative tumours are treated with chemotherapy for 12–20 weeks.
- *Recurrence:* in breast, lymph nodes and distant metastasis to any site, especially lung, liver, bone.

Breast implant-associated anaplastic large T-cell lymphoma (BIA-ALCL)

Epidemiology: incidence may be affected by significant under-reporting and underdiagnosis and is constantly changing as awareness increases.

Pathophysiology: causality has not definitively been determined, but there is a correlation with textured implants (no cases to date of BIA-ALCL have been described in patients who have only ever had smooth implants), especially salt-loss and polyurethane implants. This is thought to be related to mild chronic inflammation due to increased surface area and/or increased presence of biofilm. Patients may also have a genetic predisposition to developing the condition.

Clinical presentation: the commonest clinical presentation is ipsilateral seroma. Other presentations include capsular contracture (ipsilateral or contralateral) or a mass, with or without presence of seroma. Systemic 'B' symptoms can occur more rarely. In advanced disease states, patients may present with bulky metastatic lymphadenopathy. On average, patients present at 8 years post-surgery. 5% are bilateral.

Diagnosis and management: UK guidelines published in the *British Journal of Haematology* in 2021. Evaluate with imaging (USS breast and axilla, mammogram to exclude other pathology, and PET-CT if pathological nodes or lymphoma B-symptoms), skin biopsy if a solid mass is present, and aspiration of entire volume of peri-implant fluid sent to cytology for CD30. A solid mass should be evaluated with core biopsy. Early disease is managed by explantation with en bloc capsulectomy. Advanced cases may require chemotherapy.

Legal considerations in UK: all patients for breast augmentation should be adequately consented for BIA-ALCL as per *Montgomery v. Lanarkshire Health Board*. All breast implants should be registered on the national Breast and Cosmetic Implant Registry; this is a legal requirement. The MHRA and BAPRAS currently do not recommend routine removal of implants already in place. Some types of implants, including Allergan BioCell™ (highly textured salt-loss implant), have been voluntarily withdrawn from the market. Confirmed cases should be reported via the MHRA Yellow Card system.

Breast implant related illness
A constellation of symptoms reported by a growing group of people following insertion of breast implants. Aetiology not currently known and not currently acknowledged by WHO as a medical condition. Support networks available for patients. Bespoke management plan advised.

Breast reconstruction
Oncoplastic breast surgery guidelines in the UK stipulate providing patients with the array of possible options. Breast reconstruction options are dictated by the oncological resection.

Reconstruction following wide local excision:
• Volume redistribution in a ptotic breast in the form of a therapeutic mammoplasty. Often require 2 pedicles—one for the NAC and a second for the parenchyma to be redistributed.
• Volume replacement in a non-ptotic breast. Local flaps chosen based on tumour location:
  ○ Lateral tumours—lateral thoracic artery perforator (LTAP—perforators typically in 3–4th intercostal spaces) or lateral intercostal artery perforator (LICAP—perforators typically in 5–6th intercostal spaces);
  ○ Central tumours—LTAP or thoracodorsal artery perforator (TDAP);
  ○ Medial tumours are more challenging to reconstruct—TDAP or medial intercostal artery perforator (MICAP).

Reconstruction following mastectomy:
3 important decisions for reconstruction of the breast parenchyma:
• *Immediate vs delayed:* immediate—may have better cosmetic result by preserving skin envelope, fewer procedures, less psychological morbidity. Delayed—may be preferable if adjuvant RT planned but associated with more scar tissue and skin loss.
• *Prosthetic vs autologous:*
  ○ *Prosthetic:* remains the most common reconstructive option. May be used in conjunction with acellular dermal matrices (ADMs). Benefits of shorter operation and no donor site morbidity. Disadvantage of adjuvant RT being a relative contraindication, the likely need to replace the implant in the future and complications associated with breast implants. NMBRA reported 9% loss of implant at 3 months;
  ○ *Autologous:* advantage of replacing like with like, longevity of reconstruction and changing size with patient changes in weight. Disadvantage of a major surgery with potential for donor site morbidity. Options:
    ▪ Fat transfer—rarely performed for total parenchymal reconstruction;
    ▪ Pedicled flaps:
      • Transverse rectus abdominus (TRAM) flap;
      • Latissimus dorsi (LD) flap—can be used in combination with breast implants.
    ▪ Free flaps—donor options:
      • Abdomen: deep inferior epigastric artery (DIEP) flap is a fasciocutaneus flap and a gold standard if a suitable abdominal resource available. Muscle-sparing TRAMs may have equivalent outcomes and donor site morbidity;
      • Thigh—transverse upper gracilis (TUG) flap is a myocutaneous flap. Disadvantage of short pedicle (6–8 cm) and transgressing lymphatics; Profunda artery perforator (PAP) flap is fasciocutaneous, has a longer pedicle (10–12 cm);

- Buttocks—fasciocutaneous flaps based on superior or inferior gluteal artery perforators (SGAP/IGAP).
- *Need for contralateral breast symmetrization:*
  - Small breast can be augmented;
  - Large breasts can be reduced or reshaped (breast reduction/mastopexy).

Autologous breast reconstruction:

Operative approach is increasingly protocolized to enhance the patient journey. Considerations include:

Pre-op optimization:

- Stop smoking for minimum of a month.
- Reduce BMI.
- Optimize diabetic control.
- Carbohydrate loading.
- Stop tamoxifen 2 weeks prior to surgery.

Intra-op:

- Antibiotics.
- Prevent hypothermia.
- Consider tranexamic acid.

Post-op plan:

- Enhanced recovery after surgery (ERAS).
- Early feeding, prescribing laxatives and antiemetics if required.
- Multimodal analgesia—opiate sparing so including pregabalin and TAP block in theatre.
- Early mobilization with physio and early removal of drains and catheter.
- Support bra for 6 weeks—no wires, broad straps.

Breast reduction

A surgical technique with the primary goal of reducing the volume of breast parenchyma and a natural appearing shape of the breast. Reduction mammaplasty can be combined with mastopexy techniques to improve the lift of the breast.

Historical developments:

- *1950s:* Wise described the keyhole skin pattern adapted from brassiere design—known as the inverted T.
- *1960s:* Pitanguy described superior pedicle.
- *1970s:* Robbins described the inferior pedicle.
- *1980s:* Lassus described the superomedial pedicle, later modified by Lejour and Hall-Findlay.

Assessment:

- Establish patient goals. Ask about symptoms of back and shoulder pain, intertrigo and psychological. Ask about intention to breast feed.

- Useful measurements include:
  - Sternal notch to nipple distance—'ideal' of 21 cm;
  - NAC diameter—'ideal' of 4 cm.
- Complete oncological examination.

Techniques: The technique is a combination of two components: a skin pattern and a parenchymal pedicle:

- Skin pattern options:
  - *Periareolar:* only indicated in very small reductions as the donut skin excision facilitates limited parenchymal excision and is prone to scar widening;
  - Vertical;
  - Short inverted;
  - *Inverted T:* remains the most commonly used due to its versatility.
- Parenchymal pedicle options—of the many options available the most commonly utilised are:
  - *Superomedial pedicle:* provides excellent vascularity from internal mammary perforators, advantageous medial pole fullness, less bottoming out due to suspension of the NAC and equivalent nipple sensitivity in clinical studies. The rotation of the nipple can be technically challenging and may not be suitable for severely ptotic breasts with notch to nipple distance >40 cm;
  - *Inferior pedicle:* reliable vascularity from intercostal perforators, preserves the anatomically dominant 4th intercostals nerve branch to nipple and is applicable across a wide range of breast sizes. Criticized for creating a boxy breast and risk of bottoming out.
- Liposuction can be used as an adjunct or more rarely as the sole method for reduction.
- In significant ptosis of >40 cm notch to nipple distance can consider:
  - Free nipple grafts;
  - *Bipedicle:* inferior and superior dermal deepithelialized nipple pedicle described by McKinsey.

Principles of marking a Wise pattern reduction:

- Mark midline.
- Mark IMF.
- Mark breast meridian through the central breast mound (often more medial to the nipple). Continue under the breast so you know where T-junction will be.
- Ideal nipple position—lots of ways described. One method is IMF transposition for horizontal plane (Pitanguy point).

- Swing the breast to drop vertical limbs—do not want areola in the Wise pattern if possible. Length depends on size of breasts. Limbs from outside of the key hole will be 5–7 cm (more like 8–10 cm from the nipple position). Join vertical limbs with IMF.
- Mark areola.

Operative strategy:
- Pedicle must be incorporated to innervate and vascularize the nipple-areolar complex.
- Selected quadrants of the breast must be removed to accomplish goal of volume reduction. Send orientated specimen for histology as approximately 2% will have evidence of previously undetected malignancy.
- Excess skin envelop must be managed to minimize scarring.
- Nipple transposition.
- An aesthetic breast shape must be created.

Complications:
- Early:
  o Nipple loss—partial/total—counsel patient for potential need for free nipple graft;
  o Reduced nipple sensation;
  o Haematoma;
  o Infection;
  o Wound healing especially at the T-junction.
- Later:
  o Asymmetry;
  o Breast feeding problems—literature shows equivalent breastfeeding ability as normal population, i.e. some women will not be able to breastfeed.
  o Fat necrosis—results from focal devascularization of adipose tissue—clinically a firm area which is uncomfortable;
  o Scarring and dog ears.

Breslow thickness
- For histological staging of *Malignant melanoma*.
- The distance measured is the distance between the granular layer of the epidermis to the deepest part of the melanoma.
- This avoids the confounding effect of the variable thickness of the reticular dermis seen in *Clark's levels*.
- More precise at predicting the risk of metastatic disease and survival.
- The groupings for prognosis are 1, 2 and 4 mm.

Brewerton's view
- XR view for demonstrating involvement of metacarpal heads in RA.

- Profile second to fifth MCP joint with no overlapping of cortical surfaces.
- Reveals early erosions and occult fractures of metacarpal heads.

Broder's classification
Histological grading system of tumours:
- *Grade 1:* well differentiated.
- *Grade 2:* moderately differentiated.
- *Grade 3:* poorly differentiated.
- *Grade 4:* anaplastic.

Bromelain-based Enzymatic Debridement
(i.e. *Nexobrid*™) An effective non-surgical tool for debriding mid to deep dermal burns:
- Approved in Europe in 2013 for mid- to deep dermal burns.
- Aims to reduce blood loss, the need for skin grafting by dermis preservation. Also may reduce burn wound infection and length of hospital stay.

Indications:
- Best indicated for mixed depth mid-dermal and deeper burns because the surgeon's ability to excise mixed depth burns accurately is limited, especially when close to areas that may have capacity to heal.
- Size of burn—licenced for eschar removal <15%TBSA.

Timing of use:
- Immediate within 12 hours: most of burn still moist so does not require pre-soaking.
- Early 12–72 hours: probably the most common time it is used and enables the greatest benefit.
- Delayed: feasible but less ideal and requires more pre-soaking.

Technique:
- *Analgesia:* Nexobrid™ is painful and requires sufficient analgesia:
  o Regional anaesthesia recommended for isolated limb;
  o Local anaesthesia for minor burns.
- *Coagulopathies:* have to be managed prior to application (less of a problem for minor burns but major burns associated with coagulopathies).
- *Pre-treatment:*
  o Needs soaking as does not work in dry wounds. Chlorhexidine soaks overnight to prepare patient for treatment the following day. Needs to soak for at least 2 hours but prolonged soaking is helpful;
  o Avoid silver and copper (betadine) due to disruption of enzymatic activity.

- *Application:*
  - 4 hours or more;
  - 2g/1% TBSA—layer of approx. 1.5–3 mm thickness;
  - Barrier around the edge (paraffin) to prevent leakage;
  - Occlusive film over the top then bulky protective dressing.
- *Post-treatment:*
  - Scrape of enzyme. Soaking for at least 2 hours to avoid desiccation but prolonged better to remove remnants;
  - Assess wound 2 hours after treatment. Decision needs to be made about whether to graft or proceed conservatively. Assess colour and bleeding of tissue—if red and bleeding will heal spontaneously. Exposed fat is clear indication for grafting;
  - Grafting should be delayed for 2 days to allow enzyme removal to improve skin graft take. If conservative route opted for, skin graft at 21 days if no signs of healing.

Brow lift

A procedure to elevate the brow tissue in the setting of brow ptosis or transverse forehead rhytids.

Anatomy:

- *Zones of fixation:*
  - Temporal fusion line;
  - Supra-orbital fusion line.
- *Blood supply:* internal and external carotid via the temporal, supratrochlear and orbital arteries.
- *Sensory supply:* the supratrochlear and supraorbital nerves (divides into superficial branch and deep branch, which runs medially to temporal fusion line).
- *Muscles:*
  - *Frontalis* is main elevator of brow;
  - Opposed by corrugator supercilii, procerus and orbicularis oculi.
- Ideal brow described by Ellenbogen:
  - Brow begins medially at line running through alar base and medial canthus.
  - Brow ends medially in line with a line from lateral canthus to alar base.
  - Medial and lateral extent of brow lie on the same horizontal line.
  - The apex of the brow lies above the lateral limbus of the eye.
  - Brow arches above the supraorbital rim in females and at the rim in males.

Surgical options:

- Open:
  - *Supraciliary eyebrow lift:* gives a good lift, but leaves a visible scar. Skin, frontalis and

orbicularis excised down to periosteum. If there is a 7th nerve palsy, suture dermis to periosteum with non-absorbable sutures. If functioning, preserve the frontal nerve;
  - *Transpalpebral:* through an upper blepharoplasty incision. Suitable for minor brow ptosis;
  - *Bicoronal incision:* with plane of dissection between galea and pericranium;
  - *Hairline incision:* advocated by Tim Martin—minimal access incisions in high temporal hairline can access all elements of the forehead.
- *Endoscopic forehead lift:* make several small incisions, extensive subperiosteal dissection, release of corrugator and procerus, preserve nerves and elevate forehead and attach with screws or drill hole in outer table. There is no scalp resection, less scarring, less bleeding. Good with alopecia.

Complications:

Early:

- Scalp numbness.
- Early loss of fixation.
- Haematoma.
- Infection.
- Injury to facial nerve.

Later:

- Alopecia due to tension on hair bearing scalp.
- Asymmetry.
- Loss of brow stability.

Buccal mucosa cancer

- A disease of the elderly.
- Common in tobacco and betel nut-chewing areas. Also teeth trauma and leucoplakia. In other areas tends to be slow growing.
- Verrucous carcinoma is a well-differentiated SCC and rarely spreads. The lesions begin as flat, erythematous, roughened areas, later becoming ulcerated.
- The submandibular nodes become involved, but there may also be direct spread to the jugulodigastric, preparotid and mid-jugular nodes.

Treatment:

- T1 and T2, excision and radiation therapy are equally effective.
- Large, indurated lesions may require full-thickness resection of the cheek with a variety of flap reconstructions.
- Bone involvement will require maxillectomy or mandibulectomy.
- Radical neck dissection for positive nodes or in the N0 neck involved in the primary.
- Radiation with palliative surgery or stage III or IV disease.

Results: 5-year survival rates:
- *Stage I:* 92%.
- *Stage II:* 86%.
- *Stage III:* 65%.
- *Stage IV:* 15%.

See HEAD AND NECK CANCER.

Buerger's disease

Thrombo-angiitis obliterans.

- An idiopathic segmental inflammatory recurrent occlusive disease of small- and medium-sized arteries and veins in the extremities.
- Mostly seen in young male smokers.
- More common in Asia.
- A high percentage of patients have immune reactivity to collagen.
- Usually begins before 40 years.
- Get trophic changes, ischaemic pain at rest and venous thrombosis. Progression is slowed by cessation of smoking.
- Surgery is required for debridement and wound care.
- Sympathectomy may help, but neither cessation of smoking nor sympathectomy will reverse the arterial changes.

See VASCULAR INJURIES.

Bunnell test

- For intrinsic tightness.
- Full passive flexion of IPJ with MCPJ flexion, but not in MCPJ extension indicates intrinsic tightness.

Bupivicaine

A local anaesthetic in the amide category, developed in 1957. More potent than lidocaine with a slower onset, longer duration and higher toxicity profile. Metabolism mostly occurs in the peripheral tissues and then eliminated by the kidneys.

Maximum dose is 2 mg/kg, with or without adrenaline. Examples:

- 0.25% = 2.5 mg/ml (in average 70 kg adult – max dose = 56 ml).
- 0.5% = 5 mg/ml (in average 70 kg adult – max dose = 28 ml).

Burns—basic science

A burn is a coagulative destruction of the surface layers of the body. Improvement in burns survival has been attributed to resuscitation, early surgery, management of sepsis and nutritional support.

Epidemiology:

- Burns tend to occur to the very young, the very old and the very unlucky.

- Domestic burns are mainly scalds in children, occurring mainly in the kitchen or the bathroom.

Skin function:

- Barrier to heat loss, evaporative loss mechanical injury and infection.
- Dermal layer provides skin appendages and elasticity.
- Loss of the barrier leads to hypothermia, fluid loss, infection which is exacerbated by immunosuppression.

Pathophysiology:

Local response:

- Degree of injury relates to temperature and duration of exposure most tissue is lost from heat coagulation of protein.
- *Jackson* described three zones of injury.
- Final tissue loss is progressive and results from release of local mediators, change in blood flow, oedema and infection.
- Initial vasoconstriction followed by vasodilatation and oedema.
- Get activation of complement and coagulation systems with thrombosis, and release of histamine and bradykinin.
- Get capillary leak and vasoconstriction.
- Get release of inflammatory cytokines.
- Chemotaxis to neutrophils, which degranulate and increase injury.
- Only fluid resuscitation has been shown to have a clear benefit in reducing the injury occurring during this local response.

Systemic response:

- Seen in burns > 20% TBSA. Conceptually Jackson's outer zone of hyperaemia involves the entire body with an overspill of inflammatory mediators into the systemic circulation. Fluid loss and cytokine release lead to a characteristic systemic response. Beware of burns shock where tissue perfusion is insufficient despite adequate correction of hypovolaemia.
- Hypovolaemia, vasoconstriction and possibly cardiac dysfunction mediated by TNF.
- RBCs may be lost due to membrane fragility.
- Hypothermia from evaporative loss.
- Acute respiratory failure.
- *Bacterial translocation:* get intestinal villous atrophy, particularly if nutrition is not supplied enterally. The atrophy with capillary leak can lead to translocation of bacteria into the portal circulation. This can alter hepatic function and cause sepsis and multi-system organ failure.

- *Immune consequences:* all elements of the immune system are suppressed and sepsis is a major cause of death in large burns. Get reduced neutrophil function, skin and mucosal barrier disrupted.

Metabolic response:

- Ebb and flow phases:
  - Ebb phase in first 24–48 hours characterized by a hypometabolic response due to hypovolaemia and reduced cardiac output;
  - Flow phase follows—catabolic state characterized by hypermetabolism which can persist for years.
- Hypermetabolic response characterized by:
  - Increased cardiac output, ventilation, temperature, and decreased nitrogen balance;
  - Response proportional to burn size. Burn over 50% has a metabolic rate of twice resting;
  - Maintaining temperature is important to reduce energy expended;
  - The metabolic rate begins to return to normal when wounds are closed, but doesn't fall to normal until wound remodelling is complete;
  - Caloric requirements can be calculated with:
    - the Curreri formula, this is not very accurate;
    - the Harris–Benedict equation.
- The protein content can be estimated by using a calorie to nitrogen ratio of 100–150:1; The normal diet is 300:1. Also require fats, micronutrients;
- Weight should be monitored closely and should not fall below 10% of the ideal body weight.
- *Mediators:* catecholamines. Also increased glucagons and cortisol. All organs involved get early hypofunction and later hyperfunction.

Nutritional support:

- Aim to provide adequate calories and protein.
- Will be required for >20% burns.
- Start as soon as possible, preferably by the enteral route. This helps maintain mucosal integrity.
- May need NGT or feeding jejunostomy. Most patients with burns of over 20% get an ileus of upper GI tract, but the small bowel is usually functioning so enteral feeding should be possible. It usually resolves in 72 hours.
- Avoid TPN if possible as there is an increase of sepsis.
- Measure nitrogen balance by 24-hour urinary measurements.
- Give vitamin and micronutrient supplements.

Infections:

- Initially burns are sterile because heat kills bacteria.
- Then get colonized by gram positive initially (*Staphylococcus*) then gram negatives (*Pseudomonas*) by day 21. May be prone to MRSA.
- Burns patients are susceptible to infection due to the warm wet environment and immunosuppression. Burn patients have a large area of tissue where infection can enter, as well as a lot of invasive procedures.
- However, infection difficult to diagnose because burns patients are expected to be febrile and have erythema surrounding the burns.
- Prophylactic antibiotic use in burns is controversial—current paucity of national or international guidance.
- Antibacterial topical agents include:
  - *Flamazine:* silver sulfadiazine is active against a range of bacteria for 24 hours. Can cause leukopenia and is toxic to fibroblasts;
  - *Flammacerium:* cerium nitrate prevents bacterial invasion;
  - *Betadine:* povidone iodine is active against bacteria for a few hours but repeat application can cause iodine toxicity;
  - *Honey:* has antibacterial properties due to release of hydrogen peroxide, low PH (3.6) and high viscosity forming a barrier.

Approaches to control systemic response in burns:

- *Environment:* keep warm.
- *Nutrition:* to protect gut mucosa, preserve muscle mass, optimize wound healing. Important to correct deficiencies.
- Medications:
  - *Oxandrolone:* synthetic testosterone analogue—low virilizing effect therefore it can be used in males and females—preserves muscle mass by reducing protein catabolism;
  - *Propranolol:* reducing heart rate and benefits continue for up to 1 year;
  - Insulin;
  - Steroids.
- Control infection:
  - *Surgery:* early wound closure—reduced energy expenditure, sepsis and lower mortality.
- *Pain:* important to control. Patients with good pain control have a more stable BP and heart rate, and are less hypermetabolic with less long-term post-traumatic stress disorder. Morphine given in small frequent doses is good for the initial resuscitation period. PCAs are useful.

Burns—chemical

- Injury is by a hydrolysis which destroys bonds between proteins and this can occur via the following mechanisms:
  - *Reduction:* agents bind free electrons in tissue proteins, e.g. HCl;
  - *Oxidation:* oxidized on contact with proteins leading to toxic products, e.g. sodium hypochlorite;
  - *Corrosion:* denature tissue proteins, e.g. phenols;
  - *Protoplasmic proteins:* bind or inhibit calcium and other ions, e.g. HFl;
  - *Vesicants:* produce ischaemia with necrosis, e.g. mustard gas;
  - *Desiccants:* dehydrate and release heat, e.g. H_2SO_4.
- Chemicals are broadly classified into acids and alkalis:
  - Acids are proton donors and produce coagulative necrosis;
  - Alkalis are proton acceptors and produce liquefactive necrosis and this can enable greater depth penetration.

General first aid management:

- Remove clothing and agent.
- Irrigate copiously for 1–2 hours. However, don't use water for elemental sodium, potassium and lithium which will ignite; use a fire extinguisher or sand and cover with cooking oil. Don't use water for phenol, which penetrates more in a dilute solution.
- In the eye use normal saline if available. Manually hold the eye open as they will have blepharospasm.

Specific chemicals:

- *Tar and grease:* petroleum jelly dissolves the tar and grease. Long exposure may cause pulmonary, renal and hepatic failure.
- *Hydrofluoric acid.*
- *Sulphuric acid.*
- *Lye:* in many cleaning products—an alkali.
- *Cement:* composed of calcium carbonate, silicon dioxide, aluminium oxide, magnesium carbonate, sulphuric acid and iron oxide. Causes skin damage by allergic dermatitis, abrasions and alkali burns. Onset is insidious.
- *Ammonia:* a strong alkali base, can cause severe injury to skin, eyes, GI tract with liquefaction necrosis. One of the most devastating chemicals to injure the eye. May get rapid blindness. Distinct odour and irritant with cough. Affects upper airways only as it is very water soluble. Treat with irrigation.

- *Anilines:* from the dye industry. They cause superficial burns often violet or brown in colour. May get systemic toxicity. Get methaemoglobinaemia. Treat this with methylene blue IV 1–2 mg/kg.
- *Bleach solutions:* (sodium or calcium hypochlorite). Strong oxidizers. They are stabilized by adjusting pH and are maintained at a pH of >10. Prolonged contact may cause burns. If acid is added, chlorine gas may escape. Chlorine is a respiratory tract irritant. May produce laryngeal oedema.
- *Phosphorus:* phosphorous ignites spontaneously on exposure to air and is rapidly oxidized to phosphorous pentoxide. It is extinguished by water. Particles of phosphorous continue to burn. Treat with water irrigation followed by removal of any particles. Wash with 1% copper sulphate to form black particles, which can be seen and removed.

  See EXTRAVASATION INJURIES. *See* CHEMICAL WEAPONS.

Burns—dressings

The ideal dressing is comfortable, has no adverse effects and establishes an optimum microenvironment for wound healing. It will maintain the temperature and moisture level, permit respiration, facilitate epithelialization and prevent infection by excluding external bacteria. Despite the vast array of dressings available, there is low level evidence to support any of them over another.

Types of dressings:

- *Paraffin gauze:* long-standing use but tends to dry out (i.e. Jelonet™).
- *Silicone-coated nylon dressing:* non-stick mesh (i.e. Mepitel™ and Silflex™).
- *Polyurethane film dressing:* semi-permeable transparent adhesive-coated sheets. A barrier to water and bacteria but permeable to water vapor, oxygen and carbon dioxide. Not suitable if heavy exudate (i.e. OpSite™ and Tegaderm™).
- *Hydrocolloid dressings:* contain gelatin, pectin and sodium carboxymethylcellulose in an adhesive polymer matrix which forms a gel when in contact with exudate. Facilitates auto debridement (i.e. Comfeel™ and DuoDerm™).
- *Hydrogel dressings:* high water content gels containing insoluble polymers which enable more absorption of exudate (i.e. IntraSite™ and Solugel™).
- *Alginate dressings:* biodegradable derived from seaweed which are good at absorbing exudate. May be useful in early stages of

burns where exudate is high or on skin graft donor sites. Tendency to dry and adhere in later stages (i.e. Kaltostat™).
- Biosynthetic dressings (i.e. Biobrane™ and Suprathel™).

See INTEGRA. *See* BIOLOGICAL SKIN SUBSTITUTES.

Burns—electrical
- Two mechanisms:
  - *Thermal damage:* tissue resistance to electrical flow generates heat (Joule effect). Tissues with the most resistance will get the hottest (bone, skin and fat);
  - *Non-thermal damage:* due to depolarization. Can lead to cardiac arrythmias and brain injury leading to central respiratory arrest.
- Categorized according to magnitude of voltage:
  - Low voltage is <1,000 V—tends to occur in household electrical burns with mostly AC current. May cause fractures/dislocations due to strong muscular contractions;
  - High voltage is >1,000 V and may arc before mechanical contact. Tends to lead to muscular damage, rhabdomyolysis and myoglobinuria. Beware of compartment syndrome and arrythmias.

Assessment:
- History of being thrown suggests additional trauma.
- Neurology: altered or loss of consciousness.
- Cardiac: chest pain, palpitations.
- Entrance and exit wounds at points of contact: raised suspicion of cardiac involvement if crosses midline.
- Investigations:
  - CK, urine and renal analysis;
  - ECG and 24-hour cardiac monitoring;
  - XR for Chance fracture in cervical spine;
  - Trauma CT;
  - Ophthalmology review for corneal damage.

Treatment:
- Resuscitation:
  - Airway and c-spine immobilization due to risk of cervical spine trauma;
  - *Breathing:* risk of central respiratory suppression;
  - *Circulation:* risk of cardiac arrhythmias and arrest—prolonged CPR may be needed. Aggressive fluid resuscitation to mitigate myoglobinuria and acute renal failure,

titrated to urine output 1–1.5 ml/kg/hour rather than TBSA (which may be deceptively small).
- Fasciotomies for compartment syndrome if indicated.

Surgery:
- Non-viable skin and muscle needs to be excised. No consensus as to optimal timing.
- Early excision of frankly full thickness burnt areas can be dressed with alloderm to provide a seal, encourage wound healing and allow for further progression prior to definitive reconstruction.

Long-term sequelae:
- Cataract formation after electrical injury to the head and neck.
- *Peripheral neuropathy:* possibly due to progressive microvascular occlusion and fibrosis.
- Personality changes and post-traumatic stress.

Burns—inhalation injury
Damage to the respiratory tract following a burn:
- Inhalation is the most serious complication of thermal injury.
- It increases mortality by 40%.

Classification:
- *Supraglottic:* injury caused by dissipation of heat energy to the tissues of the larynx and pharynx. Diagnosis by direct visualization.
- *Subglottic:* injury caused by inhaled products of combustion which irritate lungs leading to bronchospasm and inflammation.
- *Systemic.*

Assessment:
- *History:* flame burn in an enclosed space, loss of consciousness at scene.
- *Symptoms:* shortness of breath, brassy cough, hoarseness, wheezing.
- *Signs:* circumoral soot, soot in the mouth, singed nasal hair, increased ventilatory effort, stridor, altered consciousness.

Investigations:
Blood gases, CO levels, CXR, bronchoscopy.

Management:
- Supportive:
  - Oxygen;
  - Secure airway.
- Nebulizers:
  - Heparin—prevent casts;
  - Salbutamol—relax smooth muscle;
  - N-Acetylcysteine—mucolytic.

- Broncholavage with fibreoptic bronchoscopy.
- Lung protective ventilation strategy:
  - Prone;
  - Small tidal volumes;
  - High-frequency ventilation;
  - PEEP;
  - Permissive hypercapnia.
- Systemic:
  - Treat carbon monoxide;
  - Treat cyanide—hydroxycobalamin.
- Tracheostomy.

Complications:
- Barotrauma.
- Tracheostomy.
- Fibrosis from ARDS.

Burns—management of major >15% TBSA
Life threatening injury:

Assessment and initial management: ATLS and EMSB principles:
- *Airway and C-spine:* consider inhalation injury. High flow oxygen. Low threshold to secure airway with endotracheal intubation. Stabilize C-spine until cleared.
- *Breathing and ventilation:* consider compromised chest compliance from chest burns and the need for escharotomies. Consider carbon monoxide and cyanide poisoning. Get ABG.
- *Circulation:* accurately fluid resuscitate. Assess depth of burn and estimate burn area. Fluid resuscitation amount commonly calculated via the modified Parkland formula of 2–4 mls/kg/TBSA calculated from the time of the burn, the first half to be given in the first 8 hours and the second half to be given in the following 16 hours.
- *Additional:*
  - Analgesia—IV Morphine 0.05–0.1mg/kg;
  - Tetanus prophylaxis;
  - Tests—bloods, crossmatch, imaging;
  - Tubes—urinary catheter to monitor fluid resuscitation and NGT to decompress stomach and start enteral feeds.

Burn depth assessment:
- *Superficial (1st degree):* involvement of epidermis only. Characterized by erythema. Heals in 1 week.
- *Partial dermal:* Involvement of papillary dermis. Characterized by blister formation due to disruption of dermo-epidermal junction. Tends to heal spontaneously by 2 weeks due to intact epithelial-lined dermal appendages (2nd degree).

- *Deep dermal:* involvement of reticular dermis. Characterized by red staining due to injury to reticular vessels in the deeper dermis. May heal by 3 weeks or will more often struggle to heal spontaneously, risking pathological scar formation.
- *Full thickness:* involves all layers of epidermis and dermis (3rd degree). Cannot heal from the base of the wound so relies on scar contraction from the periphery.

Burn area assessment methods:
- Lund and Browder chart.
- Wallace rule of 9s—in adult:
  - Head and neck—9%;
  - Anterior and posterior chest—18% × 2;
  - Upper limbs—9% × 2;
  - Lower limbs—18% × 2;
  - Perineum—1%.
- Patient palm (not including the fingers) is approximately 1%.
- Mersey Burns App.

Surgical principles:
- Minimize blood loss and keep the patent warm.
- Excise full thickness burn eschar, preferably with tangential excision, because of the benefits of early burns excision (less bleeding, infection and hypertrophic scarring) pioneered by Yankovic in Yugoslavia and later confirmed by Herndon at the Shriners—up to 50% TBSA may be safely excised in one sitting.
- Resurface prioritizing high demand areas. First excision and graft will have best take so aim to do it right first time. >40% TBSA will not have enough autologous donor sites to completely cover so will need temporary cover for some areas (i.e. allograft) and definitive re-grafting of donor areas later.

Burns—paediatric
- Mainly scalds.
- Prone to hypoglycaemia (due to limited glycogen stores) and dilutional hyponatraemia.
- Consider NAI: as much as 10% of paediatric burns may have an NAI element.
- Risk of *Toxic shock syndrome* due to paediatric population not having developed antibodies.
- Differences between adults and children:
  - *A:* airway narrower, prone to laryngomalacia;
  - *B:* diaphragmatic respiration—may need escharotomy;
  - *C:* hypovolaemia hard to assess, need higher urine output;
  - *D:* neurology difficult to assess;

- o *E:* lose heat rapidly; hypothermia may result is electrolyte and cellular changes. Particular danger when transferring a child with wet dressings;
- o *F:* Resuscitation fluid in combination with maintenance fluid;
- o *Long term:* emotional needs, growth retardation.

Burns—primary surgery
Timing:
- *Immediate:* escharotomy and tracheostomy.
- *Early:* early excision and grafting within 72 hours may produce better results.
- *Intermediate:* when depth difficult to determine. If there is little healing after a week grafting can be performed.
- *Late:* more than 3 weeks after the burn.

Escharotomy:
- Circumferential burns can prevent swelling leading to raised pressures and impaired tissue perfusion.
- In the chest, ventilation can be restricted.
- Escharotomy should be performed to maintain distal flow.
- Usually can be performed under local anaesthetic.
- Perform midlateral.
- Fasciotomies may be required with large burns or electrical burns.
- In chest perform in anterior axillary line and if bleeding is still restricted, then join incisions with a chevron-shaped incision over the costal margin.
- An occlusive dressing of cotton gauze and the biological dressings minimizes water vapour loss.
- Comfort: superficial burns are sensitive to air currents and deep burns become more sensitive as the nerves regenerate.

Excision:
- *Tangential:* excise in layers and stop when healthy tissue is found.
- *Fascial excision:* for big or deep burns as it limits the amount of bleeding.

Skin grafting:
- *Meshed graft:* can cover large areas and haematoma can be released, but gives a honeycomb appearance.
- *Full-thickness grafting:* mainly for secondary burns reconstruction. However, more durable and contract less.
- *Non-autograft options:*
  - o *Cadaveric* allograft;
  - o *Skin* substitutes.

- *Alexander 'Sandwich' technique:* meshed allograft is laid over widely meshed autograft. Useful in patients with limited donor sites.
- *Cuono technique:* take biopsy from unburned skin and culture. Place allograft. After 10 days remove the epidermis and apply the sheets of keratinocytes. The dermal elements of allograft may survive as rejection is mediated by Langerhans cells.

Upper limb:
- Excise and graft all wounds which will take >2 weeks to heal to enable early movement.
- Use a tourniquet, but don't exsanguinate as pooled blood helps guide excision.
- Use adrenaline swabs and pressure dressing to reduce haemorrhage.
- Lay meshed grafts. Use thick grafts on the palm and maintain first web space.
- For deep burns. Use pedicled or free flaps such as radial forearm fascial or fasciocutaneous, lateral arm temporalis fascial flap.
- Up to 30% of patients develop compression neuropathies. Intrinsic muscles may need decompression.
- Tendon rupture and adhesions are common, particularly of extensors. They require good quality tissue cover.
- Heterotopic calcification occurs in 10% of patients with burns of the upper extremity, particularly around the elbow.

Burns—referral
- Inhalational injury.
- Burn >10% in adults or 5% in children.
- Burn involving special area: hands, perineum, face.
- Full thickness burns greater than 5%.
- Electrical and chemical burns.
- Circumferential burns.
- Other illnesses and associated trauma.
- Social reasons (e.g. child abuse).

Burns—scar
Assessment:
- *History:* cause of burn, time course, scar symptoms and previous treatment.
- Exam:
  - o *Scar pathology:* hypertrophic or keloid;
  - o *Scar maturation:* red suggests immature whereas pale suggest mature;
  - o *Scar structure:* narrow linear band or broad band;
  - o Surrounding skin quality;
  - o Move joints to assess for extrinsic versus intrinsic contractures.

- Investigate:
  - XR for joint involvement to assess ankylosis;
  - Neck burns consider cross sectional imaging for stability of cervical spine and position of major vessels.

Multi-modal management approach:
- Prevention:
  - Splints;
  - Positioning;
  - Exercise.
- Camouflage:
  - Good for hair bearing areas and can include tattooing, wigs.
- Modulation: a multimodal approach often utilized:
  - *Pressure:* bandages, splints, masks—reduce erythema and thickness—likely due to inhibition of TGF beta release and ultimately decreased fibroblast activity;
  - *Massage:* can decrease pain and itch;
  - *Silicone:* increase elasticity and reduce itch, erythema and scar thickness;
  - *Laser:*
    - Pulse dye;
    - Fractionated CO_2 or ErYAG.
  - *Steroid injection:* inhibits inflammatory processes in dermis.
- *Surgery:* the last resort. Principles:
  - Release of contracture:
    - *Narrow linear band:* incise with fishmouth incision and local flaps:
      - Z-plasty—good in unscarred skin;
      - Multiple Zs—better in scarred skin.
    - *Broad band:* incise (if good quality skin) or excise (if poor quality skin) and resurface with SSG, FTSG, ADMs or flaps. Consider the use of tissue expansion.

Burns—surgical reconstruction by site
Scalp:
Consider tissue expansion to move non-burnt hair-bearing skin.

Face:
- Decide whether to graft by 7–10 days.
- Use good quality grafts (sheet SSG or FTSG) to reconstruct entire aesthetic units.

Neck:
- Narrow scar bands are best corrected with local flaps such as Z-plasties.
- Wide bands need resurfacing with grafts or flaps. Consider tissue expansion using lateral skin.

- Free tissue transfer for large defects and pre-expanded scapular or groin flaps can give thin pliable skin.
- Intubation may require fibre optic endoscope or emergency release or tracheotomy.

Eyelids:
- Differentiate between intrinsic scar contracture in periocular skin and extrinsic contracture from cheek scarring.
- Thick SSG or thin FTSG directly onto orbicularis.
- Extend release beyond the medial and lateral canthi in the setting of ectropion.

Eyebrows:
- Tattooing or make-up may be sufficient but difficult to get natural effect.
- Free scalp composite grafts and island flaps on superficial temporal artery.
- Hair transplant.

Ear:
- Aim to prevent suppurative chondritis—use *Mafenide*.
- If suppurative chondritis occurs, debride immediately and treat with systemic antibiotics.
- *Pseudomonas* is the most common organism.
  See EAR RECONSTRUCTION.

Nose:
- Nasal ectropion is best treated with composite grafts or turn-over flaps with a FTSG.
- Stenosis requires grafts and splints.

Lip and mouth:
- Oral *Commissure* must be symmetrical; wait for scars to mature and over-correct compared with opposite side. The commissure is not triangular in shape, but has a vertical component. Converse commisuroplasty is a Y-V mucosal advancement flap to reconstruct the commissure.
- Lip subunits can be resurfaced with full thickness skin grafts. Downward pull in lower lip can be counteracted with a fascia lata sling. Male patients may desire hair bearing skin in upper lip. Free flaps can be used to resurface entire subunits.

Axilla:
Acauer classification:
- *Type 1:* anterior or posterior fold only—local flaps, i.e. Z-plasty—often multiple. Do not transpose axillary hair outside the axilla.
- *Type 2:* both folds—local flaps.
- *Type 3:* entire axilla—will need graft or free flap.

Hands:

Identify digital nerve and arteries at the start of any procedure:

- Commonly volar contractures and linear— if extrinsic contractures amenable to Z-plasties.
- In more severe deformity with intrinsic contracture elements: need a pragmatic approach of combination of grafting and joint fusions with K-wires.
- Dorsal hand contractures: release results in extensive defects with exposure of extensor tendons that need to be covered with vascularized tissue and pinning of the joints.
- Webspace:
  ○ Proximal contractures—use local flaps:
    ■ 5-flap z plasty is the classic for 1st webspace—the advancement element should be planned on the dorsum where there is most laxity;
    ■ V-M flaps can be good for other webspace.
  ○ If approaches PIPJ—will need grafts as there will not be enough tissue—can create a dorsal rectangular flap for web base and then skin graft for uncovered

See SCAR. *See* HYPERTROPHIC SCAR.

Burow's triangles

The excessive skin at the base of an advancement flap. Can be excised to prevent standing cutaneous deformities (dog ears).

Byrd and Spicer classification of fractures

1985, classification based on the mechanism of the trauma and bone and soft tissue injury:

- *Type I:* low-energy oblique or spiral fractures, clean laceration <1 cm.
- *Type II:* medium-energy trauma; displaced or comminuted fracture, laceration >2 cm and soft tissue contusion.
- *Type III:* high-energy trauma; severely displaced or comminuted fracture; segmental fracture or bone defect, laceration >2 cm, soft tissue loss.
- *Type IV:* high-energy bursting trauma; crushing or avulsion, arterial damage requiring microvascular repair.

See LOWER LIMB RECONSTRUCTION.

Cadaveric skin

- Used as a temporary wound cover, usually for extensive burns when there are not enough donor sites from which to harvest a graft.
- Thought to be beneficial by preventing loss of water, electrolytes and proteins from the wound and encouraging angiogenesis to facilitate definitive autograft take.
- Fibrin adhesion secures the graft which typically lasts 2–3 weeks before rejection or even longer in burn patients who may be immunocompromised.
- Expensive and there are concerns about the transmission of viral infections, although stringent screening means infection risk is small.
- May increase failure rate for subsequent composite tissue transplant due to the development of antibodies to skin antigens.
- Skin can be:
  - Cryopreserved at −80°C, which may contain some viable cells;
  - Glycerol preserved, which has a longer life-span and can be stored in a normal fridge; the European bank uses glycerol preserved skin;
  - Cuono technique involves placing cultured keratinocytes on allograft dermis which is less immunogenic.

See BIOLOGICAL SKIN SUBSTITUTES. *See* BURNS.

Café au lait macules

- Pigmented benign lesions that can occur in isolation or associated with *Neurofibromatosis* when more than 6 greater than 5 mm diameter are present.
- Removal may be requested.
- Dermabrasion, salabrasion and excision can be used, but may leave scarring and permanent pigmentary changes.
- *Lasers* including Q-switched Nd:YAG (532 nm), pigmented dye laser (510 nm), and the Q-switched ruby laser (694 nm) may be effective.
- They may recur. Some lesions darken initially with treatment.

Calcifying epithelioma of Malherbe

See PILOMATRIXOMA.

Calcinosis

- Hard whitish superficial areas especially over elbows, knees and fingers.
- May discharge chalky substance.
- May require excision.
- Seen in *Scleroderma*, dermatomyositis, hyperparathyroidism, tumours and parasitic infections.
- No medical treatment. Colchicine may reduce the inflammation associated with calcinosis.

Calvarial flap

- Vascularized calvarial bone may be raised with temporoparietal fascia.
- This may be used for zygoma reconstruction.
- Place the template over parietal calvarium. Additional filler is obtained by folding the superficial temporal fascia around the bone graft. Pass the flap through a subcutaneous tunnel via a facelift excision to the zygomatic defect.

Calvarial graft

- Outer table of calvarium can be split from inner and used as a bone graft.
- Donor site morbidity is minimal and the graft can be moulded to fit the defect.
- The parietal skull is the usual site of harvest as there are no underlying venous sinuses.
- Two techniques to harvest:
  - The *in vivo* technique where the outer table is split from the inner;
  - The *ex vivo* technique, where a craniectomy is performed, the tables split and the outer table is replaced with the inner table being used for graft.

See CRANIUM RECONSTRUCTION.

Camper's chiasm

The decussation of FDS distal to where the FDP tendon pierces the two slips of FDS. Located at the level of the proximal phalanx.

See FLEXOR TENDONS.

Camptodactyly

- Flexion deformity of PIP joint, most commonly of the little finger.
- It typically presents between growth spurts which occur between age 1–4 and 10–14.
- All structures crossing the volar aspect of the finger have been implicated. The most common causes are an abnormal lumbrical insertion and an abnormal FDS insertion. Bony abnormalities in the PIPJ may occur secondarily.
- Assess whether there is extensor lag or block, the severity, whether it is progressive, the age and how many digits.
- Consider treating a contracture >50°, where conservative treatment has failed and progressive contracture.

Classification: Benson classification:

- *I:* unilateral or bilateral PIP joint contracture, otherwise healthy.
- *II:* seen in adolescence.
- *III:* other associated anomalies; usually more severe with multiple digits.

Treatment:

- Splint.
- Difficult to correct surgically. Especially if there is a narrow joint space, indented neck, flattened head of proximal phalanx. Options are explore and release soft tissue sequentially, angulation osteotomy or arthrodesis.
- Total anterior tenoarthrolysis (TATA) described by Saffar, involves releasing the entire flexor apparatus and the interphalangeal volar plates through a lateral incision with volar subperiosteal dissection.

Capillary malformation

- A subtype of vascular malformations.
- Usually present at birth as a stain of the skin.
- Can occur anywhere on the body. In the face often have a dermatomal distribution and can be associated with underlying tissue hypertrophy.
- Central capillary malformations can overlie developmental defects of neural axis such as encephaloceles or arteriovenous malformation of spinal cord (Cobb syndrome).

Management:

- Cosmetic camouflage.
- LASER photocoagulation—pulsed dye (585–95 nm) most commonly.

See PORT WINE STAIN. *See* STURGE-WEBER SYNDROME.

Capitate—fracture

- Rare.
- May be isolated or part of a perilunate injury.
- May get a fragment rotating 180° when the perilunate dislocation is reduced—scaphocapitate syndrome.
- Usually due to force transmitted through 3rd metacarpal to capitate.
- A dorsal fracture can be associated with CMC fracture/dislocation.
- If non-displaced treat with a cast; if displaced, operate.
- Reduce through a dorsal approach. Hold with a K-wire or screw. Consider bone graft.

Capsaicin

- Depletes neurones of substance P.
- Application in CRPS may cause desensitization to inflammatory agents.

Caput ulna syndrome

- End-stage destruction of the distal radio-ulnar joint.
- Get ulnar-sided wrist pain, dorsal ulnar prominence and decreased rotation.
- *Piano keyboard sign:* prominent ulnar head is volarly depressed and springs back. This should be performed gently as it can be painful.
- Ulnar prominence can lead to rupture of ulnar-sided extensors (Vaughn–Jackson syndrome).

Carbon monoxide

- Odourless, tasteless gas which binds preferentially to Hb, 210× stronger than O_2 causing displacement and shifting oxyhaemoglobin dissociation curve to the left.
- Clinically patients present with hypoxia and cherry red mucous membranes.
- Absorbs light at same wavelength as oxyhaemoglobin, therefore pulse oximetry readings may be falsely reassuring.
- If it enters the cell's cytochrome system, it impairs oxygen utilization—*Sick cell syndrome*.
- >5% COHb indicates *Inhalation*, >10% symptomatic, >20% toxic, >60% fatal.
- Diagnose by measuring carboxyhaemoglobin levels in a heparinized blood sample (arterial or venous).
- The half-life of carbon monoxide on room air is 4 hours and on 100% oxygen is 45 minutes. So treat with 100% oxygen, change when COHB levels are <10%.

Carpal tunnel
- Roof formed by *Transverse carpal ligament* spanning from scaphoid tubercle and crest of trapezium to pisiform and hamate.
- Traversed by 10 structures—FDS(4), FDP(4), FPL and median nerve.

Carpal tunnel syndrome (CTS)
- Caused by an acute intermittent or persistent increase in the pressure in the carpal tunnel.

Causes:
- *Congenital:* anomalous muscles, hypoplastic carpal bones.
- *Traumatic:* fractures and dislocations, haematoma.
- *Inflammatory:* rheumatoid tenosynovitis and nodules.
- *Infective:* pyogenic tenosynovitis.
- *Neoplastic:* lipofibroma of median nerve, lipoma.
- *Degenerative:* OA of 1st CMC joint.
- *Endocrine:* DM, hypothyroidism, acromegaly, pregnancy, menopause.
- *Metabolic:* obesity, amyloidosis, haemodialysis, gout.
- *Vascular:* haemangioma, median artery thrombosis, coagulopathy.

Most are idiopathic or multifactorial and may have an underlying genetic predisposition. No proven association between CTS and manual activities.

80% patients are >40 years old, F:M 4:1, 50% bilateral.

Symptoms: pain, paraesthesia and dysesthesia in distribution of median nerve. Loss of grip, clumsiness. Worse at night or when elevating hand.

Signs: decreased sensation, wasting of APB, *Tinel's*, *Phalen's* wrist flexion and *Durkan's* compression test.

Clinical Staging:
- *Mild:* intermittent paraesthesia and may have nocturnal symptoms.
- *Moderate:* mild thenar weakness and regular nocturnal symptoms.
- *Severe:* persistent paraesthesia and weakness with thenar muscle wasting.

Investigations: nerve conduction studies indicated if equivocal history and examination. Assess response to steroid. Image if lesion suspected.

Management:
Mild/Moderate:
- Lifestyle modification to avoid exacerbating factors.
- Splinting with wrist at neutral (Futuro™ splint).

- Steroid injection: 25 mg of hydrocortisone. For reversible CTS, e.g. due to pregnancy.

Moderate/Severe:
- Operative decompression of median nerve via release of *Transverse carpal ligament* +/− external neurolysis. May be performed:
  - Open via longitudinal palmar incision;
  - Endoscopic release.

Most surgery can be scheduled routinely but urgent surgery required if sudden progression of symptoms and clinical evidence of recent denervation.

Complications:
Persistent symptoms, 7–20%, usually incomplete release especially distally. May be due to compression more proximally (double crush), painful scar 'pillar pain', bleeding and infection (rare), nerve damage and recurrence.

Carpenter's syndrome
- Autosomal recessive inheritance with RAB23 mutation.
- Rare craniosynostosis of various sutures leading to an asymmetric head with differing shapes depending on the sutures involved. Ranges from brachycephalic to turricephalic.
- Partial syndactyly usually of the 3rd and 4th digits and pre-axial polysyndactyly of the feet.
- Low-set ears and lateral displacement of the inner canthi are also prominent features.
- Cognitive deficiency may be present.
- Congenital heart defects have been reported in as many as 33% of the cases.

See CRANIOSYNOSTOSIS.

Carpus
- *Stability:* determined by bony architecture, ligaments, TFCC and balanced musculotendinous forces.
- *Ligaments:* extrinsic (from radius and ulna to carpus), intrinsic (interconnect carpal bones, i.e. scapholunate and lunotriquetral) and collaterals.
- *Space of Poirier:* a fenestration in the capitolunate articulation where a capsular tear occurs with a lunate dislocation.
- *Assessment:* palpate for tenderness in a sequential way with knowledge of underlying anatomy. Perform provocative tests:
  - *Watson test:* scaphoid shift test; for scapholunate ligament injury;
  - *Reagan ballottement test:* for lunotriquetral ligament injury;
  - *Investigations:*
    - *XR:* AP, lateral, grip and radial and ulnar deviation of both wrists;

- *Other:* arthrography, distraction XR, bone scan, USS, CT, MRI, diagnostic arthroscopy.

Carpal instability: 'dissociative' refers to the relationship between bones in a row.

- *Carpal instability dissociative (CID):* instabilities include scapholunate and lunotriquetral ligament disruptions.
- *Carpal instability non-dissociative (CIND):* the bones maintain their normal relationships in rows but the radiocarpal and/or mid-carpal joints are disrupted.
- *Carpal instability complex (CIC):* describes greater or lesser arc injuries with lunate dislocation or fracture.

Arc injuries:
- *Greater arc:* perilunate with fracture of one or more carpal bone.
- *Lesser arc:* involves only the ligaments.
- *Inferior arc:* are spread from the radiocarpal joint with volar and dorsal radiocarpal ligament rupture with radial or ulnar styloid. Can get a pure radiocarpal dislocation.

Dislocation:
- Either volar or dorsal caused by high energy.
- 4 stages of ligamentous injury in a perilunate injury. The wrist is forced into dorsiflexion, ulnar deviation and intercarpal supination:
  - ○ *Stage I:* scapholunate ligament injury;
  - ○ *Stage II:* capitolunate disruption;
  - ○ *Stage III:* lunotriquetral joint disruption;
  - ○ *Stage IV:* volar dislocation of the lunate. If the lunate fossa is empty then the lunate has dislocated volarly. However, in volar or dorsal perilunate dislocation the lunate remains in the lunate fossa of the radius and the carpus is displaced.
- *Treatment:* dislocation should be reduced early. Varying opinion regarding open or closed treatment but results appear better for open treatment with ligamentous repair.

Scapholunate instability: *See* DISI/VISI.
- Leads to dorsal intercalated segment instability (DISI) deformity (most common dissociative pattern), i.e., the lunate 'falls' dorsally.
- Abnormal alignment of the scaphoid.
- *Terry Thomas sign,* or increase scapholunate angle of >45° due to excessive volar flexion of the scaphoid.
- *May get a cortical ring sign:* axial view of scaphoid forms a round projection.
- *Treatment:* options are splints, scapholunate repair, capsulodesis to prevent palmar flexion

of the scaphoid, intercarpal arthrodesis (4 corner, STT or scaphocapitate), proximal row carpectomy or total wrist arthrodesis.

Lunotriquetral instability:
- Leads to volar intercalated segment instability (VISI) deformity with scapholunate angle of <30°, i.e., the lunate 'falls' volarly.
- Isolated instability is rare.
- Most have perilunate injury.
- *Treatment:* options include primary repair, soft tissue reconstruction using ECU, LT arthrodesis or 4 corner arthrodesis for severe cases.

Mid-carpal instability:
- Some mobility that can be marked in young females.
- Trauma can destabilize the joint.
- If conservative treatment fails, perform limited intercarpal arthrodesis, total wrist fusion, reefing of dorsal and volar ligaments or radius osteotomy if there is malunion.

Axial instability:
- Rare injuries with dissociation of bones of the distal carpal row.
- The forces are axial and dissipate around the capitate with diastasis and possibly fractures.
- Fractures may be multiple, compartment syndrome.
- *Treatment:* often open and require debridement, fasciotomies and nerve decompression.

Ulnar translocation of the carpus:
- Rare extrinsic ligament injury with ulnar migration of the carpus.
- The lunate then sits on the ulna.
- Ligament repair gives unpredictable results and total wrist arthrodesis may be required.

Fractures:
- *Scaphoid fracture* 80%.
- *Triquetral fracture* 15%.
- Trapezium 2–5%.
- The rest 1–2%.
- Trapezoid is the least common.

Cartilage
- Hyaline (e.g. joints), elastic (e.g. ear) and fibrocartilage (e.g. intervertebral disc, tendon attachments). Hyaline cartilage dissipates loads, fibrocartilage transfers loads.
- Consists of chondrocytes in an extracellular matrix composed of proteoglycans, collagen and water.
- Cartilage does not have intrinsic blood supply but relies on diffusion of nutrients from the extracellular matrix. Chondrocytes are not

very metabolically active and divide slowly, therefore resistant to ischaemia.

- *Collagen:* type II in hyaline cartilage, type I in fibrocartilage.
- *Warping:* a tendency of cartilage to deform under mechanical stress. Mostly occurs within 60 minutes of transplantation. A delay of cartilage graft insertion for 30 minutes may help to allow the cartilage to assume its curvature prior to fixation.

Injury:
- Cartilage has a limited response to injury with slow healing.
- The inflammatory response usually results in fibrosis and scarring.
- Cartilage regeneration can only occur if bone is injured. Get fibrocartilage forming, which eventually becomes hyaline cartilage.

Cat-scratch disease
- Infection caused by the intracellular parasite *Bartonella henselae*, characterized by indolent, occasionally suppurative regional lymphadenitis occurring after being scratched by a cat. *Bartonella clarridgeiae* also implicated.
- The primary lesion is a raised slightly tender non-pruritic papule covered by a vesicle or eschar.
- Unilateral lymphadenopathy follows in a few days to weeks after.
- Systemic symptoms are mild with headache, fever and malaise lasting a few days.
- Diagnose with a skin test, which is positive after 30 days.
- No treatment is required and there is a good prognosis.

Cauliflower ear
- Particularly in pugilists or rugby players.
- Caused by direct blows, haemorrhage and fibrosis with loss of contours.
- Evacuate haematoma acutely. In chronic cases, carve and excise thickened tissue.

See EAR RECONSTRUCTION.

Causalgia
Now referred to as Type 2 CRPS.

See COMPLEX REGIONAL PAIN SYNDROME.

Cellulite
- Dimpling of the skin of the buttocks and lower limbs. Mainly in women.
- It results from hypertrophy of the superficial adipocytes.
- The superficial layer of fat is interspersed with connective tissue which attaches

the skin to the superficial fascia. These areas do not distend as the fat hypertrophies giving the dimpled appearance.
- Cellulite may also occur due to skin laxity and can be seen in weight loss. The underlying mechanism is gravity pulling on the fibrous septa. This can be corrected by tightening the skin.

See FAT ANATOMY.

Cement burn
- Forms calcium oxide with water which often causes a full thickness burn.
- Deeper penetration restricted because in fat the calcium oxide forms a deactivated soap.
- Often managed expectantly to allow opportunity for spontaneous healing and resurfaced if required.

Cephalocoele
- A herniation of intracranial contents through a cranial defect.
- If it contains meninges it is a meningocoele. If meninges and cerebral tissue are present it is a meningoencephalocoele.

Classification: Based on anatomic location:
- Sincipital (frontal), parietal, basal and occipital.
- Sincipital encephalocoeles have a great geographic variation being more common in Africa and Southeast Asia.

Surgical principles: MDT approach aided by cross-sectional imaging:
- Often combined intra and extracranial approach.
- Incision of sac to enable amputation of excess tissue to level of skull.
- Dural closure.
- Bony reconstruction.
- Skin closure.

Cephalometrics
- The science of skull measurement. Provides a quantitative method for describing dentofacial patterns.
- Useful for diagnosis, growth prediction and surgical treatment objective.
- Analysis performed using a standard lateral view of the skull. For a standard cephalogram the distance from object to XR should be 60 inches. The distance from object to film is 6 inches. The central beam is perpendicular to the ear. The head is held. This gives 10% magnification. Tracing is then performed.

- *Landmarks:* a cephalometric plane connects three or more standardized points. Cephalometric analysis is composed of skeletal, profile and dental analysis.

Skeletal analysis:
- Used to classify facial types and establish the anteroposterior relationship of the basal arches.
- SNA refers to maxillary position and SNB the mandibular position. The ANB gives the relation between maxilla and mandible.
- Measure in vertical plane. Total face height, upper and lower (100%, 45%, 55%).
- Measure anterior maxilla to cranial base, posterior maxilla to cranial base and the mandibular plane angle:
  - ○ S = sella, centre of pituitary fossa;
  - ○ N = nasion;
  - ○ A is the deepest mid-point of the maxillary alveolar process;
  - ○ B is the deepest mid-point of the mandibular alveolar process.

Dental analysis: Indicates the anteroposterior position of the teeth in relation to the bones.

Profile analysis:
- Assesses the soft tissue overlying the bones.
- Ricketts' aesthetic plane is a line drawn from nose tip to chin. The lower lip lies on this plane, the upper lip 2 mm behind.
- *Holdaway ratio:* orthodontic method to evaluate lip retrusion/prominence. Relates prominence of mandibular incisor and pogonion to the NB line. The lower incisor should be 4 mm in front of NB line and therefore so should the chin.
- Progress can be analysed by superimposing images.

Ceramics
- Three-dimensional arrays of positively charged metal ions and negatively charged non-metal ions, often oxygen.
- Probably the most chemically inert implant material.
- Low strength and brittleness limit their applications.
  See ALLOPLASTS.

Cerebral palsy
- Sequelae of irreversible perinatal brain injury associated with variable involvement of motor and sensory systems. Typical musculoskeletal anomalies:

- ○ *Shoulder:* internal rotation, spasticity and contracture;
- ○ *Elbow:* flexion deformity with spasticity;
- ○ *Forearm:* pronation due to tightness of pronator teres and pronator quadratus;
- ○ *Wrist:* flexion deformity due to tightness of FCU;
- ○ *Fingers:* flexion deformity due to tightness of FDS and FDP;
- ○ *Thumb:* thumb in palm deformity.
- Treatment options can include Botox injections, tendon releases, tendon transfers and fusions.

Cerebrospinal fluid
- In trauma, if cerebrospinal fluid (CSF) leakage is suspected check for double ring sign:
  - ○ Collect nasal drainage on paper towel. If blood separates then other component may be present. If so then blood is internal and CSF is external.
- Tau protein is only found in CSF so its presence as detected by electrophoresis is diagnostic of CSF leakage.
- Also dye can be placed in the CSF at a lumbar puncture.

Cerium nitrate-silver sulphadiazine
- Flammacerium™ is a commonly used cerium nitrate-silver sulphadiazine preparation.
- Cerium, an element has antimicrobial activity and is relatively non-toxic.
- The efficacy may be due to its effect on the immune function with improved cell-mediated immunity.
- Methaemoglobinuria is a rare problem.
  See BURNS.

Cervical radiculopathy
- Most commonly caused by spondylosis.
- Get degeneration of the cervical disc with osteophytes and impingements on spinal roots.
- Get pain in lateral neck radiating to scapula, occiput, arm or hand.
- May have sensory signs.
- May develop muscle wasting.
- XR show loss of joint space, subluxation and MRI may demonstrate reduced foramina.

Cervicofacial flaps
- A rotation flap involving the cheek and neck used to reconstruct cheek defects.
- Raised inferomedially or inferolaterally.

- Not totally reliable high on the cheek as the transverse branch of the superficial temporal artery is divided.
- It can be raised in the subcutaneous plane or to improve reliability in the deep plane beneath SMAS. It may extend beneath platysma.
- Preserve branches of facial nerve.
- Place anchoring sutures along the anterior aspect of the zygomatic arch and inferolateral orbital rim to help prevent ectropion.
- Anteriorly based flaps are useful for pre-auricular lesions.
- Primary delay can give more reliability. The base can include platysma. The lower level of the flap may be in the neck or below the clavicle.
- A larger defect may require a cervicopectoral flap based on the anterior perforators of the internal thoracic artery. It is elevated deep to platysma and to pectoral fascia. The incision extends behind the anterior trapezius border to prevent a hypertrophic scar.

See CHEEK RECONSTRUCTION.

CHARGE syndrome
- A congenital condition, usually sporadic. Mutation in CHD7 gene.
- Affects multiple organ systems, some present at birth and others becoming apparent later in life.
- Acronym: **C**oloboma of the eye (and **C**ranial nerve abnormalities), **H**eart defects, **A**tresia of the choanae, **R**estriction of growth, **G**enital anomalies and **E**ar abnormalities and hearing loss.
- Characterized by facial features of squared face, broad prominent forehead, prominent nasal bridge and associated asymmetric facial palsy and cleft lip and palate.

Charles operation
- Radical excision of lymphoedematous tissue.
- Remove skin, subcutaneous tissue and deep fascia. Skin graft over muscle.
- High morbidity and rarely used as grafts are injured easily and scar extensively.

See LYMPHOEDEMA.

Cheek advancement flap
- Used in *Nasal reconstruction* for defects of the lateral nose.
- When the inferior border of the incision is placed along the alar crease, the paranasal skin is advanced onto the nasal wall to reach the midline.
- A compensatory Burow's triangle is excised from the alar base and the nasolabial area.

- Can be used for lateral nasal defects, particularly in elderly patients.
- Up to 2.5 cm of skin from the paranasal and cheek area can be used with primary closure.
- They cause loss of the nose/cheek angle which may need correcting as a secondary procedure.

Cheek reconstruction
The cheek is the largest facial aesthetic unit with a broad, slightly convex surface. There is a relative abundance of skin laxity which provides multiple local reconstructive options, which can be selected based on characteristics of the subunits and oriented in RSTLs.

Surgical anatomy:
- SMAS and superficial muscles (orbicularis oculi, depressor anguli oris, zygomaticus major and minor, risorius) form a superficial fascial layer.
- Over parotid SMAS is adherent to parotid gland.
- The superficial mimetic muscles of midface are responsible for facial expression, and nose and mouth.
- *Aesthetic subunits:* three overlapping units.

Zygomatic:
- Skin overlying the zygomatic arch and malar eminence. Care must be taken not to distort lateral canthus or lower eyelid. Beware the temporal branch of the facial nerve traversing the mid portion of the zygomatic arch—elevate flaps in the superficial subcutaneous fat above the temporoparietal fascia.
- *Rhomboid flaps* are very useful for medium-sized defects, with the donor site scar in the relaxed skin tension line (RSTL).
- *Cervicofacial flaps* are used for more extensive defects.
- Consider tissue expansion.

Lateral:
- Pre-auricular tissue including relatively immobile tissue overlying the parotid/masseteric fascia.
- Small defects can be closed primarily with the scar in the preauricular crease. This area is often used as a skin graft donor site.
- Medium defects can be reconstructed with a variety of local flaps. Larger defects can be resurfaced with anteriorly based *Cervicofacial flaps*.
- Regional and free flaps, such as scapular flaps may be required for very large complex defects.

Medial:
- Overlying the melolabial fold.
- Small lesions amenable to direct closure over or adjacent to melolabial fold. Laxity can be

recruited from lateral and inferior areas of mobile skin via undermining.

- Medium-sized defects can be reconstructed with local flaps (such as V-Y advancement, cheek rotation or transposition) elevated in the subcutaneous plane.

Larger defects can be reconstructed using locoregional tissue via the cervicofacial rotation flap. Lower anterior cheek and reconstruction may require internal lining as well. Regional options include deltopectoral flap, pectoralis major and trapezius. Free flaps can be composite, e.g. including palmaris longus.

Cheek rotation flap

- Can be used anywhere on the face based inferiorly or superiorly.
- The optimal design places the scars at the borders of aesthetic subunits.
- It can be used for lower eyelid reconstruction with the _Mustardé flap_.
- Flaps can be elevated in the subcutaneous plane or beneath the SMAS to improve vascularity, with care to avoid injury to the facial nerve branches.
- Large cheek rotation flaps require a suspension suture to the periosteum of the bony orbital rim to help prevent ectropion.

Chemical peels

- Resurfacing technique for fine and course facial rhytids, and uneven skin pigmentation which are not effectively treated surgically.
- Pre-treatment recommended for optimal results and to minimize complications:

  ○ Avoid sun exposure and smoking cessation;
  ○ Daily skin care regime with buffing stone.

- Peels classified according to depth of action:

  ○ Superficial exfoliation in epidermis only, i.e. glycolic acid, lactic acid and salicylic acid. Causes short term rejuvenation;
  ○ _Medium peel:_ to epidermal-dermal junction causing desquamation, i.e. trichloro-acetic acid peels. End point is a foggy white frost on an erythematous base. Healing takes 5–7 days;
  ○ _Deep peel:_ to reticular dermis, i.e. _Phenol peels_. Anaesthesia may be required for pain and cardiac monitoring required for arrythmias. Re-epithelization by 14 days but erythema persists for months and can cause scarring.

- Other resurfacing techniques: _Dermabrasion_ and _Laser_.

Chemical weapons
Mustard gas:

- Used in World War I and is still the most frequently used chemical agent.
- Decontamination of the wound within 2 minutes is the only way to decrease the effects of mustard gas.
- Irrigation with dilute hypochlorite and water. Open bullae and irrigate.
- After this, treat like a burn.
- Get erythema at 4–8 hours, vesiculation at 2–18 hours.

Lewisite:

- An arsenical vesicant similar effect to mustard gas.
- Effects start in seconds. Irrigate as with mustard gas.

Phosgene oxime:

- A corrosive agent that causes severe pain.
- Erythema, urticaria and ulceration develop.
- Effects are immediate. Irrigate, but damage is irreversible due to rapid absorption.

White phosphorus:

- Used in many anti-personnel weapons and ignites when exposed to air.
- Wounds develop from ignited clothing.
- Treat as standard burn.
- Particles embedded in skin need to be debrided.

  See CHEMICAL INJURIES.

Chemodectoma

- Also known as a paraganglioma.
- Benign vascular glomus tumour arising from paraganglion cells of the carotid body. Located at the carotid bifurcation. Characteristic splaying of internal and external carotids.
- Presents as a slow growing neck mass anterior to sternocleidomastoid.
- Definitive treatment by surgical excision.

Chemotherapy

- Wound healing and tumour growth share many pathways.
- Different classes of drugs are used to treat cancer. All attenuate the inflammatory phase of healing by interfering with the vascular response.
- The fibroblast is the primary cell affected.
- If chemotherapy is delayed by a couple of weeks after surgery, then healing is not normally affected.
- The most significant effect occurs when they are used pre-operatively. Particularly alkylating agents, anti-metabolites, anti-tumour antibodies and steroids.

Cherubism

- Rare autosomal dominant familial fibrous dysplasia.
- Multiple areas of *Fibrous dysplasia* in the mandible and maxilla.
- They may occur as early as the first year.
- Usually self-limiting and may regress after puberty so any surgical intervention usually delayed until this time.
- Surgical intervention may be required in severe cases where there is functional or aesthetic concern and may include osseous contouring and orthognathic surgery.

Chest wall reconstruction
Anatomy:

- *Inspiratory muscles:* include sternocleidomastoid and scalene.
- *Expiratory muscles:* attach to the lower part of the rib cage. Include rectus abdominis, inferior and exterior oblique.
- A flail segment with paradoxical breathing may occur with >4 neighbouring ribs are excised or >5 cm of chest wall.

Indications:

- Trauma.
- Tumour.
- Radiation.
- Infection: median sternotomy infection.
- Congenital: *Poland's syndrome*, *Pectus excavatum*, *Pectus carinatum*, *Ectopia cordis*, *Sternal cleft*.

Assessment:

- Acquire details of underlying pathology, previous surgery (including viability of internal mammary arteries) and radiotherapy.
- Assess risk factors for poor wound healing.
- Assess defect for location, size, structures involved, presence of infection and existence of scars from prior surgery.
- Investigate with chest XR and CT or MRI in chronic wounds.

Pairolero classification of sternal wounds:

- *Type 1:* acute occurring within 1st week—typically serosanguinous discharge managed with antibiotics and single-stage reconstruction.
- *Type 2:* subacute occurring 2–3 weeks often involving a purulent discharge and osteomyelitis. Manage with a staged approach.
- *Type 3:* chronic occurs months to years following sternotomy with a draining sinus and osteomyelitis. Manage with a staged approach.

Management:

- MDT approach with cardiothoracic surgeons.
- Treat infection. Optimize nutrition.
- First surgical stage is debridement and wound temporization with negative pressure dressing.
- Second stage definitive reconstruction aims to obliterate dead space, fix skeleton, provide soft tissue cover with an aesthetically acceptable result.
- *Soft tissue reconstruction:* consider size, content and location of defect:

  ○ Local options: direct closure, local fasciocutaneous flap or skin graft;
  ○ Regional pedicled muscle flaps most commonly used reconstructive method including, *Pectoralis major* (pedicled either on internal mammary or thoracoacromial arteries), *Latissimus dorsi*, rectus abdominis and omentum. 'Pec-Rec' flap is bipedicled muscle advancement of the pectoralis major (based on thoracoacromial artery) and rectus abdominis (based on DIEA) raised in continuity;
  ○ Free flaps if no locoregional options available.

- *Skeleton:* stabilization may be necessary to maintain protection and function if over four ribs resected or more than 5 cm² defect.

  ○ *Autologous:* can use rib grafts with muscle flaps or free vascularized bone such as scapular;
  ○ *Synthetic:* mesh or composites, such as *Methyl methacrylate*.

Chondroblastoma

- Benign tumour of chondroblastic germ cells in the epiphysis.
- Pt <25 years old.
- Patients present with soft tissue swelling and pain with loss of range of motion.
- On XR these lesions have a thick reactive rim of bone.
- Treat by extended bone grafting or cementation.

  See BONE TUMOURS.

Chondrodermatitis nodularis helicis (CDNH)

- A painful condition affecting the ear, often pain at night waking from sleep. May be mistaken for a BCC.
- Occurs on a prominent aspect and is probably a pressure sore.
- Histological examination reveals nodular hyperplasia, fibrinoid necrosis of collagen and perichondritis.

- The condition is seen in patients who can only sleep on one side.
- Often treated surgically to exclude malignancy.
- The mainstay of treatment is relief of pressure.
- Other treatments include resection, curettage and laser, but recurrence is high.

Chondroid syringoma
- Mixed tumour of skin, salivary gland type.
- It has both epithelial and mesenchymal tissue components—sweat gland elements (syringoma) and cartilage-like elements (chondroid).
- They are deep to the epidermis and benign.
- Simple excision is performed for diagnosis.

Chondromyxoid fibroma
- Rare cartilaginous lesions that occur most commonly in the metaphyseal bone about the knee.
- They form near the anterior tibial cortex.
- The cartilaginous component is fibrocartilage not the hyaline seen in enchondromas.

  See BONE TUMOURS.

Chondrosarcoma
- Second most frequent primary malignant tumour of bone.
- Typically a low-grade malignant neoplasm with malignant chondrocytes producing cartilaginous matrix.
- Neoplastic bone is never seen.
- Primary and secondary:
  - Primary occurs in previously normal bone, usually in older patients in the axial skeleton and shoulder;
  - Secondary occurs in benign cartilage tumour, such as *Enchondroma* or *Osteochondroma*.
- Histologically, it is difficult to distinguish benign from malignant and the diagnosis is made based on the history and the imaging. Three variants:
  - *Clear cell chondrosarcoma*, rare is the malignant version of the chondroblastoma, it is low grade;
  - *Dedifferentiated chondrosarcoma* is low grade with areas of high grade, they have a poor prognosis;
  - *Mesenchymal chondrosarcoma* is high grade with islands of mature cartilage, the prognosis is better than dedifferentiated.
- CT is very helpful.

- Treatment is aggressive surgical resection. Radiotherapy and chemotherapy are not effective.

  See BONE TUMOURS.

Chordee
- Downward curvature of penile shaft.
- Mainly seen associated with *Hypospadias*.
- The mesenchyme which would have formed structures distal to the hypospadias does not differentiate normally. Instead, it becomes a layer of inelastic fibrous tissue that extends in a fan shape from the meatus to the glans. This tethers the penis and causes downward curvature with erections.

Causes:
- *Congenital:* fibrosis of corpus spongiosum, skin tethering, deficiency of Buck's fascia, hypoplastic urethra, differential corporal growth.
- *Acquired:* Peyronie's disease, peri-urethral fibrosis associated with stricture.

Treatment: surgical algorithm proposed by Snodgrass:

- Deglovie skin.
- Release ventral dartos tissue.
- Release corpus spongiosum from underlying corpus cavernosa.
- 'Fairy cuts' in surface of tunica albuginea.
- Nesbit suture to address dorsal plication.

Cierny and Mader classification
Staging of osteomyelitis.

Anatomic type:
- *Stage 1:* medullary osteomyelitis.
- *Stage 2:* superficial osteomyelitis.
- *Stage 3:* localized osteomyelitis.
- *Stage 4:* diffuse osteomyelitis.

Host type:
- *A:* normal host.
- *B:*
  - BL—locally compromised;
  - BS—systemically compromised;
- *C:* treatment for osteomyelitis worse than disease.

  See OSTEOMYELITIS.

Circumduction
Of the thumb, measured as the angle of the 2nd and 3rd MC to 1st and 2nd MC. Usually around 130°.

Clark's levels
For measuring depth of invasion of *Malignant melanoma*. Use largely superseded by *Breslow*

thickness which correlates more closely to prognosis.

- *Level 1:* tumour confined to epidermis.
- *Level 2:* tumour extending to papillary dermis.
- *Level 3:* tumour extending to junction of papillary and reticular dermis.
- *Level 4:* tumour extending into reticular dermis.
- *Level 5:* tumour extending into subcutaneous fat.

Clasped thumb

- Congenital condition with the thumb metacarpal held adducted and the proximal phalanx flexed.
- Treat by splinting in extension for 6 months.
- If there is significant adduction contracture, perform 1st web space release.
- Tendon transfers or joint fusions may be required.

Claw hand

- Seen in *Ulnar nerve palsy* due to intrinsic paralysis.
- The intrinsics pass volar to MCP joint and dorsal to PIP joint.
- They prevent hyperextension of the MCP joint.
- With extension of the MCP joint, they are placed under tension causing extension of the PIP joint.
- Paralysis leads to weakened MCP joint flexion and unopposed extension.
- As the MCP joint hyperextends flexors are placed under tension and cause unopposed PIP joint flexion. This is the *intrinsic minus position*.
- Wrist flexion worsens the clawing through tenodesis effect.
- Ulnar paradox—a more proximal ulnar nerve lesion will paralyse FDP and weaken IP flexion resulting in reduced clawing.

Cleft alveolus

Grafting of the maxilla was first performed in 1900, but not routinely carried out until 1955. It is now an accepted part of the cleft management.

Indications:

- *Odontogenic bony support:* aids tooth eruption.
- *Stabilization of the maxillary arch:* prevents the collapse of the lesser segment behind the greater segment in unilateral and the greater segments behind the premaxilla in bilateral clefts.
- *Elimination of the oronasal fistula:* prevents regurgitation into the nose.
- *Nasal bony support:* provides a platform for nasal correction.

Timing of reconstruction:

- Primary alveolar bone grafting is performed in the deciduous dental stage but is generally avoided due to detrimental maxillary growth.
- Secondary alveolar bone grafting is performed during mixed dentition, commonly just before the eruption of the canine at approximately 9–11 years of age. Common practice in the UK.
- Tertiary in adult dentition >12 years of age.

Preparation for alveolar bone graft:

- Close working with orthodontists.
- Imaging to anticipate decent of canine tooth—OPG, upper occlusal or CT.
- Remove supernumery teeth.
- Consider arch expansion to align greater and lesser segments.
- Ensure meticulous oral hygiene.

Alveolar bone graft procedure:

- Harvest cancellous bone graft (iliac crest or tibia).
- Incise and raise superiorly based mucosal flaps to open alveolar cleft.
- Repair nasal layer and oronasal fistula.
- Repair palatal layer.
- Pack in bone graft.
- Close buccal layer.

Outcome assessment following alveolar bone graft:

- Clinical assessment—healing and tooth eruption.
- Radiological assessment of bone graft take—i.e. Kindelan or Bergland scores.
- Patient reported outcomes emerging.

Cleft hand
Typical/true cleft hand:

- V-shaped cleft, familial (autosomal dominant), bilateral, middle ray absent most commonly but index and ring may be involved. Radial side more affected—monodactylous form has little finger present only.
- 1st webspace often narrowed and may have syndactyly.
- Associated with other musculoskeletal abnormalities such as:
  - Split hand split foot syndrome;
  - Ectrodactyly;
  - Ectodermal dysplasia;
  - Cleft lip and palate.
- Patients tend to have good function—a triumph of function over appearance.

Classification of typical cleft hand based on integrity of first webspace:

- Normal web.
- Mildly narrowed web.

- Syndactylized web.
- Merged web with cleft (missing index finger).
- Absent web (thumb elements suppressed).

Treatment of typical cleft hand:
- Many may not need surgical intervention if function good—intervention may risk making function worse.
- 1st web may need syndactyly to be released or web space deepening.
- Surgical techniques to close the cleft involve reconstruction of the transverse metacarpal ligament.
- The Snow–Littler technique involves raising a dorsal flap from the cleft and transposing radially to the first web but not widely used due to poor results.

Atypical cleft hand (Symbrachydactyly):
- U-shaped cleft, sporadic, usually unilateral, no foot involvement, monodactylous form has thumb present only.

Cleft lip and palate overview
- Most common congenital craniofacial anomaly.
- Fogh-Andersen (1942) established the incidence of CL/P in Denmark as 1:700 live births. This is widely used to describe the global incidence although racial differences in incidence may occur.
- Phenotypes and prevalence:
  - Cleft palate only: 40%
  - Unliteral cleft lip and palate: 30%
  - Cleft lip only: 20%
  - Bilateral cleft lip and palate: 10%
- Directional asymmetry in sidedness: left:right:bilateral 6:3:1.
- Can occur as part of a syndrome, although most non-syndromic.

Classification:
- Say what you see:
  - Involved structures—cleft of the lip, alveolus, hard and soft palate;
  - Complete/incomplete;
  - Unilateral/bilateral.
- Formal classification systems:
  - Veau classification of cleft palate involvement:
    - *Type 1:* incomplete cleft of secondary palate;
    - *Type 2:* complete cleft of secondary palate;
    - *Type 3:* complete unilateral cleft lip and palate;
    - *Type 4:* complete bilateral cleft lip and palate.
  - Kernahan classification (striped Y);
  - LAHSHAL described by Otto Kriens—a palindrome.

Embryology:
- A cleft lip is a failure of fusion between the medial nasal process and maxillary prominence in the primary palate anterior to the incisive foramen occurring in week 4–8.
- A cleft palate is a failure of the palatal shelves to fuse in the secondary palate posterior to the incisive foramen in weeks 8–12.

Aetiology: Complex aetiology involving inter-play between multiple environmental and gen-etic factors. Suggests a threshold over which the cleft phenotype is expressed.

Cleft lip and palate (*CL/P*) should be con-sidered separately from cleft palate only (CPO) due to distinct genetic profiles and patterns of presentation.

CL/P:

- More common in males.
- Less commonly associated with syndromes—*Van de Woude's syndrome* is one of the few to be associated with CL alone.

CPO:

- More common in females.
- More commonly associated with other abnormalities as part of a syndrome. Associated with *22Q*, *Treacher Collins*, *Stickler's*, *Apert's*, *Crouzon's*, *Down's*, *Pierre Robin*.

Management pathway for cleft lip and palate: Patients born with a CL/P are best managed by a specialist cleft multidisciplinary team. Care begins antenatally and continues through to adulthood.

- Infant:
  - The Specialist Cleft Nurse helps babies born with a cleft palate with feeding due to an inability to create negative intra-oral pressure. Assisted feeding can be provided using a soft bottle (i.e. MAM with a latex orthodontic teat for parent-controlled milk flow) or a rigid bottle (i.e. Dr Brown's with a non-return valve to allow baby-controlled milk flow);
  - Patients will usually undergo primary reconstruction for cleft lip and palate in infancy;
  - Infants are assessed for hearing, early speech sounds and genetics.
- Childhood:
  - Children are assessed by MDT members including speech, dentistry and audiology and psychology. Interventions if required;

o Secondary alveolar bone graft surgery planned with the orthodontist and timed according to development of adult teeth;
o Revisional surgery for speech or fistula repair if required.
• Adolescence:
o Assessment by orthodontist, maxillofacial surgeon and restorative dentist for orthodontic devices and orthognathic surgery if required;
o Definitive septorhinoplasty and lip revisional surgery if required at the completion of facial growth.
• Adulthood:
o Adult patient can return to the cleft team for further interdisciplinary care if required.

Sequence of unilateral cleft lip and palate reconstruction: Many sequences described with common options being:

• Two stage reconstruction with lip and hard palate (vomer flap) reconstruction at the first stage and soft palate repair at the second stage (often termed the Oslo protocol and is the standard sequence used in the UK).
• Two stage reconstruction with lip and soft palate reconstruction as a first stage and delayed hard palate reconstruction as a second stage (Gothenburg or Malek protocol).
• Two stage reconstruction with lip reconstruction at the first stage and the simultaneous reconstruction of hard and soft palate at a second stage (commonly used in North America).
• Single stage reconstruction of lip, hard and soft palate.

Timing of surgical reconstruction: Ideal timing of primary reconstruction is controversial.

• *Cleft lip:* earlier repair helps with maternal bonding but this is balanced against anaesthetic risk. Commonly reconstructed at 3–6 months of age.
• *Cleft palate:* a balance of achieving good speech outcomes (which may benefit from earlier repair before the child starts babbling) and avoiding damage to maxillary growth (which may benefit from later repair). Cleft palates are commonly reconstructed between 6–18 months.

Cleft lip
A congenital anomaly of the embryological primary palate anterior to the incisive foramen, characterized by discontinuity of the upper lip skin and muscle +/− the underling alveolar ridge. There is an associated nasal deformity.

Cleft lip embryology:
• Medial nasal prominences at the leading edge of the frontonasal prominence are pushed together by medially expanding paired maxillary prominences and fuse to form primary palate anterior to incisive foramen including:
o Premaxilla and upper four incisors;
o Prolabium;
o Philtrum.
• Maxillary prominences merge with lateral and medial nasal prominences and mesenchymal cells from the first arch migrate into primary palate.
• Lateral nasal prominences form into alar.

Normal lip anatomy:
From top to bottom:
• Philtral columns:
o Paired vertical linear protuberances—dermal thickenings, perhaps influenced by decussating fibres of orbicularis oris;
• Philtrum (aka philtral dimple or groove):
o Central depression between the columns—perhaps due to fewer muscles fibres in this area.
• White roll:
o Inferior cutaneous skin border with vermilion. Its anterior projection is due to pars marginalis of underlying orbicularis oris.
• Cupid's bow—described the curve of the vermilion-cutaneous border as it said to resemble the bow of the ancient roman god of love:
o Peaks at the bases of the philtral columns;
o Central trough (nadir).
• Vermilion (aka dry vermilion):
o Keratinized mucous membrane of stratified squamous epithelium—on outer lip;
o Median tubercle—central plumping of the dry vermilion.
• Red line:
o Wet/dry border.
• Mucosa (aka wet vermilion):
o Non-keratinized mucous membrane of stratified squamous epithelium—on inner lip.

Unilateral cleft lip:
Anatomy:
• Skin:
o Medial element:
▪ Cupid's bow and white roll is preserved;
▪ Medial lip height is deficient;
▪ Vermilion height is deficient.

- ○ Lateral element:
  - Noordhof's point—where cutaneous roll and vermilion-mucosal junction start to converge medially;
  - Lateral lip height is different to medial lip height; excessive in incomplete and short in complete;
  - Transverse length of the lateral lip is short.
- Muscle—orbicularis oris is misdirected:
  - ○ Medial element—muscle goes vertically to columella and periosteum of piriform aperture;
  - ○ Lateral element—muscle inserts on ala and nasolabial fold.
- Nose:
  - ○ Columella and caudal septum pulled to non-cleft side;
  - ○ Angle between medial and lateral crura increased on cleft side, with apparent shortening of medial crura and lengthening of lateral crura;
  - ○ Cleft side alar base pulled postero-laterally.
- Bone:
  - ○ +– alveolar cleft.

Timing of reconstruction:
- Earlier repair helps with maternal bonding but this is balanced against anaesthetic risk. Commonly reconstructed at 3 months of age.

Surgical principles:
- Lengthen medial lip element.
- Retain normal landmarks such as Cupid's bow, Noordhofs point and place scars along anatomical subunit boundaries such as the philtral column.
- Orbicularis muscle reconstruction.
- Equal nostril margins without violating growth potential of the nose. Controversy exists about how aggressive to be with the nose at primary lip repair.

Surgical techniques:
- *Straight line:*
  - ○ *Rose and Thompson:* slight length increase was achieved by curving the incision.
- *Lower lip Z-plasty or inferior triangle technique:*
  - ○ *Le Mesurier-Hagedorn* provided a quadrangular flap to recreate Cupid's bow;
  - ○ *Tennison-Randall* provided the same with a triangular flap. So both these brought tissue from laterally and recreated Cupid's bow:
    - Fisher—described anatomical subunit technique which combines lengthening from a Rose-Thompson effect and a

lower triangle placed above the white role. Scars are placed along anatomical subunit boundaries.
- *Upper lip Z-plasty or superior triangle technique:*
  - ○ *Millard* introduced the concept of rotation-advancement, placing incisions under the nose where they are more hidden;
  - ○ Mohler brings the incision into the columella to achieve a more rectangularly shaped philtrum.

Bilateral cleft lip:
Anatomy:
- Skin—prolabium (derivative of frontonasal process) are separate from the lateral lip (derivative of maxillary prominences):
  - ○ Cutaneous portion devoid of philtral elements, has poor quality white roll and inadequate vermilion;
  - ○ Labial sulcus is shallow or absent.
- Muscle:
  - ○ No muscle in prolabium—mesenchymal cells from the 1st brachial arch have not been able to migrate.
- Nose:
  - ○ Wide, broad and depressed nasal tip with flared alar—tending to be symmetrical;
  - ○ Angles between crura increased with medial crura appearing short and lateral long—columella appears short.
- Bone:
  - ○ Premaxilla protrusive.

Timing of reconstruction:
- Variable timing as some surgeons perform initial lip adhesion followed by definitive lip reconstruction whereas others utilize presurgical orthopaedics (i.e. NAM) to align alveolar segments and premaxilla prior to definitive lip reconstruction.

Surgical principles:
- BCL are less common than UCL but more challenging to reconstruct and achieve good post-operative outcomes:
  - ○ The surgical principles are similar to UCL but there is an advantage of symmetry;
  - ○ Muscle comes from the lateral elements into the prolabium—this requires wide undermining to mobilize muscles sufficiently.
- *Premaxilla:* protrusion can be controlled by non-operative means with a head cap, tapes or acrylic plates or operative means, such as fixed pin traction, lip adhesion or surgical setback.

Surgical Techniques:
- Reconstruction techniques differ in their philosophy to the prolabial vermilion with some techniques preserving it and other techniques discarding it and recruiting vermilion from lateral lip elements instead.
- Preservation of prolabial white roll:
  - *Manchester repair:* uses the prolabium vermilion to which the lateral lip elements are attached.
- Discarding prolabial white roll:
  - *Millard repair:* prolabium marked and elevated. Vermilion turned down to create sulcus. Lateral flaps are elevated as forked flaps. Lateral lip segments come to midline bringing white roll to the prolabium. Muscle brought to midline.
  - *Mulliken repair:* makes a much narrower prolabial flap. Intercartilaginous incisions are made to superiorly advance the lateral alar cartilages before suturing them overlapped with the upper lateral cartilages. The alar base flaps are medially transposed.

Cleft lip revisional surgery
Unilateral cleft lip:
- *Assessment:* look at lip symmetry, length discrepancies, Cupid's bow and white roll alignment. Assess dynamic lip function asking the patient to purse the lips.
- *Vermilion asymmetry:* due to scar, poor alignment of muscle or vermilion. Treat with local tissue transposition procedures:
  - White roll mismatches can be corrected with Z-plasty or excision;
  - Superficial notching can be corrected with a simple V–Y advancement;
  - Severe deficiencies may require full lip revision.
- *Short or long upper lip:* with asymmetry in the vertical lengths of the repaired cleft lip segments. Due to poor planning or scar contracture. In either case the treatment is full lip revision.
- *Muscular diastasis:* requires resuturing of muscle layer.
- *Mucosal anomalies:* Z plasties.
- *Loss of Cupid's bow:* triangular skin excision above the mucocutaneous line. The excision is then is closed horizontally.

Bilateral cleft lip:
- *Assessment:* problems relate to the size, shape and positioning of the premaxillary and prolabial segments, which are generally hypoplastic and anteriorly displaced. The buccal sulcus narrow.
- *Whistle tip deformity:* soft tissue deficiency in the central portion of lip vermilion, but with an adequate prolabium:
  - Small defects are treated by local mucosal V–Y flaps or Z-plasties;
  - Moderate deformities use *Kapetansky flaps*;
  - Severe deformities: full lip revision or use an *Abbé flap*.
- *Short upper lip:* reflects a composite central lip deformity. The cause is the hypoplastic lip. First re-operate that allows correction of prolabial width, reorientation of muscle and scar resection. This can be accompanied by lateral vermilion advancement.
- *Constricted upper lip:* with vertical and horizontal deficiency. Reconstruct with an *Abbé flap*.
- *Long upper lip:* This can be corrected by using a curved elliptical excision below the nasal sill.

Cleft orthognathic surgery
Hypoplasia of maxilla and class 3 malocclusion may be present in a patient born with a cleft. Managed in collaboration with orthodontist, restorative dentist, speech therapists and psychology.

Assessment:
- Patient expectations and desires.
- Clinical analysis of facial proportions.
- Occlusal relationships and intra-arch features.
- Radiological analysis:
  - 2D cephalometry traditional;
  - 3D virtual planning: the CAD/CAM approach is rapidly replacing traditional cephalometric analysis and mock surgery on models. Surgeon can plan incisions fixation, need for bone grafts and removal of overlapping bone segments.

Surgical procedures:
Based on severity of maxillary retrusion:
- <6 mm—can do a conventional LeFort 1 osteotomy to advance the maxilla the most common type of osteotomy used for CLP.
- >6 mm or there is significant scarring or hypoplastic bone segments with compromised vascular supply—consider distraction osteogenesis with an external device.
- >10–14 mm consider bimaxillary procedure.

Cleft palate
A congenital anomaly of the embryological secondary palate posterior to the incisive foramen,

characterized by an abnormal communication between the oral and nasal cavities that can variably involve both the hard and soft palate.

Embryology:

- In the 7-week-old embryo, the two palatal shelves lie vertically.
- The neck straightens, the tongue drops posteriorly, and the shelves rotate superiorly to a horizontal position.
- They fuse by a series of biological processes including cell migration, epithelial-mesenchymal transition and apoptosis of medial edges. Fusion occurs from the incisive foramen, anterior to posterior, by 12 weeks.

Normal palate anatomy:

- The incisive foramen behind the incisors is the point where the lateral maxillary bones meet the premaxilla.
- The hard palate is composed of palatal process of maxilla anteriorly and palatal bones posteriorly.
- The soft palate contains five muscles:
  - *Tensor veli palatini:* originates around the Eustachian tube and passes around the hamular process of the pterygoid plate to insert into palatine aponeurosis; tenses the palate;
  - *Levator veli palatini:* originates around the Eustachian tube and descends down to insert into the palatine aponeurosis in the middle third; elevates the palate and important for velopharyngeal closure;
  - *Muscularis uvulae:* lies within the uvula at the centre of the palate and thickens the centre of the soft palate;
  - *Palatoglossus:* forms the anterior tonsillar pillar. Arises in the palate aponeurosis and inserts in lateral tongue. Depresses soft palate;
  - *Palatopharyngeus:* forms the posterior tonsillar pillar. Arises in palatal aponeurosis and inserts in upper border of thyroid cartilage. Depresses soft palate and pulls posteriorly towards pharynx during swallowing.
- The greater palatine artery passes anteriorly and medially from the greater palatine foramen situated at the posterolateral border of the palate and provides the main blood supply for the hard palate. The soft palate gets vascular supply from the lesser palatine artery, ascending palatine branch of the facial artery and palatine branches of the ascending pharyngeal artery.

Cleft palate anatomy:

- Hard palate—characteristic discontinuity of the bones and mucoperiosteum:
  - *Unilateral hard palate:* the vomer is attached to the palatal shelf on the non-cleft side;
  - *Bilateral hard palate:* the vomer is attached anteriorly to the premaxilla but remains free from the palatal shelves.
- Soft palate—discontinuity in the mucosa and malpositioning of the musculature:
  - Levator veli palatini arises normally from the skull base but inserts abnormally anteriorly into the cleft margin. Usually attaches in a muscular sling in the middle 2/3 of the plate;
  - Fibres of palatopharyngeus and palatoglossus also attach anteriorly and can go to the hard palate in a fanning out pattern;
  - Tensor veli palatini tendon attaches to the lateral aspect of the hard palate instead of forming the palatal aponeurosis in the anterior third of the palate.

Goals of palate reconstruction:

- Prevent nasal regurgitation by separating oral and nasal cavities.
- Optimize resonance by reconstruction of the velopharyngeal valve and repositioning of the soft palate muscles.
- Minimize growth disturbance and minimizing scarring.

Timing of reconstruction:

- Timing is a balance between ensuring safety of the operation (when the child has a big enough airway), optimizing speech outcome (earlier surgery believed to be beneficial to establish continuity before babbling commences) and minimizing maxillary growth disturbance (later surgery believed to be beneficial to avoid damage to growth centres).
- Lack of international consensus on optimal timing. Most surgeons would reconstruct between 6–18 months.

Surgical techniques for hard palate reconstruction:

- *Bardach's two-flap repair:* single pedicle flaps based on the greater palatine artery.
- *Veau–Wardill–Kilner push-back repair:* with 4 flaps, 2 close off the region of the incisive foramen, and 2 are pushed back to lengthen the palate. Has been associated with significant scarring.

- *Von Langenbeck's repair:* bipedicled flaps are raised to enable closure with lateral releasing incisions. Each flap receives its blood supply from the greater palatine vessels.
- *Vomer flap:* can be used variably as a single-layered closure when performed simultaneously with cleft lip reconstruction or as the nasal layer in a double-layered closure in conjunction with a soft palate reconstruction.

Surgical techniques for soft palate reconstruction:

- *Intravelar veloplasty:* marginal incisions in the cleft palate to reposition the musculature. Originally described by Kriens. Sommerlad advocated radical IVVP with wide dissection of the soft palate musculature to enable them to lie at the posterior aspect of the soft palate and also the use of the operating microscope.
- *Furlow double opposing Z-plasty:* aims to achieve muscle retro-positioning and to lengthen the palate. Used for primary repair and also for velopharyngeal incompetence.

Cleft secondary speech surgery
See VELOPHARYNGEAL DYSFUNCTION.

Cleft septorhinoplasty
Surgical procedure to address the cleft nasal deformity associated with unilateral or bilateral cleft lip may be performed primarily or secondarily.

Approach to nose during primary cleft lip repair:

- Controversy in how much to do to the nose primarily. Approaches include:
  - *Conservative approach:* a belief that intervention in the nose at primary lip repair will damage cartilages and growth potential of nose. Delayed correction performed in teenage years;
  - *Foundation approach:* advocated by Tse. Avoids tip dissection but instead centralizes septum to midline;
  - *Use of existing lip repair incisions:* i.e. McComb. Skin undermined over lower lateral cartilages and dorsum and external suspension sutures;
  - *Use of additional incisions:* i.e. Tajima. U-shaped rim incisions and wide skin undermining with internal interdomal suspension sutures.

Secondary (definitive) septorhinoplasty:

- Controversy as to optimal timing but tends to be performed at skeletal deformity and following completion of orthognathic procedures when the bony foundation is set.

- Challenging surgically as reconstruction has to overcome scarring and deformational forces of the cleft deformity.
- The multifaceted procedure often involves septal repositioning and reconstruction of the dorsum and tip with a combination of cartilage graft and suture techniques.

Cleft speech characteristics
CSCs are a UK framework approach to speech error analysis which is globally adopted.
  Can be broadly categorized as:

1. *Active:* errors are equated with compensatory behaviour. Speech therapy to modify place, manner or airflow direction.
2. *Passive:* errors are equated with obligatory behaviours. Surgery required:

- *Anterior:* a consequence of altered oral anatomy. Amenable to orthodontic treatment:
  - *Dentalization:* part of normal development—only relevant if persist into elder ages;
  - *Lateralization:* airflow over lateral part of tongue;
  - *Palatalization:* sounds too far back behind alveolar ridge instead of tip of tongue.

- *Posterior (backing):* errors of place of articulation (sound is produced further back in oral cavity). Either active or compensatory. Amenable to speech therapy:
  - *Double articulation:* correct place articulation coupled with more posterior placement at same time;
  - *Backing* to velar or uvular.

- *Non-oral (glotto-pharyngeal):* active compensatory errors—attempt to achieve air pressure by using glottal articulation. Not resolved after surgery—required therapy. Loss of place of articulation, loss of manner—plosives replaced with fricatives, Marking of place of articulation with silent gesture with accompanying glottal realization:
  - *Pharyngeal fricatives:* fraction made in pharynx;
  - *Glottal fricatives:* may have correct manner but placement is too proximal;
  - *Active nasal fricatives:* sound is produced in the nasal cavity—sounds like nasal emission but actually the nasal sound is replacing the oral sound rather than accompanying it:
    - *Active nasal fricative:* complete structure in oral cavity—no audible oral release—a behavioural phenomenon in mislearning when the child is sending the air into the nose to make the fricative;

■ *Passive nasal fricative:* sounds the same but when you pinch the nose then an 's' comes out through the mouth.
• *Passive:* strongly associated with VPI—sounds that are made involuntarily due to nasal air escape:
  ○ *Weak or nasalized consonants:* weak pressure on the pressure consonants;
  ○ *Nasal realization of plosives/fricatives:* sounds like hypernasality;
  ○ Absent pressure consonants;
  ○ Gliding of fricatives/affricatives.

Cleland's ligaments
• These originate from the digital skeleton and pass laterally to attach to the digital skin.
• The major bundles are around the PIP joint. They arise from the distal third of the proximal phalanx and the base of the middle phalanx, diverging away from the joint to be attached to the skin.
• The minor bundles are short strong fibres originating from the lateral aspect of the DIP joint and insert into the skin laterally and dorsally.
• They all pass dorsal to the neurovascular bundles.

See GRAYSON'S LIGAMENT. *See* RETINACULAR SYSTEM.

Clinodactyly
• Inherited condition (usually autosomal dominant).
• The finger deviates in the radial-ulnar plane.
• Most often bilateral little fingers.
• Usually caused by a delta phalanx of the middle phalanx so called because it is triangular (Δ)—a longitudinal bracketed epiphysis.
• The growth plate is C-shaped.
• Worsens with growth.
• Most cases managed conservatively. Surgery may be indicated for functional reasons with marked shortening and angulation via a wedge osteotomy—closing wedge if long and opening wedge if short. In the immature skeleton, physiolysis can be performed which aims to remove the tethering on the short side of the bone by inserting a fat graft. May require soft tissue reconstruction with advancement flap or full thickness skin graft.

CMC joint arthritis thumb
• Two key ligaments are palmar (ulnar) ligament (beak ligament) that holds trapezium to MC and dorsal intermetacarpal ligament which holds 1st metacarpal to 2nd.
• Ligaments stressed in opposition and pinch. Once the ligaments are disrupted arthritis can follow.
• Hypermobility may lead to early OA.

Assessment:
• Pain and weakness in thumb.
• One-third of patients with CMC OA also have carpal tunnel syndrome. Tenderness over joint. Locate with 1st MC in adduction.
• *Torque test (grind test):* axial rotation in distraction and compression.
• *Crank test:* axial loading while passively flexing and extending the metacarpal base. Prominent MC base and laxity with crepitus.
• *Swan neck deformity:* get radial subluxation leading to adduction contracture. Compensatory MCPJ hyperextension occurs to allow adequate thumb positioning during grasp.
• XR changes: <u>Eaton-Littler classification</u>.

Treatment:
• *Non-operative:* splints, steroid injection, analgesia.

Surgery:
• <u>Basal osteotomy</u>. Uncommonly performed as disease is usually too far advanced.
• <u>Arthrodesis</u>. E.g. for young, manual workers. The thumb will be fixed out of the plane of the palm, and patients should be warned they will be unable to do press ups.
• <u>Trapeziectomy</u> with or without ligament reconstruction and tendon interposition is the commonest procedure and considered the gold standard.
• <u>Arthroplasty</u> is increasing in popularity for select patient groups.

Coagulation cascade
• Essential for haemostasis. Results in the formation of fibrin clot.
• Coagulation factors circulate as inactive precursors (zymogen). These are converted into enzymes that activate the next zymogen causing amplification to finally produce thrombin and then fibrin.
• The classic description is of an extrinsic pathway stimulated by injury and exposure of tissue factor and an intrinsic pathway activated when blood contacts a foreign surface. Both converge on factor 10 and then have a common pathway.
• Intrinsic cascade begins with factor 12 and is evaluated by the activated partial thromboplastin time (aPTT).
• Extrinsic cascade starts with factor 7 and is evaluated by the prothrombin time (PT).

- Heparin, low molecular weight heparin (LMWH) and novel oral anticoagulants (NOACs) regulate the common factor 10a to have their anticoagulation effect. Heparin also regulates thrombin (factor 2a).
- Warfarin impacts the intrinsic and extrinsic pathways by inhibiting clotting factors 9, 10, 7 and 2 (prothrombin).
- Tranexamic acid prevents the breakdown of fibrin by inhibiting plasmin formation.

Cobb syndrome
Capillary malformation in the midline scalp overlying an encephalocele.

Cocaine
- First local anaesthetic discovered.
- A crystalline alkaloid derived from coco leaves, first isolated in 1860.
- Local anaesthetic, vasoconstrictive and sympathomimetic.
- It blocks reuptake of noradrenaline and adrenaline centrally and peripherally.
- Most commonly used for topical anaesthesia, particularly in nasal surgery and laceration in children.
- The safe maximum dose for nasally administered 4% cocaine solution is 1.5 mg/kg. Each drop of 4% cocaine solution has approximately 3 mg cocaine.

See LOCAL ANAESTHETICS.

Cold intolerance (TICAS)
TICAS: trauma-induced cold-associated symptoms.

- A collection of acquired symptoms resulting in an aversion to cold with:
  ○ Pain/discomfort;
  ○ Stiffness;
  ○ Altered sensibility;
  ○ Colour change.
- Half of patients experience these at the time of injury, the rest after a lag period once the cold weather comes.
- Symptoms generally improve after 2 years.

Collagen
- An elastic protein that due to cross-linking can withstand shearing forces. Play a structural role to provide tensile strength in skin and resistance to traction in ligaments. Makes up 30% of total body protein.
- Collagen can withstand a static load of 20 kg per 1 mm fibre.
- There are 28 types of collagen. Procollagen is produced by fibroblasts. This is excreted from the cell and forms tropocollagen. The common structural feature is a triple helix of polypeptide chains (alpha chains).

- Collagen formation is inhibited by colchicine, penicillamide, steroids, vitamin C and iron deficiency.
- Normal dermis mainly composed of type I collagen (90%). Type III collagen is produced by the foetus and in early stages of wound healing. By week 2 type I collagen is again produced. During remodelling type III collagen is replaced by type I.
- Collagen production in a healing wound peaks at 6 weeks though accumulation is maximal at 3 weeks. Rates of synthesis remain elevated for up to a year. Reduced scar strength is due to lack of organization not lack of quantity.
- Collagen type by tissue:
  ○ *Type I:* in skin, bone, tendon;
  ○ *Type II:* hyaline cartilage and cornea;
  ○ *Type III:* healing tissue, foetal wounds;
  ○ *Type IV:* basement membrane;
  ○ *Type V:* also basement membrane.
- Many disorders are caused by mutations in the genes coding for collagen alpha chains such as osteogenesis imperfecta (COL1A1), Ehlers-Danlos syndrome (COL1A2 and COL3A1) and Stickler syndrome (COL2A1).

See WOUND HEALING. *See* FOETAL WOUND HEALING. *See* SKIN.

Collagen: injectable
- Injectable collagens shrink as they extrude water and biodegrade.
- Primarily type I collagen.
- Bovine collagen was developed in 1981 and has the antigenic peptide end regions removed.
- The main concern with injectable collagens is the immune response so perform skin testing first.
- Cross-linkage with glutaraldehyde gives a longer lifespan.
- Re-injection required up to 6 monthly.

Types of injectable collagen:
- *Zyderm™ 1:* bovine collagen, 35 mg/ml. For fine wrinkles.
- *Zyderm™ 2:* as above, but 65 mg/ml. For more coarse wrinkles.
- *Zyplast™:* cross-linkage of collagen with glutaraldehyde. Firmer than the above and used for coarse wrinkles.

See ALLOPLASTS.

Collar-button abscess
- An infection commencing superficially between skin and palmar fascia.
- It erodes through the fascia and then spreads quickly in the underlying loose space.

- A poor understanding of the anatomy may lead to incomplete drainage.

Collateral ligament

- True collateral ligament of phalanges arises from condyle of proximal bone and inserts into palmar third of distal bone.
- Accessory collateral ligament inserts into lateral margin of volar plate distally.

  See PROXIMAL INTERPHALANGEAL JOINT. *See* METACARPOPHALANGEAL JOINT DISLOCATION.

Coloboma

- From the Greek meaning 'curtailed'.
- Refers to a defect in or around the eye. Can involve any structure including eyelid, lens, macula, optic nerve etc.
- An eyelid coloboma is a notch or cleft of the eyelid of varying degree. Associated with Treacher Collins syndrome. In a *Tessier* 3 cleft they are found medial to the punctum of the lower eyelid.

Commissure reconstruction

- Converse described the three-flap mucosal technique:

  o A triangular wedge of scar is excised with the apex at the desired point for the commissure;

  o Three flaps of oral mucosa are created the centre of which is everted laterally to form the small vertical component of the commissure;

  o The superior and inferior mucosal flaps are folded outward to fill the defect of the upper and lower lateral lip elements.

- Z-plasties, double opposing Z-plasties, vermilion transposition flaps and bilobed mucosal flaps have been described.

  See LIP RECONSTRUCTION.

Common peroneal nerve

- L4–S1.
- Winds round head of fibula then enters peroneal compartment.
- The deep peroneal nerve supplies tibialis anterior, extensor digitorum longus, extensor hallucis longus, extensor digitorum brevis and the skin to the 1st web space.
- The superficial peroneal nerve supplies peroneal muscles and sensory supply to lateral lower leg and dorsum of foot.
- Compression leads to foot drop and paraesthesia but not usually pain.

Compartment syndrome

- Vascular compromise and tissue necrosis in a compartment resulting from sustained rise in intracompartmental pressure.
- Normal pressures 0–8 mmHg.
- Increase compartment pressure raises venous pressure. Capillary flow is reduced leading to ischaemia. When compartment pressure exceeds venous pressure there is no perfusion.

Aetiology:

- Most common is fracture.
- Decrease of compartment size, e.g. constrictive dressings, casts and burns.
- Increase fluid content, e.g. crush, reperfusion, bleeding, electrical injury venepuncture.

Diagnosis:

- Clinical diagnosis is the primary method. Balakrishnan described the 6 P's:

  o *Pain:* out of proportion: the most important clinical sign.

  o Passive stretch exacerbating pain by raising intra-compartmental pressure.

  o *Paraesthesia:* a late sign.

  o *Paralysis:* a late sign.

  o *Palpation:* tense and tender.

  o *Pulseless:* a late sign.

- Pressure measurement can be performed with a Stryker device or manometry. Useful if clinical diagnosis uncertain or paediatric or moribund patient. A difference of 30 mmHg or less between compartment pressure and diastolic blood pressure considered suggestive of compartment syndrome.

Management:

Urgent fasciotomy to decompress the osseofascial compartment.

Forearm:

- *Three compartments:* volar, dorsal and mobile wad. The compartments are interconnected so they can be decompressed by releasing the volar compartment though the dorsal compartment may also require decompression.
- *Volar forearm:* should include release of carpal tunnel. Carry incision towards the ulnar border then centrally. This avoids injury to radial artery and median nerve, and the radial flap covers the tendon. Incise fascia. Examine superficial and deep compartments. The deeper compartments should be particularly examined in electrical injuries as the most injured muscles are adjacent to bone.
- Complete release will usually also release mobile wad and dorsal compartment. If they remain tense then incise dorsally.

The hand:

- *Ten separate non-communicating compartments:* 4 dorsal interossei, 3 volar interossei, hypothenar, thenar and a separate compartment for adductor pollicis. Each must be released separately. Test by abducting and adducting the fingers. The finger has tight fascia which can cause a localized compartment syndrome.
- Release interossei through two dorsal incisions along 2nd and 4th MC.
- Incise over thenar and hypothenar muscles.
- Digital decompression is indicated if blood supply is compromised. Mid-axial incision, ulnar side of index, middle, and ring and radial side of little finger.

Lower limb:

- Four compartments in the lower leg, anterior, lateral and deep and superficial posterior. Two incisions are required to decompress.
- Incise 2 cm medial to tibial border to release anterior and deep compartments.
- Incise 2 cm lateral to tibial border to release lateral compartment.

Untreated compartment syndrome results in *Volkmann's ischaemic contracture*.

Complex combined vascular malformations

- Include CVM, CLM, CLVM and CLAVM.
- They are often associated with soft tissue and skeletal hypertrophy.
- Like the 'pure' *Vascular malformations*, complex-combined anomalies can be categorized as either slow flow or fast flow.

Slow-flow complex-combined malformations:

- *Klippel–Trenaunay syndrome*.
- *Proteus syndrome*.

Fast-flow complex-combined anomalies:

- These anomalies are uncommon.
- CAVM, CAVF or CLAVM correspond to the old term *Parkes Weber syndrome* (capillary, arterial, venous and lymphatic malformation).
- Cutaneous warmth, bruit, and thrill are pathognomonic.
- MRI or arteriography in young children usually shows only diffuse hypervascularity of the limb; multiple AVFs become obvious later, occurring throughout the affected limb, particularly near the joints.
- Assess leg length.

- Muscles and joints are not usually involved in fast flow anomalies.
- MR angiography and MR venography are useful to detect arterial feeders.

Treatment:

- Conservative:
  - Compression stockings;
  - Shoe raise;
  - sclerosis of superficial veins.
- Surgical:
  - Epiphyseal stapling for length discrepancy;
  - Staged resection;
  - Amputation.

Complex regional pain syndrome (CRPS)

- Previously called reflex sympathetic dystrophy (type I) or causalgia (type II).
- A debilitating, painful condition in a limb associated with sensory, motor, autonomic, skin and bone abnormalities, commonly arising after injury or surgery to that limb. However, there is no relationship to the severity of trauma, and in some cases, no history of precipitating trauma (9%).

Classification:

- *CRPS Type I:* more common. Develops in absence of a lesion to a major nerve.
- *CRPS Type II:* develops in the presence of a lesion to a major nerve.

Incidence:

- 20–4/100,000 person years.
- Most commonly in the upper and lower extremity, but has been reported in other areas.
- M = F, usually 30–60 years of age.
- It may occur in children where it usually has a shorter duration and a better prognosis.

Prognosis and outcome:

- Complete remission is rare. Great variations between different studies.
- Approximately 15% will have unrelenting pain and physical impairment 2 years after CRPS onset.

Diagnosis:

- Diagnosis of exclusion.
- Clinical diagnosis according to the Budapest criteria:

A-D must apply:

A. The patient has continuing pain which is disproportionate to any inciting event.
B. The patient has at least one sign (found on clinical examination) in two or more of the below categories.
C. The patient reports at least one symptom (problem reported by patient) in three or more of the categories.
D. No other diagnosis can better explain the signs and symptoms.

Category	Signs/Symptoms
Sensory	Allodynia (pain on light touch and/or temperature sensation and/or deep somatic pressure) and/or hyperalgesia (to pinprick) and/or hyperesthesia.
Vasomotor	Temperature asymmetry ($>1°C$) and/or skin colour changes and/or skin colour asymmetry.
Sudomotor/ oedema	Oedema and/or sweating changes and/or sweating asymmetry.
Motor/ trophic	Decreased range of motion and/or motor dysfunction (weakness, tremor, dystonia) and/or trophic changes (hair/nail/skin).

Aetiology:

- No unifying hypothesis explains the disproportionate pain with vasomotor, inflammatory and dystrophic changes:
  - Neurogenic inflammation with a role for substance P has been mooted;
  - Previously thought to be related to sympathetic nervous system disfunction, but this theory is now obsolete.
- *Peripheral basis:* E phase theory suggests that artificial synapses occur at the injury site with efferent fibres directly activating afferent fibres. This leads to abnormal sensitization.
- *Spinal cord level:* suggests that peripheral nerves could activate internuncial neural pool in the spinal cord, which spreads to sympathetic neurons. Nociceptors are activated leading to excitation of wide-dynamic range (WDR) neurons. These then respond to all afferent stimulation. Sympathetic activity is increased. Also get failure of inhibitory mechanisms.
- *Psychophysiologic mechanisms:* previously thought that there may be a predisposing psychological make-up in some patients. This theory is now also considered obsolete.

- *Opioid pain-control system:* endorphins have an inhibitory effect on substance P production. They may have a role in the strong placebo effect in CRPS.

Treatment:

- Royal College of Physicians produced guidelines in 2018 incorporating contributions from 28 professional bodies/organizations, including BAPRAS (British Association of Plastic, Reconstructive and Aesthetic Surgeons) and BSSH (British Society for Surgery of the Hand):

  - Treatment rests on four pillars: physical, psychological, patient educational and pain relief (medications and interventions);
  - (Plastic) surgical involvement should include timely diagnosis, referral for intensive (hand) physiotherapy, simple analgesia (paracetamol, NSAIDs and weak opiates), +/- low dose tricyclic drugs and/or gabapentin/pregabalin. If not improving, refer to pain clinic, to be seen within 3 months of onset;
  - Surgical treatment: insufficient evidence but recommended to consider surgery in setting of Type 2 CRPS, i.e. where there is an identifiable and remedial nerve lesion driving the abnormal pain response (e.g. nerve compression, neuroma formation, acute nerve transection or a post-operative nerve deficit);
  - Amputation: does not cure pain—literature reports recurrent symptoms at some level in all cases (CRPS may continue in amputation stump (27%), migrate to other limbs or present as phantom pain (77%)). May be considered in an MDT setting in context of intractable infection or ulceration. RCP guidelines suggests waiting at least 24 months from diagnosis unless life-threatening emergency;
  - There is insufficient evidence to support any preventative treatments including ascorbic acid (vitamin C) and aspirin;
  - There is insufficient evidence to support sympathectomy or guanethidine blocks (two randomized controlled trials have shown no benefit);
  - Elective surgery and (past) CRPS: recurrence is relatively uncommon ($<15\%$). Recommended to wait 1 year after resolution or 2 years from onset prior to further surgery if possible.

Component separation

- A surgical technique for the mobilization of abdominal wall tissues in the reconstruction of myofascial defects of the abdominal wall such as hernias.
- Anterior component separation as described by Ramirez in 1990—release of external oblique fascia at the linea semilunaris which is just lateral to the rectus abdominis to allow the medialization of the rectus. Theoretically allows mobilization of 3–5 cm at epigastrium, 7–10 cm at umbilicus and 1–3 cm at suprapubic line. Good for superior defects of the abdominal wall, technically easy to perform and remains the most common type of component separation.
- Posterior component separation described since 2011 and involves Rives-Stoppa approach behind rectus and TAR (transverse abdominis release). Avoids raising large subcutaneous flaps, provides space behind the rectus muscle for mesh placement and useful for repairing lateral hernias.
- Can do posterior on one side and anterior on the other side. But do not do both on the same side as you will get very thin unstable muscles that will bulge later.
- Sneiders et al. 2019 cadaveric study comparing amount of movement between anterior and posterior component separation showed significantly more medialization with the posterior component separation technique.

Composite grafts

- Composite grafts commonly contain skin, as well as other tissue such as fat or cartilage.
- Useful in _Nasal reconstruction_ and ear reconstruction.
- In general, any composite graft >5 mm distant from a vascular bed is at risk for necrosis of skin and fat.
- Initially, a graft is white then cyanotic from venous congestions with a change to a pink colour after 3–7 days.
- Improve take of a graft by maximizing the contact of the graft with vascularized tissue.
- Post-operative cooling initially may improve.

Composite tissue allografts

- Transplantation of composite blocks of tissue which may include skin, bone, muscle, nerves, vessels etc. These tissues originate from different embryological tissues.
- Major advances in this field made possible by evolving immunosuppressive regimes.
- Acute rejection categorized by _Banff classification_.

See TRANSPLANTATION. _See_ FACE TRANSPLANT. _See_ HAND TRANSPLANT.

Congenital hand differences

Incidence:
- 1:600.
- Most isolated. Radial congenital hand differences have a higher incidence of associated congenital anomalies.

Embryology:
- Limb bud is an outgrowth of somatic mesoderm and starts at 4 weeks. 33 days hand paddle. 50 days digital separation. 50 days full bony structure.
- Complete development at birth except for myelination which is complete by 2 years.
- There are three axes of development, each with a signalling centre which secretes ligands which go on to activate transcription factors:
  ○ Proximal/distal axis: signalling centre is apical epidermal ridge (AER) and ligand is fibroblast growth factor (FGF);
  ○ Radial/ulnar axis: signalling centre is zone of polarizing activity (ZPA) and ligand is sonic hedgehog (SHH);
  ○ Dorsal/ventral axis: signalling centre is dorsal ectoderm and ligand is wingless-type mouse mammary tumour (WNT7a).

Classification: 2 classification systems have been in common use. The first is Swansons IFSSH classification and the latter is the Oberg Manske Tonkin (OMT) classification. Neither is perfect and both are here for comparison.

Swanson IFSSH classification of congenital hand anomalies. Seven types:
1. Failure of formation (developmental arrest):
   - Longitudinal arrest: pre-axial:
     ○ Pre-axial deficiency, _see_ RADIAL CLUB HAND;
     ○ Central ray deficiency, _see_ CLEFT HAND;
     ○ Post-axial deficiency, _see_ ULNAR CLUB HAND.
   - Transverse arrest:
     ○ Complete deficiencies;
     ○ Intercalated deficiencies.
2. Failure of differentiation:
   - Soft tissues:
     ○ _Syndactyly_;
     ○ _Camptodactyly_;
     ○ _Trigger thumb and finger_;
     ○ _Clasped thumb_.
   - Skeletal:
     ○ C_linodactyly_;
     ○ _Symphalangism_;
     ○ _Arthrogryposis_.

3. Duplication:
   • Ulnar *Polydactyly*.
   • Central polydactyly.
   • Radial polydactyly.
   • Ulnar dimelia.

4. Overgrowth:

   • *Macrodactyly*.

5. Undergrowth:

   • Hypoplastic fingers (*Symbrachydactyly*).
   • *Brachydactyly*.
   • *Thumb hypoplasia*.

6. Congenital construction ring.
7. Generalized skeletal deformity.

OMT classification:
1. Malformations:

   • *Axis formation entire limb:*
     ○ *Proximal distal axis:* symbrachydactyly, brachydactyly and transverse deficiencies;
     ○ *Radial/ulnar axis:* duplications, ulnar dimelia;
     ○ *Dorsal/ventral axis:* nail-patella syndrome.
   • *Axis formation hand:*
     ○ *Radial/ulnar:* polydactyly, triphalangeal thumb;
     ○ *Dorsal/ventral:* dorsal dimelia, hypoplastic nail.
   • *Handplate formation:*
     ○ *Soft tissue:* syndactyly, camptodactyly;
     ○ *Bone:* brachydactyly, clinodactyly, Kirners;
     ○ *Complex:* cleft hand, Apert hand.

2. Deformations:

   • Constriction ring.
   • Arthgryosis.
   • Trigger digits.

3. Dysplasia:

   • *Hypertrophy:* macrodactyly.

4. Syndromes.

Principles of assessment of the congenital hand:
• *History:* determine functionality of hand, family history and associated syndromes.
• *Examination:* mostly observational:

   ○ Examine parents' hands for size and anomalies;
   ○ Examine face, feet and contralateral hand;
   ○ Examine entire upper limb for chest wall anomalies and stiff joints;
   ○ Examine hand to classify and assess function.

• *Investigation:* XR possible from 6 months due to ossification.

Principles of surgical management in congenital hand differences:
• Restore fundamental hand functions of grasp and precision pinch.
• Minimize restriction to growth.
• Cosmesis is important alongside function.

Congenital naevus
• Any *Naevus* present at birth.
• A *Naevus* refers to abnormal growth. Most are congenital melanocytic naevi (CMN).
• Melanoblasts migrate early from the neural crest to differentiate into melanocytes. When this migration is disturbed, the result is an ectopic population of cells.
• Histologically congenital naevi differ from acquired in being deeper into the dermis with nests of melanocytes.

Size:
• *Small:* <1.5 cm diameter.
• *Medium:* >1.5 cm <20 cm diameter.
• *Giant:* (GHN) many definitions, >20 cm diameter, >100 cm², >5% surface area. <1:20,000 newborns.

Clinical features:
• Untreated CMNs tend to lighten spontaneously with age.
• Most are raised with follicular, pebble stone surface.
• May develop hairs as the lesion matures.
• Giant (GCMN) may be associated with underdevelopment of underlying tissue. They are more common on the lower back or thighs, *Neurocutaneous melanosis*.
• Head and neck naevi may be associated with epilepsy. Over the spine there may be underlying spinal defects.

Malignancy:
• There is an association between giant naevi and melanoma.
• The quoted risk is variable, ranging from 0 to 40% and is likely distorted by reporting bias. Largest studies show lifetime risk to be between 0.5 and 3%. Highest risk is in childhood and adolescence.
• Excisional surgery of the cutaneous lesion is not thought to reduce the risk of malignancy because malignant potential tends to occur in cells along the melanoblast migration pathway deep to the dermis.

Treatment:
• MDT setting.
• Conservative management involves serial photographs to document spontaneous lightening.

- Facial CMNs may benefit from excisional surgery for cosmetic reasons. A single small solitary lesion may be excised completely whereas larger lesions may require serial excisions, expansion or resurfacing with skin grafts.

Consent
In England:
- Consent is supported decision making. It is not a one-off event and patients have the right to change their minds.
- For consent to be obtained, the patient must have capacity, must give consent voluntarily and must be informed.
- Assume every adult has capacity to make a decision and assist capacity where needed. Assess capacity by seeing if patient can:
  - Understand information;
  - Retain information;
  - Use information;
  - Communicate decision.
- Adults with capacity have the right to make unwise decision or refuse treatment.
- If an adult lacks capacity, no one else can give consent on their behalf but advanced statement of legal power of attorneys can guide decisions about refusal to life-sustaining treatments. Treatment is given based on the best interests of the patient as judged by the treating healthcare professionals. Independent advocates (IMCAs) can be used to make decisions about best interest.
- *Children:* over 16, individuals are presumed to have capacity. Younger children can also give consent if they understand fully and are deemed to be Gillick competent. If not, someone with parental responsibility can give consent on the child's behalf unless they can't be reached in an emergency. A parent cannot override a competent child who consents. Legally, a minor under 16 years does not have the right to refuse medical treatment but competent refusal is complex and legal advice should be sought.

Constricted ear
See LOP EAR.

Constriction ring syndrome
- Probably due to premature rupture of amnion causing strands of amniotic tissue, which create tight bands leading to ischaemia in limbs.
- Incidence 1:15,000.
- May get compromised vascularity and oedema.

- Sporadic.
- Assess urgency, assess circulation and neurology. Note intrinsic muscles.

Classification:
Patterson described 4 types:
- *Group 1:* simple, a groove in the skin.
- *Group 2:* distal deformity +/- lymphoedema, acrosyndactyly, but no vascular compromise.
- *Group 3:* progressive lymphaticovenous or arterial compromise.
- *Group 4:* intrauterine amputations.

Treatment:
- Release early when oedema gross use circumferential Z-plasties.
- Amputation may be required.
- If thumb is shortened the structures proximally are normal; may need phalangization, metacarpal lengthening, toe-hand, digital transfer.

Converse flap
See SCALPING FLAP.

Copper
Needed for lysyl oxidase used for collagen metabolism.

Cormack and Lamberty: fasciocutaneous flaps
Classification of *Fasciocutaneous flaps:*
- *A:* multiple perforators, direct and indirect, e.g. Pontén flap.
- *B:* single perforator, usually direct, which runs along the axis of the flap; e.g. *Scapular* and parascapular.
- *C:* segmental perforators—from same source vessel, e.g. *Radial forearm flap*, *Lateral arm flap*.

Coronal synostosis
Unilateral coronal synostosis:
- 8–10% of *Craniosynostosis.*
- Premature fusion of one of the coronal sutures results in anterior plagiocephaly (a Greek term meaning oblique skull).
- 1 of 10,000 live births.
- Superior growth elongates the forehead.
- Inferior growth deforms the middle cranial fossa and bows the greater wing of the sphenoid causing proptosis and the *Harlequin* sign.
- There is a bulge of the ipsilateral temporal bone.
- The fused suture is ridged.
- Surgical options:

○ Bifrontal craniotomy and supra-orbital rim osteotomy with fronto-orbital advancement (FOAR). The frontal bone is reshaped and fixed;

○ Minimally invasive unilateral remodelling within first year of life.

Bilateral coronal synostosis:

• 9–20% of synostosis, many are syndromic.
• Tower-shaped, but short, head: turribrachycephaly.
• Surgical:

○ Anterior advancement: fronto-orbital advancement (FOAR);

○ Posterior advancement: provides more intracranial volume per mm of movement than anterior surgery. Can be performed statically with advancement and fixation or dynamically with distraction.

Cortical ring sign

• Seen in scapho-lunate advanced collapse (SLAC).
• Palmar tilting of the scaphoid results in a ring appearance on a PA.
• Also get *Terry-Thomas sign*.

See CARPAL INSTABILITY.

Cosmetic camouflage

• *Counteract:* with neutralizers or colour correctors. A yellow colour negates red (neutralizer); colour correctors act as a primer and are followed by foundation.
• *Cover:* camouflage cream. These cover any scars, pigmentation, etc., that foundation won't hide being thicker and more opaque.
• *Create:* using contour shadow. Correct the brows, eyes and lips.

Cottle sign

• To assess the internal nasal valve which is typically the narrowest part of the nasal airway and is formed between the septum and upper lateral cartilages.
• If lateral cheek traction improves airway obstruction (positive Cottle sign), then spreader grafts may be of benefit.

Coup de sabre

• From the French meaning 'by a strike of the sword'.
• Sharp linear depression in forehead seen in *Hemifacial atrophy*.
• Can have an atrophic shiny plaque overlying it.
• Surgical management: may be appropriate when condition has stabilized:

○ Mild defects can be amenable to lipofilling or fillers;
○ More complex defects may require bone grafts or implants.

Cowden syndrome

• Autosomal dominant condition. Mutation of PTEN gene.
• Characterized by multiple hamartomas— typically multiple *Tricholemmomas* and mucosal papillomas.
• Associated with increased risk of breast, thyroid and endometrial cancer.

Crane principle

• Described by Millard in 1969 to provide a platform for complex soft tissue reconstructions.
• A flap is transposed to cover the defect.
• The flap is then split into two lamina with the skin and outer lamina being returned to the original site after a delay period.
• The soft tissue now adherent to the wound providing a stable platform for skin grafting.

Cranial bones

• *Five bones:* 2 frontal, 2 parietal and occipital.
• *Intramembranous ossification:* a centre of osteogenesis develops first into cancellous bone and then into compact bone. They grow until they touch adjacent bones at the sutures. Once they contact, they only grow at the sutures. The metopic suture ossifies in the second year, but the rest ossify in the 30s. After the age of 8 the single plates of bone become two plates of compact bone separated by cancellous bone.
• *Endochondral ossification:* the method of bone formation in the cranial base. Cartilage models are replaced by bone and they articulate with cartilage—synchondrosis.

Craniofacial clefts (also known as atypical clefts)

• A soft tissue and a bony disruption in the normal growth pattern of the face.
• Sporadic incidence and occurs 1:25,000 births.
• Aetiology multifactorial. Viruses, toxoplasmosis, teratogens such as anticonvulsants and steroids, and metabolic disorders have been implicated.
• Some overlap between clefts and other hypoplastic syndromes. Treacher Collins is hypoplastic and also Tessier 6, 7, 8 cleft.

Classification: *Tessier*.

Pathogenesis: theories include:

• *Failure of fusion:* this theory suggests that the face is the site of union of the free ends of the facial processes. After contact penetration by the mesoderm completes the fusion. Disruption leads to a cleft.

- *Mesodermal migration and penetration:* suggests that there are no free ends, but instead the face is a continuous sheet, demarcated by epithelial seams. Mesenchyme migrates into this. The craniofacial skeleton is derived from neuroectoderm. If the neuroectoderm fails to penetrate then the epithelium breaks down. Partial penetration will lead to a partial cleft.
- *Amniotic bands:* with intrauterine compression.

Surgical principles:

- *Optimize facial function:*
  - ○ Eyelid reconstruction is a priority to protect the eye;
  - ○ Oral competence and speech optimization.
- *Separation of cavities:* oral, maxillary sinus, nasal, orbital.
- *Cosmesis:* reconstruction is facilitated by wide surgical exposure.
  - ○ *Skeleton:* can be reconstructed by:
    - ▪ Removal of abnormal elements;
    - ▪ Transposing skeletal components—i.e. *Distraction osteogenesis*;
    - ▪ Bone grafting;
    - ▪ Alloplastic implants.
  - ○ Muscle repair is the foundation of the dynamic reconstruction—can be reattached anatomically by transposition and fixation. Serves to animate face and stimulate growth.
  - ○ *Soft tissues:* can be reconstructed with local tissue advancement and rearrangement with or without prior expansion. Scars should be positioned within boundaries of aesthetic units and subunits if possible.

Craniofacial genetics
Orofacial clefts:

- Over 200 syndromes, but most clefts are isolated events.
- CL with or without CP is distinct from isolated CP.
- There may be two forms of CP. An autosomal dominant type and a non-familial, which is caused by environmental factors.

Orofacial cleft syndromes:

- *DiGeorge sequence/Velocardiofacial syndrome:* diagnosis has been aided by molecular genetic techniques, especially fluorescently tag DNA probes, which shows only one signal as opposed to two when the deletion is present.
- *Stickler syndrome.*
- *Robin sequence.*
- *Van der Woude's Syndrome.*

Craniosynostosis:

- Premature fusion can occur alone or with other anomalies.
- Most *Apert's* are sporadic with a few cases of autosomal dominance.
- Two-thirds of *Crouzon's* are familial.
- Both result from mutations of fibroblast growth factor receptor 2 (FGFR2) localized on chromosome 10.
- Most syndromic cases are confined to the coronal suture.

External ears and face:

- *Mandibulofacial dysostosis* (*Treacher Collins syndrome*): the genetic defect is localized to the long arm of chromosome 5 (5q32–q33.1). The gene has been labelled *TCOF1*, which codes a protein called treacle. This protein probably has a role in early human facial development.
- *Craniofacial microsomia/Goldenhar syndrome:* most are sporadic.

Craniofacial microsomia

- Previously known as hemifacial microsomia.
- Second most common craniofacial congenital anomaly following cleft lip and palate.
- Involves structures of first and second branchial arch and characterized by underdevelopment of facial structures. Correlated with Tessier Atypical Cleft 7.
- Considered as part of oculo-auriculovertebral spectrum, which includes *Goldenhar syndrome*.
- 1:4,000 births. 80% are unilateral. Bilateral are asymmetric.
- M:F 3:2.
- Most are sporadic though autosomal dominant and recessive have been reported. Variable expression:
  - ○ May be caused by vascular disruption of the primitive stapedial artery (a temporary embryonic collateral of the hyoid artery)—on which the 1st and 2nd branchial arches are dependent.

Presentation:

- Characteristically affects the ears (microtia), mandible (hypoplasia), eyes and mouth (macrostomia).

- Ocular abnormalities include blepharoptosis, anophthalmia or microphthalmia. Epibulbar tumours are found in 1/3.
- Cranial nerves V and VII may be involved.
- The zygoma, maxilla and temporal bone may also be hypoplastic.
- Skin tags may be present between the first and second branchial arch.
- Muscles of mastication may be hypoplastic especially the lateral pterygoid muscle, which moves the mandible to the contralateral side.
- Cleft lip and palate may be present.
- Radial ray defects occur in 10%.
- Other abnormalities include lung, renal and congenital heart disease.

  See GOLDENHAR SYNDROME.

Classification:

- *OMENS* plus classification: orbits, mandible, ear, nerve, soft tissues, plus extra-cranial features.
- Also *Harvold classification* and *Prozansky classification*.

Treatment:

Before 2 years:

- Fit hearing aids.
- Remove auricular appendages.
- Correct macrostomia—closure is either as a straight line or Z-plasty.

2–6 years:

- Osseodistraction of mandibular ramus: this is the commonest technique used for skeletal correction. There are many devices, including internal ones to prevent scarring. Advance by 1 mm per day. Aim to over-correct in the growing child. Get associated elongation of the soft tissues, particularly the inferior alveolar nerve. The biggest problem is that an absent TMJ is not restored and an absent zygoma is not addressed. It also does not correct the medial displacement, but only elongates an abnormally placed mandible.

6–14 years:

- Orthodontic treatment.
- Orthognathic those with mild involvement and an intact TMJ have a Le Fort I and a bilateral sagittal mandibular osteotomy.
- Ear reconstruction.
- Soft tissue reconstruction:
  - Fat grafting for mild and free tissue transfer for major;
  - Facial reanimation—may not be needed if residual function.

  See CRANIOFACIAL GENETICS. *See* TESSIER CLEFTS.

Craniopagus

- Rare anomaly seen in 1:600 twin births and 1:60,000 live births.
- It consists of identical twins joined at the skull, brain and/or scalp.
- It may be partial or total.
- Problems with separation include the complex sharing of brain and particularly venous drainage. Skin separation has been facilitated by tissue expansion.

  See SCALP RECONSTRUCTION.

Craniosynostosis

- First described by Hippocrates in 100 BC.
- Virchow described the condition in 1851.
- Premature fusion of one or more cranial suture *in utero* or shortly after birth. Growth perpendicular to the suture is restricted and parallel to it is increased.
- 1:2200 live births.
- Most are sporadic.
- 50% involve the sagittal suture.
- Syndromes often associated with malformations of limbs, ears, and heart.

Anatomy *See* CRANIAL BONES.

Pathogenesis:

- The stimulus for growth is the expanding brain. It is 50% of the adult volume at 6 months of age.
- The primary problem is probably in the cranial suture although the cranial base may be the site of the primary problem.
- The causes may be multifactorial—in non-syndromic metabolic, such as vitamin D deficiency or brain malformations, in syndromic chromosomal abnormalities.
- The biomechanical model suggests that there are fibre tracts running through dura from cranial base to suture. Abnormalities in the cranial base result in transmission of abnormal stresses to the vault resulting in premature fusion.
- The model may be more biochemical, but the dura seems to be important.
- Lots of factors have been shown to be important in this process such as FGF and TGF-β. TGF-β1, 2 and 3 appear to play different roles with perhaps TGF-β2 inducing fusion and TGF-β3 aiding suture patency.
- At least 5 genes have been identified which, when mutated lead to craniosynostosis—MSX2, FGFR1–3, TWIST.

Radiology:

- *CT:* requires GA so only if a procedure is planned.

- Plain XR look for primary and secondary signs but not sensitive.

Primary signs:
- Partial or total suture absence.
- Indistinct zones along the suture.
- Perisutural sclerosis.

Secondary signs:
- Calvarial shape.
- *Harlequin sign:* ipsilateral elevation of the lesser wing of sphenoid causing an abnormally shaped orbit with unicoronal synostosis.
- Hypotelorism with metopic suture.

Clinical progression:
- *Raised intracranial pressure:* up to 60% of Crouzon's, which present later. Note papilloedema and *Thumb-printing/copper beaten* XR sign.
- *Eye signs:*
  - Exorbitism with corneal exposure;
  - Papilloedema and optic atrophy;
  - Ocular motility problems and strabismus.
- *Hydrocephalus:* particularly with Apert's syndrome. It may be due to increased venous pressure in the sagittal sinus secondary to obstruction of the venous outflow.

Classification:
Characteristic skull shape depending on which suture is involved:
- *Metopic:* triangular—trigonocephaly.
- *Sagittal:* elongated keel shape—scaphocephaly.
- *Unilateral coronal:* twisted anteriorly—anterior plagiocephaly.
- *Unilateral lambdoid:* twisted posteriorly—posterior plagiocephaly.
- *Bilateral coronal:* anterior brachycephaly.
- *Bilateral lambdoid:* posterior brachycephly.
- *Sagittal and bilateral coronal:* oxycephaly.
- *Multiple:* clover leaf—Kleeblattschädel.

Non-syndromic craniosynostosis:
- 94% of craniosynostosis. Usually single suture ICP not raised.
- *Sagittal suture synostosis:* the commonest.
- *Lambdoid synostosis:* rare but must be differentiated from deformational plagiocephaly.
- *Deformational/positional plagiocephaly:* results from extrinsic forces making the back of the head flattened. These can be intrauterine or post-natal

positioning, more common following the 'back to sleep' campaign. Characteristic parallelogram skull shape with ear pushed forward, commonly associated with torticollis. There is an absence of facial scoliosis.

Management:
- Managed within MDT.
- Vault remodelling timing: if before 12 months then cranial bines pliable and takes advantage of brain expansion to drive skull shape, if after 12 months safer complication profile.
- Sagittal synostosis options:
  - Minimally invasive options performed within the first year include endoscopic strip craniectomy assisted with helmet or the use of springs;
  - Total calvarial remodelling usually at 10-18 months aims to address the multiple elements of deformity.
- Metopic synostosis options:
  - Minimally invasive option of endoscopic strip craniectomy;
  - Fronto-orbital advancement.
- Unicoronal synostosis:
  - Minimally invasive option of endoscopic strip craniectomy of the unilateral fused suture;
  - Fronto-orbital advancement.

Syndromic craniosynostosis:
- More complex as many sutures including the base of skull and face are involved.
- The problems are not easily correctable and require multiple procedures.
- Syndromic craniosynostosis include:
  - *Apert's;*
  - *Saethre-Chotzen;*
  - *Carpenter's;*
  - *Pfeiffer's;*
  - *Crouzon's;*
  - Jackson-Weiss.

Management:
- Aim to correct functional problems and improve appearance.
- *Ocular:* topical protection, tarsorraphy, fronto-orbital advancement.
- *ICP:* shunts, treat airway obstruction, vault expansion.
- Vault expansion:
  - *Anterior:* fronto-orbital advancement;
  - *Posterior:* achieves more volume per unit of advancement.

- Midface hypoplasia can be addressed with Le Fort osteotomies and advancement with bone grafts or distraction osteogenesis. A monobloc advancement advances the fronto-orbital and Le Fort 3 segments as one block.

Complications:

- Intra-op:
  - Hypovolaemia;
  - Sagittal sinus injury and significant bleeding;
  - Dura and brain injury.
- Early:
  - SIADH;
  - Air embolism;
  - Infection—meningitis;
  - CSF leak;
  - Death.
- Later:
  - Relapse to the primary deformity;
  - Secondary deformity including scarring and temporal hollowing;
  - Recurrent raised ICP.

Cranium reconstruction

- *Split cranial bone graft*.
- *Rib graft*.
- Alloplastic materials such as *Methyl methacrylate*, infection is a problem. Contraindicated when there is exposure to sinuses or nasal cavity.

See SCALP RECONSTRUCTION.

Creep

- Refers to the permanent stretching seen in *Tissue expansion*.
- Collagen is convoluted and allows stretching up to a certain point after, which there is sudden resistance. Recoil is due to elastin fibres.
- Prolonged loading causes irreversible extension.
- During creep there is a change in collagen fibre bonding and collagen fibre realignment.
- Creep may also be due to displacement of water from the ground substance.

CREST

- **C**alcinosis.
- **R**aynaud's.
- **E**sophageal problems.
- **S**clerodactyly.
- **T**elangiectasis.

   Two out of the 5 are needed for a diagnosis of CREST.

Critical ischaemia time

- The maximum period of ischaemia that tissues can withstand and remain viable.
- It is temperature and tissue dependent.
- Skin grafts can survive 3 weeks at 3–4°C.
- Digits can last over 24 hours when hypothermic.
- Normothermic skin flaps have a CIT_{50} (time when 50% of flaps would necrose) of 9 hours.
- Muscle has a higher metabolic requirement and is more sensitive, as is bowel.

Cross-finger flap

- Vascularized pedicle flap from dorsum of one finger to volar aspect of the adjacent finger. Pedicle is divided after 2 weeks.
- For dorsal digit defects, a reverse cross-finger flap can be used which consists of de-epithelialized tissue that is then covered with a skin graft.
- Side cross-finger flap is useful for thumb tip injuries. A proximally based flap is raised from the side of the donor digit and rotated 90° to inset it. The donor site can be on the ulnar side.

Technique:

- Draw a pattern of the defect on the dorsum of the middle or proximal phalanx.
- The flap is based laterally along the midlateral line and elevated above the level of paratenon.
- Preserve veins near the base.
- Cleland's ligaments need to be divided to mobilize the flap.
- Suture the flap in place and immobilize the finger by suturing together.
- Graft the defect and divide the flap 3 weeks after the surgery.

See FINGERTIP INJURIES.

Crouzon's syndrome

Bicoronal synostosis, midfacial hypoplasia with exorbitism and normal hands.

- A syndromic *Craniosynostosis*.
- Bicoronal, but may also include sagittal and lambdoid cranisynostosis.
- Midface hypoplasia.
- Shallow orbits, and ocular proptosis (defining feature) may get exposure keratitis, poor vision and blindness.
- Development is normal in 95% of patients.
- Usually present after 2–3 years.
- Conductive hearing loss in over 50% of cases.
- Incidence is 1:25,000 with variable expression.

- Two-thirds are familial, the rest are sporadic.
- Mutation in fibroblast growth factor receptor 2 (FGFR2).
- Similar to *Apert's syndrome*, but without the hand anomalies.

    See CRANIOFACIAL GENETICS. *See* CRANIOSYNOSTOSIS.

Cryptotia
- Congenital anomaly of the ear where the upper pole of ear is buried beneath the scalp.
- More common in Japanese.
- Non-surgical treatment is with splints.
- Surgical treatment is used to create sulcus with SSG or flaps.

    See EAR RECONSTRUCTION.

CSAG cleft lip and palate
- *CSAG:* clinical standards advisory group commissioned by UK government in 1996. Led to the establishment of centralized cleft care in the UK.
- Study into the quality of the UK cleft service was triggered by Eurocleft results where UK had the worst maxillary growth results (speech outcomes not assessed).
- Survey of UK centres performing cleft repairs auditing 647 patients with UCLP in 2 cohorts: 5- and 12-year-olds.
- Results and recommendations:
    - Revealed fragmented decentralized services that were achieving low standard of clinical care in certain areas such as occlusion, maxillary growth and dental health:
        - Recommended centralized care from a single regional centre equipped with a comprehensive specialist cleft team;
        - Surgeons to operate on at least 40 new cleft cases per year.

CT scan
- Computerized tomography.
- Differentiate from MRI as the bone is white.
- Scout films show the levels and spacing of the cuts.
- Bone weighted scans are darker and demonstrate bone architecture.
- Lymph nodes are significant if >1 cm. Malignant nodes have a radiolucent core and a radio-opaque periphery.
- Spiral CT is fast. Five separate scanners move along the body. A chest can be scanned in 10–15 seconds.

- *Advantages:* good for bones, quick, cheap, easily accessible, better for ill patients.
- *Disadvantages:* artefacts from bones, patients receive dose of radiation.

Cubital tunnel syndrome
- *Ulnar nerve compression* at the elbow.
- Second commonest compression in the upper limb.
- Distinguish from compression in Guyon's canal by assessing sensation on the dorsum of the little finger as the dorsal branch of the ulnar nerve commences proximally to Guyon's canal.

Anatomy:
- Fibro-osseous tunnel beginning at the humeral condyle with the medial epicondyle anteriorly.
- Lateral border and floor is the medial collateral ligament and elbow joint.
- Medial border is head of FCU.
- The roof is a fibrous aponeurotic band—Osborne's ligament.

Compression points:
- Arcade of Struthers (fascial band above the elbow).
- Compression of overlying muscles (medial head of triceps).
- Arcuate ligament (fascial arcade of FCU).
- Local mass effect (osteophytes, tumour).
- Osborne's ligament (roof of cubital tunnel).
- Cubitus valgus.

Management:
- *Get nerve conduction studies:* see velocities <50m/sec across elbow.
- *Cubital tunnel release method:* controversial—no evidence to suggest simple decompression is inferior to medial epicondylectomy or transpositions.
- *Simple decompression:* approach nerve by a longitudinal incision in the midpoint between medial epicondyle and the olecranon. Find the nerve proximally before it enters under Osborne's ligament.
- *Medial epicondylectomy:* only partially resected to avoid destabilization of elbow.
- Anterior transposition of the ulnar nerve can be:
    - Subcutaneous;
    - Submuscular deep to flexors;
    - Intramuscular.

Cup ear *See* LOP EAR.

Cup size: bra

- Measure in centimetres or inches.
- First measure under the breasts at the level of the inframammary fold—the underband.
- Next measure around the breast at the most prominent point—the overbust.
- Round up to the nearest unit.
- The back size is the underband—add 4 inches if even and 5 inches if an odd number.
- For the cup size compare overbust to back size. If equal it is an A, then for every inch over the cup size increases. If less it is an AA.

Curreri formula

- Used for assessing nutritional requirements in burns patients.
- The adult daily caloric requirement is 25 kcal/kg + 40 kcal/% TBSA burn.
- For children, the formula is 60 kcal/kg + 35 kcal/% TBSA burn.
- This formula appears to be accurate in assessing moderate-sized burns in young healthy patients.
- Caloric requirements are overestimated with this formula in large burns or in the elderly.

See BURNS.

Cutaneous horn

- Arise from underlying epidermal lesions, usually *Actinic keratosis*.
- Up to 10% may have an underlying *SCC*.
- It may also be associated with keratoacanthoma, sebaceous adenoma or Kaposi's sarcoma.
- Excise for histology.

Cutis hyperelastica

See EHLERS–DANLOS SYNDROME.

Cutis laxa

- Degeneration of elastic fibres in the dermis. The patient has coarse drooping skin.
- Due to a deficiency of lysyl oxidase.
- Wound healing normal. May benefit from facial rejuvenation.
- Associated with pulmonary infections, cor pulmonale, diverticuli.

Cutis marmorata telangiectatica congenita (also known as van Lohuizen syndrome)

- Get dilated dermal capillaries and veins.
- Usually localized on trunk and extremity.
- May get ulceration.

- The condition improves over the first year of life, but the cutaneous atrophy, vascular staining and venous ectasia persist.

See TELANGIECTASIS.

Cutler–Beard bridge flap

- Upper *Eyelid reconstruction* with a pedicled flap from the lower lid.
- Two-stage reconstruction for large full-thickness defects of the upper lid.
- Create the defect then pull edges together to judge the width.
- Draw horizontal line 5 mm inferior to lash line on lower lid.
- Draw vertical lines to orbital rim. Incise full thickness (including conjunctiva) and lift up flap under lower lid. Suture in 3 layers place, leave for 6 weeks, then divide.

Cyanide poisoning

- May occur in flame burns due to incomplete combustion of substances containing nitrogen.
- Usually presents with neurological disturbance in combination with carbon monoxide poisoning and is dose dependent. Cyanide has a higher affinity to haemoglobin than oxygen, shifting the oxyhaemoglobin curve to the left.
- It is metabolized in the liver by rhodanese and converted to thiocyanate which is excreted in urine.
- Manage with oxygen and an antidote such as hydroxycobalamin, sodium thiosulphate or sodium nitrite which chelates the cyanide.

See HYDROGEN CYANIDE.

Cyanoacrylates

- The cyanoacrylates are quick-setting, biodegradable, polymeric tissue adhesives.
- Useful tissue-bonding agents and haemostatic.
- They work well on a moist surface.
- Histoacryl is butyl-2-cyanoacrylate.
- Degradation of the cyanoacrylates yields the tissue toxic metabolites, alkyl cyanoacetate and formaldehyde.
- The longer alkyl chain compounds, such as histoacryl degrade more slowly than the methyl and ethyl cyanoacrylates, and therefore cause less tissue toxicity.

See ALLOPLASTS.

Cyclic loading

A method of intra-operative *Tissue expansion* with 3–5 minutes of stretch followed by 2 minutes rest.

Cylindroma: turban tumour

- Solitary or multiple, pink nodules up to several centimetres occurs.
- Predominantly on the scalp or forehead.
- Slow-growing in adulthood.
- Autosomal dominant form associated with trichoepitheliomas covers the scalp like a turban.
- Treatment—excision.

Cytokines and growth factors
Summary:

- Cytokines and growth factors are essential for wound healing and host defence.
- They are polypeptide regulatory molecules crucial in initiating, sustaining and regulating the post-injury response.
- They are also implicated in impaired wound healing and abnormal scarring.
- The term cytokine is used for polypeptides essential for host defence and growth factors are primarily concerned with cell maturation, but these activities are often very similar.

Pro-inflammatory cytokines:
Tumour necrosis factor-α (TNF-α):

- Released by macrophage-monocyte.
- Initiates immune cascade in response to injury or bacteria.
- Involved in maturation of cellular component of inflammation.
- Excess TNF-α is associated with multisystem organ failure.
- High levels of TNF-α have been found in non-healing chronic venous ulcers.

Interleukin-1:
- Similar to TNF-α.
- Also promotes other cells to secrete pro-inflammatory cytokines.
- May be responsible for long-term host defence.

Interleukin-2:
- Produced by T lymphocytes.
- Involved in T-cell activation.

Interleukin-6:
- Wide variety of effects.
- B and T-cell activation.
- Found early after injury and stays around for over a week.
- Stimulates fibroblast proliferation.
- Less in foetus that may contribute to scarless healing.
- May be used as a marker for severity of wound.

Interleukin-8:
- Secreted by macrophages and fibroblasts.
- Increase neutrophil and monocyte chemotaxis.
- Elevated in psoriasis and reduced in foetus.

Interferon-γ:
- Important in tissue remodelling.
- Reduces wound contraction.

Anti-inflammatory cytokines:
Interleukin-4:

- Inhibition of pro-inflammatory cytokines.
- Increased in scleroderma where it may be implicated in fibrosis.

Interleukin-10:
- Inhibits synthesis of major pro-inflammatory cytokines.
- Found in high concentrations in chronic venous ulcers.

Growth factors:
Platelet-derived growth factor (PDGF):

- Essential in initiating and sustaining wound-healing response.
- PDGF is released from platelets early.
- Causes activation of immune cells and fibroblasts.
- PDGF is then secreted by macrophages and stimulates collagen synthesis.
- Found to be decreased in non-healing wounds.
- Recombinant PDGF improves healing in acute and chronic wounds. Approved for use in diabetic neuropathic ulcers.

Transforming growth factor-β (TGF-β):
- Released by platelets, macrophages and fibroblasts.
- Central for wound healing.
- Effects include fibroblast migration, maturation and extra-cellular matrix synthesis.
- Elevated levels are found in fibroproliferative states, such as keloid scars.
- TGF-β appears to play an important role in tissue fibrosis.
- Three iso-forms. Type 1 and 2 promote wound healing and scarring. Type 3 decreases wound healing and scarring.
- Not present in foetal wounds.

Fibroblast growth factor (FGF):
- Important mediator of angiogenesis and epithelialization.
- Ten members of the family isolated.

Keratinocyte growth factor (KGF):
- Member of the FGF family.
- Important regulators of keratinocyte proliferation.

Epidermal growth factor (EGF):
- Secreted by keratinocytes and directs epithelialization.
- Important in wound remodelling.

Vascular endothelial growth factor (VEGF):
- Released by keratinocytes.
- Levels rise steadily.

- Potent angiogenic factor.
- It is elevated in ischaemia.

Insulin-like growth factor (IGF):
- Produced primarily in the liver, but also found in wounds.
- Stimulates fibroblasts and keratinocyte production, and collagen synthesis.

Treatment: PDGF licensed. Anti-TNF for sepsis, anti-TGF for scarring.

Dacrocystorhinostomy to Dystopia

Dacrocystorhinostomy

A procedure performed to bypass nasolacrimal duct obstruction and allow tear drainage directly into the nasal cavity from the canaliculi by removing a portion of nasal bone adjacent to the lacrimal sac and incorporating the lacrimal sac with the nasal mucosa.

Darrach procedure

Resection of distal ulnar head for _DRUJ instability_ in Rheumatoid arthritis.

Operative procedure:

- Incise proximally over ulnar head, preserve dorsal cutaneous branch of ulnar nerve. Find ECU and mark out a flap with the base radially and the distal end running along ECU. The flap should be big enough to split proximal half for use as a sling and distal half to take under tendons to cover ulna bone after head excision.
- Incise extensor retinaculum on ulna border to enter 6th compartment (ECU). Enter 5th compartment and preserve EDM. Reflect and preserve joint capsule, perform synovectomy. Place Howarth and Mitchell trimmer around head of ulna and resect with oscillating saw. Avoid ulnar nerve and artery deep to head. Take only head, resect approximately 1 cm of ulna. Perform synovectomy.
- Close capsule over ulnar head. While doing this, flex elbow and supinate to bring ulna in volar direction. Ask assistant to apply gentle pressure to ulna. Split extensor retinaculum into two. Pass one half under ECU and suture to capsule to hold head down. Pass other half around ECU and suture retinaculum to itself to bring ECU dorsally over ulna to assist in holding ulna down. Insert size 8 drain. Close skin. Apply above elbow backslab with volar slab at wrist in supination.

Modifications:

- Swanson caps ulna, flap of ulnar capsule sutured to dorsal ulnar stump. Ulnar stump can be tethered with distally based strip of ECU.

See ULNA, DISTAL: ARTHRITIS.

Debridement

- Usually refers to the surgical removal of dead tissue and foreign material from a wound. More appropriately termed 'wound excision' by some. Can also be:
  - _Autolytic:_ using digestive enzymes;
  - _Chemical:_ enzymes such as streptokinase and collagenase; also lava therapy;
  - _Other mechanical:_ such as pulsatile jet lavage and saline gauze.

Deep circumflex iliac artery (DCIA) flap

- Described by Taylor 1979.
- Can provide large skin flap, long pedicle and good bone height to facilitate osseous implants in mandibular reconstruction.
- Based on deep circumflex iliac artery, originating from external iliac artery.

Flap raise:

- Supine with sand bag under hip.
- Landmarks:
  - Iliac crest;
  - ASIS;
  - Inguinal ligament;
  - Mid-inguinal point—femoral artery.
- Mark:
  - Incision 1 finger breath above the lateral half of the inguinal ligament to locate perforator;
  - Skin paddle centred over the iliac crest.
- Raise:
  - Start in mid-inguinal region;
  - Incise through external oblique and internal oblique fascia to expose transversalis fascia. Locate the DCIA vessels at the medial part of the incision at their origin and trace laterally towards the ASIS in the substance of the transversalis fascia. You will encounter lateral cutaneous nerve of thigh—preserve if possible;
  - If taking a skin paddle:
    - Raise the superior skin paddle over the external oblique. Take a 2–3 cm cuff of muscle over the iliac crest to preserve the perforating vessels to skin. Visualize iliacus

muscle on medial surface of iliac bone—
incise the muscle medial to the pedicle to
expose medial surface of bone for
osteotomy;

- Raise inferior skin paddle sub fascial and
  release muscles (gluteus maximus, gluteus
  medius and TFL) of the iliac crest to expose
  lateral surface of bone for osteotomy;
- Mark osteotomy sites and perform
  osteotomy.

See ILIAC CREST.

Deep inferior epigastric perforator (DIEP) flap

Currently considered the gold standard for autologous breast reconstruction due to reliability,
durability, ability to withstand radiotherapy,
similarity of abdominal tissue to natural breast
parenchyma (warm, soft and ptosis with age
similar to native breast), low donor site morbidity and aesthetic enhancement of the donor
site. Pre-operative CTA is usually performed to
map out vascular anatomy and select most
favourable perforator(s).

Blood supply:

- *Arterial supply:* Deep inferior epigastric artery
  (DIEA) from external iliac.
- *Venous drainage:* Deep inferior epigastric
  vein (DIEV in 90%) and/or superficial inferior
  epigastric vein (SIEV dominant in 10%)

Classification: Moon and Taylor classified
DIEA branching pattern:

1. Single DIEA.
2. DIEA that bifurcates below the level of the
   umbilicus.
3. DIEA that splits into three or more branches
   below the level of the umbilicus.

Operative technique for breast reconstruction:

- Position—supine.
- Landmarks:
  - Midline;
  - Umbilicus;
  - ASIS;
  - Pubic symphysis.
- Identify perforators—using CTA map and
  doppler.
- Marking:
  - Lower incision in suprapubic crease from
    ASIS to ASIS;
  - Pinch test—upper incision should be
    placed just above the umbilicus.
- Raise:
  - Inject LA except for position of SIEA/V
    4–8cm lateral to midline;

- Make lower incision—identify SIEV and
  dissect out desired length. Can also identify
  and dissect out SIEA as a supercharge
  option;
- Choose which side to start—make the
  upper incision and dissect laterally to
  medially above deep fascia to the
  semilunar line—then identify perforators;
- Dissect the perforator—incise rectus sheath
  and split the rectus abdominis muscle
  fibres to follow the perforator. Muscle
  relaxant is helpful to reduce muscle fibre
  contraction and avoid damaging pedicle;
- Then raise contralateral side;
- Neurotized DIEP flaps have been
  described in which a sensory nerve
  entering the flap is preserved and a length
  raised. This is then anastomosed onto an
  intercostal nerve found running just
  inferior to costal cartilage.

- Prepare recipient site:
  - Preparation of IMA/IMV described here,
    but anastomosis can also be done onto
    thoracodorsal vessels. Advantage is no risk
    of pneumothorax or haemorrhage, and no
    need to resect rib which some feel gives a
    divot. Disadvantage is difficulty having an
    assistant under microscope and loss of
    salvage option (latissimus dorsi flap);
  - Following mastectomy, pectoralis major
    muscle fibres are split to expose costal
    cartilage of 3rd rib (4th can be used, e.g. in
    nipple-sparing mastectomy);
  - Anterior perichondrium is incised and
    costal cartilage is dissected free of posterior
    perichondrium then removed entirely to
    sternocostal joint;
  - Posterior perichondrium is carefully
    dissected away to expose IMA and IMVs
    (usually a lateral and medial IMV at this level);
  - It is also possible to use a large perforator
    as a recipient without resecting costal
    cartilage.

- Anastomoses:
  - 8-0 or 9-0 nylon and/or venous coupler.

- Close:
  - Rectus sheath with or without mesh deep
    to muscle;
  - Rectus divarication plication can be done if
    needed;
  - Transversus abdominis plane (TAP) blocks;
  - Scarpa's and skin.

- Second stage procedures:
  - *Nipple reconstruction* +/− areolar tattooing;
  - Symmetrising reduction and/or mastopexy;
  - Flap reduction and/or mastopexy;
  - Lipofilling to improve contour.

Options for increasing the vascularity in a DIEP flap:
- Multiple ipsilateral perforators.
- Bipedicled, with a perforator from contralateral DIEA or SIEA supercharge.
- Additional anastomosis can be in series (one artery on to a side branch of another) or in parallel (antegrade or retrograde on to the recipient internal mammary artery).

Options for managing venous congestion in a DIEP flap:
- 5-20% of DIEP flaps rely on a superficial dominant venous draining system. The SIEV can be preserved during the flap raise and anastomosed to one of the following options if the flap appears congested intra-operatively after DIEA/V anastomosis is complete:
  - Superficial outside-flap shunt procedure—cranial extension of DIEV to facilitate superficial outside flap shunt;
  - Cephalic turn down;
  - Internal mammary vein—either 2nd IMV (often a medial and lateral IMV is present) or retrograde onto 1st IMV;
  - Thoracodorsal vein, lateral thoracic vein or intercostal vein;
  - 2nd DIEV from pedicle.
  - Large side branch of pedicle.

Deep palmar arch
- Formed at the level of metacarpal bases by the anastomosis of radial artery and deep branch of ulnar artery.
- It gives off metacarpal branches to 2nd–4th intermetacarpal spaces and dorsal perforating branches to join the dorsal metacarpal arteries.
  See SUPERFICIAL PALMAR ARCH.

Degloving injuries
Avulsion of skin from the underlying fascia, muscle and bones.
  See ARNEZ AND TYLER CLASSIFICATION. *See* RING AVULSION INJURIES.

Delaire cleft lip and palate philosophy
- French orthodontist.
- Advocated closure of the lip and soft palate as a first stage at 6 and 9 months of age.
- Delayed hard palate repair between 12 and 18 months of age.
- The rationale is an attempt to improve facial growth by delaying hard palate repair.

Delay phenomenon
- The delay procedure is where a portion of the vascular supply to a flap is divided before the definitive elevation and transfer of the flap.

- This extends the longitudinal reach of the flap's vascular pedicle as there is improved flap perfusion.
- *Tagliacozzi* used delay with his nasal reconstruction.
- Milton experimented on pigs to find that a bipedicled incision was the most effective.
- The flap is usually raised definitively 10-14 days after the delay.

Mechanism of action:
- Multifactorial.
- *Sympathectomy:* an alteration of sympathetic tone producing vasodilatation.
- Reorientation of the blood supply along the length of the flap.
- Dilation of choke vessels.
- *Tolerance to ischaemia:* cells become conditioned to a hypoxic state after the initial delay procedure. Less tissue necrosis occurs after the second operation.
- *Hyperadrenergic state:* which results in vasoconstriction. This would not be as severe in a delayed flap.

Deltopectoral flap
- Described by Bakamjiam in 1965.
- Outlined along the inferior border of the clavicle, beginning at the sternum and extending lateral to acromion process. Returning at the level of 5th rib.
- *Blood supply:* sternal border to deltopectoral groove supplied by first 4 perforating branches of the internal mammary artery, particularly the 2nd and 3rd. At the upper portion of the groove, the thoracoacromial artery supplies the upper mid portion. The area of flap overlying deltoid is supplied by perforating vessels. This portion of the flap is, therefore, a random pattern supply. This may require delay to improve reliability.

Flap raise:
- *Position:* supine;
- Landmarks:
  - Sternal midline (medial aspect);
  - Clavicle (superior aspect);
  - 4th rib (inferior aspect);
  - Deltopectoral groove (lateral aspect).
- *Locate perforator:* 2nd intercostal space will probably be biggest—2 cm lateral to border of sternum;
- Marking:
  - Incorporate a pedicle in 2nd or third intercostal space;
  - Superior margin in parallel to clavicle;

○ Extend towards deltopectoral groove—if you go beyond this, a delay procedure will be required.
• Raise:
  ○ Incise down to pectoral fascia—fascia usually raised with the flap;
  ○ Raise from lateral to medial;
  ○ Do not venture within 2 cm of medial sternal edge.
• Close in layers.

De Quervain's disease
• Stenosing tenosynovitis of first dorsal compartment, involving APL and EPB sheaths at the radial styloid.
• Inflammation, oedema, adhesions and fibrosis restrict tendon glide.
• Get local tenderness and moderate swelling of the extensor retinaculum over first dorsal compartment and positive *Finklestein's test*.
• May occur through repetitive use of the wrist and hand.
• Most common in women between 30 and 50 years.
• *Get crepitus:* the *Wet leather sign*.
• APL and EPB pass through a tight canal 1 cm long. There is variation with number of APL tendon slips and presence of subsheaths within 1st compartment potentially separating APL and EPB.
• *Differential diagnosis:* CMC OA, scaphoid fracture, *Intersection syndrome*, *Wartenberg's syndrome*.

Treatment:
• *Conservative:* rest, immobilize, NSAIDs. Steroid injections do not tend to be successful if APL and EPB in separate subsheaths within 1st compartment.
• *Operative:* release of the first dorsal compartment at wrist via longitudinal or transverse incision. Preserve branches of SBRN. The sheath can incised or excised or leave a radially-based flap attached to the radius, incise dorsal ligament over EPB. This may help prevent subluxation on wrist flexion.

Complications:
• SBRN neuroma, radial artery injury, tendon subluxation, scar tenderness, CRPS, failure to release all subcompartments.
  See TENOSYNOVITIS.

Dercum's disease
• Also known as adipose dolorosa. Autosomal dominant condition characterized by multiple lipomata, which are sometimes indirectly painful due to nerve compression or mass effect on deep fascia.
• Trunk and limbs most commonly affected.
• More common in women (20:1) and is usually associated with obesity.
• Management tailored for symptoms. Surgery may have a role to excise lesions but may also stimulate inflammation-induced recurrence.

Dermabrasion
• An abrasive process to remove epidermis and superficial dermis to smooth contours.
• Good for perioral rhytids.
• It has less bleaching and the contrast between treated and untreated skin is less than for *Chemical peels*.
• Not as effective as phenol for rhytids but more effective for acne scarring.
• Patients usually require 2–3 sessions.

Technique:
• Acyclovir is given if there is a history of herpes simplex. Topical treatment with tretinoin may hasten re-epithelialization.
• Dermabrasion is usually performed with a motor-driven instrument attached to either wire brushes, cylinders of sandpaper or steel burrs. When driven at relatively low speeds, a superficial- to medium-depth plane is produced. The correct level is determined by the multiple fine bleeding points.
• After abrasion the area is irrigated with saline and a moist gauze placed on top. The appearance during healing is similar to *Phenol peels*.

Dermagraft™
Human neonatal dermal fibroblasts seeded onto a synthetic mesh.
  See BIOLOGICAL SKIN SUBSTITUTES.

Dermal angiomyoma
See VASCULAR LEIOMYOMA.

Dermatochalasis
• Horizontal redundancy of skin of the eyelids caused by ageing.
• Herniation of intra-orbital fat.
• Common bilateral conditions.
• M=F.
  See BLEPHAROPLASTY.

Dermatofibroma
• Also called nodular subepidermal fibrosis, fibroma simplex, sclerosing haemangioma, noduli cutanei, fibroma durum and histiocytoma.
• Papule or nodule, usually in the extremities.

- Usually solitary, but 20% of patients have more than one.
- Slow growing, attached to the skin. Vary from 1 to 2 cm.
- Histologically composed of proliferating fibrocytes, collagen, vessels and monocytes.
- Either no treatment or excise.

See MESODERMAL TUMOURS.

Dermatofibrosarcoma protuberans (DFSP)
- Considered a malignant form of fibrohistiocytic tumour. Locally aggressive but metastasis is virtually unknown. Tendency to local recurrence.
- Usually arises in the dermis of the trunk and proximal extremities.
- More common in men. Peak incidence in the 30s.
- Presents as a firm plaque-like bluish-red nodule with a keloid-like appearance.
- May remain unchanged for years and then develop a rapid growth phase to form a multinodular mass.
- Histologically, there is a characteristic 'cartwheel' pattern of fibrous bundles in a non-encapsulated tumour that extend finger-like processes into adjacent subcutis and fascia. Mitotic figures may be numerous.

Management:
- Lack of consensus guidance on surgical margins.
- Peripheral margins of 2–3 cm usually recommended to reduce risk of local recurrence.
- Slow Mohs may be appropriate. CK staining is required in addition to H&E staining.
- Radiotherapy may be considered for inoperable disease.

See MESODERMAL TUMOURS. *See* SARCOMA.

Dermatosis papulosa nigra
- *Seborrhoeic keratosis* in dark-skinned individuals.
- Occur most frequently on the upper cheeks, and are small, pedunculated and heavily pigmented with minimal keratosis.

Dermoid cyst
Two types, congenital inclusion dermoid and acquired implantation dermoid.

Inclusion dermoid:
- Subcutaneous cysts present at birth.
- Situated along embryonic lines of fusion, where ectodermal tissue becomes sequestered.
- Contain well-defined epidermoid structures.

See also EPIDERMOID INCLUSION CYST.

Scalp:
- Assess carefully for relation to cranial sutures as they may extend intracranially, particularly if over a fontanelle or lambdoid suture.

Lateral brow:
- Commonest site.
- Asymptomatic, slow growing, usually superficial.
- May be fixed deeply, particularly in the area of the frontozygomatic suture.
- CT scan is not usually necessary unless it feels fixed.
- Excise through an upper lateral lid incision or lateral brow incision.

Frontonasal:
- Usually have a cranial origin.
- Situated from glabellar to nasal tip.
- Due to incomplete obliteration of a tract from the foramen caecum to nasal tip or foramen caecum through the frontonasal suture.
- Any failure of obliteration will leave both ectodermal and glial tissue.
- A CT scan is essential.
- A midline dermoid may have a pit possibly with hair and a wide nasal dorsum.
- The child may present with a brain abscess.
- Simple cysts can be approached through a dorsal nasal incision.
- If there is an intracranial extension, approach through a small frontal bone flap.

See EPITHELIAL CYSTS.

Dermolytic bullous dermatitis
The most severe subtype of dystrophic epidermolysis bullosa, which results in hand fibrosis and syndactyly.

Desmoid tumour
- Unencapsulated accumulation of fibrous tissue arising from the musculo-aponeurotic layers to the torso.
- Usually females in 30–50s, often after pregnancy.
- They are histologically benign, but locally invasive and recurrence after resection is high.
- International consensus guidelines published in 2020. No difference in long term outcomes between patients managed initially with surgery and those undergoing observation. Commence active treatment for progressive and/or symptomatic disease and/or disease close to critical structures.
- Adjuvant RT may reduce recurrence.

See ABDOMINAL WALL RECONSTRUCTION.

Dexon™
- Synthetic suture composed of polyglycolic acid.
- It is degraded by hydrolization.
- It loses its strength by 3 weeks and is absorbed by 3 months.

See ABSORBABLE POLYMERS.

Dextran
- A low molecular weight polysaccharide available as 40,000 and 70,000.
- It is a product of the fermentation of sucrose.
- It has anti-platelet and anti-fibrin functions. The exact mechanism is unknown.
- It may work by the formation of a negative charge on the platelet surface or inactivation of von Willebrand's factor.
- It also is a plasma expander.
- Need to give a test dose of Dextran-40.
- Give 15–25 ml/hour for 3 days.
- Generally used in microsurgery if there has been a complication.
- There is a lack of evidence supporting its routine use.
- There are some significant complications associated with its use including anaphylaxis and ARDS.

See MICROSURGERY.

Diabetes
Wound healing:
- *Wound healing* is significantly impaired in diabetes.
- Diabetic rats have diminished wound tensile strength which correlates with hydroxyproline content.
- Glycosylated collagen is less stable.
- Get impaired epithelialization and neo-vascularization.
- Leucocyte function is impaired, which will diminish inflammatory response and higher infection rates.
- Capillary basement membrane thickens in all organs causing hypoperfusion.

Diabetic Foot
20% of diabetic admissions are with foot problems, 50% of non-trauma amputations are in diabetics.

Pathophysiology:
- Multifactorial.
- *Neuropathy:* get segmental demyelination. Compression neuropathies are increased. Compression and double crush may account for some symptoms. Get motor, sensory and autonomic which leads to arch collapse and a dry insensate foot.

- *Vascular disease:* diabetics develop peripheral vascular disease which may start earlier and be more distal. Get pedal sparing.
- *Haemorheology:* blood flow is reduced and viscosity increased with increased platelet aggregation.
- *Immunology:* PMNs and T cells have reduced functions. Raised glucose encourages bacterial growth. Fissures provide an entry for infection.

Biomechanics:
- *Charcot foot:* joint collapse from trauma caused by insensitivity to pain. Collapse of the arches, gait disturbance, ulceration and infection.
- *Achilles tendon:* may be tight with reduced ankle movement which contributes to Charcot's joint. Lengthening may be required.

Assessment:
- Glucose control over last 3 months is assessed with HbA1C which is a measure of glycated haemoglobin and is reported as a percentage with <6% being in normal range.
- Radiology to assess bones and presence of osteomyelitis.
- MRI is the most useful investigation. Vascular studies.

Management:
- Optimization with glucose control, analgesia and treatment of infection.
- Vascular optimization with angioplasty of bypass if indicated.
- Staged reconstruction:
  - Tumour-like wound excision with deep wound biopsies and wound temporization. Excision may need to be of an entire angiosome;
  - Definitive reconstruction:
    - Autologous reconstruction—if vascularization adequate. If free flap required, anastomosis should be away from zone of injury. If 1st and 5th metatarsal heads and calcaneum is present—foot is stable for ambulation and can be salvaged;
    - Amputation if vascularization inadequate.

30–40% of amputees will require contralateral amputation.

DiGeorge sequence
- Associated conditions are *Velocardiofacial syndrome*, 22q11.2 deletion syndromes.
- Generally sporadic.
- 90% have a specific deletion of 22q11.2.

- Composed of:
  - Aortic coarctation;
  - Thymic aplasia;
  - Parathyroid abnormalities with low calcium.

Disability
According to the WHO:

- Dysfunction inside the person is impairment.
- Dysfunction of the person affecting activities is disability.
- Dysfunction outside the person affecting the role in life is handicap.
- Disablement is the negative impact of the injury-healing process. This is a dynamic process.

Discoid lupus erythematosus (DLE)
- A chronic dermatitis that results in extensive atrophic scarring.
- The lesions may occur on the scalp, face, arms and trunk.
- They are often induced by exposure to sunlight.
- Treatment is with topical steroids and anti-malarial drugs.
- Persistent scarring and deformity of the nose and face may occur.
- The lesions are usually discrete, and can be excised and reconstructed with skin grafts.
- Previously radiotherapy was used to treat DLE leading to a high incidence of SCC. Chronically active DLE lesions should be excised.
- Sun protection is important.

DISI/VISI
- Dorsal and volar intercalated segmental instability.
- Refer to the static posture of the lunate on a true lateral XR.
- *DISI:* lunate dorsal, seen in scapholunate ligament degeneration. This is the most common carpal instability pattern. Scapholunate angle >45 degrees.
- *VISI:* lunate volar, lunotriquetral rupture. Scapholunate angle <30 degrees.
  See CARPUS.

Dissecting cellulitis of the scalp
See PERIFOLLICULITIS CAPITIS ABSCEDENS ET SUFFODIENS.

Distal interphalangeal joint
Anatomy:
- Similar to *Proximal interphalangeal joint.*
- ROM from −20 to 80°.
- Angulation of each is slightly different.
- Ligamentous support is similar to PIPJ, but also the insertion of flexor and extensor increase stability. Dislocation is less common.

Dislocation:
- More common dorsally.
- Reduction may be prevented by FDP getting trapped behind a condyle or volar plate interposition.
- Treat with reduction and splint.
- If dislocated for more than 4 weeks surgery is required to reduce. Release volar aspects of collateral ligaments and a dorsal capsulotomy. Fix with K-wire.

Arthritis:
- OA affects the DIP joint most commonly.
- It is rarely functionally disabling.
- They may be associated with a *Mucous cyst.*
- Osteophytes are termed *Heberden's node.*
- Pain, deformity and instability may require *Arthrodesis.*

Distraction osteogenesis
- Formation of new bone from the gradual separation of osteotomised fronts.
- Popularised by *Ilizarov* in 1950s for long bones and McCarthy for the craniofacial skeleton in 1990s.
- A stable device, usually a distraction frame is required during three stages:

  - Latency 1–7 days allowing callus formation;
  - Activation of distraction usually at 1 mm per day to stimulate osteogenesis;
  - Consolidation—to allow maturation and remodelling.

Dog ear
- Also known as standing cutaneous deformity.
- Forms at the end of a closed wound when either the ellipse is made too short or one side of the ellipse is shorter than the other.
- They may flatten but primary correction is best.
- Either the ellipse can be lengthened or the dog ears excised as two triangles.

Dorsal carpal arch
- Formed from radial and ulnar dorsal carpal arteries on dorsum of wrist.
- Also a branch from the anterior interosseous artery.
- It gives off dorsal metacarpal branches to the 2nd–4th intermetacarpal spaces.
- The 1st dorsal metacarpal artery supplying the thumb and index finger usually arises from the radial artery before it passes between the two heads of the 1st dorsal interosseous muscle.

Dorsal infections: upper limb
- *Dorsal subcutaneous space:* overlies the dorsum of the hand and communicates with the palm through the web space.

- *Dorsal subaponeurotic space:* lies below extensor retinaculum.
- Drain by incisions over the 2nd metacarpal and between the 4th and 5th metacarpal.

See INFECTION.

Dorsalis pedis flap
- Not very frequently used because there is a high rate of donor site problems.
- The skin is thin and pliable, and supplied by the superficial peroneal nerve.
- It can be harvested with underlying metatarsal bone or MTP joint.
- Based on the dorsalis pedis artery (DPA), which is 2–3 mm in diameter, a continuation of the anterior tibial artery as it passes beneath the extensor retinaculum.
- The first dorsal metatarsal artery within the deep interosseous muscle supplies periosteal circulation to the second metatarsal and articular branches of the joint capsule.

Technique:
- Centre skin over DPA distal to extensor retinaculum and no further than the interdigital web space.
- Incise over extensor retinaculum, and isolate DPA, venae comitantes and deep peroneal nerve.
- Include extensor hallucis brevis with the flap as it lies between skin and the 1st dorsal metatarsal artery (DMTA). Include some interosseous muscle.

Double crush phenomenon
Compression at one point of a peripheral nerve lowers the threshold for compression neuropathy at another site. Pathophysiology uncertain but patients with compressive neuropathies should be evaluated for a dual proximal lesion.

Doughnut circumareolar mastopexy
See BENELLI MASTOPEXY.

Down's syndrome
Facial characteristics:
- Epicanthus.
- Oblique lid axis.
- Strabismus.
- Hypoplastic nose.
- Hypoplastic jaw.
- Macroglossia.
- Lip ectropion.
- Microgenia.
- Submental fat collection.
- Protruding ears.

Dressings
- The ideal dressing should:
  - Provide a sterile moist environment;
  - Remove necrotic material;
  - Promote healing;
  - Protect the wound;
  - Be cheap.
- *Low adherent dressings:* e.g. Melolin, Inadine, paraffin gauze-based dressing such as jelonet and Bactigras.
- *Semipermeable films:* permeable to gas and vapour, but impermeable to liquids and bacteria, e.g. omniderm, opsite, tegaderm.
- Hydrogels.
- Hydrocolloids.
- Alginates.
- *Synthetic foams:* usually used in concave wounds. They conform to the cavity, obliterating dead space. They are suitable for heavily exuding wounds. An example is lyofoam.
- VAC dressing.

See BURNS DRESSINGS.

DRUJ
- Distal radioulnar joint consists of the articular surface of the radius sigmoid notch and the ulnar head.
- It is separated from the radiocarpal joint by the triangular fibrocartilage complex (TFCC).
- Stability is due to TFCC, ECU sheath, interosseous membrane, pronator quadratus and the shape of the bones.
- *Rotation:* supination and pronation occur by rotation of radius around a fixed ulna.

Dislocation:
- Described by the position of the ulnar head relative to the distal radius.
- In a dorsal dislocation the ulna head is dorsal to the radius.
- Dorsal dislocation occurs by forced pronation.
- Reduce by supinating the wrist.
- The reverse is true for palmar dislocation. A long arm cast is applied.
- Chronic dislocation may require ligament reconstruction.

See GALEAZZI FRACTURE.

DRUJ instability
- Prevent with splinting, steroid and synovectomy.
- Treat with:
  - Darrach procedure;
  - Sauvé-Kapandji procedure;
  - Resection hemiarthoplasty.

Du Pan syndrome
Thumb hypoplasia with a constriction band at the base.

Duchenne's sign
- In *Ulnar nerve palsy*.
- Ring and little finger clawing due to loss of intrinsics and inability to flex at MCPJ, and unopposed flexion at PIPJ.

Duckett procedure
- Preputial skin island flap to treat *Hypospadias* with a one-stage procedure.
- Use when meatus is too proximal for more distal procedures or when there is significant chordee.
- Uses a vascularized flap of prepuce on a pedicle which is tubularized.
- Either split the glans or tunnel.
- Urethral plate can be preserved, and the flap sutured to it.
- Skin coverage is obtained using Byars flaps— dorsal preputial skin that is split in midline and redistributed.

Dufourmental flap
- Variation of rhomboid flap in which the angles differ from standard 60/120°.
- Usually use angles of 30/150°.
- Use for coverage of defect in shape of rhomboid rather than rhombus. A rhomboid has acute angles of varying degrees.
- Diagonals are not of equal length.
- Planning is more complex and it is often easier to convert the rhomboid into a rhombus.
- A line is drawn as a continuation of the short diagonal and another line is a continuation of one of the sides. This angle when bisected is the side of the flap.
- The length of the edge is the same as the length of the side.
- The other edge of the flap is made with an incision parallel to the long axis.
  See RHOMBOID FLAP.

Dupuytren's contracture
- First described by Sir Astley Cooper then by Dupuytren in 1831.
- Proliferative fibroplasia of palmar and digital fascia leading to nodules, cords, and flexion contracture of MCP and PIP joints.
- Normal fascia is called a band, when abnormal it is a cord.
- Commonest in the little and ring finger.

Incidence:
- Affects 1–3% of the population in North Europe and USA.
- M:F 10:1. Incidence increases with age.

- 10–44% have a family history. Autosomal dominant with variable penetrance.

Anatomy: *see* RETINACULAR SYSTEM.
- In the palm, the fascia involved are pretendinous band and natatory ligament.
- Transverse fibres of the palmar aponeurosis are usually uninvolved.
- In the finger the involved fascia is the spiral band of Gosset, *Grayson's ligaments* and retrovascular tissue.
- MCP joint contracture is caused by the pretendinous cord.
- PIP joint contracture is caused by the central, spiral and lateral cords.
- The spiral cord combines the distal prolongation of the pretendinous cord through the spiral band, which comes dorsal to the NVB at the MCP joint. It joins the lateral digital sheet and distally joins Grayson's ligament.
- DIP joint contracture is caused by the retrovascular cord, located dorsal to the neurovascular bundle, palmar to *Cleland's ligaments*. It arises from the periosteum of the proximal phalanx and attaches to the side of the distal phalanx.
- The NVB is displaced superficially and towards the midline by the spiral cord.

Association:
- Diabetes (more radial, probably due to microangiopathy).
- Alcoholism (often thickening of the palmar aponeurosis without significant contractures though can be severe).
- Liver disease.
- Epilepsy (probably due to barbiturates).
- Smoking.
- Chronic lung disease.
- HIV.
- *Occupation:* trombonists, jockeys, vibrating tools.

Diathesis: Aggressive. Starts early, strong family history. Often with bilateral disease, knuckle pads (Garrod's pads), plantar disease (Ledderhose's disease) and penile (*Peyronies disease*).

Pathology:
- *Intrinsic theory:* begin with activity in the perivascular fibroblast within normal fascia. The cords form along normal fascial bands (except the central cord).
- *Extrinsic theory:* Hueston suggests that the fibrous tissue starts superficial to palmar fascia and the cords overlay the aponeurosis.
- *Synthesis theory:* suggests that nodules arise de novo and cords from normal fascia.

- *Murrell's hypothesis:* age, genetics and environment create microvessel stenosis, localized ischaemia and free radical generation. This causes fibroblast proliferation.
- The fibroblast changes to become the myofibroblast. The actively contracting fascia is seen in the proliferative phase and the dense network in the involutional phase, In the residual phase myofibroblasts are replaced by more dormant fibrocytes. Type III collagen predominates in the early phases of the disease. The proportion of type I collagen increases as the disease progresses.
- Microtrauma may be a cause for Dupuytren's. In genetically predisposed individuals, tension causes rupture of the collagen with healing by hypertrophic scarring.

Classification—BSSH:

- *Mild:* no functional problems and MCPJ contracture less than 30°:
  - Observe and follow-up in 6–12 months—take measurements plus or minus clinical pictures perhaps.
- *Moderate:* functional problems and MCPJ 30–60° +/− PIPJ <30° +— first web contracture:
  - Consider needle fasciotomy for isolated MCPJ contracture;
  - Limited fasciectomy.
- *Severe:* functional problems and MCPJ >60° and PIPJ >30°:
  - Consider limited fasciectomy or dermofasciectomy.

Non-surgical treatment:

- *Observation:* suitable for disease that does not affect function or quality of life.
- Exercises and splinting are not supported by evidence.
- Radiotherapy is currently used primarily in a research setting.

Relative indications for surgery:

- *MCPJ contracture more than 30°:* correlates with positive Heuston table top test.
- *Any PIPJ contracture:* because shortening of the collateral ligaments in PIPJ is difficult to manage and may need a capsuloligamentous release.
- Adduction contracture of 1st webspace.

Surgery:

- Nodules can be painful and may require limited excision.
- Limited or regional fasciectomy:
  - *Incisions:* Brunner, Z-plasty, Y-V, McCash. Skoog—transverse palmar incision with extensions into the fingers;

- Subcutaneous fasciotomy can be used in patients unfit for more extensive surgery, can be performed percutaneously;
- *Fasciectomy:* regional excises all diseased fascia retaining transverse fibres, a limited regional fasciectomy excises diseased fascia in a digit and a radical fasciectomy involves removal of all palmar fascia;
- Dermofasciectomy for skin involvement.
- Joint release sequentially to minimize joint instability:
  - Check-rein ligaments;
  - Partial release of proximal volar plate;
  - Accessory collaterals;
  - Flexor tendon sheath.
- Joint replacement or arthrodesis.

Complications:

- *Intraoperative:* NVB division, ischaemia.
- *Early post-operative:* haematoma, flap necrosis, graft failure, infection.
- *Late post-operative:* decreased movement, extensor block, CRPS, recurrence, scar related.

Durkan's test

- Test for *Carpal tunnel syndrome*.
- With the forearm supinated the examiner presses his/her thumb into the median nerve.
- Numbness or tingling within 30 seconds is a positive result.

Dysaesthesia

Abnormal unpleasant sensation whether spontaneous or evoked.

Dysgeusia

Distortion or absence of sense of taste.

Dysplastic naevus

- Larger than ordinary naevi with more ill-defined borders.
- >5 mm diameter.
- Variegated, flat, but with palpable dermal component.
- Mainly trunk and extremities. Usually acquired in adolescence.
- May be familial or sporadic.
- Syndrome is described if >100 dysplastic naevi are present.
- Familial are at increased risk of developing melanoma.
- Sporadic has less risk.
- Patients should be examined regularly and excision recommended for changing naevi.

See MELANOMA. See NAEVUS.

Dystopia

See ORBITAL DYSTOPIA.

Eagle–Barrett syndrome
See PRUNE BELLY SYNDROME.

Ear—anatomy
- Normal adult ear 5.5–6.5 cm. Width 55% of height. 85% of ear development occurs in 1st 3 years. Position is one ear length posterior to lateral orbital rim, lateral protrusion of helix is 1.5–2.0 cm. Inclination of the ear is 20°.
- Blood supply from branches of external carotid artery:
  - *Superficial temporal artery:* lateral surface;
  - *Posterior auricular artery:* main blood supply to posterior surface and lobe;
  - *Occipital artery:* minor contribution;
  - Venous flow is to the posterior auricular, superficial temporal and retromandibular veins.
- Nerve supply:
  - *Great auricular nerve:* inferior half of ear;
  - *Auriculotemporal nerve:* lateral aspect of superior half;
  - *Lesser occipital nerve:* medial aspect of superior half;
  - *Arnold's nerve (auricular branch of vagus):* conchal bowl.

See CONSTRICTED EAR. *See* STAHL'S EAR. *See* CRYPTOTIA.

Ear reconstruction
Indications:
- *Cancer:* 9:1 ratio M:F. SCC equals BCC. SCCs have high recurrence rate and metastatic potential, higher than any other site.
- Trauma.
- *Microtia:* incidence—1:7,000. M:F = 2:1. A component of first and second branchial arch syndrome (*Hemifacial microsomia*). Possibly linked with viruses, drugs, and inheritance. Congenital ear anomalies classified by *Tanzer.*

Surgery:
- Reconstruction for microtia.

- Helical rim algorithm:
  - <1 cm—wedge excision with triangles;
  - <2 cm Antia-Buch helical advancement;
  - Up to 25% helical length—conchal cartilage graft with post-auricular flap (2 stage);
  - >25% helical length—rib cartilage with post-auricular flap (2 stage);
  - Total or near total—formal ear reconstruction (skin envelope over cartilage structure).
- Lower third—earlobe:
  - Use soft tissue flap from behind or below the ear;
  - *Split earlobe:* from traumatic avulsion of ear ring—either close the defect completely or use the lining of the cleft to create a tunnel for future ear ring use.

Total ear reconstruction:
- Trace normal ear and reverse. Tape template in position to find correct place.
- *First stage:* This involves making and inserting the cartilage framework. This is most reliably obtained from rib, though alloplastic and prosthetic frames have been used.
  - Rib is taken from contralateral rib. Remove through an oblique incision just above the costal margin;
  - Helical rim is fashioned separately. Ribs 6 and 7 provide enough cartilage for the main block;
  - Aim to fabricate a framework with an exaggerated rim and distinct details of the anti-helical complex. It is achieved with scalpel blades and a rounded wood-carving chisel;
  - Create the pocket with an anterior incision;
  - Cartilage remnant is excised. Used suction to prevent haematoma and oppose the skin to the cartilage. Infection can be treated with an antibiotic drip irrigation into the pocket.
- *Second stage:*
  - The posterior auricular groove is developed and the ear is kept in position with a

posterior cartilage block. Temporoparietal fascia is used to cover the posterior ear, covered with a SSG. If it had already been used in the first stage then deep parietal fascia can be used.

- *Subsequent stages:*
  - ○ *Rotation of the lobule:* performed more accurately as a separate procedure. This is accomplished by Z-plasty transposition of a narrow inferiorly based triangular flap;
  - ○ *Tragal construction and conchal definition:* this can be performed in a single operation. A crescent-shape conchal cartilage graft is harvested as a composite graft and placed as a shelf to recreate tragus;
  - ○ *Detaching the posterior auricular cartilage:* separate the ear from the head and apply a thick split skin graft;
  - ○ *Managing the hairline:* this may need to be removed from the ear at a later stage by electrolysis.

Ear replantation
- Practised in seventeenth century following punitive amputation. Prynne, a lawyer had his ears amputated (for publishing an offensive book). When brought before a tribunal a second time the judge was surprised to see two normal-looking ears.
- Anastomose posterior auricular artery and posterior auricular vein.
- Small segments can be placed as composite grafts. Larger pieces are unlikely to survive.
- Partial avulsion on a narrow pedicle may succeed due to the good blood supply.
- Cartilage can be banked, but tends to flatten.
- Posterior skin can be excised and lifted later, and cartilage can be fenestrated.

Eaton classification of volar plate avulsion
For PIP joint *Hyperextension injuries.* Proposed by Eaton and Malerich in 1980:

- *Type I:* volar plate avulsion, usually distally. Opposing joint surfaces remain congruent. Can usually be managed conservatively with extension blocking splint.
- *Type II:* dorsal dislocation of PIPJ with avulsion of volar plate and complete tear of collateral ligaments. May require joint stabilisation if inherently unstable.
- *Type III:* fracture dislocations where the volar plate is attached to the fragment. These tend to be stable if <40% of articular surface because dorsal collateral ligament is intact and unstable if >40%.

Eaton-Littler classification: 1st CMCJ OA
Grades the XR changes.

- *Stage 1:* widening of joint space.
- *Stage 2:* narrowing of joint space, osteophytes <2 mm.
- *Stage 3:* severe narrowing of joint space, osteophytes >2 mm.
- *Stage 4:* as for stage 3 but with scaphotrapezial joint arthritis.

  See CMC JOINT ARTHRITIS.

Eccrine acrospiroma
Clear cell hidradenoma or nodular hidradenoma.

- May occur anywhere on the body, usually as a single, solid or cystic nodular lesion.
- Flesh-coloured or reddish and most often 1–2 cm in diameter.
- A few are tender on pressure, and a few show drainage or ulceration.
- Treated by simple excision.
- Rarely malignant variants have been reported. Eccrine glands.

  See SWEAT GLANDS.

Eccrine hidrocystoma
- May resemble *Syringoma* in distribution, but the lesions are translucent.
- Situated on the face of older women.
- They are exacerbated by the heat and reduce in a cool environment.
- The lesions are obstructed sweat ducts.
- Treatment involves a cool environment and puncturing of the lesions.

Eccrine poroma
- Usually occurs on plantar or palmar skin.
- Firm red nodular tumour.
- Can be confused with pyogenic granuloma, amelanotic melanoma or Kaposi's sarcoma.
- Treatment is excision for histology.

Eccrine spiradenoma
- Can be tender.
- Severe pain may lead to confusion with glomus tumour.
- Usually solitary lesions on the upper body.

Eccrine tumours See:
- *Syringomas.*
- *Eccrine hidrocystoma.*
- *Eccrine acrospiroma.*
- *Eccrine poroma.*
- *Eccrine spiradenoma.*
- *Cylindroma.*

Ectopia cordis
- Very rare anomaly, may be seen prenatally, with varying degrees of abdominal

involvement. The heart is located in an abnormal position.

- Thoracoabdominal defect, if any pressure on a dressing will get a tamponade.
- Usually lethal.
- Cover heart with Biobrane™, custom-made expanders and a silicone cage.

Ectropion

Eversion of the lid margin producing scleral show. May lead to significant exposure keratinization.

Causes: Paralytic, involutional, cicatricial, mechanical.

Surgery:

- *Cicatricial:* release tethered structures and reconstruct with flap or graft.
- *Involutional:* caused by laxity of eyelid. The best method for reconstruction depends on the site of laxity and stability of canthal tendons. If medial laxity and the medial canthus stable then perform a medial wedge excision. If lateral laxity and the lateral canthus is stable, perform *Kuhnt–Szymanowski* procedure. If lateral laxity and lateral canthus unstable then perform a lateral canthal sling procedure.

See EYELID RECONSTRUCTION.

Ehlers–Danlos syndrome

- Group of connective tissue disorders with hypermobile joints, hyperextensible skin and fragile connective tissues.
- Genetically transmitted.
- They have defects in cross-linkage of collagen.
- This leads to decreased wound strength and delayed healing.
- May be associated with bleeding.
- Caused by inadequate production of the enzyme lysyl oxidase.
- These patients are at great risk of wound healing complications from surgery.

Elective lymph node dissection (ELND)

- Refers to lymphadenectomy of the primary lymphatic basin when clinically negative. Referred to as completion lymph node dissection (CLND) if done following a (positive) sentinel lymph node biopsy.
- The presumed advantage is clearing disease *if* it has spread to the lymph nodes.
- The disadvantage is the morbidity. 80% of intermediate thickness *Melanoma* (Breslow thickness 1–4 mm) will be node negative.
- WHO trial—no difference in survival.
- Large retrospective review by Sydney melanoma group—no difference.
- United States Cooperative reported by Balch (Intergroup Melanoma Trial) studied ELND for

intermediate thickness elective lymph node dissection for intermediate-thickness melanomas. For patients with tumour thickness of 1.1–2.0 mm who were 60 years old or younger, a 96% 5-year survival was demonstrated for those who had elective node dissection, compared with 84% for those who did not.

- MSLT-I and MSLT-II were large, international randomized-controlled trials of completion lymphadenectomy in melanoma. No survival benefit was found although CLND increased disease-free survival.
- With head and neck melanomas it was noted that involved LNs were always in adjacent nodes.

Head and neck cancer:

- Use ELND to stage disease or if there is a >20% incidence of occult LN metastasis. If occult it should be selective.
- High-risk primaries can be judged by:
  ○ *Site* tongue, floor of mouth;
  ○ *Thickness:* >4 mm have high incidence of metastasis;
  ○ Character of tumour histologically.
- Also non-compliant patients, or patients who cannot attend follow-up or have thick necks are considered for ELND.

Embolization and sclerotherapy

- Used in the treatment of *Vascular malformations*, usually just prior to surgical excision to reduce blood loss and the morbidity of surgery.
- Superselective catheterization of 1 mm vessels is possible. The flexibility of the catheters is improving. The success depends on the number of loops of the vessel as with each loop, friction increases. Materials used are either solid or liquid.
- *Solids:* particles of polyvinyl alcohol foam (PVA) are irregular and adhere to the vessel wall. 30% ethanol can be added which increases occlusion but also necrosis. Occlusion is not permanent so this is used pre-operatively. Coils made of platinum can be used for permanent occlusion. Their thrombogenicity is increased by attaching fibres to the coils.
- *Liquids:* silicone can be made radiopaque by adding tantalum, bismuth or tungsten powder. It solidifies after injection. Tissue necrosis is greater. Hydroxy-ethylmethacrylic glue solidifies after contact with blood so it can be used for occluding A–V fistulae. Pure ethanol is a good sclerotherapy agent when used in slow flow lesions. There is a risk of tissue necrosis. Use with venous angiomas. Do not inject intra-arterially.

Embryology

Branchial apparatus:

- Branchial arches are paired swellings, which lie along the developing neck. There are six paired swellings. The first and second are the most important in facial development. The grooves are branchial clefts, their inner surface is called pharyngeal pouch. The branchial cleft between the first and second arch becomes the external auditory meatus.
- The paired branchial arches decrease in size from cranial to caudal, with each pair merging midventrally to form 'collars' in the cervical region.
- Each branchial arch contains four essential tissue components:

  ○ *Cartilage;*
  ○ *Aortic arch artery:* these arteries course through the pharynx, joining the heart, which is ventrally located, to the aorta, which is dorsally located;
  ○ *Nerve:* these comprise both sensory and motor fibres from the respective cranial nerves;
  ○ *Muscle*.

- The embryological origin of muscles can be determined by their nerve supply and, although they may be intimately associated, two muscles may migrate from different origins, e.g. tensor veli palatini supplied by trigeminal nerve and levator veli palatini by vagus. Also muscle development and innervation are closely linked as seen in *Möbius' syndrome*.
- The branchial arches are separated by a series of clefts, which are termed 'branchial grooves'. All are obliterated except the dorsal end of the first branchial groove which deepens to form the external acoustic meatus.
- When the second, third or fourth branchial grooves are not completely obliterated, this can result in a branchial fistula, sinus or cyst.

First branchial arch: gives rise to:

- Maxillary and mandibular prominences.
- The maxilla, zygoma and squamous portion of temporal bone form by intramembranous ossification.
- The trigeminal nerve supplying the muscles of mastication, anterior belly of digastric, mylohyoid and tensor veli palatini.

Second branchial arch:

- Facial nerve comes from 2nd branchial arch.
- The muscles are the muscles of facial expression, posterior digastric, stapedius, stylohyoid.

Facial development:

- The frontonasal process is not a branchial arch derivative. Get paired placodes on the inferior border. Medial part forms medial nasal process, lateral part forms lateral nasal process and between the two is the nasal pit which becomes the nostril.
- Merging of the medial nasal prominences forms the philtrum and Cupid's bow region of the upper lip, the nasal tip, the premaxilla and primary palate, and the nasal septum. The lateral nasal prominences form the nasal alae.
- The frontonasal process merges with the paired maxillary and mandibular processes.
- Merging of the paired mandibular prominences produces the lower jaw.
- Failure of fusion of maxillary process and medial nasal process results in cleft lip.
- Failure of fusion of maxillary process and lateral nasal process results in a cleft along the alar margin—*Tessier 3* cleft.
- Failure of fusion of maxillary and mandibular process results in macrostomia, a Tessier 7 cleft.
- A median cleft lip is due to incomplete merging of the medial nasal prominences in the midline and is associated with midline furrowing of the nose, and a bifid nose—a number 0 Tessier cleft.
- Failure of the mandibular prominences to unite in the midline produces a central defect of the lower lip and chin, which is referred to as a number 30 cleft by the Tessier classification.

The palate:

- The palate represents both the frontonasal (median) and maxillary (lateral) prominences—the primary and secondary palates.
- All 3 elements are widely separated with the tongue in between.
- At week 8 the lateral palate elements move from a vertical to a horizontal position.
- The jaw protrudes forward to give space to the descending palate and tongue.
- The medial edge of the palatal shelf undergoes apoptosis to enable fusion.
- The nasal septum also fuses with the palate.
- The median palatine process subsequently gives rise to the premaxillary portion of the maxilla and forms the primary palate; the lateral palatine processes give rise to the secondary palate.
- The primary palate and anterior secondary palate ossifies to become the hard palate and the posterior part of the secondary palate becomes the soft palate.

- Cleft palate results from failure of the lateral palatine processes or the medial nasal prominences to meet and fuse with each other—resulting in a cleft of the primary or secondary palate.
- Delay in elevation of the palatal shelves from vertical to horizontal is part of the underlying mechanism of cleft palate formation.
- In Pierre Robin sequence with micrognathia, glossoptosis and cleft palate, the tongue fills the oropharynx because the mandible is small, so the shelves can't meet.
- *Epstein's pearls:* midline palatal microcysts occur along the median raphe of the hard palate and at the junction of the hard and soft palates during the process of apoptosis due to cystic degeneration of the epithelial remnants. The external ear.

The ear:

- The auricle arises from the first and second branchial arches.
- Three anterior hillocks of the first branchial arch form the tragus, helical crus and superior helix.
- Three posterior hillocks of the second branchial arch form the anti-helix, anti-tragus and lobule.
- The external acoustic meatus develops from the dorsal aspect of the cleft between the first and second branchial arches, or the first branchial groove.
- Although the auricle and external acoustic meatus begin in the cervical region, they migrate cranially to reach their normal location.
- Patients with microtia or partial arrest in auricular development may have a caudally placed ear with respect to the contralateral normal ear.
- Spread of lymphatics follow embryology. Cancers of former origin drain to parotid nodes, the latter drain to mastoid nodes. Cancers of concha and meatus drain to both.

Chest wall and breast:

- Skin from ventral portion of embryonic head fold.
- Ribs and muscles from ventral migration of dorsal mesoderm.
- The sternum is paired midline mesodermal bars which fuse in the 7th week.
- Mammary ridges disappear from the 4th week.
- The breast bud is a downgrowth of epidermis into the mesenchyme.

Reproductive organs:
Internal organs:
   Arise from:

- *Paramesonephric duct:* also known as Müllerian duct. In the female this develops into the fallopian tubes, uterus, cervix and upper part of vagina. In the male it degenerates to form the appendix testes.
- *Mesonephric duct:* also known as the Wolffian duct. It forms the majority of the internal sexual organs in the male. In the male the Sertoli cells within the gonad secrete a testosterone analogue, which acts as a Müllerian-inhibiting factor. The Leydig cells secrete testosterone, which stimulates development of the mesonephric duct and genital tubercle. In the male the mesonephric duct gives rise to the epididymis, the ductus deferens, the seminal vesicles and the ejaculatory ducts.
- Mullerian Female → internal organs, Wolffian Male → internal organs.

External organs:

- *Indifferent stage:* mesenchyme cells migrate around cloacal membrane to form cloacal folds. These unite cranially to form the genital tubercle. Caudally they become urethral folds and anal folds. On either side of these, genital swellings become visible and become scrotum or labia majora.
- *Male:* genital tubercle elongates to form the phallus. It pulls the urethral fold forward to form the urethral groove. This does not reach the distal part of the glans. The groove forms the urethral plate. They close over to become penile urethra. The most distal part is formed in the 4th month from ectodermal cells of the tip which becomes the external urethral meatus:
  - *Timing:*
    - 3/52—cloacal fold forms on cloacal membrane and the anterior part is the genital tubercle;
    - 6/52—cloacal membrane → urogenital and anal membrane; cloacal fold → urethral fold and anal fold;
    - 6–11/52—genital tubercle → phallus with urethral folds;
    - 12/52—urethral folds form over groove to form urethra;
    - >13/52—urethra canalized;
    - 7/12—testes descend.
  - *Hypospadias:* results from incomplete closure of the urethral folds during the 12th week of development;
  - *Epispadias:* urethral meatus is found on the dorsum of the penis. The genital tubercle seems to form in the region of the

urogenital septum, so a portion of the cloacal membrane is found cranial to the genital tubercle and when this membrane ruptures the outlet of the urogenital sinus comes to lie on the cranial aspect of the penis;

○ *Exstrophy of bladder:* with epispadias. The abdominal wall is normally formed in front of the bladder by primitive streak mesoderm, which migrates around the cloacal membrane. When this migration does not occur, rupture of the cloacal membrane extends cranially creating extrophy;

○ *Micropenis:* insufficient androgen stimulation;

○ Bifid or double penis occurs if the genital tubercle splits.

• *Female:* stimulated by oestrogen. Genital tubercle elongates slightly to form the clitoris. Urethral folds don't fuse but become the labia minora. Genital swellings become labia majora. Urogenital groove opens to form the vestibule.

Upper limb:

Embryogenesis is complete by the 8th week, but differential growth occurs until birth. Most congenital deformities occur between 3 and 8/40. Skeletal, then muscle, then nerve development.

Upper limb formation:

• *Proximal-distal sequence, apical ectodermal ridge (AER):* small buds of mesenchymal cells covered with ectoderm. Forms in response to signal from flank mesoderm. Initial bud formation is not cell proliferation, but decrease in cell proliferation. AER plays important role. *Progress zone* of undifferentiated mesenchyme at the end of the AER. Without the AER, mesoderm doesn't differentiate. AER controls limb-growth sequencing, but not the type of structure which is determined by mesenchyme. The time cells spend in the progress zone determines what they turn in to. So if they are in the PZ for short periods they will become more proximal structures.

• *Dorsal-ventral development (front to back):* controlled by ectodermal signals and interactions between ectoderm and the underlying mesenchyme. Dorsal structures are signalled by expression of WNT-7A, which is found in limb dorsal ectoderm. When it is inhibited, a double ventral pattern is produced.

• *The anterior-posterior axis (head to tail):* controlled by signals from the *zone of polarizing activity* (ZPA). A region of mesenchymal cells on the posterior margin of the limb bud. Substances are produce which in high concentrations produce posterior structures and in low concentrations produce anterior substances. Sonic hedgehog protein and BMPs may be responsible. Mirror hand results from duplication of the ZPA.

Hand and phalangeal formation:

• The AER becomes flattened distally.
• Portions of rim degenerate forming web spaces.
• Tissue beneath AER condenses to become digits.
• *Programmed cell death* (PCD) is important in development in modelling the digits. PCD clears the web spaces and prevents extra digits forming. Digits are seen by 8th week.

Genetic encoding and molecular response:

Several regulatory molecules are expressed by genes of the AER.

• *FGF:* important for initiation of limb growth. FGF appears to have a significant role in signalling between the AER and the mesenchyme. FGF-4 appears to maintain proliferation and polarizing activity. FGF-8 appears to be a key regulator of limb induction initiation and development.

• Signals from the AER control several regulatory proteins, e.g. MSX-1 and MSX-2. Changes in expressions of these genes occur rapidly supporting the idea of a continuous interplay between AER and mesenchyme during growth.

• Signals from AER are necessary for the proper expression of *HOX* genes. There are 38 *HOX* genes, which encode proteins responsible for the establishment of cell identity along the AP axis. The position of gene on the chromosome correlates with the axial level of the limb bud, where they are expressed. They determine timing and extent of local growth rates.

• *Retinoic acid:* found in high concentration in undifferentiated buds. It plays a role in limb development though its role is not well understood.

• *Sonic hedgehog (SHH):* a segment polarity gene. SHH is the endogenous polarizing signal. It is expressed in the posterior mesenchyme of limb buds. It patterns the AP limb axis. It may maintain the progress zone of the AER, while acting as a positional signal along the AP axis.

Encephalocoele
Frontonasal encephalocoele:
- Present at birth and can become huge. They change in size with crying.
- Much of the dural sac is CSF filled. It may contain herniated frontal lobe.
- The herniation is through the open foramen caecum and patent frontonasal suture.
- They may also herniate caudally through defects in the sphenoids and ethmoids with presentation in the mouth, associated with a wide cleft palate and midline cleft lip.
- Imaging is required prior to surgery.

Enchondromas
- Most common benign hand *Tumour*.
- 50% found in hand.
- They may arise from misplaced islands of cartilage, which are shed into the medullary substance.
- Usually in the 20s to 30s.
- Well-defined lucent lesion in diaphysis or metaphysis with sclerotic rim. Cartilaginous. Often expansile. May have internal calcification.
- Extraosseous chondromas may occur in joints, tendon sheaths or bursa.
- Most common site is the proximal phalanx.
- Usually found incidentally.
- Occasionally present with pain or fracture. Treat fracture by curettage with bone grafting.
- Lesions in the hand often require treatment, whereas in other sites they often change from an active stage 2 to a latent stage 1 lesion at skeletal maturity. Risk of malignant change is minimal.
- Syndromic enchondromas such as *Ollier's disease* and *Maffuci's syndrome* usually present earlier in life and have a more aggressive histology. There is a malignant transformation rate of 30–50% usually after 30 years of age.

Endoscopic plastic surgery
The rod-lens endoscope was introduced by Hopkins in 1953. Composed of rod glass lenses with intervening air spaces. It is still the main scope for most plastic surgical procedures. Computer chip video camera has enabled the image to be displayed on a monitor.

Benefits:
- Scar reduction and placement in hidden areas.
- Good illumination with magnification.

Applications:
- Correction recti diastasis if skin excess is not great and patients wish to avoid large scar. Combine it with liposuction.
- Endoscopic neck lift and brow lift can avoid a long scar.
- Endoscopic breast augmentation through an axillary or an umbilical port.
- Carpal tunnel release to avoid a palmar scar.
  See BREAST AUGMENTATION.

Endotoxin
Components of the wall of Gram-negative bacteria, released upon lysis and can stimulate cytokine secretion.

Enneking's system
- For staging tumours of muscoloskeletal system.
- Allows selection of treatment, assessment of prognosis and evaluation of results.
- Based on histology, anatomy and metastasis.

Benign:
- *Stage 1 inactive:* may heal spontaneously, indolent course. Well encapsulated, often incidental finding. Can be observed.
- *Stage 2 active:* progressive growth. Well encapsulated, but may deform the boundaries. Require resection to prevent bone destruction. More aggressive treatment, sometimes with a margin of normal tissue.
- *Stage 3 aggressive:* locally invasive. Extend beyond natural boundaries. Some such as chondroblastoma may metastasize.

Malignant: I–III. Each split into A and B if intra- or extracompartmental. Staging is determined by grade (G), tumour site (T) and metastasis (M).

- *IA:* low-grade intracompartmental sarcoma.
- *IB:* low-grade extracompartmental.
- *IIA:* high-grade intracompartmental.
- *IIB:* high-grade extracompartmental.
- *III:* regional or distant metastasis.
  See SARCOMA. *See* BONE TUMOURS.

Enophthalmos
- Posterior displacement of the eye.
- It could also be due to loss of volume, but in the post-traumatic patient is principally due to an enlarged orbit.

Assessment: Check visual fields, extra-ocular range of motion, forced duction testing and exophthalmometry. Image with CT and XR.

Surgery:
- Complete exposure of the zygomatic complex and orbital walls is important.

- If severe scarring of the peri-orbital tissue is present, it can be incised to allow anterior movement of the globe.
- For mild deformities, the volume of the orbital contents can be increased with autogenous rib cartilage.
- Soft tissue repositioning is important.
- The lateral canthal ligament needs to be repositioned in a slightly overcorrected position.

See ORBITAL FRACTURES.

Entropion
Inward rotation of the lower eyelid towards the globe. Trauma to the globe from the lid margin and eyelashes results in pain and corneal scarring.

Causes:
Congenital, involutional, cicatricial (CIC).

Surgery:
- Cicatrical entropion is caused by vertical deficiency in the posterior lamella. It is treated by releasing cicatricial bands and grafting the resultant defect.
- Can also use everting sutures, transverse fracture of the tarsal plate and everting wedge excisions.

Ephelis
- Also known as a freckle.
- Defined as a pigmented lesion without an increase in the number of melanocytes, which disappears in the absence of sunlight.

Epiblepharon
Anomaly common in children of Asian descent where the eyelashes are in contact with the cornea.

Epicanthal folds
- Prominent vertical skin folds over the medial canthus.
- They occur in Down's syndrome, *Blepharophimosis*, people of Asian descent.
- They may be released with a jumping man flap.

See EYELID RECONSTRUCTION.

Epidermal naevus
- Benign hamartoma, with hyperkeratosis, acanthosis and hypertrophy.
- 60% occur at birth. M = F.
- Lesions are hyperpigmented, linear or papillomatous.
- Naevus verrucous is a solitary lesion present at birth.
- Naevus unius lateralis are extensive forms of epidermal naevus, which can cover more than half the body.

- Ichthyosis hystrix are widespread epidermal lesions in irregular patterns.
- Inflammatory naevi can be misdiagnosed as psoriasis.
- Epidermal naevi with other anomalies is called *Epidermal naevus syndrome*.

See NAEVUS.

Epidermal naevus syndrome
- *Epidermal naevi* with other anomalies.
- Get skeletal anomalies, CNS abnormalities and ocular abnormalities.
- May uncommonly get malignant degeneration.
- Vitamin A analogues can be used to treat.

Epidermodysplasia verruciformis
- Wart-like lesions on the face, neck, hands, feet and trunk.
- Autosomal recessive cell-mediated immunity disorder.
- Several subtypes of human papillomavirus induce verrucous lesions with transformation to *SCCs*.

Epidermoid inclusion cyst
- Present as slowly growing palmar lesions due to implanted epidermal skin elements.
- The cyst is filled with white material.

Epidermolysis bullosa
- Epidermolysis bullosa (EB) is a group of inherited bullous disorders.
- Formation of blistering after minor trauma (Nikolksy sign), healing with scarring.
- Excessive epidermal collagenase activity, which breaks down papillary dermal collagen fibres, where blister formation begins.
- The digits become cocooned in atrophic scar.
- There are varying degrees of clinical expression.
- There is no effective treatment.
- Topical steroid therapy may reduce blistering and scar formation.
- The most severe subtype is dermolytic bullous dermatitis (DBD), which results in hand fibrosis and syndactyly.
- Correction of hand deformities is usually short-lived.

Epignathus
- An oropharyngeal teratoma composed of cells from ectodermal, mesodermal and endodermal layers.
- Epignathi arise from the palate or pharynx and protrude through the mouth.
- They often cause airway obstruction.
- Failure of fusion may lead to a midline nasopharyngeal teratoma.

Epispadias

- 1 in 30,000. M:F 4:1.
- Abnormal development of cloacal membrane with failure of rupture and abnormal growth.
- Leads to failure or blockage of normal development of the dorsal surface of penis, abdomen and anterior bladder wall. These defects are considered as part of the same disorder.
- *Exstrophy* with epispadias most common.
- Penis is short, wide and stubby, with flat cleft glans and a dorsal chordee. There is divarication of the recti, wide symphysis. Females have a short vagina, wide separation of the labia and a bifid clitoris.
- Epispadias distal to bladder neck are continent.

Reconstruction:

- The reconstruction of the epispadias is similar to hypospadias (also need chordee release).
- If the epispadias encroaches on the bladder neck then a Young–Dees–Leadbetter bladder neck reconstruction is performed. Bladder is released from symphysis and wedges of bladder neck excised to elongate urethra. Urethra is closed and sphincter muscle wrapped around. Ureters may need reimplanting and the bladder may need augmenting.

Secondary surgery: often required because of persisting chordee and inadequate penile length. W flap technique—exposes base of penis. Persistent bowing is usually due to inadequate urethral length. Divide distally. May need dermal graft to tunica albuginea. Urethral reconstruction with full thickness skin graft or flap.

Epithelial cysts

- Most epidermal (sebaceous) cysts arise from occluded pilosebaceous follicles. Get a small keratin-filled punctum. Asymptomatic.
- Histologically the cysts are lined with true epidermis that forms a granular layer and keratin. The keratin forms laminated layers within the cysts.
- Malignant degeneration can occur.
- *Pilar cysts:* also called *Tricholemmal cysts,* occur in the scalp derived from the outer root of a hair follicle. Clinically indistinguishable from an epidermal cyst.
- *Milia:* or whiteheads. Tiny epidermal cysts occurring on the face. They may follow skin trauma or burns. Treatment is to incise the top and express the contents.
- *Steatocystoma multiplex:* autosomal dominant, multiple intradermal nodules in upper trunk. They contain oily fluid and lanugo hairs.
- *Dermoid cysts.*
- *Gardner's syndrome:* multiple cysts.

Epstein's pearls

Midline palatal microcysts, which are commonly located along the median raphe of the hard palate, and at the junction of the hard and soft palates. *See* PALATE EMBRYOLOGY.

Erb-Duchenne palsy

See BRACHIAL PLEXUS INJURY—OBSTETRIC. Palsy of C5–6.

Erb's point

Point at which the spinal accessory nerve exits from behind sternocleidomastoid at its midpoint. *See* NECK DISSECTION.

Erythema nodosum

- Painful, palpable, blue-red lesions on the calves and shins.
- Due to lymphocytic vasculitis.
- Usually women.
- Usually a tissue reaction to streptococcal infection, drug ingestion, sarcoidosis and other infections.

Erythroplasia of Queyrat

- *Bowen's disease* of mucous membranes.
- Most often affects the glans penis.
- Seen in the 50s to 60s, mainly in uncircumcised men.
- Get solitary or multiple erythematous lesions.
- It is more likely than Bowen's disease to become invasive with tendency to metastasize.

Essex–Lopresti injury Longitudinal radioulnar instability with:

- Displaced fracture of the radial head.
- Disruption of the interosseous membrane and distal radioulnar ligament.
- Proximal migration of the radius.
  See ULNOCARPAL IMPACTION SYNDROME.

Estlander flap

- Useful for *Lip reconstruction* with medium-sized lateral defects of the upper and lower lip, which include the commissure.
- It can be performed in one stage.
- Based on the superior labial artery for reconstructing lower lip defects involving commissure.
- Include 1/2 dimension of the defect.
- It is a laterally-based switch flap.
- Get indistinct commissure, but acceptable oral competence.

Ethics
The philosophical inquiry into the nature and ground of morality.
- *Normative ethics:* the ethics involved in hand's-on reasoning.
- *Applied normative ethics:* the ethics of medicine also called medical ethics.
- General theories of normative ethics are:
  - *Teleological:* assess right and wrong by consequence (utilitarianism);
  - *Deontological:* suggests that an act is inherently right or wrong regardless of consequences.
- *Teleology:* utilitarianism states that moral rightness can be measured by the amount of good. Good is measured by terms such as wealth, health and pleasure. These are non-moral. So utility assesses morality by balancing the positive and negative non-moral good that the action achieves— 'the greatest good for the greatest number'. Utilitarians differ on which good should be sought. Action's morality is judged by outcome. The problem is that different outcomes may conflict in medicine, e.g. long life and wholeness. Also whose good is being considered? One may need to consider consequences for individual, family, community or mankind. The main criticism of utilitarianism is that there are no unchangeable rights and wrongs.
- *Deontology:* actions are morally right or wrong. So a disabled child has moral worth. The grounds for deontological theories is reason. Kant said that the capacity and freedom to act rationally are human in nature and we should respect other persons. Kant looked at actions and tried to determine whether they can apply universally. If so then they were moral. Different moral criteria have been defined. Again these can come into conflict. For example, beneficence and patient autonomy. The other problem is one of absolutes. If something is morally good is it an absolute rule, e.g. preserving life?

Moral problem-solving: Often the two methods and variations of them are merged when making decisions.

Cardinal principles of medical ethics (Neauchamp and Chidress):
- *Justice:* fair, equitable treatment.
- *Non-maleficence:* obligation not to intentionally harm or impose risks of harm through negligence.

- *Autonomy:* individual freedom and capacity for intentional action.
- *Beneficence:* acts performed for the welfare of others.

Code of ethics in medicine:
- *Self-regulation:* code of medical ethics form part of the structure of self-regulation. Principles that determine the doctor's duties to others are external norms. Working for the patients good is part of the code, but the problem comes in defining it. If a doctor imposes treatment this is paternalism, if the patient decides this is autonomy. Autonomy has become more important. Codes related to others in the profession are internal norms.
- *Conflicts with norms:* problems arise when an external norm conflicts with an internal norm or when two external norms conflict. Advertising is an example. This conflicts with internal norms by drawing patients away from other physicians, but gives patients more choice. It does, however, also conflict with medicine's altruism, putting commerce above all. The fee structure frequently causes conflict of interest.
- As the profession becomes more divided in itself, it is less able to self-regulate and external regulation is required. In plastic aesthetic surgery, the economic model becomes more prominent than the medical model. Patients are consumers, surgeons are businessmen.

Plastic surgery and medical ethics—applied ethics:
Many of the areas of difficult ethical dilemmas don't affect the plastic surgeon such as life and death decisions. *Tagliacozzi* recognized the psychological elements and this aspect distinguishes the plastic surgeon from other doctors. Ward breaks down ethics of plastic surgery into:
- *Bedside ethics:* day-to-day matters of patient care.
- *Armchair ethics:* involves the aspects of running a business, providing a service, sharing resources. This area relies less on clinical proficiency. The physician acts as the patient's advocate.
- *Ethics of the technological imperative:* this states that what can be done technologically should be done.

See BOLAM CASE. *See* BOLITHO CASE. *See* MONTGOMERY V. LANARKSHIRE HEALTH BOARD.

Ewing's sarcoma
- Primitive malignant *Bone tumour* with small cells with round nuclei and without distinct cytoplasmic border.

- Probably of neuroectodermal origin.
- Occur in 20s to 30s.
- Found in the upper limb in 20% of patients, the humerus is the most common site.
- Present with pain, raised ESR, anaemia, raised white count and low-grade fever. Mimic osteomyelitis.
- The tumour infiltrates the Haversian canals without diffuse cortical destruction.
- *XR:* mottled radiolucent lesion, poor boundaries, onion peel periosteal reaction.
- Most are stage IIB. Patients have chromosome 11-22 translocation.

Treatment:
Excision with wide margin with ray amputation with neoadjuvant chemotherapy and/or radiotherapy.

Exophthalmos

- Excess orbital contents in a normal bony orbit.
- The most common cause is Graves' disease.
- Also orbital tumours, invasive sinus mucocoeles, and post-traumatic haematomas.

Examination:
- Get extraocular muscle dysfunction, eyelid retraction, and peri-orbital and conjunctival oedema.
- The Hertel exophthalmometer is useful in measuring the distance from the lateral orbital rim to the corneal apex. The normal range is 16–18 mm.
- Computed tomographic scan imaging pre-operatively demonstrates skeletal and peri-orbital tissue abnormalities.

Treatment:
- It is difficult to alter the globe position by removing peri-orbital fat.
- Therefore, with moderate to severe exophthalmos, a three-wall orbital expansion is the best treatment for surgical correction.

Exorbitism

- Normal orbital soft tissue in the presence of decreased bony orbital volume.
- There is a risk of corneal exposure and the development of keratitis, pain, infection, ulceration and blindness.
- If severe, urgent surgery is required.

Causes:
- Craniofacial dysostosis, such as Crouzon's, fibrous dysplasia, osteoma, meningioma, frontal sinus mucocoele and traumatic bony fragments.

Surgery:
- With congenital hypoplastic orbits and normal globes, e.g. Crouzon's, treat by fronto-

orbital advancement followed by Le Fort III osteotomy or monobloc frontofacial advancement.
- For acquired exorbitism, make an osteotomy in the zygoma to rotate it outwards and increase space by a 'blow out' medially and inferiorly.

Exotoxin

- Proteins secreted by bacteria.
- TSST-1 is an exotoxin released by *Staphylococcus aureus* in <u>toxic shock syndrome</u>.
- Cause blistering and erythema when released by *Staphylococcus aureus* in scalded skin syndrome.
- Botulinum toxin is an exotoxin produced by *Clostridium botulin*.

Exstrophy/epispadias

See HYPOSPADIAS. *See* EPISPADIAS. *See* EMBRYOLOGY.

Get divergent rectus with exposed bladder plate, low umbilicus, widened symphysis pubis, anterior anus, short penis with dorsal meatus (epispadias), short urethra, short vagina, bifid clitoris. Exstrophy results from failure of cloacal membrane to rupture which prevents development of the lower abdominal wall.

Surgical goals: abdominal wall closure, bladder closure with good capacity, continence, preservation of renal function, cosmesis and functional considerations. More serious abnormality than epispadias. If untreated get infections, renal impairment and bladder cancer. Most are reconstructable, 5% require urinary diversion.

Functional closure: bilateral iliac osteotomies, free bladder and close. Close abdominal wall. Leave with suprapubic catheter. Females have better chance of continence.

Extensor carpi radialis brevis

Origin: lateral epicondyle. Passes between ECRL and EDC. Through 2nd extensor compartment.

Insertion: base of 3rd metacarpal.

Nerve supply: radial nerve.

Action: wrist extensor. Doesn't produce any radial or ulnar deviation.

See MUSCLES.

Extensor carpi radialis longus

Origin: distal 1/3 of lateral supracondylar ridge of humerus and lateral epicondyle. It passes radial to ECRB and through the 2nd extensor compartment radial to Lister's tubercle.

Insertion: base of 2nd metacarpal. It may give a slip with ECRB.

Nerve supply: radial nerve.

Action: wrist extensor, radial deviator. Acts as a reciprocal antagonist with FCU.
  See MUSCLES.

Extensor carpi ulnaris

Origin: common extensor origin and dorsal aspect of ulna. A long muscle with short fibres. It enters the hand through the 6th extensor compartment. It passes through a groove dorsal to the ulnar styloid.

Insertion: ulnar aspect of the base of the 5th metacarpal.

Nerve supply: posterior interosseous nerve.

Action: wrist extensor, ulnar deviator. Stabilizes the head of the ulna.
  See MUSCLES.

Extensor compartments of wrist

Radial to ulnar:
1. APL, EPB on radial styloid.
2. ECRL, ECRB through floor of anatomical snuffbox.
3. EPL separated from compartment 2 by Lister's tubercle.
4. EDC, EIP.
5. EDM.
6. ECU, over head of ulna.

Extensor digiti minimi

Origin: the common extensor origin and intermuscular septum.

Insertion: little finger. It passes through the 5th extensor compartment. It is larger than EDC tendon and often has two or more slips. It passes ulnar to EDC and unites with it just proximal to MCPJ.

Nerve supply: posterior interosseous nerve.
  See MUSCLES.

Extensor digitorum communis Most radial of the superficial group of tendons.

Origin: the lateral epicondyle.

Insertion: it divides into 4 slips in the distal third of the forearm. They enter the 4th dorsal wrist compartment. The tendons are interconnected on the hand by the *Juncturae tendinum*. The tendons insert into the dorsal hood of index to little finger. The tendon to little finger is variable and may only be a fine slip.

Nerve supply: posterior interosseous nerve.

Action: extends the MCPJ and, in conjunction with intrinsics, the PIPJ.
  See MUSCLES.

Extensor indicis proprius

Origin: dorsum of distal 1/3 ulna and interosseus membrane.

Insertion: passes with EDC in 4th extensor compartment. Passes on the ulnar side of the index finger with EDC into extensor hood. It may be absent and may give a slip to middle or ring finger.

Nerve supply: posterior interosseous nerve.

Action: independent index extension. Weak muscle.
  See MUSCLES.

Extensor pollicis brevis

Origin: dorsum of radius distally to APL and interosseous membrane. It runs obliquely distal then dorsal to APL. They pass superficial to ECRL/B and brachioradialis. It passes through the 1st extensor compartment.

Insertion: base of proximal phalanx of thumb and extensor hood, and base of 1st metacarpal in 20%. It is often in its own compartment which should be released in *De Quervain's disease*.

Nerve supply: posterior interosseous nerve.
  See MUSCLES.

Extensor pollicis longus

Origin: dorsum of middle third of ulna and interosseous membrane. Passes through the 3rd extensor compartment. It curves around Lister's tubercle, crossing ECRL/B. It receives an insertion from APB and AP.

Insertion: base of distal phalanx of thumb.

Nerve supply: posterior interosseous nerve.

Action: extends IP and MCPJ. Adducts and extends 1st CMC joint. It supinates the thumb MC. Radial deviates the wrist. It pulls the whole thumb towards the plane of the hand (retroposition). Test by placing palm on table and lifting up thumb (retropulsion) as this isolates EPL.
  See MUSCLES.

Extensor pollicis longus tenosynovitis

• Pain on moving the thumb, swelling, tenderness, crepitus just distal to Lister's tubercle.
• Symptoms should be treated urgently to prevent tendon rupture.
• Rupture is called Drummer's palsy.
  See TENOSYNOVITIS.

Extensor retinaculum

• Thickened distal portion of antebrachial fascia, 2–3 cm long and 4–6 cm wide.
• Radially it covers FCR and base of thenar muscles.
• Ulnarly it attaches to the pisiform and triquetrum.

- It has two layers. The deep layer forms the floor of the tendinous tunnel. It acts as a powerful pulley.
- It also stabilizes ECU tendon and _DRUJ_.

See EXTENSOR COMPARTMENTS OF WRIST.

Extensor tendon zones
- Tendon divides at proximal half of proximal phalanx into 3 slips, one central and two lateral. Wing tendons form from interossei on the ulnar side and interossei and lumbricals on the radial side.

Zones:
- _Fingers:_ I–IX. I, III, V over joints. VI over metacarpals, VII beneath retinaculum, VIII in distal forearm and IX over muscles.
- _Thumb:_ 5 zones with V being over wrist.
- _Extensors:_ most commonly injured over metacarpal—zone IV in thumb and VI in finger.
- _Zone VII injuries:_ more like the flexor injuries as each tendon runs in its own sheath and repair has to be carefully performed to prevent triggering.

See SAGITTAL BAND. See TRIANGULAR LIGAMENT.

Extravasation injuries
See CHEMICAL INJURIES. Most occur during intravenous injections, mostly in upper limb. Get inflammation followed by sloughing and ulceration. Get demarcation within a week.

Agents:
- _Osmotically active agents:_ hypertonic solutions, such as calcium and potassium cause osmotic imbalance and cell death.
- _Ischaemia inducing agents:_ such as catecholamines, dopamines cause cell death by ischaemia.
- _Cellular toxicity agents:_ such as chemotherapy (commonly doxirubicin, vincristine, mithramycin), digoxin, sodium bicarbonate.

Presentation: an inflammatory reaction, which may progress to necrosis, eschar and infection. The _Recall phenomenon_ is the extension of necrosis following recommencing administration of the toxic substance (mostly seen with doxorubicin).

Treatment: Varying advice.
- _Remove agent,_ remove line (though may keep it in to aspirate and administer antidote).
- Apply _cold_ to cause vasoconstriction (varying effect on chemicals, reducing toxicity of doxorubicin, but increasing vinca alkaloids).
- _Warm:_ may help to dissipate chemical and reduce toxicity.
- _Antidotes:_ phentolamine opposes vasopressors.
- _Saline flush:_ after injecting hyaluronidase, make several stab incisions and using a blunt cannula flush copious volumes of saline to dilute the chemical.
- _Excision:_ a well-circumscribed injury may require excision, and graft or flap.

Outcome: most isotonic extravasations don't require special management. Most osmotically active and vasoconstrictive agents need non-operative treatment, and a few only need surgery.

Eyelid anatomy
- Each eyelid is bilamellar, divided by the orbital septum.
- Anterior lamella of upper and lower lid: skin and orbicularis oculi.
- Posterior lamella of upper and lower lid: tarsus, levator aponeurosis and Müller's muscle (upper), capsulopalpebral fascia (lower), conjunctiva.
- The orbital septum is a fascial membrane.

Orbicularis oculi.

Tarsus: forms structural framework. Upper is 10 mm, lower is 4 mm. Dense fibrous tissue with meibomian glands.

Levator palpebrae superioris: the principal retractor of upper eyelid. Striated muscle supplied by the 3rd cranial nerve. Originates from the superior/posterior orbit, broadens into levator aponeurosis, which inserts into tarsal plate posteriorly and orbicularis oculi muscle and skin anteriorly. It is tented over Whitnall's ligament. The length is 55 mm of which 15 mm is tendon. In some people of Asian descent the levator only attaches to tarsal plate so the lid doesn't have a fold.

Whitnall's ligament: the superior sheath of levator condenses to form the superior transverse ligament of Whitnall, a check ligament. This attaches medially to the pulley of superior oblique muscle and laterally to the lacrimal gland. It functions as a pulley to facilitate the change in direction of the levator action from horizontal to vertical.

Müller's muscle: smooth muscle with sympathetic innervation. Situated in the posterior lamellar of the upper lid and attaches to levator and tarsus. Origin—posterior border of levator. Insertion—superior border of tarsus. It is 10-12 mm long and 15 mm wide. It is adherent to conjunctiva.

Lateral canthus: composed of a number of structures. Lockwood's ligament (inferior suspensory ligament), lateral extension of levator aponeurosis, continuations of pretarsal and preseptal muscles and check ligament of lateral rectus. This attaches to the lateral orbital wall at Whitnall's tubercle.

Medial canthus: the tendon is a complex structure which attaches onto the medial part of the orbit in a tripartite manner. Closely associated with the lacrimal pump mechanism. The lacrimal sac lies between the anterior and posterior insertions of the medial canthal tendon.

Supratarsal fold: corresponds to dermal attachments of the levator aponeurosis. Approximately 10 mm above the eyelid margin. In ptosis, a high-positioned supratarsal fold may suggest a levator defect.

Fascial framework: supports the globe and allows coordinated movement of the orbit. Consists of Tenon's capsule, fascial layers of the extraocular muscles, check ligaments.

Palpebral fissure: vertical height of 10–12 mm and width of 28–30 mm. Upper eyelid rests 2 mm below the upper corneoscleral limbus. The lower lip rests at the lower corneoscleral limbus.

Orbital septum: a thin sheet of fibrous tissue that lies deep to the preseptal portion of orbicularis. It is a protective barrier and restricts protrusion of orbital fat. It spreads from periosteum to tarsal borders. In the upper eyelid it fuses with levator aponeurosis 2–3 mm above the upper border of tarsus. They then insert into the lower anterior surface of tarsus. In the lower eyelid the orbital septum attaches directly to inferior border of tarsus.

Peri-orbital fat: between orbicularis and periosteum over the lateral half of the orbital rim. Also preaponeurotic (post-septal) fat between levator and orbital septum of the upper eyelid. Two pockets are found in the upper eyelid—medial and central and 3 on the lower eyelid—medial, central and lateral. Preseptal fat lies between septum and orbicularis oculi—retro-orbicularis oculi fat (ROOF) in upper eyelid and suborbicularis oculi fat (SOOF) in lower eyelid.

Lower lid: similar structure to upper lid. The retractor of the lower lid is known as the capsulopalpebral ligament and is continuous posteriorly with Lockwood's ligament.

Blood supply: ophthalmic branch of internal carotid and facial branch of external carotid.

Nerve supply: sensation to upper eyelid is through trigeminal nerve. The ophthalmic branch divides into lacrimal, frontal and nasociliary. The frontal nerve gives supra-orbital and supratrochlear. Lower eyelid is supplied by infra-orbital.

Eyelid reconstruction

Assessment:
- Separate the component portions of the defect into deficiencies of:

  o The anterior and posterior lamella;
  o Upper and lower lid;
  o The support structures of the medial and lateral canthus.

- Posterior lamella defects may require reconstruction of the tarso-ligamentous sling with shared tarsoconjunctival flaps, mucoperichondrium or cartilage grafts.
- Anterior lamellar defects may require local flaps or grafts.

Pathology: trauma, *Eyelid tumours*, *Coloboma*.

Skin graft:
- The best site for lower lid is upper lid. Take equal amounts from both sides.
- *Post-auricular skin:* the sulcus should bisect the planned defect. Needs to be thinned. The graft can be extended laterally and medially to act as a sling.

Lower eyelid algorithm based on width of defect:
- <1/3 eyelid consider direct closure with pentagon excision.
- >1/3 eyelid consider Tenzel flap and canthotomy (posterior lamella advancement achieved from mucosal laxity).
- >2/3 eyelid need flap for one lamella and graft for the other. Consider:
  o Anterior lamella flap, i.e. cheek rotation, Fricke flap or orbicularis flap and posterior lamella graft, i.e. hard palate mucosa;
  o Posterior lamella flap, i.e. Hughes tarsoconjunctival flap and anterior lamella graft (FTSG).

Upper eyelid algorithm based on width of defect:
- <1/3 eyelid consider direct closure with pentagon excision.
- >1/3 eyelid consider Tenzel flap and lateral canthotomy.
- >2/3 eyelid consider lower lid switch or cutler beard flap.

Posterior lamellar reconstruction:
- *Sliding tarsoconjunctival flap:* isolated defects of the medial or lateral upper eyelid can be reconstructed with a sliding tarsoconjunctival flap taken from the under-surface of the remaining upper lid. A trans-position flap is created based on adjacent conjunctiva for blood supply and lining. Base flap 4 mm superior to the inferior edge of remaining tarsal plate. Extend incision laterally and angled superiorly to the border of the tarsal plate. Transpose laterally. The anterior lamella can be reconstructed with a flap or graft.
- *Free tarsoconjunctival graft:* shallow defects of lower lid can be reconstructed with a free tarsoconjunctival graft from the upper lid. The upper lid is everted and a graft is taken preserving 4 mm of inferior lid margin. Separate tarsal plate from the overlying

Müllers muscle. The graft is sutured in place and a skin muscle flap advanced.

- *Ear cartilage:* provides support. The exposed surface becomes epithelialized by conjunctiva in a couple of weeks. It should be harvested from scaphoid fossa as concha is too curved. Through a posterior incision an incision is made into cartilage 5 mm from helical rim.
- *Hard palate mucosal graft:* useful as it has both support and mucosal lining. Good for large defects of the lower eyelid. Also for cicatricial ectropion. The keratinized mucosa transforms to non-keratinized mucosa in several weeks. Prior to this it may be irritating and cornea should be well lubricated. Too thick for upper lid. Take mucosa lateral to the midline. Leave periosteum intact. Beware the palatine artery.
- *Oral mucosa graft:* if thin mucosal lining is required it can be harvested from upper or lower lip or buccal mucosa. Use to line musculocutaneous flaps. Split thickness grafts can be used to reconstruct episclera. Avoid *Stensen's duct* in the buccal recess.
- *Septal chondromucosal grafts:* a graft 25 mm square can be harvested and indications include total upper and lower eyelid reconstruction. The septal is infiltrated and the graft outlined and an angled incision made parallel to the dorsum and caudal septum, preserving 10 mm of septum as an L strut. Contralateral cartilage is separated. The graft is removed. Any perforations should be repaired. A lateral rhinotomy incision (full thickness incision in the alar groove) is usually required to gain adequate access to the septum.

Medial canthal reconstruction:
- Loss of the medial canthus leads to loss of medial support and, to correct this, the tarsoligamentous sling needs to be reattached to bone.
- If there is residual tendon, it can be directly reattached.
- The point of fixation should be posterior to the lacrimal sac.
- If there is no tendon, a nasal periosteal flap can be elevated. This is posteriorly based.
- If bone is also lost, a Y-shaped miniplate can be used and the tarsal plate is sutured to an empty hole in the plate or use Mitek™ bone anchor. Alternatively use transnasal wiring.

Lateral canthal reconstruction:
- Lateral canthotomy is achieved by an incision in the lateral palpebral fissure with subsequent detachment of the lower limb of the lateral canthal tendon, which allows relaxation of the lateral portion of the lower lid and adjacent cheek skin.

- For reconstruction use separate points of fixation for the anterior and posterior lamella to the lateral orbital rim.
- The lower lid is adynamic and fixation supports it. The upper lid is dynamic and fixation provides the fulcrum point.
- If tendon is resected, a lateral periosteal flap can reconstruct it. It is released from the junction of deep temporal fascia. Tarsal plate is sutured to this. If upper and lower limbs are missing, use crossed lateral periosteal flaps. If periosteum has been resected, use drill holes for fixation. Lower lid may require a fascial sling, and fascia lata is the best option. This is passed along the margin of the lower lid and attached to periosteum.

Anterior lamellar reconstruction:
- *Tenzel flap.*
- *McGregor cheek flap.*
- *Mustardé flap.*
- *Subperiosteal cheek advancement:* the cheek lift is particularly useful in patients with midfacial aging and tissue laxity. The cheek flap is anchored to the deep temporal fascia lateral to the orbital rim.
- *Hughe's flap.*
- *Hewe's tarsoconjunctival transposition flap.*
- *Cutler–Beard.*
- *Fricke flap.*
- *Mustardé lid switch.*
- *Tripier flap.*
- *Glabellar flap.*

Eyelid tumours
Benign: seborrhoeic keratosis, benign pigmented naevus, dermoid cysts and hamartomas.

Malignant:
- *BCC:* most often on the lower eyelid and medial canthus. Most are nodular.
- *SCC:* <2% of all lid tumours. typically arising in sun-damaged skin, but also on the inner conjunctival surface. Those on the inner surface or arising after RT have a much higher metastatic potential.
- *Sebaceous cell carcinoma:* third most common eyelid tumour.
- *Melanoma:* lentigo maligna, or malignant melanoma *in situ*, accounts for about 1% of all lid lesions and is treated by excision with a 5-mm margin.

Benign	Malignant
SK	BCC
Pigmented naevi	SCC
Dermoid	Sebaceous ca
Hamartoma	MM

Face lift to Furlow technique

Face lift
Anatomy:
- Skin.
- Subcutaneous tissue—thicker in nasolabial area known as the malar fat pad and the retinacular fibres are longer and more prone to weakness.
- Musculoaponeurotic—continuous layers over head and neck:
  - *Scalp:* galea aponeurotica;
  - *Forehead:* frontalis;
  - *Temporal area:* superficial temporal fascia (temporoparietal fascia);
  - *Orbits:* orbicularis oculi;
  - *Face:* SMAS;
  - *Neck and lower face:* platysma.
- Loose areolar layer—on the scalp this is a simple mobile layer which can be easily dissected but in the face it is a complex layer containing:
  - Retaining ligaments:
    - *True:* between dermis and periosteum:
      1. Orbicularis retaining ligament—from orbital margin;
      2. Zygomatic retaining ligaments—from zygoma (McGregor's patch);
      3. Mandibular ligament—from parasymphyseal region.
    - *False:* no bony attachments—from dermis to fascia:
      1. Platysma-auricular fascia;
      2. Masseteric ligaments.
  - *Spaces:* areas devoid of attachments between bone and overlying soft tissue allowing mobility. Bounded by retinacular ligaments for stability:
    - *Prezygomatic space:* between orbicularis and zygomatic retaining ligaments—bulging causes malar mounds;
    - *Premasseter space:* between auricular and masseteric ligaments—bulging forms jowls;
    - *Masticator space:* medial to masseter and contains the buccal fat pad—bulging deepens the labiomandibular fold.

- *Facial nerve branches:* branches of the facial nerve enter the face in the parotid and exit on the surface of masseter. Initially protected by the masseter fascia. Branches become at risk when they come superficially to supply the musculoaponeurotic layer and this happens at a vertical line of retaining ligaments—zygomatic, masseteric and mandibular. Frontal and mandibular branches most at risk:
  - *Frontal branch:* leaves parotid just inferior to zygomatic arch. Initially is in the parotid-masseteric fascia (underneath the musculoaponeurotic layer)—it then passes superficial to the arch in the mid-third, sandwiched between superficial temporal fascia and deep temporal fascia (in the parotid-temporal fascia). Safe dissection is deep to it by going directly onto the deep temporal fascia;
  - *Mandibular branch:* classically described as running 1-2 cm inferior to mandible but this increases with ptosis of lower face. At risk where it is fixed against a ligament:
    1. Platysma-auricular fascia posteriorly;
    2. Mandibular ligament anteriorly.

  Protect it by dissecting superficial to platysma:
- Periosteum and deep fascia—in the lateral face, periosteum is continuous with masseteric and deep temporal fascia as these deep muscles of mastication take their origin from bone:
  - 2 cm superior to zygoma, the deep temporal fascia splits into 2 laminae to envelop the superficial temporal fat pad:
    - superficial lamina of deep temporal fascia inserts onto anterosuperior surface of zygomatic arch;
    - Deep lamina of deep temporal fascia inserts onto posterosuperior surface of zygomatic arch.

History: ask about smoking, BP, medication, healing disorders, DM, RA, psychological disorders.

Examination: look at distribution of skin excess, wrinkling, skin type and quality, facial movement, hair.

Surgical options:

- Incisions:
  - *Standard:* hairline → preauricular → post auricular → mastoid hairline. Facilitates lateral vector of pull;
  - *Short:* inverted L incision. Hairline → preauricular. Facilitates vertical vector.
- Plane of dissection:
  - *Subcutaneous:* skin-only facelift associated with early recurrence. Can be combined with SMAS procedures to enhance impact and longevity;
  - *Sub-SMAS: Deep plane face lift:* under SMAS and skin not dissected separately. The composite flap is tightened. Indicated in smokers as the flap is thicker;
  - *Subperiosteal:* soft tissues are dissected in the subperiosteal plane through a number of open incisions. Can be performed open or endoscopically.
- Approach to the SMAS:
  - *SMASectomy:* for excess tissue;
  - *SMAS plication:* for thin faces if need tissue fullness:
    - MACS type lift as described by Tonnard 2002 through a short scar via a vertical vector. Permanent or slowly resorbing sutures 1-0 PDS round are woven into SMAS like a purse string (SMAS not undermined) anchored to deep temporal fascia above zygomatic arch away from facial nerve:
      - Simple—2 sutures for neck and lower face;
      - Extended 3rd suture to malar fat pad.
- *Approach to the neck:* get divarication of platysma. Debate about open versus closed approaches to the neck. Options include Botox™ for dynamic platysmal bands, defatting by liposuction, corset platysmoplasty with plication of medial borders of platysma, resection of platysmal bands. Also laser resurfacing.

Complications:

- Early:
  - Bleeding;
  - Skin necrosis;
  - Infection;
  - Parotid gland pseudocyst;
  - Wound dehiscence.

- Later:
  - Alopecia;
  - Scarring:
    - Hypertrophic or keloid;
    - Ear distortion—Pixie ear;
    - Steps in hairline.
  - Asymmetry;
  - Recurrence over time;
  - Skin pigment change.

Facial fractures

Classification:

- Closed or open, or by the anatomic region.
- Anatomic areas in the upper face consist of the frontal bone, frontal sinus and supra-orbital areas.
- The orbit is divided into the rim and the internal orbit. Rim fractures are classified in three sections: supraorbital, zygomatic and nasoethmoidal. The internal orbit is classified into four areas.
- The maxilla, the nose and the mandible are the other anatomic areas.
- Fractures tend to occur in patterns as the bone demonstrates weak areas that fracture first despite the source or location of the impact.

Management principles: trauma assessment and resuscitation to identify and treat concomitant c-spine and brain injury and internal breathing threatening the airway. Fractures need accurate diagnosis, early single stage surgery, good exposure, rigid fixation, bone grafting where needed, soft tissue reconstruction.

Radiology:

- Straight PA views.
- *Caldwell views (forehead on plate):* inclined PA views with 23° head extension.
- *Water's views (chin on plate):* inclined PA views with 37° head extension.
- *Towne's views:* AP views with XR tube rotated 30° in a caudal direction.
- *Reversed Towne's views:* as above with tube and film reversed.
- CT and 3D CT.

Incisions:

- Through existing lacerations if present.
- Bicoronal incision for access to frontal sinus and nasal bridge.
- Lower eyelid: to access orbital floor:
  - Transconjunctival;
  - Subciliary;
  - Mid-lid;
  - Junction of eyelid and cheek.
- Upper or lower buccal incision for access to mandible and maxillary fractures.

- Dingman's lateral brow incision for access to zygomatic fractures.
- Risdon's retromandibular incision for access to mandibular angle and ramus fractures.
- Lynch's medial canthus incision for access to naso-orbitoethmoidal fractures.
- Gilles' incision in the temple hairline to facilitate a Gilles lift in an isolated zygomatic arch fracture.

Management of soft tissue injuries:
- *Skin:* good blood supply so debride minimally. Excise edges.
- *Facial nerve:* repair branches lateral to lateral canthus, but medial branches are too small to repair. Muscle will often reinnervate spontaneously.
- *Infra-orbital nerve:* numbness suggests fracture of the floor of the orbit or zygoma. If the zygoma fracture is impacted into the nerve canal then decompression is advised. A branch of the nerve travels to the maxilla and supplies the teeth so numbness here suggests partial injury.
- *Parotid duct:* (*anatomy*) closely related to buccal branch of facial nerve. If in doubt place a probe in the opening at maxillary 2nd premolar. If divided, repair over a thin stent, otherwise risk of salivary collections, fistulae, duct stenosis and parotiditis.
- *Lacrimal apparatus:* injuries to canaliculi, lacrimal sac or duct should be repaired over a silastic stent, which should be inserted along the length of the lacrimal system and tied externally to each other.

Timing: other major injuries take priority. Fracture fixation can be:
- *Early:* preferred if the patient is stable.
- *Delayed primary:* 10 days after injury once swelling has settled, indicated if multiple injuries.
- *Secondary:* try to avoid late surgery as soft tissues contract making realignment difficult.

Immediate management of pan-facial fractures:
- *Airway:* stabilize cervical spine, remove loose teeth, clean vomit and blood from airway. If the patient is not maintaining the airway, distract mandible forward. It may be improved by relocating maxilla upwards and forwards. Obstruction may be due to swelling. Unrelieved obstruction may require intubation, cricothyroidotomy or tracheostomy. Never attempt nasotracheal intubation with midface fractures as brainstem may be impaled. Place gastric tube orally.
- *Breathing:* look for chest injury, and adequate ventilation.

- *Circulation:* significant haemorrhage is usually associated with upper Le Fort or naso-ethmoidal fractures. Insert large bore cannula, start infusion. Send bloods (including drug and alcohol screen). Reduce bleeding by reduction of fractures, nasal packing. If still profuse, give blood, correct coagulopathy, take the patient to theatre, reduce fractures and hold with K wires. Consider facial bandaging, by packing nose and mouth followed by circumferential bandages. If it continues consider external carotid artery ligation through an incision behind the ramus of the mandible or endoscopically through the maxillary sinus or embolization.
- *Other injuries:* once stabilized exclude other injuries. 10% of patients with facial fractures have cervical spine fractures, and 10% have eye injury—need opthalmological assessment.

See also: MANDIBULAR FRACTURES. ZYGOMATIC FRACTURES. MAXILLARY FRACTURES. ORBITAL FRACTURES. NASAL FRACTURES. NASO-ETHMOIDAL FRACTURES. FRONTAL SINUS FRACTURES.

Facial nerve
CN VII. Arises from the 2nd brachial cleft arch and is the motor to muscle of facial expression. It leaves the stylomastoid foramen and passes through the parotid gland.

- Intratemporally the facial nerve has sensory, as well as motor fibres:
  - The superficial petrosal nerve supplies the lacrimal gland;
  - The chorda tympani provides sensation to the anterior 2/3 of the tongue; parasympathetic nerves of facial nerve travels with the trigeminal nerve;
  - Tympanic nerve is a small sensory branch;
  - The nerve to stapedius—if not functioning get hyperacusia.
- As it leaves it gives off:
  - The posterior auricular nerve to the occipital muscles and sensation behind the ear lobe (sensory fibres travel with the auricular branch of vagus);
  - A muscular branch to the posterior belly of digastric and stylohyoid;
  - *Five branches:* temporal (frontal) zygomatic, buccal, mandibular and cervical.
- As it leaves the foramen, it passes anterior to posterior belly of digastric, lateral to styloid process and external carotid artery, and posterior to the facial vein. Find frontal branch on *Pitanguy's line*.
- The facial nerve runs quite superficial, but always below the SMAS. In the midface there are communications between branches.

- Identify nerve by mobilizing the tail of the parotid, bring anterior sternocleidomastoid muscle laterally to find posterior belly of digastric. Follow the muscle up, separate parotid from cartilage of external auditory canal. Facial nerve lies 1 cm deep to tragal pointer.

Temporal branch: frontal branch is deep to SMAS, but lies superficially over the zygomatic arch, lying between periosteum and temporo-parietal fascia (TPF). Superior to the zygomatic arch it lies within or under TPF, superficial to the deep temporal fascia. The nerve enters frontalis on its deep surface where orbicularis oculi intersects with the lateral aspect of frontalis 1.5 cm above the lateral point of the eyebrow.

Zygomatic branch: supplies orbicularis oculi. Division results in inability to close the eye.

Buccal branch: divides into multiple branches, which travel along the parotid duct. They supply buccinator muscle and the muscles of the upper lip. Division causes difficulty emptying the cheek.

Marginal mandibular: runs 1–2 cm below border of mandible deep to platysma and superficial to facial vein. Supplies lower lip. Division results in elevation of the corner of the mouth.

Cervical branch: runs downwards into the neck to supply the platysma muscle. There is significant cross-over between buccal and zygomatic branches of the facial nerve. Injury to either is compensated for. There is little cross-over with frontal and marginal mandibular nerves, and there is little compensation if they are injured.

Muscles: posterior belly of digastric, stapedius. Muscles of facial expression—the muscles levator anguli superioris, mentalis and buccinator lie deep, and therefore are innervated on the superficial surface. All other muscles lie superficial to the plane of the facial nerve and receive their innervation on the deep surface.

Facial danger zones: all the nerves are below SMAS apart from frontal branch within SMAS.
- *6.5 cm below external auditory canal:* great auricular nerve.
- *Pitanguy's line:* temporal branch.
- *Midmandible 2 cm posterior to oral commissure:* marginal mandibular.
- *Anterior to parotid and posterior to zygomaticus:* zygomatic and buccal.
- *Superior orbital rim:* supra-orbital and supratrochlear nerve.
- *1 cm below inferior orbital rim, mid-pupil:* infra-orbital nerve.
- *Mid-mandibular below 2nd premolar:* mental nerve.

Facial re-animation

History: particularly note onset. A slow onset is indicative of tumour, acute with infection, trauma, medication or vascular. Also note changes in hearing, taste and dizziness.

Aetiology: congenital or acquired:
- *Congenital:* facial musculature doesn't develop. This is usually not complete. Usually unilateral and more rarely bilateral. See MÖBIUS SYNDROME.
- *Acquired:* most common is <u>Bell's palsy</u>, which usually has spontaneous complete recovery (71%). Also trauma, neoplasm and post-infective, e.g. Ramsay–Hunt syndrome:
  - *Intracranial:*
    - Vascular abnormalities;
    - Central nervous system; degenerative diseases;
    - Tumours of the intracranial cavity;
    - Trauma to the brain;
    - Congenital abnormalities and agenesis.
  - *Intratemporal:*
    - bacterial and viral infections (Ramsay Hunt syndrome accounts for 10% of unilateral causes and Lyme disease is the commonest cause of bilateral palsy);
    - cholesteatoma;
    - trauma;
    - longitudinal and horizontal fractures of the temporal bone;
    - gunshot wounds;
    - tumours invading the middle ear, mastoid, and facial nerve;
    - iatrogenic causes.
  - *Extracranial:*
    - malignant tumours of the parotid gland;
    - trauma (lacerations and gunshot wounds);
    - iatrogenic causes;
    - primary tumours of the facial nerve;
    - malignant tumours of the ascending ramus of the mandible pterygoid region, and skin.

Grading: House-Brackman scale; evaluates gross facial appearance, facial symmetry and tone at rest, and motion of the forehead, eyes and mouth.
- *1:* normal.
- *2:* mild: normal symmetry at rest with weak mimetic muscles.
- *3:* moderate: slight asymmetry at rest with weak mimetic muscles.
- *4:* moderately severe: obvious asymmetry at rest with incomplete eye closure.

- *5:* severe: as above with only slight movement of mimetic muscles.
- *6:* total paralysis.

Sunnybrook scale is more objective and sensitive to small changes, and evaluates:
- Resting symmetry (eye, cheek, mouth).
- Symmetry of voluntary movement (brow, eye, smile, frown, kiss).
- Synkinesis (severity with movements of brow, eye, smile, frown, kiss).
- Normal patients score 100 on the Sunnybrook scale.

Examination:
- Upper motor neuron lesion presents with ipsilateral lower face paralysis as the upper face is supplied by both sides from the cerebral cortex.
- Intratemporal lesions involve sensory, as well as motor fibres. Test for intratemporal lesions with:
  - *Schirmer's test* (for tear production);
  - the stapedius reflex test;
  - the electrogustatory test for the tongue.
- Look for scars, movement of upper eyelid. Test strength of eyelid closure, perform lower eyelid snap test, assess nasal valving and examine temporalis muscle.

Investigations:
- Plain XRs, CT, MRI and serologic tests to establish the cause.
- Electroneuronography (ENoG) is most accurate test to determine prognosis in early stages of Bell's Palsy. Stimulates facial nerve at stylomastoid foramen and measures action potentials near nasolabial fold. Performed after 72 hours of symptom onset. Degree of axonal degeneration is expressed as a proportion of the normal side's amplitude. Less than 90% degeneration is associated with 80-100% recovery rates.
- Electromyography (EMG) is useful in planning late reanimation surgery to determine if facial muscles are viable and could have useful function after reinnervation.

Anatomy: 17 facial muscles. Three sphincters—eye, nose and mouth.

Treatment:
Non-operative:
- Protect eyes with eye drops, glasses, taping closed at night.
- Ectropion can be taped.
- *Botulinum* toxin into the normal side may equalize the face.

Static operations:
Indicated in older patients where more complex procedures are less likely to be successful.

- Around the eye include temporary or permanent *Tarsorrhaphy*.
- The *Kuhnt-Szymanowski* procedure for ectropion.
- Lateral canthopexy.
- Insertion of gold weights or springs, brow lift or forehead skin excision.
- Around the mouth include unilateral face lift procedures and static slings with fascia lata.

Dynamic operations:
Neurotise native facial muscles if the motor plates are viable:
- *Nerve repair:* if nerve divided, attempt immediate repair (maximum 3 weeks post-injury) for good results. Beyond a line dropped from the lateral canthus, repair may not be required due to the numerous anastomoses.
- *Nerve graft:* to bridge gaps between proximal and distal stumps following resection. Require a good bed for the tissues. Donors include great auricular nerve, cervical plexus from ipsilateral or contralateral side or sural nerve. Return of facial movement occurs between 6 and 24 months. First tone improves then movement in the middle third of the face.
- Neurotization from a new source indicated when proximal segments of facial nerve are irreversibly damaged but in the presence of intact distal branches:
  - *Cross-face contralateral facial nerve graft:* first described by Scaramella in 1970s. Sural nerve graft used to go onto intact facial nerve the contralateral side onto a branch that produces pure smile without eye closure or grimace. Advantage of this technique is spontaneous movement (smile, blink). Disadvantages are weakness on the normal side;
  - *Masseter nerve transfer:* identify via a transverse incision in parotid gland 1 cm below zygomatic arch and 3 cm anterior to tragus. Then blunt dissection (to avoid facial nerve branch damage) to reach masseter muscle surface—use nerve stimulators to identify nerve. Descending branch of masseter nerve divided—this leaves some branches intact so the masseter muscle can partially function and does not atrophy. Good for power but not good for spontaneity or resting tone (only the facial nerve is highly modulated by the limbic system producing emotionally mediated spontaneous mimetic facial motion).

Recruit new muscle when motor end plates on native facial muscles not viable:

- *Regional muscle transfer:* uses muscles innervated by trigeminal nerve and is applicable for partial, complete and bilateral facial paralysis patients—masseter and temporalis most common. Quick and easy but function not synchronized.
  - *Labbé procedure* (*lengthening temporalis myoplasty:* a one-stage surgical re-animation with no revascularization or reinnervation). Temporalis is partially released from its insertion on temporal crest to lengthen it—Labbé describes with a temporal approach, zygomatic arch osteotomy and coranoidectomy;
  - *Masseter:* transposed to orbicularis oris;
  - Anterior belly of digastric can also be used for lower lip. Results are rapid but require more effort than free flap transfer to activate muscles of mastication to achieve smiling.
- *Free-muscle transfer:* has become the standard for patients with long-standing permanent facial paralysis. Offers surgeons the ability to design precise origin, insertion and tension. Procedure of choice in congenital palsy due to lack of muscle and facial nerve. There is a common need between techniques for a donor muscle and recipient nerve supply. Reconstructions can be in 1 or 2 stages. Can result in excellent contour and strong movement but longer operative time, potential vascular complications, delay in muscle functions and a final result at about 2-years post-operatively.
  - A one-stage transfer on to the nerve to masseter muscle may be appropriate for bilateral facial paralysis in children or unilateral paralysis in adults >30 years. 98% success rate but no resting tone;
  - A two-stage procedure is commonly used for unilateral long standing facial palsy in younger patients (20% failure rate):
    - Cross facial nerve graft from contralateral side produces a bilateral emotion response. You can follow the progress of the facial nerve through the graft with an advancing Tinel sign;
    - Second stage involves a free-muscle transfer when the donor nerves have matured. Potential donors include gracilis, pectoralis minor, latissimus dorsi (bulky), serratus anterior, ECRB, rectus abdominis. Facial artery and vein and often used as recipient vessels due to proximity and size match.

Eyelid and Lower lip:
- *Eyelid:* determine whether the upper or lower lid needs correction. A lower lid ectropion needs support using a tendon, such as palmaris longus. For the upper lid use a gold weight or an eyespring, which gives a better result but is more troublesome to fit. Local and free muscle transfer with CFNG can be used.
- *Lower lip:* if mandibular nerve cannot be coapted, use direct coaptation of hypoglossal nerve or use a muscle transfer with platysma or digastric. Platysma is preferred as it gives co-ordinated movement being supplied by facial nerve, but if also paralysed digastric muscle with CFNG can be used.

Falconer's test
- Test for *Thoracic outlet syndrome*. Costoclavicular compression.
- Perform with patient standing. Military brace position with shoulders pushed back, arms behind the back and shoulders depressed. (Like a diving falcon.)
- Feel both radial pulses and apply downward traction.

Fanconi's anaemia
See RADIAL CLUB HAND.

- Autosomal recessive aplastic anaemia presenting end of first decade.
- Associated with abnormal repair of damaged DNA.
- The carrier frequency is 1:300.
- Death is by bone marrow failure, leukaemia and solid tumours.
- The average life expectancy is 30 years.
- Associated with altered skin pigmentation, thumb and radial anomalies, abnormal male gonads, microcephaly, developmental delay.
- The thumb is usually present with this form of radial club hand.

Fasanella–Servat operation
- Tarso-Müllerectomy via a posterior approach to shorten Müller's muscle.
- For correction of moderate eyelid *Ptosis*.
- Upper eyelid is everted. Conjunctiva and lower end of Müllers muscle is held in a clip. A row of sutures is placed above the clip. Tissue held by clip is excised.

Fascia
See RETINACULAR SYSTEM.

Fascia lata graft
Useful in facial reconstructions when intrinsic support systems are absent or stretched. Used for lower lid ptosis, 7th nerve palsy, static sling.

Technique:
- Several transverse incisions are made over the middle 1/3 of the lateral thigh on a line between the greater trochanter and lateral condyle.
- Parallel incisions are made in the fascia lata and the fascia lata harvested directly or with a stripper.

Fasciocutaneous flap
- A flap containing skin and deep fascia to augment the blood supply.
- Fascia has subfascial, fascial and suprafascial network of vessels.
- The suprafascial network is the most significant and lifting fascia ensures this network is protected.
- Fascial perforators can be direct—going straight to skin—or indirect—ending in skin after supplying deeper structures.
- Fasciocutaneous perforators arise from septa and occur mainly in extremities.
- *Axis of flap:* determined by the predominant direction of flow—longitudinal in the extremities and oblique in the torso.

Classification:
- *Cormack and Lamberty* (CandL): perforators are multiple, solitary or segmental.
- *Nahai-Mathes* (NandM): perforators are direct, septocutaneous or musculocutaneous.

To increase the length of pedicle of a flap:
- *CandL A:* dissect indirect perforators through muscle, e.g. periumbilical flap includes the deep inferior epigastric, but not muscle.
- *CandL B:* follow the perforator through septum to origin, e.g. circumflex scapular artery leads to the subscapular artery.
- *CandL C:* include entire source vessel, such as the radial forearm flap.

See NEUROCUTANEOUS FLAPS. *See* PONTÉN FLAP.

Fat anatomy
Fat cells arise from mesodermal adipoblasts. In children, accumulation of fat is by increase in number of adipose cells (hyperplasia) for the first 5 years and again during adolescence. After adolescence, no new adipocytes are formed, but the size of the cells enlarge (hypertrophy).

Adipose tissue is composed of:

- *Mature adipocytes:* sensitive to trauma.
- *Pre-adipocytes:* spontaneously differentiate to mature adipocytes—fat graft survival is largely dependent on pre-adipocyte differentiation.
- *Adipose-derived stem cells (ADSCs):* can differentiate into any cell type.

Subcutaneous fat divides to three layers:

1. *Apical layer:* immediately deep to reticular dermis—surrounds sweat glands, hair follicles, blood and lymphatics so injury results in seroma, erythema, pigment change and skin necrosis.
2. *Mantle layer:* consists of columnar fat cells within a vertical fibrous stroma. There is no mantle layer in eyelids, nailed dorsum of nose or penis.
3. *Deep layer:* between mantle layer and deep fascia—thickness varies by sex, genes and diet—this is the main target for liposuction. With weight gain there is a disproportionate enlargement of the deep fat.

Anatomy of fat is specific in certain areas:

- *Neck:* fat deposits in a 'wattle' deformity—fat can be removed from the subcutaneous/supraplatysmal plane via liposuction. Fat deep to platysma is better to remove via direct excision due to risk of nerve injury.
- *Abdomen:* fat is divided by:
  - Camper's fascia—consists of fat within a loose fibrous meshwork;
  - Scarpa's fascia in lower abdomen defines an additional deep layer of fat.
- *Flanks:* fat divides into superficial and deep by the superficial fascial system:
  - Zones of adherence connect the superficial fascial system to muscle fascia and should not be transgressed by liposuction as they define android and gynaecoid patterns of fat deposition:
    - *Males:* adherence along iliac crest;
    - *Females:* adherence is lower so fat is localized over the crest.
  - Additional zones of adherence exist in gluteal crease and distal thigh.

See LIPOSUCTION.

Fat graft
- Also known as lipomodelling, lipofilling, fat transfer.

Indications:
- Breast: post-reconstruction or contour defects.
- Breast augmentation.
- Scar management.
- Pre-conditioning.
- Post-radiotherapy.

Generally, 50% of transferred fat cells will survive so tendency to overfill to compensate.

Theories on graft survival:
- *Cell survival theory:* depends on number of surviving cells in the graft.

• *Host replacement theory:* depends on recruitment of host adipocytes.
• *Niche theory:* cells physiology is regulated by its microenvironment.

Technique: Originally described by Coleman. Aim is to minimize trauma by harvesting intact parcels of fat small enough to inject but large enough to preserve architecture:
• *Harvest:* most commonly from abdomen, flanks and medial thighs. 1 ml dilute LA and adrenaline infiltrated for each 1 ml of aspirate. Use a blunt 3 mm harvesting cannula.

• Refinement via centrifuge, sedimentation, filtration or washing—separation of aspirate into:
  ○ Supernatant of oil released from damaged adipocytes;
  ○ Middle layer of fatty tissue;
  ○ Subnatant of blood, water and infiltration fluid.
• *Placement:* refined fat is injected into target area—aim to maximize contact between fat parcels and recipient tissue.

Complications:
• Infection.
• Swelling and bruising.
• Intravascular injection—PE, stroke, blindness.
• Over-/undercorrection and contour irregularities.
• Fat absorption with calcification and oil cysts.
• All potential complications of liposuction at donor site (i.e. visceral perforation).

Felon
• Infection in the digital pulp which is inhibited from side-to-side spread by the tight network of vertical fibres attaching to the skin of the distal phalanx.
• Spread occurs by erosion of the walls one by one. Progression can lead to osteomyelitis.
• Characterized by rapid onset throbbing pain and swelling of pulp which does not extend beyond DIPJ.

  2 incisions commonly used for drainage:

• Classic dorsal midaxial incision down to periosteum—then blunt dissection of the vertical septa. Put the incision on the non-contact side.
• Central longitudinal incision—avoids the neurovascular bundle and usually heals well. Described by Conolly and Kilgore.

Femoral nerve: anatomy
• L2–4. Lies behind fascia iliacus, lateral to femoral artery.

• Terminates 4 cm below inguinal ligament. Divides into anterior and posterior branch. Supplies muscles of anterior compartment.
• Anterior division has 2 cutaneous branches (medial cutaneous nerve of the thigh and the intermediate cutaneous nerve of the thigh), and 2 muscle branches (sartorius and pectineus).
• Posterior division has 1 cutaneous (saphenous nerve to ball of big toe).
• Muscles of anterior compartment are sartorius, iliacus, psoas, pectineus, and quadriceps femoris (rectus femoris, vastus lateralis, vastus medialis and vastus intermedius).

Femoral triangle
Boundaries: inguinal ligament, medial border of sartorius laterally, medial border of adductor longus medially, and the apex is where the two converge (some take the boundary as the lateral border of adductor longus). The floor consists of iliopsoas, pectineus and adductor longus.

Contents: the femoral artery and vein lie anterior to the fascia. Femoral and lateral cutaneous nerve lie deep to fascia.
See GROIN LYMPH NODE DISSECTION.

Ferguson–Smith syndrome
Condition linked to a single gene mutation in West of Scotland 200 years ago. Autosomal dominant. Multiple self-healing epitheliomas, which look like *KAs*.

Fibrillation potentials
• An action potential of a single muscle fibre.
• Arises from a spontaneously contracting muscle and is recorded with a needle electrode.
• Usually suggestive of denervation though they can be seen in healthy muscles. Fibrillations may indicate a lower motor neuron lesion such as arising from the anterior horn cell, nerve root or peripheral nerve. Also in muscular dystrophy or polymyositis.
• After nerve injury it usually takes 14 days before fibrillation potentials are seen due to the delayed onset of denervation hypersensitivity.
See NERVE CONDUCTION STUDIES.

Fibrin glue
Prepared by a mixture of cryoprecipitate, calcium and thrombin. It has been shown to decrease subgraft haematoma rate and increase wound healing.

Fibroblast Growth Factor (FGF)-receptor
A family of tyrosine kinase receptors sharing a common protein structure. Binding of FGF to

the receptor results in activation of the tyrosine kinase signalling pathways for cell replication and differentiation.

Fibroma of tendon sheath

Fibromas of tendon sheaths are difficult to distinguish from cysts. They are treated by excision with a small amount of sheath.

- *Juvenile aponeurotic fibroma:* a rapidly growing firm irregular mass on the sole of foot or palm of hand in children. They require conservative excisional surgery. Histologically, there may be infiltration into surrounding muscle, but no mitotic activity. Initial frequent recurrences become less frequent with age.
- *Recurring digital fibrous tumour of childhood:* occurs as multiple smooth masses on the dorsum of the fingers and toes of infants and children. They may appear simultaneously on several digits. Intracytoplasmic inclusion bodies are seen suggesting a viral origin. Treatment is conservative unless there is interference with function. Local recurrence occurs in >50% of cases.

Fibrous dysplasia

- A benign disease of bone representing 2.5% of all bone tumours.
- Normal bone matrix is replaced with fibroblastic proliferation, which contains irregular trabeculae of partially calcified osteoid.
- Its aetiology remains unclear, but it appears to be a congenital anomaly, which produces dysplastic growth of bone with incomplete maturation of mesenchymal tissue.
- It may be monostotic (one site) or polyostotic. Monostotic are more common and tend to involve ribs, femur, tibia and craniofacial.
- A subset have <u>Albright's syndrome</u>. Also <u>Cherubism</u>.

XR:

- *Variable:* central metaphyseal or diaphyseal lesion with mild cortical expansion. Ground glass appearance.
- *3 types:*
  - ○ *I:* pagetoid;
  - ○ *II:* sclerotic;
  - ○ *III:* cystic.

Histology: immature trabeculae giving a Chinese letters appearance.

Craniofacial fibrous dysplasia:

- Ranges from a painless local swelling to a gross deformity. May get proptosis, optic atrophy and vision loss.

- May be confused with ossifying fibroma, Paget's and meningioma.
- *Malignancy:* rare. Risk greatest in males with polyostotic disease. The most common malignancy is osteosarcoma. Never use RT for fibrous dysplasia.
- *Treatment:* curettage and cortical strut grafting. Options are observe, contouring or radical resection.
- Fibrous dysplasia divided by location into:
  - ○ *Zone 1:* around the orbit; may get displacement of the globe and this causes the greatest cosmetic problem; may require radical resection; perform en bloc excision of all involved bone; reconstruct with cranial grafts (inner cortex), rib grafts or iliac bone;
  - ○ *Zone 2:* hair-bearing cranium; can be hidden;
  - ○ *Zone 3:* cranial base; resection hazardous and, therefore, conservative treatment if asymptomatic;
  - ○ *Zone 4:* teeth-bearing areas of maxilla or mandible; resection would require dentures.

See BONE TUMOURS.

Fibrous tumours

- <u>*Dermatofibroma*</u>.
- <u>*Pseudosarcomatous lesions*</u>.
- <u>*Dermatofibrosarcoma protuberans*</u>.
- <u>*Angiofibroma*</u>.

Fibula flap

- Free fibular flap. Described by Hidalgo 1989.
- Can achieve a bone length of 26 cm, has a thick cortex, gives good structural strength, and minimal donor morbidity.
- Blood supply from peroneal artery via both a dominant nutrient artery, which enters 14 cm from proximal end of fibula, and segmental periosteal supply, which facilitates multiple osteotomies.
- Skin can be harvested reliably along with the bone.

Technique:

- Intra-operative position—sandbag under hip so that hip is internally rotated and triangle under knee to flex it.
- Mark the fibula on the surface of the skin.
- Define the perforators with a Doppler at posterior border of fibula:
  - ○ Mark skin paddle to incorporate the perforators.
- Start with anterior skin incision—avoid the superficial peroneal nerve:
  - ○ Dissect down through fascia to expose peroneus longus;

○ Subfascial dissection to reach the posterior crural septum—perforators can be identified.

- Take the peroneal muscles off the posterior crural septum.
- Take the peroneal muscles off the lateral fibula (leave the periosteum in place).
- Divide the anterior crural septum.
- Dissect the extensor digitorum longus and extensor hallucis longus off the anterior aspect of the fibula—this allows you to see interosseous membrane.
- Make the posterior skin paddle incision—subfascial dissection to posterior crural septum and follow the septum down—will need to divide the multiple branches from the perforator to the soleus muscle. Dissect soleus and FHL off the posterior crural septum.
- Mark distal osteotomy site on fibula—6–8 cm proximal to lateral malleolus to maintain ankle stability.
- Mark proximal osteotomy (leave 7 cm proximal to take care not to damage common peroneal nerve).
- Perform proximal and distal osteotomies, ensuring pedicle protection. Use bone hooks in intramedullary canal to place traction on fibula which aids visualization of interosseous membrane—incise this under tension to reveal tibialis posterior muscle underneath it.
- Division of the tibialis posterior muscle fibres will reveal the peroneal artery and venae comitantes. Clip and divide distal end of it so that dissection of the pedicle can proceed distal to proximal until the flap is islanded on the peroneal vessels.
- 4 cm skin paddle width can close directly.

See MANDIBULAR RECONSTRUCTION.

Fillet flap

- A technique using 'spare parts' to reconstruct using tissue of amputated or non-salvageable limbs.
- Axial pattern flaps that function as composite tissue transfers.
- Can be pedicled or free.
- Examples include finger, toe and 'fillet of sole' (plantar surface of foot).
- Fillet of sole flaps (pedicled or free) are useful to give durable, potentially sensate weight-bearing surface to a lower limb amputation. Particularly useful if the additional skin coverage afforded allows knee joint to be preserved.

Finasteride

- Finasteride is a competitive inhibitor of 5-alpha reductase, which converts testosterone to dihydrotestosterone.
- It is licensed for treatment of androgenic alopecia in men.
- It is contraindicated in women of child-bearing age due to the impaired androgenization of the male foetus.
- It has been used for *Hydradenitis suppuritiva*.

Fingertip injuries

- Distal pulp is divided by radial fibrous septa, which create a multipyramidal structure of fibroadipose tissue compartments.
- Digital nerve trifurcates at the level of the DIP joint.
- Determine the level and angle of tissue loss and what is left.

Non-operative:

- If no exposed bone and <1 cm diameter, leave to heal by secondary intention. Use an occlusive dressing to maintain a moist wound healing environment. Healing occurs in 3–6 weeks. It may lead to loss of pulp volume and pulp sensitivity but gives good sensory return.

Operative:

- *Primary closure:* limited bone shortening may be required. If there is significant loss of terminal phalanx, germinal matrix should be excised.
- *Skin graft:* SSG or FTSG. Return of sensation is better with thicker graft. Sharply amputated tissue can be replaced as a graft.
- *Kutler lateral V-Y flaps.*
- *Atasoy volar V-Y flap.*
- *Moberg volar neurovascular flap.*
- *Cross finger flap.*
- *Thenar flexion crease flap.*
- *Littler neurovascular island flap.*
- *Venkataswami flap.*
- *Homodigital island flap.*

Finklestein's test

A test used to help diagnose *de Quervain's disease*. The patient grasps own thumb within ipsilateral palm. Pain elicited when patient's wrist moves from radial to extreme ulnar deviation.

Finochietto–Bunnell test

A test used to help diagnose contractures of interosseous muscles in the hand. With MCP joint in extension, PIP joint flexion is prevented due to a contracted interosseous. Flexion of MCP joint releases PIP joint.

Fistula (oronasal in cleft palate)

- A communication between oral and nasal cavities following cleft palate reconstruction.
- Risk factors include tension at the repair site which is increased in wider cleft palates and post-operative infection or hematoma.
- Assess with speech therapist to determine whether symptomatic for speech and nasal regurgitation.

Classification: Pittsburgh based on anatomical location of the fistula.

- *Type 1:* uvular
- *Type 2:* soft palate
- *Type 3:* hard/soft palate junction
- *Type 4:* hard palate
- *Type 5:* junction of primary/secondary palate at the incisive foramen
- *Type 6:* lingual-alveolar
- *Type 7:* labial-alveolar

Management:

- Conservative may be suitable for small asymptomatic fistulae.
- Surgical techniques depending on size and location of fistulae.
  - *Re-repair in two layers:* suitable for soft palate fistulae and hard palate fistulae, where turn down flaps can be used for nasal layer and advancement of oral mucoperiosteum can close oral layers with lateral releasing incisions;
  - *Recruit vascularised tissue:* buccinator flaps useful for junctional fistulae, FAMM and tongue flaps useful for anterior hard palate fistulae;
  - *Tissue substitutes:* acellular dermal matrix has been used for an additional third layer for robustness.
- Palatal obturator for patients not fit or willing for surgery

Fitzpatrick skin types

Six different skin types based on colour and reaction to sun exposure:

1. *Very white or freckled:* always burn.
2. *White:* usually burn.
3. *White to olive:* sometimes burn.
4. *Brown:* rarely burn.
5. *Dark brown:* very rarely burn.
6. *Black:* never burn.

Five-flap Z-plasty

See JUMPING MAN FLAP.

Five Year Old's Index

- An occlusal index used for assessing facial growth in patients born with a unilateral cleft lip and palate at 5 years of age during deciduous dentition.
- Based on the GOSLON index and so retains the format of 5 categories.
- Raters need to be trained and calibrated.

Flag flap

Axial flap using skin from the dorsal index or middle fingers at the proximal phalanx based upon the dorsal metacarpal artery. It can be used to resurface skin loss over the base of the adjacent index or middle finger.

Flap

- A unit of tissue which retains its own blood supply whilst being transferred from a donor site to a recipient site.
- *Composite flap:* contains more than one tissue layer.
- *Blood supply of skin:* arises from either fasciocutaneous vessels, musculocutaneous perforators or direct cutaneous arteries. These supply a deep plexus at the junction of deep dermis and subcutaneous tissue and a superficial layer at the junction of papillary and reticular dermis.
- *Regulation of blood flow:* extrinsic and intrinsic factors affect flow and can either be due to the vessel, the blood or a combination.

Classification: 5 Cs, circulation, composition, contiguity, contour, conditioning.

- *Circulation: Random, Axial.*
- *Composition:* cutaneous, fasciocutaneous, fascial, musculocutaneous, muscle, osseocutaneous, osseous.
- *Contiguity:* local, regional, distant (pedicled and free).
- *Contour:* the method in which they are transferred into the defect. *Advance flaps, Transposition, Rotation, Interpolation, Crane principle.*
- *Conditioning:* by *Delay.*

Fleur-de-Lis abdominoplasty

- *Abdominoplasty* technique when lateral and vertical skin excision is required, usually with central tissue excess after significant weight loss.
- The operation takes its name from the pattern generated when the first key stitch is placed to bring the skin flaps together.

Flexor carpi radialis

Origin: medial epicondyle and common flexor pronator origin lateral to PT. Tendinous in midforearm. It crosses the wrist under the crest of trapezium.

Insertion: volar aspect of base of 2nd MC. Sometimes it inserts into flexor retinaculum if there is no PL.

Nerve supply: median nerve.

Action: wrist flexor, weak elbow flexor and radial deviator.

See MUSCLES.

Flexor carpi radialis tendonitis

Pain and tenderness over FCR just proximal to the scaphoid tubercle and trapezoid crest. Worsened by resisted flexion.

Treatment: rest, NSAIDs and steroids. Surgical release is performed by opening the fibro-osseous tunnel from 3 cm proximal to wrist to the insertion of FCR.

See TENOSYNOVITIS.

Flexor carpi ulnaris

Origin: humeral head arising from the common tendon attached to the medial epicondyle of the humerus and an ulnar head from the medial aspect of the olecranon process of the ulna and the posterior border of the ulna. The two heads are united by a tendinous arch—Osborne's ligament. Long fleshy muscle with short fibres running into tendon almost to the insertion.

Insertion: into the pisiform bone and by two ligaments, the pisohamate and pisometacarpal ligaments into the hook of hamate and base of 5th metacarpal. Some fibres form a roof for ulnar artery and nerve.

Nerve supply: ulnar nerve.

Action: powerful flexor and wrist ulnar deviator. Stabilizes the wrist. Can be used in radial nerve palsy to restore wrist extension.

See MUSCLES.

Flexor carpi ulnaris tenosynovitis

Volar wrist pain worsened by flexion and ulnar deviation.

Differential diagnosis: pisiform fracture, Pisotriquetral arthritis, ulnar neuritis.

See TENOSYNOVITIS.

Flexor digitorum profundus (FDP)

Origin: volar and ulnar aspect of proximal 2/3 ulnar, septum that separates profundus from FCU and ulnar half of interosseus membrane, occasionally from the radius. Independence decreases from the radial to ulnar with the index finger being the most independent. It lies beneath FDS. Lumbricals arise from the radial side in the palm.

Insertion: distal phalanx.

Nerve supply: radial half anterior interosseous nerve from the median nerve, ulnar half ulnar nerve.

Blood supply: muscle belly by ulnar anterior interosseous and common interosseous arteries. Tendons at the wrist by branches of the superficial palmar arch. In the sheaths the digital arteries supply the tendons. The only tendon to flex the DIPJ. To test, immobilize the PIPJ in extension and for maximal effect with wrist and MCPJ also in extension. Any flexion is caused by FDP.

See MUSCLES.

Flexor digitorum profundus avulsion

- Forced avulsion from the insertion is the next common tendon injury after laceration.
- FDS can be avulsed, but is rare.
- Most occur in the ring finger. A common muscle belly may make it more susceptible to hyperextension. Also the insertion is weaker and the ring finger is longer in flexion.

Classification: *Leddy and Packer.*

Treatment:
- Repair is easier with early diagnosis and treatment.
- Ultrasound can locate the tendon.
- It should be retrieved and passed through the tunnel and inserted into the distal phalanx.
- Raise a periosteal flap and suture through drill holes to a button tied over the nail. A Mitek™ bone anchor can also be used. A bony fragment large enough to take a screw should be fixed.

Flexor digitorum superficialis

Origin: three heads—humeral from medial epicondyle, ulnar from coronoid process and radial from oblique muscular line of the radius. An aponeurotic arch connects radial to ulnar head and passes over median nerve and ulnar artery. The muscle divides into 4 distinct bundles. Four tendons, superficial are ring and middle, deep are index and little. Pass under TCL.

Insertion: FDS inserts into the volar aspect of the middle phalanx and flexes the PIPJ. FDP also flexes the PIPJ so FDP needs to be blocked to test FDS. FDP has a common muscle belly so holding the other fingers in extension will prevent contraction of FDP on the finger to be tested. As the PIPJ flexes due to FDS action the DIPJ remains extended as the FPD can't function. This may not occur in the index finger as the FDP may function separately. FDS to little finger may not appear to function because 15% are absent, 15% are not functional and some are adherent to the FDS ring thus blocking flexion if the ring is in extension.

Nerve supply: median nerve.

Blood supply: muscle is supplied by branches of the ulnar artery, as well as contributions of radial artery. Tendons at the wrist are supplied by branches of the superficial palmar arch. Digital arteries supply tendons in the sheath. To test FDS to index finger ask patient to squeeze a piece of paper between the index and thumb. If the FDS is functional the finger is held in the pseudo-boutonniere. If absent the finger is held in the pseudomdal position.

See MUSCLES.

Flexor digitorum superficialis tenodesis

See PROXIMAL INTERPHALANGEAL JOINT. For chronic hyperextension injury. Take radial slip of FDS and fix to bone with interosseous wire or Mitek™ bone anchor.

Flexor pollicis brevis

Origin: two heads. Superficial from anterior TCL, FCR tendon sheath and crest of trapezium. Deep originates from anterior surface of trapezoid and capitate. They unite, forming an arch for the passage of FPL. They insert into the lateral sesamoid and lateral tubercle of the base of the proximal phalanx.

Nerve supply: mainly median nerve, but deep fibres have dual innervation.

See MUSCLES.

Flexor pollicis longus

Origin: middle 1/3 of radius. An accessory belly may originate from the coronoid process—the accessory muscle of Gantzer. It passes through the carpal tunnel on the radial side of median nerve, bends around trapezium, runs between two heads of FPB, between the two sesamoids. May have an attachment to FDP—*Linburg's syndrome*.

Insertion: *distal* phalanx of thumb.

Nerve supply: median nerve.

Blood supply: muscular perforators from the radial artery. It is usually supplied by two distinct vincula in the tendon sheath of the thumb.

See MUSCLES.

Flexor sheaths

The flexor sheaths of the thumb and little finger are contiguous with the radial and ulnar bursa. That of the index, middle and ring finger originate at the metacarpal neck. Double-walled fibro-osseous tunnel sealed at both ends. Inner visceral and outer parietal layer. Floor is composed of periosteum and volar plate. The system of annular and cruciate *Pulleys* holds the tendon close to the bone. The sheath forms a closed cavity.

Flexor sheath infection

- Usually caused by a penetrating injury especially over the volar joint creases where skin and sheath are close. Also secondary spread from felons, palmar space infections and haematogenous spread. Most commonly seen in index middle or ring finger.
- Flexor tendon sheath infection of the thumb and little finger can spread proximally because the tendon sheath is in relation with the radial and ulnar bursae which is continuous with the space of Parona in the forearm (between PQ and FDP).
- Clinically test for *Kanavel's signs*.

1. Fusiform swelling of finger.
2. Finger held in semi-flexed position.
3. Exquisite tenderness over the flexor aspect.
4. Increased tenderness with passive extension—most reliable sign.

- Early (emergent) surgical drainage improves outcomes.
- Perform tendon washout through minimal access incisions at proximal and distal ends of the flexor sheath. If there is evidence of tissue necrosis, the entire tendon sheath is exposed via an extended incision (e.g. Bruner's) along the entire digit. Delayed tendon reconstruction performed in the presence of tendon necrosis.

Classification: Michon:

- *Type 1:* increased serous fluid in sheath—washout through minimal access incisions in a single stage.
- *Type 2:* pus in sheath with granulomatous synovium—washout through minimal access incisions with low threshold for return to theatre in 24–48 hours for second look.
- *Type 3:* necrosis of the tendon, pulleys or tendon sheath—wide exposure required and consideration for staged tendon reconstruction.

See TENOSYNOVITIS.

Flexor tendons

Anatomic relationship:

- In arm, FDP is deep to FDS with median nerve in between.
- *FDS:* middle and ring finger volar to index and little in wrist, but in the palm they lie in the same plane. At the distal palmar crease each FDS splits to wrap around FDP. The two slips merge deep to FDP then insert along middle phalanx. The decussation distal to where the FDP tendon pierces the two slips is called Camper's chiasm.

Pulleys: A2 and A4 most important for function.

Flexion: starts at PIPJ. FDP is the prime flexor. MCP joint flexion is resisted by the extensors. Flexion of PIP joint increases intrinsic tension which causes MCP joint flexion. Flexion of DIP joint is limited by ORL tightness. Flexion of PIP joint relaxes ORL allowing for DIP flexion.

Blood supply: from 3 sources:

- Point of bony insertion.
- The _Vinculae_ and vessels in the palm.
- In the palm they are surrounded by paratenon containing vessels from the palmar arch.

Nutrition:

- Vascular perfusion (vincula).
- Diffusion of nutrients from synovial fluid (predominant system). Diffusion is probably more important within the tendon sheath than vascular perfusion.

Healing: Healing occurs via:

- _Intrinsic:_ depends upon blood flow through long and short vinculae and diffusion of nutrients from synovial fluid proliferation of epitenon cells producing collagen and endotenon.
- _Extrinsic:_ by fibrous attachments forming between tendons sheath and tendon.
- _Histology:_ three overlapping phases of inflammation, proliferation and remodelling. Invasion of white cells with granulation tissue (inflammation). Fibroblasts produce matrix (proliferation). Endotenocytes and epitenocytes migrate into gap. After 6 weeks remodelling occurs with maturation of tissue and realignment of cells.

Flexor tendon repair:

Incisions:

- Incisions commonly incorporate laceration and are extended to enable visualization. Can be Bruner or midlateral.

Retrieval:

- Retrieve through the sheath in the least traumatic manner usually through funnel-shaped incisions in the cruciate pulleys proximal and distal to A4 pulley.
- Core sutures can be placed in each tendon through the closest window to assist retrieval.
- Milk tendon or blind retrieval.
- If it can't be retrieved, incise in the palm for fingers or wrist for FPL. A feeding tube can be used to feed tendon through pulleys.

Suture repair:

- Two types of suture, the core suture and the epitendinous suture.

- The strength of repair is proportional to the number of strands in the core suture. There are multiple methods described for core sutures. The BSSH recommends a 4-strand repair as these have the initial strength to withstand the 20N force required to undergo early active mobilization.
- The epitendinous suture increase strength, decreases bunching (thus promoting glide) and resists gapping. Depth of penetration 1/4 diameter of tendon with 2 mm bites from edge of repair. Common techniques include simple running or locking Silfverskiöld stitches.

Approach to pulleys:

- Differing views with some advocating venting pulleys to facilitate glide with others advocating preservation of pulley system.
- A2 and A4 pulley integrity widely regarded as most important for preventing bowstringing.
- More recent literature (e.g. Jin Bo Tang and others) suggests all of A4 (and A3) can be released if at least part of A2 is preserved, and that all of A2 can be released if other pulleys are preserved.

Post-operative therapy: tensile strength decreases for 7–10 days. A number of regimes used:

- Immobilization—usually reserved for young children.
- Controlled passive motion (Duran and Houser). Wrist and fingers are held in dorsal blocking splint.
- Passive flexion and active extension (Kleinert).
- Early active motion—thought to be advantageous due to accelerating fibroblast proliferation and reducing adhesions. Promotes intrinsic tendon healing over extrinsic. Popular regimes include Belfast and Manchester short splint.

Partial tendon laceration: <60% mobilize without tenorrhaphy.

Outcome measures used:

- Measurements of flexion include: distance from pulp to palm, extension deficit, composite joint flexion, flexion minus extensor lag at each joint. Strickland excludes MCP joint function, which is more dependent on intrinsics and measures flexion at DIP joint and PIP joint minus extension loss.
- Functional assessments—DASH score.
- Patient-reported outcome measures.

Complications:

Early complications:

• Infection.
• Rupture—most likely to occur at day 10 when repair site is weakest.

Late complications:

• Adhesions.
• Tenolysis—6%. 91% within the first year.
• Joint contracture.
• Bowstringing.
• *Quadriga*—due to a common muscle belly, functional shortening of the FDP to small, ring or middle results in restricted flexion of all profundus tendons and weakened grip.

Late reconstruction:

Indications:

• Immediate repair or tendon graft may not be possible if there is significant trauma, infection, delay or failure of previous operation. Pulleys may have been lost.
• New sheath formation by the insertion of a silicone rod, developed by Hunter seems the most effective reconstruction.
• The ring and little finger require full flexion for strong grasp.
• The radial fingers require less flexion as they are used more for pinch.
• The thumb requires a stable post so full flexion is less important.

Tendon grafting: one-stage grafting is indicated for acute trauma with segmental loss, otherwise perform in two stages.

Operation:

• *Choice of motor unit:* contracture of the motor unit which is being replaced may prevent it from being used. A minimum of 2–3 cm amplitude is required. FDS is independent and should be used over FDP if available. FDP needs to be tensioned correctly to prevent the quadriga effect.
• *Donor tendon selection:* PL and *Plantaris*, or toe extensors (*EDL*).
• *First stage:* expose the pulleys in the finger from A1–A5 with Bruner incisions. Remove FDP. Pulley reconstruction may be required. Make a wrist incision and pass a 4-mm Hunter silicone rod through the carpal tunnel then through the pulleys. Suture to periosteum. Suture to FDP in the wrist to help at the second stage. Perform the second stage in 3–4 months.
• *Pulley reconstruction:* use fascia lata, PL or extensor retinaculum. Use a single, double or triple loop encircling the phalanx or attach to volar plate. Double loop will need 10 cm of graft.

• *Second stage:* Harvest tendon and perform Pulvertaft weave to proximal end. Distal the tendon can be attached with a pullout suture or Mitek™ bone anchor. Alternatively, the tendon can be passed through the pulp, tensioned and suture to the nail.

Flexor tendon zones

Zones:

• *I:* insertion of FDS (middle of middle phalanx) to FDP insertion.
• *II:* A1 (distal palmar crease) to FDS insertion (middle of middle phalanx).
• *III:* distal to carpal tunnel to A1 (distal palmar crease).
• *IV:* carpal tunnel.
• *V:* proximal to carpal tunnel.

Thumb also has 5 zones:

• *I:* distal to IPJ.
• *II:* A1 to IPJ.
• *III:* thenar eminence.
• *IV and V:* as above.

Described by Verdan. Zone II was described as 'no man's land' by Bunnell reflecting the historically poor results of tendon repair at this site.

Flexor tenolysis

Indicated if lack of movement is due to excessive scar formation. Adhesions are released followed by intensive hand therapy.

• *Operation:* perform under LA. Expose the sheath, preserve pulleys. Make transverse incisions between pulleys. Release scars to improve ROM. Steroid injection gives a higher rate of rupture. Active mobilization postoperatively.
• *Complications:* tendon rupture. If pulleys significantly damaged then staged reconstruction may be better. *CRPS* will compromise function obtained.

Flip-flap urethroplasty

Described by Mathieu for distal *Hypospadias*.

• Use if no chordee and meatal opening is adequate and if urethral plate flat and narrow and can not be tubularized.
• Use ventral shaft skin to make ventral wall by flipping over with closure over this by glans wings.
• Devine and Horton modified the flip-flap with triple glans flaps. If the native urethra is more proximal, FTSG is used to reconstruct the anterior urethra beyond the limits of the flip-flap.

Floor of mouth cancer

Present around 60 years. Related to smoking and alcohol. The area between tongue and inner surface of mandible. Most are anterior. Tumours may involve Wharton's duct (excretory duct of submandibular gland) causing submandibular gland enlargement. It begins as an inflamed ulcer.

Treatment:
- Small lesions can be treated with surgery or RT. Stenosis of Wharton's duct may lead to submandibular enlargement and confusion with lymphadenopathy.
- If they abut the mandible perform a rim mandibulectomy.
- Advanced lesions require a partial mandibulectomy.
- High incidence of neck disease so >T1 require neck dissection, surgery and RT.

Results:
- Stage I and II lesions have 70–90% 5-year cure rates with excision and interstitial radiotherapy. Large lesions have a much poorer prognosis, ranging from 30 to 60%.
- The overall 5-year survival rate has been reported as 65%.

  See HEAD AND NECK CANCER.

5-Fluorouracil
- Commonly known as Efudix™ cream.
- An analogue of thiamine—inhibits thymidylate synthase leading to cell death.
- Used to treat superficial malignant and pre-malignant skin lesions.
- Applied thinly 1–2 times a day for 3–4 weeks.
- Warn patients that their skin will initially get red and inflamed in the first 2 weeks.

Foetal surgery
Prenatal diagnosis:
- By ultrasound, amniocentesis, umbilical blood sampling and chorionic villus sampling.
- Foetal cleft lip and palate can be diagnosed at 15–20 weeks of gestation.
- Foetal MRI is developing.
- A thorough assessment of all organs is required before a surgical intervention. A careful risk–benefit assessment is required for non-lethal conditions. Also accuracy must be 100%. Some conditions such as clefts are associated with undetectable syndromes.

Maternal risk:
- Particularly in having two GA operations in a short space of time.
- Tocolytics to prevent preterm labour have their risk.
- Pulmonary oedema can occur from magnesium sulphate.

- Hysterotomy can cause uterine rupture.
- There is a potential risk of infertility.

Foetal risk:
- All human subjects have delivered prematurely.
- Seven out of 33 foetuses had neurological injury.

Foetal surgical techniques:
- In experiments with monkeys, surgical procedures were performed through a hysterotomy in the upper segment of the uterus.
- *Open surgery:* US is used to localize placenta. Classic hysterotomy is used. Irrigate the foetus. Restore amniotic fluid with normal saline. Three layer closure to reduce amniotic leak.
- *Foetal endoscopy:* potentially less invasive. Requires CO_2 insufflation as cautery doesn't work in amnion. The magnification allows earlier surgery. It may be useful for clefts, neural tube defects and amniotic bands.
- *Foetal surgical interventions:* performed for diaphragmatic hernia, obstructive uropathy, hydrocephalus.

Foetal indications in plastic surgery: there are presently **no** indications in plastic surgery.

- *Cleft lip and palate:* repair *in utero* may allow scarless healing. A rabbit model has shown good repair with normal midface growth. Endoscopic cleft repair has been performed on a lamb.
- *Craniosynostosis:* the pathology was created by performing a strip craniectomy and inserting demineralized bone matrix to cause fusion. Repair was then performed by excising the area, and the margins were wrapped with Gortex. All had open craniectomy sites.
- *Amniotic band syndrome:* constrictive bands. Lambs had limbs banded and two limbs were released, the other two left banded. The released limbs had normal development, whereas the unreleased limb showed gross changes.
- *Myelomeningocoele:* May be caused by failure of mesoderm migration with exposure and damage to the spinal cord. Lamb models have been performed with latissimus dorsi distally-based flap. Though there was a high mortality, those that survived had near normal neurology.

Foetal wound healing
Scarless *Wound healing* up to the early third trimester. Not all foetal tissues heal without scar. Doesn't follow adult pattern and normal tissue architecture restored by 5–7 days. There are many extrinsic and intrinsic differences.

- In adults, the inflammatory process is orchestrated by the macrophage. In the foetus, there are few inflammatory cells and the healing process is controlled by the foetal fibroblast and epidermis.
- Wound repair occurs by the rapid deposition of type III *Collagen* with a ratio of 3:1, which remains unlike adult wounds where it is replaced with type I.
- The extracellular matrix also differs (ECM). Hyaluronic acid is elevated which aids fibroblast movement and favours scarless healing.
- Fibronectin is rapidly laid down providing a good scaffold for cells.
- Amniotic fluid plays a role, inhibiting foetal and adult fibroblast contraction.
- *Growth factors* differ in foetal wounds. Some, such as TGF-β1, PDGF, bFGF are reduced. TGF-β3 may be increased and have and anti-scarring effect.

Foot: anatomy
Four layers of muscles.

- Flexor digitorum brevis, abductor hallucis, abductor digiti quinti.
- Flexor hallucis longus, flexor accesorius, lumbricals.
- Flexor digiti quinti brevis, flexor hallucis brevis, adductor hallucis.
- Tibialis posterior, peroneus longus, interossei.

Foramen caecum
A blind opening formed between the frontal crest and the crista galli, which sometimes transmits a vein from the nasal cavity to the superior sagittal sinus.
  See DERMOID CYST.

Forced duction test
Detects true entrapment of extraocular muscles e.g. due to orbital fractures (as opposed to weakness of extraocular muscles). Performed by injecting local anaesthetic into conjunctival fornices, grasping inferior rectus tendon with a forceps through the inferior fornix and rotating the globe upwards. Resistance to globe movement indicates mechanical restriction of movement.

Fordyce's spots
See SEBACEOUS HYPERPLASIA. Ectopic sebaceous glands on the vermilion border of the lips and oral mucosa.

Forehead flap
- Commonly used in *Nasal reconstruction*. Described in detail by Menick and considered the gold standard skin coverage for large defects of the nose.

- Forehead is supplied by supraorbital, supratrochlear, infratrochlear and dorsal, nasal and angular vessels.
- A vertically-designed paramedian forehead flap is an axial flap based on the supratrochlear vessels. The raise can be considered in thirds: the distal 1/3 of the flap is raised thinly (skin and subcutaneous fat), the middle 1/3 is raised with frontalis (supraperiosteally) and the proximal 1/3 is raised subperiosteally. The flap can be extended into the scalp with this area thinned and hair bulbs clipped.
- Pedicle can be divided at 3 weeks, but also it can be lifted as a bipedicled flap, attached at ala and still attached to forehead.
- Lateral forehead can be transferred on the unilateral superficial temporal artery.
- Forehead flaps can be expanded or delayed prior to raising.
  See GULLWING FLAP.

Forehead rejuvenation
- *Botulinum toxin:* 1/2 ml is injected into each corrugator. Ask the patient to frown. Palpate the muscle. Mark the injection site that is the medial end of the eyebrow at the supra-orbital rim. Inject at one site only. Paralysis usually lasts 4–6 months.
- *Fat graft*.
- *Transpalpebral corrugator resection:* if there is no ptosis, but significant frown lines, corrugator resection can be performed through the upper eyelid. Corrugator is exposed cephalad to the orbital rim. Nerves are protected. Muscle is removed completely. Procerus is transected if active. Fat is placed in the space.
- *Brow lift*.

Forme fruste
Also called microform *Cleft lip*. Very mild or incomplete cleft lip. May have:

- A kink in the alar cartilage.
- A notch in the vermilion.
- A fibrous band across the lip.

  Management depends on assessment of the vertical lip height:

- If same as non-cleft side can do small procedure to modify the imperfections.
- If difference is >1–2 mm—reconstruction is same as a complete cleft lip but more difficult to get post-operative satisfaction due to marginal gains.

Foucher flap
- A flap based on the first dorsal metacarpal artery and using skin from the radial side of the proximal dorsum of the index finger.

- The dominant branch of the radial artery travels in the base of the anatomic snuff box before giving off terminal branches to the dorsal carpal arch and first dorsal metacarpal artery.
- The first dorsal metacarpal artery courses within the fascia and occasionally within the belly of first dorsal interosseous muscle adjacent to the second metacarpal bone.
- There is an anastomotic communication within the first web space with the palmar vessels.

- Veins run more superficially and venae comitantes run with the artery.
- It can also be raised with the vessel to resurface the thumb.
- Extend the incision proximally, and include superficial veins and fascia overlying first dorsal interosseous muscle.
- This tissue contains the first dorsal metacarpal artery and branches of the radial nerve.
- The flap can be tunnelled to the thumb defect. Particularly useful for dorsal thumb defects to maintain length. Can be used for pulp reconstruction but 2-point discrimination is 12–15 mm so other options may be preferable if available.

See FLAG FLAP. *See* MARUYAMA FLAP.

Four-flap Z-plasty

- Useful for correcting thumb-index web space and axillary contractures.
- Use 90° or 120° angle *Z-plasty*.
- Convert to four flaps by bisecting the angles.
- This produces greater lengthening (124%) with less tension on the flaps.
- Flaps ABCD become CADB (therefore known as the Cadbury Flap).

Fractures: metacarpal and phalangeal

Instability: the primary problem leading to surgery. Leads to displacement. Get angulation, shortening or rotation. Rotation and lateral angulation are poorly tolerated. Shortening and dorsal angulation are better tolerated.

Pathology: an unstable fracture cannot be held in the functional position without fixation. Muscle balance causes dorsal angulation of metacarpal and volar angulation of phalangeal fractures.

Goals: anatomic reduction, stability, early movement.

Free flap science

Anticoagulation: the role has not been clearly defined. There is no definite indication in elective free tissue transfer. It may reduce the risk of anastomotic thrombosis, but will increase the

risk of haematoma. Indicated following re-exploration. Aspirin, dextran and heparin used.

Reperfusion injury: free radicals normally play a role against bacteria. Free radicals accumulate in the free flap when it is devascularized. When a flap is reperfused:

- Endothelial cell damage.
- Endothelial cell swelling.
- Increased capillary permeability.

No-flow phenomenon: failure to perfuse tissue after re-establishing a blood supply. Related to endothelial injury, platelet aggregation, and leakage of intravascular fluid. Relates to ischaemic time.

Occlusion: if arterial the flap is pale with sluggish refill. If venous it will be bluish with a brisk refill.

Vessel healing following anastomosis: platelets are deposited on the injured intima. Pseudointima forms within 5 days. By 2 weeks new endothelium covers the anastomosis. Platelet deposition only leads to fibrin deposition and thrombosis if there is extensive intimal exposure.

Spasm: topical lidocaine may relieve it. Papaverine dilates small vessels (acts as a phosphodiesterase inhibitor increasing levels of cAMP). Epidural and other regional blocks may block sympathetically-mediated spasm.

Management of a non-flowing anastomosis in theatre:

- Apply a vasodilator (lidocaine, papaverine) over the anastomosis.
- Optimize the patient:
  - ○ Ensure warm and well-hydrated;
  - ○ Not receiving vasopressors;
  - ○ Good BP.
- Leave the anastomosis to rest for 15 minutes.
- If still bad:
  - ○ Extrinsic checks:
    - ▪ Twisting/kinking;
    - ▪ Compression.
  - ○ Intrinsic checks:
    - ▪ Vascular Allen's test with micro forceps to assess refill of vessel;
    - ▪ Assess pulse pressure from recipient artery;
    - ▪ Can use Fogarty catheter for thrombectomy of recipient vessels but care not to damage intima.
- With repeated thromboses you can consider thrombolytic therapy.
- With refractory no-flow, disseminated intraflap microthrombosis may have occurred. Consider new free flap.

Post-op monitoring: viability easier to assess with skin-bearing flaps. Assess colour, capillary refill, warmth, turgor. Can check dermal bleeding if diagnostic uncertainty. Surface Doppler also commonly used to monitor although can be misleading if a recipient vessel is nearby. Muscle flaps without a skin paddle can be monitored for all but skin colour/capillary refill. If a skin graft is adherent to the muscle flap it is almost certainly viable. Also fluorescein, implantable Doppler, temperature probes, *Laser Doppler flowometry*, tissue pH, pulse oximetry and direct tissue oxygen measurements.

Free flap salvage

• Assess a patient with a failing free flap:

  o Understand the background, patient factors and flap factors to understand what flap and its function;

  o Assess and optimize the patient to ensure well filled, analgesia and warm;

  o Assess and optimize the flap by release of tight dressings, asses for haematoma and consider releasing stitches.

Operative management: Prepare theatre staff and anaesthetist for potential second free flap. Keep theatre warm and warm fluids:

• Raise flap away from metalwork and near pedicle to gain access.

• Inspect for extrinsic factors leading to compromise:

  o Haematoma and any obvious bleeders— use warm saline to gently wash away;

  o Trace vessels from flap to anastomosis to assess for kinking, twisting or tethering;

  o Anastomosis:

    ▪ Patency of vein anastomosis—is it compressible, is it draining?

    ▪ Patency of arterial anastomosis—is it pulsing, is it filling?

• If problem with the anastomosis identified, take down anastomosis to assess recipient and flap vessels. Can always take out a few stitches to assess flow. Can always use a vein graft or vein loop if recipient vessels are not adequate.

• Consider simplifying the anatomy of the flap by discarding anything that is not essential.

• Consider use of anti-thrombotic to clear the flap. Can inject into an arterial branch (clamp inflow) and can let flow out of vein—you must not allow systemic injection. Then release artery first to allow to flush through the vein:

  o Urokinase 100,000 units in 5 mls of saline—max 400,000 units;

  o Streptokinase 10,000 units–max 60,000 units in 1 hour;

  o Tissue plasminogen activator.

• If an intrinsic problem in the flap (i.e. disseminated intraflap microthrombosis) you cannot do anything—consider second free flap—immediately or temporise wound and do another day.

Free radicals

Atoms or molecules with unpaired electrons in the outer orbit.

French gauge

Measurement for catheters—diameter measured in millimetres.

Frey's syndrome

• Gustatory sweating related to parotid surgery or infection.

• Post-ganglionic parasympathetic nervous system (PNS) secretomotor fibres destined for the parotid hitch-hiking on the auriculotemporal nerve.

• Trauma of parotidectomy divides PNS branches of the nerve which degenerate to the level of the cell bodies in the otic ganglion and regenerate along the auriculotemporal nerve within divided sympathetic nerve fibres to the sweat glands.

• Subsequent eating with activation of the salivation nerves induces sweating in the distribution of the auriculotemporal nerve.

• Incidence is 10–40%.

• Treatment:

  o *Conservative:* antiperspirants;

  o *Medical:* topical scopolamine or 1% glycopyrrolate (paraympatholytic) or Botox™;

  o *Surgical:* re-elevation of skin flap and placing temporalis fascia or dermofat grafts. Jacobsen's tympanic neurectomy of division of preganglionic parasympathetic nerve fibres in middle ear.

Fricke flap

• A flap designed with the base at the lateral canthus and the limb extending above the eyebrow (inferiorly-based). It can be used for lower eyelid reconstruction.

• *Modified Fricke flap:* superiorly based: also for eyelid reconstruction.

Frohse: Arcade of

See RADIAL TUNNEL SYNDROME. A fibrous band on the surface of supinator. One of the structures implicated in compression of the radial nerve at the elbow.

Froment's sign

• In *Ulnar nerve palsy*.

• Pinch between index finger and thumb only achieved with thumb IPJ flexion. Indicates paralysis of first dorsal and second palmar interosseus and adductor pollicis muscles (ulnar nerve innervated), meaning pinch can only be achieved by FPL (median nerve innervated).

Frontal sinus fractures

- 'Le Fort IV' fractures.
- Often associated with other fractures as the force required to fracture the frontal bone is great.
- The frontal sinuses are small in children and really expand from age 7, therefore they are less likely to be involved in children.

- A blow associated with depression of the bone, CSF rhinorrhoea, supra-orbital anaesthesia, crepitus are all suggestive of frontal sinus involvement.
- Complications are due to obstruction of the nasofrontal duct and mucosal tears. Can get meningitis, sinusitis, osteomyelitis and cerebral abscesses.

Symptoms and signs:
- Bruising and swelling.
- Palpable bony step.
- CSF rhinorrhoea.
- Frontal lobe injury.
- Pneumocephalus and orbital emphysema.
- Visual loss.

Management:
- *Conservative:* if undisplaced, no CSF leak, intact posterior wall and unaffected drainage system.
- *ORIF anterior wall:* if displaced anterior wall, no CSF leak, intact posterior wall, unaffected drainage system.
- *ORIF anterior wall and obliteration of frontal sinus:* if displaced fracture, no CSF leak, intact posterior wall, damaged drainage system. Obliteration of frontal sinus is performed by complete removal of nasal lining, followed by spontaneous osteogenesis or bone graft.
- *Cranialization of frontal sinus:* if displaced fracture of anterior wall, CSF leak, minimally displaced fracture of posterior wall. Cranialization is achieved by complete removal of mucosal lining, plugging nasofrontal duct with bone graft, removing posterior wall, allowing brain and dura to expand into the resultant dead space.
- *Cranialization of frontal sinus with dural repair:* if displaced fracture, CSF leak, displaced fracture of posterior wall.

Frontalis
Origin: from epicranial aponeurosis at the anterior hairline.

Insertion: into the dermis of the skin.

Nerve supply: temporal branch of facial nerve.

Action: to elevate the eyebrow.
See BROW LIFT.

Frostbite
- Three types of cold injury are tissue-freezing injury (frostbite), non-tissue freezing injury (trenchfoot, chilblain, pernio) and hypothermia.
- Frostbite occurs when the temperature falls to −2°C resulting in intracellular and extracellular ice crystals and microvascular occlusion.

Chilblain: high humidity and low temperature without freezing, particularly in mountaineers.

Trenchfoot: extremities exposed to a damp environment at temperatures of 1–10°C. Heat is lost as it is wet and vascular flow is poor. Get numbness, tingling, pain and itching. Skin is red and oedematous then grey-blue. Symptoms resolve in 3–6 weeks, but get cold intolerance.

Cold urticaria: urticaria and angio-oedema due to exposure to cold temperatures, especially with aquatic activities. Anaphylaxis may occur. May be familial or acquired.

Aetiology: temperature, wind, humidity, protection and mental state.

Pathophysiology: tissue damage from direct cellular damage or vascular compromise. 3 phases:

- With reduced temperature get peripheral vasoconstriction but periodic cold induced vasodilatation to protect the periphery until the core temperature drops when the peripheral circulation shuts down by closing the A-V shunts.
- Direct cellular trauma by freezing. Intra- and extracellular ice crystals. With rapid cooling get intracellular crystals, which are lethal to the cells unless they are small as in supercooling. With slow cooling get extracellular crystals, and an osmotic gradient with cell dehydration.
- With rewarming there is microvascular damage and a reperfusion injury. Endothelial cell damage leads to oedema and hypoxia. O_2-free radicals are released by neutrophils and thromboxane causes vasoconstriction.

Clinical: 4 degrees, 1 and 2 are superficial, 3 and 4 are deep. Get initial swelling and erythema followed by white waxy skin. With thawing there is vasodilatation with a purple colour, pain and blisters. Oedema in the region with deeper areas developing dry gangrene which demarcates over several weeks.

Treatment:
- Rapid rewarming. Immerse body in water at 40–42°C. Lower temperatures aren't as effective and higher will cause a burn. 15–30

minutes are required to restore core temperature. Painful so provide analgesia: ibuprofen is recommended but aspirin is less useful due to blockade of prostaglandins which may expedite wound healing.

- A number of treatments to improve the circulation have been tried with varying results:
  - Dextran and heparin have been effective in some trials;
  - Streptokinase was significantly beneficial;
  - Recombinant tissue plasminogen activator (r-tPA) is fibrinolytic;
  - Prostaglandin and thromboxane blockers may improve tissue survival.
- Give analgesia. Don't massage. Debride clear blisters, elevate, apply topical thromboxane inhibitor (aloe vera), systemic anti-prostaglandin, tetanus, whirlpool treatment.

Surgery: not in acute management. Relieve constricting eschar. Amputation may be required, but wait until demarcation.

Other treatment: alpha blocker to relieve spasm. Nifedipine for chilblains, heparin and streptokinase.

Late sequelae: arthritis, cold sensitivity, hyperhydrosis.

Fungal hand infections

Most are treated by local or systemic antifungal agents. Surgery is generally not required though *Coccidiomycosis* may cause tenosynovitis, and blastomycosis and brucellosis may cause septic arthritis or osteomyelitis. *Aspergillosis* is an exception, and surgery may be requested to rule out neoplasm.

Furlow technique

- Technique of soft palate reconstruction for management of primary cleft palate and also used as a treatment of *VPI*.
- Double-opposing Z-plasty technique.
- The technique lengthens the soft palate and attempts to place the muscle in a more posterior position.
- A Z-plasty of the oral layer includes the muscle on the posteriorly based flap.
- A Z-plasty of the nasal layer is performed in the opposite direction with the muscle again included on the posterior flap on the opposite side.
- The hard palate can be reconstructed with any chosen technique such as a vomer flap.

Galeazzi fracture to Gynaecomastia

Galeazzi fracture
Fracture dislocation with fracture to the radius shaft and dislocation of the distal radioulnar joint.
See DRUJ.

Gamekeeper's thumb
Chronic attritional change to ulnar collateral ligament in MCPJ of thumb. Name refers to the prevalence of the injury in Scottish game-keepers because of the technique of killing rabbits by twisting the head and neck.

Ganglion
The most common hand mass.

Pathogenesis:
- Herniation of fluid from a joint or tendon sheath. The cyst has a stalk which can be a one- or two-way valve.
- Ligament strain with mucinous degeneration.
- Embryological remnants of synovial tissue.

Site:
- Dorsal wrist ganglia most frequently arise from the articulation of lunate and scaphoid.
- Volar wrist ganglia may be adherent to radial artery and arise from radiocarpal or joint.
- Mucous cysts arise from the DIPJ in association with OA. They may arise from tendon sheath.

Presentation: 20s–40s. F:M 3:1.

Signs and symptoms: Many are asymptomatic or present with a dull ache.

Dorsal wrist ganglia:
- 60–70% of hand ganglia. They arise from the scapholunate ligament (SLL). The pedicle arising from SLL usually emerges between EPL and EDC. Occult SLL ganglia may cause pain by pressure on the SLL. Diagnose with USS.
- *Conservative treatment:* 40% resolve spontaneously. Cysts can be aspirated and injected with sclerosants or steroids.
- *Surgery:* dissect down to the SLL and excise ganglion off SLL. Recurrence rates of up to 40% are reported, so surgery is discouraged for asymptomatic ganglia.

Volar wrist ganglia:
- *20% of hand ganglia:* originates from the scaphotrapezium-trapezoid joint (STT). They pass superficially radial to FCR. They may be attached to radial artery.
- *Treatment:* excision is usually recommended. Aspiration may injure the radial artery.

Flexor sheath ganglia:
- Also called volar retinacular ganglia. 10% of hand ganglia. Occur at the proximal palmar sheath, arising from the A1 pulley. Most commonly in the middle finger.
- *Treatment:* needle rupture and steroid injection can be tried prior to surgery. If resected this is done with a small portion of A1 pulley.

Mucous cyst:
Nuances of management:
- Capsular cysts also called daughter cysts may be a cause for recurrence.
- Ganglions should be traced as far down the stalk as possible and tied off at base.
- After resection some surgeons advise closure of the capsule.
- Arthroscopic excision has been described.
- Carpal ganglia are more difficult to treat and extensive resection may lead to capsular instability.
- Ganglion cysts may arise on the ulnar side of the wrist from the pisohamate joint or TFCC. They can stretch the dorsal branch of the ulnar nerve giving pain.
  See SOFT TISSUE TUMOURS.

Gantzer: accessory muscle of
An accessory belly of *Flexor pollicis longus*, which originates from the coronoid process.

Gardner's syndrome
- Multiple *Epithelial cysts*.
- Polyposis coli.
- Osteomas of the jaw.
- Intestinal desmoid tumours.

Associated with increased risk of desmoid-type fibromatosis.

Garrod's pads
- Benign fibrofatty pads on dorsal aspect of IPJs on digits.
- Associated with _Dupuytren's diathesis_.
- Usually asymptomatic but may be tender.
- Usually treated conservatively.

Gas gangrene
- Similar presentation to _Necrotizing fasciitis_. Characterized by the present of gas in gangrenous tissue and usually caused by exotoxin-producing _Clostridium_ species.
- Patient presents critically unwell with surgical emphysema.
- _Clostridium perfringens:_ is the most common pathogen (Gram-positive bacilli).

Clostridial myonecrosis:
- Seen in _Abdominal_ infections as a post-operative complication.
- Get rapid progression of sepsis with crepitus. Patient is very toxic.
- Polymicrobial with _Clostridium,_ usually _C. oedamatiens or C. septicum._ The most important exotoxin is lecithinase.
- With myonecrosis get a small amount of gas and severe toxicity.

Gastric pull-up
- Surgical procedure used for _Pharynx_ reconstruction.
- Largely replaced by free jejunal transfer or free fasciocutaneous flaps that have less morbidity and mortality.
- May be indicated for reconstruction of a pharyngolaryngeal defect when the inferior end extends into the superior mediastinum and when there are skip lesions.
- The viability of the stomach depends on the preservation of right gastric and right gastroepiploic arteries, as well as the entire gastroepiploic arcade.
- The spleen is left. The left gastric artery and branches are divided. The hiatus is enlarged and the lower oesophagus mobilized. Kocher manoeuvre and pyloromyotomy is performed. The oesophagus is removed by blunt dissection and the stomach passed up and anastamosed to the pharynx.

Gastrocnemius flap
- Proximally-based flap of one head of gastrocnemius useful for soft tissue cover of the knee and upper tibia.
- Loss of one head of gastrocnemius still allows good ankle function due to action of the remaining head and soleus muscle.

- Medial head has a longer reach than the lateral head, as it is longer at its insertion and lateral head has to pass around fibula.
- Fibres of the two may decussate in the midline.
- _Arterial supply:_ Type 1 muscle with dominant branch from the popliteal artery which enters the muscle proximally.

Flap Raise:
- _Position:_ Supine with hip adducted and knee flexed.
- _Landmarks:_ Palpate Longitudinal raphe in the popliteal fossa.
- _Incision:_ a lazy S from medial aspect of popliteal fossa to the midline inferiorly.
- _Raise:_ medial head of gastrocnemius:
  - Incise down to muscle—identify lesser saphenous vein and sural nerve and retract laterally;
  - Incise the midline raphe and locate the pedicle and trace under the muscle;
  - Divide muscle proximally first around the pedicle so it is protected whilst the muscle is tensioned. Then divide distal end.
- Close in layers.

Gastroschisis
- A full thickness congenital defect of abdominal wall, which occurs lateral to the umbilical ring usually on the right side with cord in the normal position.
- The viscera are not covered by amnion. The bowel is not rotated and the midgut is short with a small peritoneal cavity. It lacks a covering sac and the intestines are usually matted and shortened.
- Mortality usually from sepsis, respiratory insufficiency and a prolonged ileus.
- 20–25% of patients with gastroschisis and omphalocoele have intestinal atresia, malrotation and volvulus.

Treatment: primary closure if it doesn't produce too high intra-abdominal pressure. Otherwise slowly close on Teflon sheets.
See ABDOMINAL WALL RECONSTRUCTION.

Giant cell tumour of bone
- Found in long bones. 50% occur around the knee.
- In the upper limb, it is most commonly found in the distal radius. In the hand, they are mainly in the phalanges.
- 1/3 are aggressive stage 3 lesion with cortical breakthrough and a soft tissue component.
- 5% of patients develop lung metastasis.
- Excision frequently leads to local recurrence.

XR: expansile eccentric radiolucent lesion involving epiphysis and subchondral bone of distal radius. Cortex thinned with sclerotic margin. May get pathological fracture.

Histology: numerous giant cells.

Differential diagnosis: chondroblastoma, non-ossifying fibroma, brown tumour, fibrosarcoma, osteogenic sarcoma.

Treatment: curettage with adjuvants such as polymethylmethacrylate cement, liquid nitrogen or phenol, +/- bone grafting. Vascularized fibular graft.

See BONE TUMOURS.

Giant cell tumour (PVNS)
Also call pigmented villonodular tenovaginosynovitis (PVNS).

- Benign soft tissue tumour seen over the palmar aspect of the fingers which slowly increase in size.
- Firm, nodular and maybe mobile.
- Treatment is excisional biopsy.
- Recurrence rate of 10-30%.
- Commonly occur in middle-aged women.
- They occur along tendon sheaths and other sites where synovial fluid is formed.

See SOFT TISSUE TUMOURS.

Giant condyloma acuminatum
- A fungating growth usually on the prepuce of an uncircumcised male.
- Locally destructive and may transform to a verrucous *SCC*.
- Frequently mistaken for condyloma (viral wart) and verrucous SCC.
- It probably has a viral origin.
- Recurrence is common following excision.

Gibson's principle
Of interlocking stress: Cartilage moves away from the scored surface.

See PROMINENT EAR CORRECTION.

Gillies fan flap
- Used for *Lip reconstruction*.
- Fan-shaped rotational advancement flap based on the superior labial artery, for defects over 50% of lower lip.
- Flap made around nasolabial fold with 1 cm back-cut.
- Extended version of the *Estlander flap*.

Gillies lift
- Used in the treatment of *Zygomatic fractures*.
- For reduction of displaced fractures of the zygomatic arch.
- Make a radial incision above and anterior to the ear. Deepen through temporoparietal fascia (superficial temporal fascia). Incise the deep temporal fascia and insert a Gillies elevator between it and temporalis muscle. This leads under the zygomatic arch. Elevate the fracture by lifting. Pivoting the elevator on temporal bone may result in a secondary fracture.

Gillick competence
- Competence of a child below aged 16 to consent for a medical procedure if they have sufficient understanding and intelligence.
- Children from 13 years of age can consent to treatment (but cannot refuse it) if they are considered Gillick competent.
- Following case of Gillick vs West Norfolk and Wisbeth Health Authority 1985.

Gilula's lines
Two parallel, smooth, curved lines on AP XR made by the proximal and distal carpal row. Disruption can indicate dislocation or fracture of the carpus.

Glasgow Coma Scale
- Eye opening (1-4):
  - *1:* none;
  - *2:* to pain;
  - *3:* to speech;
  - *4:* spontaneously.
- Best verbal response (1-5):
  - *1:* none;
  - *2:* incomprehensible sound;
  - *3:* inappropriate words;
  - *4:* confused;
  - *5:* orientated.
- Best motor response (1-6):
  - *1:* none;
  - *2:* pain extension;
  - *3:* pain flexion;
  - *4:* pain withdrawal;
  - *5:* pain—localizes;
  - *6:* obeys command.

Highest score 15.
Lowest score 3.

Glioma
- Nasal gliomas are uncommon, smooth, non-compressible masses present at birth or early childhood. Either extra- or intranasal.
- Lack of change in size with crying distinguishes it from an encephalocoele.
- If extranasal it may penetrate the bone in the frontonasal suture area and may have a broadened nasal root.
- Intranasal gliomas present with nasal airway obstruction.
- Need imaging prior to excision.

Glomus body

A glomus body is an arteriovenous anastomosis in the reticular layer of the dermis involved in thermoregulation. Glomus bodies are numerus in the fingers and toes.

Glomus tumour

- Benign vascular hamartomatous derivative of the glomus body—a normal intradermal arteriovenous anastomosis that arises from the normal neuromyoarterial glomus.
- Derived from smooth muscle cells and are usually solitary, occurring in nail bed and less commonly on the pulp. They can occur at other sites.
- *Presentation:* usually present in adults. They are tender blue-red 1–2 mm papules. The lesions may be single or multiple and most characteristically occur on the hands and feet, especially subungually. Glomus tumours have also been reported on the face.
- *Signs and symptoms:* they are very painful and sensitive to temperature change. *Hildreth sign* (pain relief on application of a tourniquet proximally) is considered pathognomonic. Also assess with *Love's sign*.
- *Treatment:* of symptomatic lesions requires complete excision, which dramatically relieves the severe episodes of pain. Subungual, highly sensitive lesions may be small and difficult to locate visibly but can be detected on MRI.
- Multiple glomus tumours are inherited as autosomal dominant with incomplete penetrance. They develop 10–15 years earlier than solitary tumours. Pain is not as severe as in solitary glomus tumours. They can present as regional, disseminated or congenital plaque-like.
- *Haemangiopericytoma* may resemble a painless glomus tumour.

  See FAMILIAL GLOMANGIOMATOSIS.

Glossectomy

- Most commonly required for *Tongue carcinoma*.
- Tongue mobility is important for speech and food propulsion.
- With partial glossectomy, the goal of reconstruction is to preserve mobility, restore shape and volume and sensation. Need adequate bulk and mobility.
- If >30% of the tongue remains, a thin, pliable flap e.g. radial forearm flap is used to keep the tongue mobile. It can also be made sensate. It is useful for tongue and floor of mouth as a sulcus can be created.
- If less tongue remains, a bulkier flap is used such as the anterolateral thigh flap or

rectus abdominis flap to fill dead space. Sometimes there is too much bulk in these flaps, in which case skin and fat is excised leaving just muscle which can be grafted or left to re-epithelialize.

- Midline posterior tumours which require total glossectomy may be treated by brachytherapy to reduce the debilitating nature of the surgery.

Gluteal flap

- Can be a muscle flap (type III) or a fasciocutaneous flap.
- Useful for sacral pressure sores as a pedicled or rotation flap, if surgical reconstruction indicated.
- Free fasciocutaneous SGAP or IGAP perforator flaps can be used in breast reconstruction.

Blood supply: superior (SGAP) or inferior (IGAP) gluteal artery (terminal branches of internal iliac artery). Pass out of pelvis by passing above and below the piriformis muscle

Flap raise for sacral pressure sore:

- Position: prone.
- Landmarks:
  - Posterior Superior Iliac Spine (PSIS);
  - Ischial tuberosity;
  - Greater trochanter;
  - Coccyx.
- Perforators: confirm with doppler:
  - SGAP: junction of medial/middle third of line between PSIS and greater trochanter;
  - IGAP: junction of middle/inferior third of line between PSIS and ischial tuberosity.
- Markings: wide arc for rotation.
- Flap raise:
  - Incise down to muscle;
  - Undermine flap. Keep at least one of SGAP or IGAP.

Gluteus maximus rotation flap:

- As above, but raise in plane between gluteus maximus and medius.
- Divide origin from ilium to rotate into defect. If arc of rotation limited by superior gluteal vessels, these can be divided.

  See RECONSTRUCTION. See PRESSURE SORES.

Gluteus maximus

Origin: lateral sacrum and posterior superior iliac crest.

Insertion: greater trochanter of femur. Rotates and extends the hip.

Blood supply: type III muscle with two dominant pedicles—superior and inferior gluteal arteries.

Nerve supply: superior and inferior gluteal nerves. The inferior is more dominant.

See MUSCLE.

Gold

Gold is resistant to corrosion, but has a low tensile strength. It is used primarily as an upper-eyelid weight to facilitate eye closing in *Facial palsy*. *See* ALLOPLASTS.

Goldenhar syndrome

Craniofacial microsomia associated with epibulbar ocular dermoids and vertebral anomalies. Occurs in less than 5% of craniofacial microsomia.

Gorlin syndrome

Also called basal cell naevus syndrome.

- Get multiple basal cell naevi with malignant change to *Basal cell carcinoma* by puberty. The naevi are reddish brown and papular.
- Autosomal dominant though 20–30% are due to *de novo* mutations.
- Traced to a mutation in a suppressor gene located at 9q23.1–q31—the Patched gene (PTCH).
- Also jaw cysts (adontogenic keratocysts), pitting of the palm and soles, calcification of the falx cerebri by 20 years of age, pseudohypertelorism, frontal bossing, syndactyly and spina bifida.

GOSLON index

- Developed by Michael Mars to assess malocclusion in patients born with a unilateral cleft lip and palate in late mixed and early permanent dentition. Assesses anteroposterior, vertical and transverse relationships of jaws.
- Five models of malocclusion were made based on previous patients. These were graded 1–5. Dental models are assessed by this yardstick and graded.
- Grades 1-2 indicate a favourable occlusion whereas Grades 4–5 indicate maxillary retrusion and are more likely to require orthognathic surgery.
- *Advantage:* patients scored in early permanent dentition phase when skeletal and occlusal problems are evident.
- *Disadvantages:* raters must be trained and calibrated to ensure standardization and patients must be at least 10 years old, so may have had orthodontic treatment or alveolar bone graft. Only tested on a cohort with unilateral cleft lip and palate, so may not be applicable to patients born with bilateral clefts.

Gout

- M:F 8:1.
- High levels of uric acid with precipitation of sodium urate in the joint.

Aetiology:

- *Primary hyperuricaemia:* increased dietary intake (red wine and meat), enzyme abnormalities.
- *Secondary hyperuricaemia:* is caused by diuretics and myeloproliferative disorders.

Acute gout:

- Painful synovitis.
- 90% of attacks are self-limiting.
- 60% are of 1st MTPJ. It can involve wrists and fingers.
- *Tophi:* deposits of sodium urate in joints and periarticular tissues. With chronic gout get extra-articular deposits.

Diagnosis:

- Identification of monosodium urate monohydrate crystals by polarized light microscopy.
- High uric acid levels are not diagnostic.
- Most patients with hyperuricaemia do not have gout.
- XR show punched-out erosions away from the joint margin.

Treatment:

- *Acute:* high-dose NSAIDs, colchicine.
- *Chronic:* low-purine diet, allopurinol (xanthine oxidase inhibitor), probenecid (uricosuric drug).

See PSEUDOGOUT.

Gracilis

Origin: inferior margin of symphysis pubis, inferior ramus of pubis and adjacent ramus of ischium.

Insertion: medial surface of tibial shaft, posterior to sartorius.

Action: flexes knee, adducts thigh and medially rotates tibia on femur.

Nerve supply: anterior division of obturator nerve.

Blood supply: medial circumflex femoral artery from profunda femoris.

See MUSCLE.

Gracilis flap

Thin strap-shaped muscle with consistent pedicle. Minimal morbidity. Donor site can be closed. Can be innervated by including the anterior branch of obturator nerve. Can be used for facial re-animation.

Blood supply:
- Dominant supply is the medial circumflex femoral artery from the profunda femoris.
- The pedicle runs from medial to lateral entering the under surface of the muscle 10–12 cm inferior to the pubic tubercle.
- A 6-cm pedicle length can be achieved in adults.

Flap raise:
- *Position:* supine, thigh abducted and knee flexed.
- *Identify landmarks:*
  - Pubic symphysis;
  - Adductor longus.
- *Mark:* axis of muscle (2-3 fingers breadth behind and parallel to adductor longus) and position of perforator (10cm inferior to pubic symphysis). May need a second small incision over insertion in knee if whole length of muscle needed.
- *Raise:*
  - Incise down to muscle and locate septum between gracilis and adductor longus. Identify pedicle and nerve proximal to it. There will be a large branch going up into adductor longus;
  - Free muscle of all attachments. Detach proximal end first whilst tensioned so as not to injure pedicle. Then detach distal end;
  - If using as a functioning muscle flap, before dividing, place muscle under maximum physiological stretch and mark every 5 cm with a suture.
- Wound closed in layers over a drain.

Graft

Tissue that is separated completely from the donor bed. It depends on the ingrowth of vessels from the recipient bed for survival.
- *Autograft:* tissue transplanted within the same individual.
- *Isograft:* a graft exchanged between genetically identical individuals.
- *Allograft:* graft exchanged between genetically different individuals.
- *Xenograft:* interspecies graft.
- *Orthotopic:* transplant is transferred into an anatomically similar site.
- *Heterotopic:* transplant is transferred into a different site from its origin.

Granular cell myoblastoma
- Uncertain origin, but may come from Schwann cell sheath.
- Most common in 40–60 years in dark skin.

- 1/3 are on the tongue, 1/2 are on the head and neck.
- Usually solitary.
- Treatment is excision.

See MESODERMAL TUMOURS.

Granulation tissue
- The tissue underlying a healing wound consisting of inflammatory cells, capillary loops and fibroblasts. It is collagen-rich connective tissue with a plentiful blood supply that serves as a bed for tissue repair. Soft to touch and moist.
- The extracellular matrix (ECM) of granulation tissue is formulated by fibroblasts. Initially the structure is type III collagen (as this can be rapidly produced by the fibroblasts)— this is later replaced by the standard type I collagen.
- In ischemic wounds, contraction of the granulation tissue is impaired due to faulty myofibroblasts.

Grayson's ligaments
- Present in the digits, these fibres pass transversely from the volar aspect of the flexor tendon to the skin.
- They lie in the same plane as the natatory ligament.
- They form the palmar wall of the compartment through which the neurovascular bundle passes and prevents them from bowstringing.
- They also stabilize the palmar skin in grasp.
- They form part of the spiral cord in *Dupuytren's contracture*.

See CLELAND'S LIGAMENT.

Great auricular nerve

Branch of cervical plexus. Emerges from behind sternocleidomastoid 6.5 cm below tragus. It supplies sensation to the inner and outer aspect of lower half of ear.

Groin flap
- Type B (i.e. solitary perforator) *Cormack-Lamberty* fasciocutaneous flap.
- Fed medially by the superficial circumflex iliac artery and the superficial inferior epigastric artery and laterally from the deep circumflex iliac artery. Many variations in this configuration.
- The donor site is well hidden. Flaps up to 15 cm wide can be harvested. The flap is fairly thin and hairless. Good for the dorsum of the hand and thumb web space. However, the pedicle length is short.

Flap Raise:

- *Position:* supine.
- *Identify landmarks:*
  - Sartorius muscle;
  - Inguinal ligament;
  - Anterior superior iliac spine (ASIS).
- *Identify pedicle with doppler:* 1 finger breadth below the inguinal ligament.
- *Markings:* draw skin paddle over the inguinal ligament—ensure it can close by using a skin pinch test.
- *Raise:*
  - Incise in the superolateral portion first down to deep fascia—at ASIS, identify the sartorius and potentially the lateral femoral cutaneous nerve as it exits the deep fascia to become superficial—may need to be transected if involved in flap;
  - Sartorius is key—when reached, the dissection needs to proceed deep to fascia overlying the sartorius—the pedicle will be in this fascia and you will need to ligate any branches going into the muscle;
  - Follow the pedicle to the origin (either femoral or external iliac vessels).
- Close defect primarily (after undermining of skin if required).

Groin lymph node dissection

- Superficial lymph node dissection (LND) removes a block of tissue below the inguinal ligament in the femoral triangle.
- Radical groin LND involves division of the inguinal ligament with proximal dissection and possibly retroperitoneal dissection to the obturator-ilial, hypogastric and para-aortic nodes.
- Operation:
  - *Position:* supine;
  - *Incision:* lazy S longitudinal at midpoint of inguinal ligament. Raise skin flaps beneath superficial fascia and preserve lateral femoral cutaneous nerve;
  - *Define borders of femoral triangle:* medial border of sartorius, medial border of adductor longus and inguinal ligament;
  - *Identify vessels:* skeletonize femoral artery and vein. Secure saphenous vein by double ligation at saphenofemoral function;
  - Removal of superficial lymph node contents including Cloquet's node;
  - *Closure:* in layers over a drain.

Growth factors

Polypeptides whose primary role is cell maturation. Involved with cytokines in wound healing and host defence.

See CYTOKINES.

Gullwing flap

- Design of *Forehead flap* for larger defects of the nasal tip, infratip and lobule designed by Millard.
- Transverse extensions are created on the standard paramedian flap. These can be used to cover extensive bilateral lobular defects.
- The donor site frequently can be closed primarily.

See NASAL RECONSTRUCTION.

Gunshot wounds

- Degree of injury depends on mass and speed.
- Kinetic energy = mass $\times$ velocity^2/2G. Doubling the velocity squares the kinetic energy.
- Low-energy deposits travel at <1,000 feet/second and include hand guns.
- Shotgun pellets have a larger mass so are intermediate. They travel at 1,200 feet/second.

Gustilo-Anderson score

Scoring system for open lower limb fractures. Wounds can only be classified after definitive wound excision and debridement. High inter-observer variability but commonly used as simple to remember and communicate.

- *I:* wound <1 cm, minimal muscle contusion, simple fracture.
- *II:* wound >1 cm, moderate soft tissue injury and stripping.
- *IIIA:* high energy, segmental or highly comminuted fracture, wound >10 cm, extensive soft tissue injury but adequate soft tissue coverage of bone.
- *IIIB:* as above but without adequate soft tissue coverage of bone. Requires flap coverage or amputation.
- *IIIC:* any fracture with associated vascular injury. Requires emergent exploration with a view to repair neurovascular structures as well as debridement, wound excision and skeletal stabilization.

See LOWER LIMB RECONSTRUCTION. *See* BYRD CLASSIFICATION.

Guyon's canal

- The tunnel through which the *Ulnar nerve* and artery passes across the wrist.
- It begins at the level of the proximal edge of the wrist.

- Transverse carpal ligament and pisohamate ligament forms floor, the volar carpal ligament the roof and the pisiform and FCU the ulnar wall. The radial wall is formed by the hook of the hamate.
- The ulnar artery is radial to the nerve in the canal.
- To release the tunnel, use carpal tunnel incision. Incise more distally to find the superficial palmar arch. Follow the ulna branch, which will lead to ulnar nerve.

Gynaecomastia

- Excessive development of male breasts.
- No relationship with breast cancer.
- *Idiopathic* occurs in newborns (due to the transplacental passage of oestrogens), pubertal boys and adult men.
- Gynaecomastia may be unilateral, bilateral or asymmetrical. Usually asymptomatic.

Examination:
- *Breasts:* thickened breast tissue, if irregular mass suspect carcinoma.
- *Testes:* if small, perform chromosome study. If asymmetric, look for tumour.
- *Liver:* hepatomegaly, ascites.
- *Thyroid* enlargement, *nutritional status.*

Aetiology: due to the increase in effective oestrogen-testosterone ratio.

- *Physiological:* newborn—60%, puberty—64% and old age—30%.
- *Pathology:* cirrhosis, malnutrition, hypogonadism, Klinefelter's, neoplasm (testicular, adrenal, pituitary, lung), renal, hyperthyoidism, hypothyroidism.
- *Pharmacological—mnemonic:* some (spironolactone) men (marijuana) can (cimetidine) develop (diazepam) rather (reserpine) excessive (oestrogens) thoracic (theophylline) diameters (digoxin).

Resolution: gynaecomastia of puberty often regresses spontaneously within 2 years.

Drug-related gynaecomastia may regress after cessation of drug.

Pseudo gynaecomastia: increased breast size due to fat deposition.

Medical treatment: most effective during the active proliferative phase.

- Testosterone used for gynaecomastia secondary to testicular failure.
- Tamoxifen for middle-aged men.
- Danazol is a gonadotrophin inhibitor and reduces the pain and extent of gynaecomastia.

Indication for surgery: for adolescent males with enlargement for over 18 months, symptomatic patients with fibrotic gynaecomastia, risk of carcinoma (e.g. Klinefelter's).

Classification: by *Simon.*

Surgical technique:
- *Grade 1–2:* excise breast tissue through semi-circular areola incision (Webster) or transverse incision in axilla.
- *Grade 2–3:* skin resection is necessary with nipple transposition based on a superior pedicle. The nipple can be raised on a dermal bipedicled attachment and a horizontal extension either side to resect skin. Skin can be excised with a circumareolar incision or a Lejour vertical incision procedure can be performed.
- *Grade 3:* in massive gynaecomastia skin and breast tissue is excised and free nipple grafting performed. The graft is placed over the fifth rib.
- *Liposuction:* used in conjunction with surgery. Most successful with fatty breasts. Often leave a nubbin of firm breast tissue if used alone. Ultrasound assisted liposuction increases the scope for liposuction without open surgery.

Complications: haematoma, seroma, nipple necrosis, nipples adherent to fascia if too much tissue resected.

Haber's syndrome

Familial variant of _Bowen's disease_ with rosacea-like eruption of the face and Bowen's lesions on the covered areas of the body.

Haemangioma

Congenital:

- Present fully formed at birth.
- Less common than infantile haemangioma and do not tend to proliferate as rapidly. Large lesions can cause high-output cardiac failure.
- GLUT1-negative.
- Can be categorized as:
  - RICH—rapidly involuting congenital haemangioma;
  - NICH—non-involuting haemangioma.

Infantile:

- A benign vascular tumour, which typically has rapid growth followed by involution.
- Usually appear in the first couple of weeks of birth.
- 10% have multiple lesions. Consider liver involvement.
- F:M 3:1.
- Cells often have oestrogen receptors and grow with hormonal changes.
- Haemangiomas are more commonly seen in Caucasians.

Pathology:

- GLUT1-positive.
- Mast cells containing prostaglandins and leukotrienes are present.
- Each lesion is supplied by a single afferent arterial vessel. Regression occurs with thrombosis of the feeder vessels. Outflow is by multiple veins.
- The behaviour is variable, though when there is association with tissue, such as lymphohaemangiomas, they are less likely to resolve.

Natural history:

- Proliferating phase (0–1 year). See rapid division of endothelial cells. Upregulated angiogenesis thought to be driven by VEGF and FDF expression.

- Involuting phase (1–5 years). See decreased proliferation, increasing apoptosis and fibrofatty replacement. Suppressed angiogenesis by TIMP-1.
- Involuted phase (>5 years)—50% have involuted by age 5, 70% by age 7 with no change after age 12. In general, normal skin is restored in 50% patients.
- 10% ulcerate (most common complication)—usually the very large ones in the proliferating phase.

Differential diagnosis:

- Port-wine stain, AVM, _Pyogenic granulomas_, _Tufted angiomas_.
- A deep haemangioma can be confused with a lymphatic malformation and USS or MRI will differentiate.

Associated malformations: there are some rare associations.

- A large cervicofacial haemangioma may be accompanied by ocular abnormalities (microphthalmia, congenital cataract, optic nerve hypoplasia).
- Also other conditions such as sternal non-union, supraumbilical raphe.
- _Cutaneovisceral malformations:_ seen where there are multiple cutaneous haemangiomas, particularly intrahepatic. The baby may present with congenital cardiac failure (CCF), anaemia and hepatomegaly. Tumours may also occur in the GI tract and CNS. Babies may also get CCF from a large solitary cutaneous or intrahepatic haemangioma.

Complications:

- _Ulceration:_ most common complication.
- _Bleeding and thrombocytpenia:_ may result from platelet-trapping coagulopathy—_Kasabach–Merritt syndrome._
- Infection.
- _Visual obstruction:_ upper eyelid haemangioma can cause amblyopia and failure to develop binocular vision. Can also deform the cornea and produce astigmatism. This can occur with even a small haemangioma.

- *Airway or luminal obstruction:* beware haemangioma in the 'beard distribution'.
- *Cardiovascular decompensation:* A–V shunting leading to high-output congestive heart failure. Also with multiple lesions. Symptoms usually develop within 2–8 weeks.
- Skeletal distortion.

Examination:
- Lesion characteristics—site, size, colour, complicated (ulcer, bleeding, infection).
- Involvement of organs—airway and eyes.
- Evidence of systemic involvement—multiple lesions, hepatomegaly, sacral region.

Investigation:
- Serial clinical photos.
- USS—soft tissue mass with fast-flow, decreased arterial resistance and increased venous drainage.
- MRI—T1 = isodense tumour and T2 = hyperdense tumour.

Treatment:
- 90% will not need intervention and can be managed with observation only. Ulceration and infections can most commonly be treated with wound care and dressings.
- *Pharmacological:*
  - Oral propranolol (non-selective beta-blocker) inhibits noradrenaline release and induces apoptosis leading to accelerated involution. Originally described in NEJM 2008 at 2mg/Kg/day but follow local guidance with paediatric and cardiology input. Usually started at 4 months of age and continued for entire proliferating phase to prevent rebound. Side effects include hypoglycaemia, bronchospasm, hypotension, hypothermia;
  - Topical timolol (beta-blocker) for superficial haemangiomas where systemic propranolol is contraindicated;
  - Steroids. May be indicated to manage life-threatening haemangiomas in the beard-distribution around the airway.
- *Minimally invasive:*
  - Laser—for telangiectasia following involution.
- *Surgical:*
  - Proliferating phase—if haemangioma obstructing structures (eyes, airway) or for control of bleeding;
  - Reconstructive surgery to improve disfiguring fibrofatty residual tissue should be delayed to involuted phase if possible and may require a staged approach.

See VASCULAR MALFORMATIONS. *See* SALMON PATCH.

Haemangiopericytoma
- Rare vascular tumour originating from pericytes.
- May resemble a *Glomus tumour*.
- May grow up to 10 cm in size.
- Treatment is excision.

Haines–Zancolli test
- Test for *Oblique retinacular ligament* tightness.
- Flexion of DIPJ is limited when PIPJ is in extension due to tension in ORL.

Hair
Three types:
- *Lanugo hair:* soft and fine, unpigmented and without a medulla. It is found on the foetus and is usually shed by the 8th month of gestation.
- *Vellus hair:* soft and unmedullated. Short, rarely exceeding 2 cm in length and may be pigmented. It replaces lanugo hair in the postnatal period and is spread over the entire body surface.
- *Terminal hair:* longer, coarser, pigmented and medullated. It replaces vellus hair at specific sites.
- Bald scalp has normal number of hair follicles though they are smaller and the hair is absent.
- The average scalp contains more than 1 million hair follicles with 100,000 terminal hairs. 90% are in anagen (growing) phase lasting 1,000 days and 10% are in telogen (resting) phase lasting 100 days. Humans shed 50–100 hairs a day.

Hair anatomy
- A pilosebaceous unit consists of a hair follicle, a sebaceous gland and an arrector pili muscle.
- Each hair shaft has a medulla, cortex and outer cuticle. The shaft cuticle is encased in the inner root sheath (derived from epidermis) which shapes the hair as it grows. Finally, the outer root sheath (derived from dermis) encases the entirety.
- The hair follicle consists of the infundibulum in the upper portion from the epidermal surface to the opening of the sebaceous duct, the isthmus centrally to the arrector pili muscle and the bulb inferiorly to the base of the follicle.
- Several sebaceous glands drain into each follicle. Discharge from these glands is aided by contraction of erector pili muscles.
- The living cells at the base of the hair follicle show active mitotic growth. A zone of keratinization forms above the dividing cells. The cells become dehydrated and are converted to a mass of keratin. The keratin filaments are cemented together by a matrix rich in cystine.

Hair growth

- Anagen—growth phase lasting 3–10 years. Rapid cell division occurs in the hair bulb. 90% of hair is in this phase at any one time.
- Catagen—transition phase lasting 2–3 weeks.
- Telogen—resting phase lasting 2–3 months during which hairs are shed.

Hair restoration with flaps

Classification: *Juri*. Also Norwood classification.

Scalp reduction flaps:

- *Advancement flaps:* multiple procedures are necessary. Most create undesirable scars.
- *Bilateral occipitoparietal flaps (BOP):* useful for vertex balding. There is extensive undermining of the hair-bearing scalp. It will remove a width of bald scalp of 5–8 cm from the vertex. The superficial temporal artery should be Dopplered and protected as it will provide the majority of the blood supply. The whole scalp is mobilized to the nape of the neck and to the ear. It is advanced and the overlapping tissue is excised. Excessive tension may lead to necrosis. This is repeated several times often with hair transplantation. Some surgeons delay the flap by first ligating the occipital arteries.
- *Bitemporal flaps:* for midline alopecia but often performed 3 months after BOP flap to complete the excision.

Random flaps:

- *Temporoparietal short flap:* this is not delayed and narrower than the Juri flap and aims to create half of a frontal hairline. The larger delayed flap may give better results.
- *Nataf flap:* superiorly based to maintain natural hair direction and delayed. It rarely reaches the midline.

Temporoparieto-occipital flaps: *Juri flap:* 4 cm wide, based on the superficial temporal artery. It is long enough to extend across the entire width of the bald forehead. It uses 2 de-lays. The first cuts the superior and inferior border. After 1 week the distal quarter of flap is raised. The occipital vessels are divided. One week later the flap is transposed.

Scalp expansion: the advantage is to be able to move more tissue with tension free closures. It does, however, take more time with a cosmetic deformity for the duration of treatment, and hair follicles will be more widely spaced.

Hair transplantation

Hair transplantation is the most common cosmetic procedure performed on men for male pattern baldness (MPB) and is based on the principle of donor dominance. If a graft is taken from an area destined to be permanently hair-bearing, and is transplanted into an area of MPB or future MPB, it will continue to grow hair in its new site for as long as it would have in its original one.

Classification: *See* JURI.

Operations:

- *Grafts:*
  - *Micrografts:* one or two hair grafts are sectioned from larger grafts or strip grafts and placed in holes created by 16–18-gauge needles;
  - *Minigrafts:* harvested using a trephine, scalpel or laser and sectioned into smaller grafts containing 3–6 hairs and can be round, linear or square; size is <2 mm;
  - *Standard grafts:* round or square containing 8–30 hairs, harvested with a trephine;
  - *Strip grafts:* more than 10 mm in length;
  - *Follicular unit grafts:* 1–5 hairs, each graft consists of a single hair follicle;
- *Planning:* design and placement are crucial. The hairline should not be placed too low as it will look unnatural in later years.
- *Recipient area:* with mini- and micrografts, smaller spaces are left between grafts leaving a more natural result. However, increased density is sacrificed for decreased detectability. Mini-slits can be made and they should be at the correct angulation.
- *Graft preparation and insertion:* the graft is kept moist. The strip is sectioned with the blade parallel to the follicles. Glue helps to keep them in place.
- *Scalp reduction:* this can be performed before or between hair transplantation procedures. This can be accompanied by prolonged acute tissue expansion where an expander is placed and inflated and deflated over 2 hours, thus allowing 200% more tissue removal.

Halo naevus

- Benign skin lesion characterized by a depigmented halo around a *Naevus*, thought to be due to immune-mediated destruction of nevus cells.
- May be mistaken for a melanoma with halo-like depigmentation that has undergone regression.
- Halo naevi typically occur on the back of young adults and children (mean age 15 years) and are exaggerated by a suntan.

- It is associated with atopic dermatitis and autoimmune disorders such as vitiligo and thyroid disease.
- Evaluate with dermatoscope. Most can be managed conservatively but excision biopsy if any doubt.

Hamartoma
- Congenital malformations consisting of normal tissue found in excessive amount or in abnormal relationship with surrounding structures. The cells usually retain normal histology and function. Malignant degeneration may occur.
- *Ectodermal hamartomas:* also called *Naevi*.
- *Neuroectodermal hamartomas:* arise from the neural crest. Two primary disorders—*Neurofibromatosis* and *Melanocytic naevi*.
- *Mesodermal hamartomas: Vascular malformations*.
- *Mixed origin hamartomas: Dermoid cyst*, Nasal gliomas, Frontonasal encephalocoeles.

Hamate fracture
Uncommon, 3 types.
- *Body:* direct trauma. Also part of axial carpal instability injury.
- *Hook:* direct injury in golf or racket sports, or avulsion by the TCL by falling on the outstretched hand. May get non-union that requires excision or bone grafting and fixation.
- *Marginal fractures:* associated with fracture dislocation of ring and little metacarpals.

Hamate hook
Find hook by deep palpation over tip of hamular process in the palm by the examiner's thumb with dorsal/ulnar pressure with index and middle finger. Slide finger 2 cm distal from pisiform to locate hamular process. Running along the ulnar aspect of the base of the hook is the motor branch of the ulnar nerve. This can be injured in hook fractures. Usually the sensory portion is unaffected.

Harlequin deformity
The characteristic XR findings in unicoronal synostosis. Ipsilateral elevation of the lesser wing of sphenoid causes an elevation of the superolateral orbit. *See* CRANIOSYNOSTOSIS.

Harris–Benedict equation
- An equation to calculate daily calorie needs based on basal metabolic rate.
- Equation includes sex, age, weight and height.

- Can be adjusted by multiplying by 1.5 to calculate calorie requirements in the burn patient.
- This method may well underestimate the caloric requirement for a given patient. In contrast, the *Curreri formula* may overestimate caloric needs.

See BURNS.

Harvold classification
For *Craniofacial microsomia*.
- *Ia:* classic type with unilateral facial underdevelopment.
- *Ib:* Ia with microphthalmos.
- *Ic:* bilateral asymmetrical type.
- *Id:* complex type, which doesn't fit Ia–c.
- *II:* limb deficiency type.
- *III:* frontonasal type with hypertelorism.
- *IVa:* unilateral Goldenhar with ocular dermoids +/- upper lid coloboma.
- *IVb:* bilateral Goldenhar.

Hatchet flap
Also known as a sickle flap.
- A local rotation-advancement flap with a Z-plasty in the tail to allow direct closure.
- Design flap adjacent to the defect with an arc two times the diameter of the defect. Place a backcut in the tail.
- Good for defects on dorsum of hand and nose. If using to resurface dorsum of proximal phalanx, hatchet must extend past MCPJ to recruit lax skin from dorsum of hand.
- The *Marchac dorsal nasal flap* is a large version of the flap which can be rotated towards the tip of the nose.

Head and neck cancer
Incidence:
- Most are squamous cell carcinomas.
- 3/4 are oral cavity and pharynx.
- Highest incidence in Melanesia (Papua New Guinea), West Europe and South Central Asia.

Aetiology:
- *Human papillomavirus:* linked to oropharyngeal cancer determined by surrogate marker P16. A leading cause of oropharyngeal cancer globally. HPV-associated oropharyngeal cancer associated with improved outcomes compared to HPV-negative disease.
- *Smoking:* stopping smoking reduces the risk to that of non-smokers after 15 years. Pipe smokers have a higher incidence of oral cavity cancer. Users of smokeless tobacco develop cancers on the alveolar ridge or buccal mucosa.

- *Alcohol:* is associated with a sixfold increase in aerodigestive cancer compared with that in non-drinker. It may also upregulate enzymes of cytochrome p450 system required to convert procarcinogens to carcinogens.
- EBV associated with nasopharyngeal cancers.
- *Other factors:* genetic susceptibility, areca (betel) nut chewing, marijuana, diets high in animal fats and low in fruits and radiotherapy.

Diagnosis:
Presentation depends on site.

- Frequently identified incidentally.
- Nasopharynx cancer may present with epistaxis or nasal obstruction, also cranial neuropathies and posterior cervical lymphadenopathy.
- Oral cancers may present with pain, ulcers or ill-fitting dentures.
- Oropharynx and hypopharynx cancers typically present late.
- General symptoms may include otalgia due to referred pain, hoarseness, dysphagia, weight loss.
- Oral cancers are a surgical disease. Surgery for cancers of the nasopharynx is less common. These are more often treated with radiotherapy.
- 25% present with a neck mass.
- Get tissue diagnosis with FNA.
- PET-CT in common use for staging evaluation for both primary and nodal disease. Also require axial imaging of primary tumour site—either contrast-enhanced CT or MRI.

General principles of AJCC staging for Head and Neck Cancer 8th Edition:
- *TX:* primary tumour cannot be assessed.
- *T0:* no evidence of primary tumour.
- *Tis:* carcinoma *in situ.*
- *T1:* tumour 0–2 cm in greatest dimension.
- *T2:* tumour >2–4 cm in greatest dimension.
- *T3:* tumour >4 cm in greatest dimension.
- *T4:* tumour invades adjacent structures (e.g. through cortical bone, into deep muscle of tongue maxillary sinus, skin).
- *NX:* regional lymph nodes cannot be assessed.
- *N0:* no regional lymph node metastasis.
- *N1:* single ipsilateral lymph node 0–3 cm.
- *N2a:* single ipsilateral lymph node >3–6 cm.
- *N2b:* multiple ipsilateral nodes 0–6 cm.
- *N2c:* contralateral or bilateral lymph node(s) 0–6 cm in greatest dimension.
- *N3:* lymph node >6 cm in greatest dimension.
- Recognition of extranodal extension in lymph node staging in all subtypes except nasopharynx and high-risk HPV oropharyngeal cancers.
- Nodal designation for above and below lower border of cricoid.
- *MX:* distant metastasis cannot be assessed.
- *M0:* no distant metastasis.
- *M1:* distant metastasis.

Specific anatomical staging variations

	Oral cavity Oropharynx	Nasopharynx	Hypopharynx	Larynx	Maxillary sinus
T1	Diameter 0–2 cm and DOI 0–5 mm	Confined to subsites (nasopharynx, oropharynx or nasal cavity)	1 subsite (piriform sinus, post-cricoid region, posterior pharyngeal wall)	1 subsite (epiglottis, AE folds, arytenoids)	Antral mucosa
T2	Diameter 0–2 cm and DOI >5 mm or Diameter >2–4 cm and DOI <10 mm	Invasion of parapharyngeal space or adjacent soft tissue	>1 subsite, no-fixation of hemilarynx	Invades mucosa of adjacent subsite	Bone below Ohngren's line
T3	>4 cm or DOI >10 mm	Bony involvement	Fixed hemilarynx or oesophageal invasion	Cord fixation	Bone above Ohngrens line
T4	Invading through cortical bone	Intracranial extension	Invades surrounding soft tissue	Invades surrounding soft tissue	Adjacent structures

DOI = depth of invasion

Clinical staging

Stage 0	Tis (in situ)	N0	M0
Stage 1	T1	N0	M0
Stage 2	T2	N0	M0
Stage 3	T3	N0	M0
	T1-3	N1	M0
Stage 4a	T4	N0-1	M0
	T1-4	N2	M0
Stage 4b	T1-4	N3	M0
Stage 4c	T1-4	N0-3	M1

Prognosis: Survival curves are calculated for each individual anatomical area and stage in AJCC 8th Edition. 5-year overall survival for Stage 1–2 is typically 70–90% and for Stage 3–4 40%.

Treatment: Best managed with a multimodal approach within a specialised head and neck cancer MDT. Usually combines surgery with radiotherapy.

• Primary surgical intervention should aim for en bloc resection with clear margins >5 mm whilst obtaining good function, aesthetic outcome and quality of life.
• Primary resection often accompanied by ipsilateral neck dissection due to risk of metastases. Bilateral neck dissection considered for midline tumours or base of tongue tumours. Efficacy of SLNB for early-stage head and neck cancer is being investigated in RCTs.
• Reconstruction is a key element of surgical management and varies from simple skin grafts to vascularized free flaps. Free flaps (i.e. radial forearm, ALT) tend to be first choice because they provide a consistent blood supply, which allows more aggressive contouring and better wound coverage than the regional flaps that used to be commonly used. Free flaps also provide opportunity to reconstruct the bony architecture with fibular flaps and iliac crest and scapular.

Sites of head and neck cancer:
• *Oral cavity:* the most common site of head and neck cancer. Bordered by lip vermilion, junction of hard and soft palate and anterior tonsillar pillar. Tumours frequently invade maxilla or mandible. Surgery remains primary strategy with adjuvant RT +/− chemotherapy reserved for advanced disease.
• *Oropharynx:* bounded by the junction of hard and soft palate anteriorly to the hyoid bone, including soft palate, uvula, tonsil and

pharyngeal wall. Often poorly differentiated and frequently has nodal metastasis. Transoral robotic surgery (TORS) may be appropriate for HPV-associated disease with minimal neck involved (N0-1) to reduce morbidity.
• *Larynx:* most frequent site after oral cavity. Three anatomic areas. *Supraglottic larynx* is composed of epiglottis, aryepiglottic fold and false vocal cords. These are occult and present very large. They metastasize early. If present early treat with supraglottic laryngectomy or RT. If larger, need total laryngectomy, RT and neck dissection. *The glottis* comprises the true vocal cords. There are few lymphatics. Patients present early with hoarseness without neck metastasis. If early treat effectively with RT. T2 and T3 give CT and RT. The *subglottic larynx* is an infrequent site of laryngeal cancer. They are difficult to diagnose and present late. Treat with surgery and RT. Prognosis is poor.
• *Nasopharynx:* common in China and Asia. Most present with nodal metastasis in the posterior neck. Lymphoepithelioma has a better prognosis than SCC. They are highly radiosensitive and RT is the treatment of choice.
• *Base of tongue:* posterior to the circumvallate papillae. Often occult. 75% present with nodal spread. Surgery is difficult and morbid. 5-year survival is 50% for stage I and 10% for stage IV.
• *Hypopharynx:* from hyoid to the lower border of cricoid cartilage split into larynx and hypopharynx. Most are seen in the piriform sinus. Occult until large and metastasized. 66% have LN, often bilateral. Require laryngopharyngectomy, bilateral neck dissection and RT.
• *Paranasal sinuses:* rare. Most commonly in the maxillary sinus, then the ethmoid sinus. Most are epidermoid, 10% are salivary, 10% are lymphomas, sarcomas or melanomas. T1 and T2 lesions treat with surgery or RT.

Nerve involvement:
• Symptoms of numbness, facial palsy and facial pain suggest nerve involvement.
• Usually due to perineural lymphatic invasion.
• Involvement of the trigeminal ganglion is deemed irresectable.

Management of occult metastatic LN (unknown primary):
• Often presents as a neck lump in level 2 or 3. Location can give clue as to primary (i.e. level 1 will more likely be oral cavity whereas 6 would be in keeping with thyroid, larynx or cervical oesophagus).

- *History:* general symptoms like weight loss, and local symptoms for primary.
- *Examination:* cachexia and secondaries. Extra-oral skin examination, Intraoral examination.
- *Investigations:* biopsy—FNA or open. CXR, MRI, PET-CT, panendoscopy with biopsy of suspicious lesions. On MRI, involved nodes are >1 cm, round not oval and have central necrosis.
- Bilateral tonsillectomy.
- *Treatment:* led by MDT. Neck dissection and RT to neck and likely primary sites.

Heberden's node
Bony spurs on the dorsal aspect of the *DIPJ*. The most common clinical manifestation of OA. 10–20× more common in women. Rarely they may produce pain and require debridement or joint fusion.

Hemifacial atrophy
- Also called *Romberg's disease* and *Parry-Romberg's disease.*
- Usually unilateral. Sporadic. Unknown aetiology. Possibly viral or abnormality of sympathetic nervous system.

Clinical features: get gradual wasting of one side of face and forehead, typically in a trigeminal dermatome distribution. Usually starts between 5 and 20 years of age. It continues for several years before stopping. Get permanent tissue deficiency.

- *Skin:* localized atrophy.
- *Hair:* pigment changes.
- *Iris:* pigment changes.
- *Forehead:* sharp depression—coup de sabre.
- *Cheek:* soft tissue atrophy.
- *Skeleton:* hypoplasia.

Treatment: avoid intervention when the condition is active and progressive. Reconstruction is performed once the condition is stable for at least 6 months. Options include:

- Synthetic implants.
- Fat and dermofat grafts.
- Temporoparietal fascia and temporalis muscle transfers.
- Free-tissue transfer—commonly scapular, parascapular, omentum.
- Osteotomies for skeletal abnormalities.

Hemifacial microsomia
See CRANIOFACIAL MICROSOMIA.

Heparin
- Action is to inactivate thrombin in the clotting cascade by increasing the effect of anti-thrombin III.

- In *Microsurgery* in a multicentre trial into the use of heparin, dextran and aspirin in free flaps, only heparin given as DVT prophylaxis showed any difference to flap survival. Give a bolus intra-operatively if the anastomosis is redone or a clot develops.

Hereditary haemorrhagic telangiectasia
See TELANGIECTASIS.

Hermaphrodites
Outdated term referring to individuals with characteristics of both sexes. True hermaphrodites have both ovarian and testicular tissue and is the only correct usage of this word. *See* AMBIGUOUS GENITALIA.

Herpetic whitlow
- Herpetic whitlow is a superficial viral infection of the fingertip.
- Medical and dental personnel are at the highest risk.
- Present with vesicles containing turbid fluid with local erythema and may also have fever and lymphangitis. Usually last 2/52.
- Do not perform incision and drainage. Severe cases may require systemic acyclovir.

Heterotopic ossification
Formation of bone in extraskeletal tissue and can occur following trauma and burns. Most commonly located adjacent to joints. May be associated with raised alkaline phosphatase. Can be excised if symptomatic.

Hewe's tarsoconjunctival transposition flap
- Used for lower *Eyelid reconstruction*. Not to be confused with the Hughes tarsoconjunctival flap.
- For defects involving the lateral half of the lid margin.
- A single-stage, laterally-based tarsoconjunctival flap is moved from upper to lower lid to reconstruct the posterior lamellar.
- The skin muscle flap is advanced over this.

Hidalgo and Shaw classification
Classification of foot injuries into:

- *Type 1:* soft tissue.
- *Type II:* major soft tissue, with or without distal amputation.
- *Type III:* soft tissue loss with fracture of ankle, calcaneous or bimalleolar.

See LOWER LIMB RECONSTRUCTION.

High-pressure injury
- Significant injuries, which may appear trivial initially.
- Often occur in the upper limb.

- The hand will rapidly swell in hours.
- Undetected or untreated it may lead to ischaemia and tissue necrosis.

Treatment:
- Is a surgical emergency. XRs may help establish the extent of injection. Give antibiotics, perform wide exposure with debridement followed by serial debridement and aggressive hand therapy with early movement.
- There is a poor prognosis with delay, oil-based solvent, finger injection, high pressure or high volume.

Highet's scale for sensory testing
- *S0:* no sensation.
- *S1:* sensation to deep pain.
- *S1+:* sensation to superficial pain.
- *S2:* sensation to light touch.
- *S2+:* hyperpathia.
- *S3:* 2PD >15 mm.
- *S3+:* 2PD 7–15.
- *S4:* full.

Hildreth's sign
See GLOMUS TUMOUR. Reduction of pain on ex-sanguination of the affected part using a prox-imally-placed tourniquet.

Histiocytosis
- The benign reticuloendothelioses are a group of diseases including eosinophilic granuloma, Hand-Schuller-Christian disease and Letterer-Siwe disease.
- Eosinophilic granuloma is the most common lesion.
- Get aggregates of xanthomatous histiocytes.
- Solitary lesions heal spontaneously.

See BONE TUMOURS.

History of plastic surgery
Plastic is derived from the Greek word *plastikos*—able to be moulded or given form. The word was first used by *Von Graefe* in 1818 in his Rhino-plastik. Goal of plastic surgery is the restoration of normal form and function and the enhance-ment of form.

Egypt: the Edwin Smith papyrus dated at 3000 BC contains description of the management of facial trauma and fractures.

India: the first recorded scripts of actual plastic surgery were recorded in Sanskrit texts 2,600 years ago. This was required due to frequent acts of facial mutilation during conflict and for unfaithfulness. *Sushruta* wrote in the Samhita (encyclopaedia) about the forehead or cheek flap for nasal reconstruction. The Koomas

caste of tile and brick makers may also have used full thickness skin grafts.

Roman: Celsus the Roman medical writer in-cluded similar techniques to repair mutilated lips, ears and noses in his medical text. Oriba-sius the fourth-century Byzantine physician de-voted two chapters to the repair of facial defects including the use of flaps. He described bipedi-cle flaps and wound undermining.

Turkish: in the fifteenth century Şerafeddin Sabuncuoğlu described treatment of gynaeco-mastia and eyelid surgery. He may be the first to describe a purely cosmetic procedure.

Italy: the nasal reconstruction was developed with a pedicle from the arm. It was performed by the Branca family in the fifteenth century and the technique kept a secret. This was learnt (not developed) by *Tagliacozzi* in the sixteenth century.

Europe: the forehead flap was reported in the *Gentleman's Magazine* when a British bullock driver had his nose mutilated as punishment for transporting supplies for the British East Indian forces. His nose was reconstructed by a man from the brickmaker caste, observed by two British surgeons. The report was read and tried by Carpue and *Von Graefe*.

Dieffenbach: also described rhinoplasty, and was one of the first to use anaesthesia.

Microsurgery:
WW1: great advances were made in reconstruc-tion, particularly with the use of pedicled flaps. Gillies developed a unit in Sidcup, Kent.

WWII: at the start of WWII there were only 4 plastic surgeons in the UK—Gillies, Kilner, Mowlem and McIndoe. With control of infec-tion, early closure of facial wounds was advo-cated. Hand surgery developed during WWII led by Sterling Bunnell.

HIV
Currently recommended post-exposure prophylaxis regimen is triple therapy with:
- Zidovudine 200 mg BD.
- Lamivudine 150 mg BD.
- Inidavir 800 mg TDS.

Start as soon as possible and continue for 4 weeks. A negative test 6 months later suggests HIV infection is unlikely.

Holoprosencephaly
- A disorder caused by the failure of the *prosencephalon* (the embryonic forebrain) to sufficiently divide into the double lobes of the cerebral hemispheres.
- This results in a single-lobed brain structure and severe skull and facial defects.

- Often the malformations are so severe that babies die before birth.
- In less severe cases, babies are born with normal or near-normal brain development and facial deformities that may affect the eyes, nose and upper lip.

Classification:
- *Alobar:* in which the brain has not divided at all, is usually associated with severe facial deformities.
- *Semilobar:* in which the brain's hemispheres have partially divided, causes an intermediate form of the disorder.
- *Lobar:* in which there is considerable evidence of separate brain hemispheres, is the least severe form. In some cases of lobar holoprosencephaly the baby's brain may be nearly normal.
- *Premaxillary agenesis:* or median cleft lip, the least severe of the facial anomalies.
- *Cyclopia:* the most severe facial anomaly with a single eye located in the area normally occupied by the root of the nose, and a missing nose or a proboscis (a tubular-shaped nose) located above the eye.
- *Ethmocephaly:* the least common facial anomaly, in which a proboscis separates closely set eyes.
- *Cebocephaly:* characterized by a small, flattened nose with a single nostril situated below incomplete or underdeveloped closely set eyes.

Surgical Management:
- May be indicated to reconstruct a cleft lip, palate or nose. Cleft palate reconstruction only indicated if patient physiologically well enough and demonstrates speech ability.

Holt–Oram syndrome
- The most common heart-hand syndrome.
- Autosomal dominant.
- Usually have an abnormal scaphoid with extra carpal bones and absent radius.
- Thumb is abnormal. Consider in radial congenital limb defects.
- Get cardiac septal defects.

Horner's syndrome
Consists of ptosis, meiosis and anhydrosis. Due to the interruption of the sympathetic supply to the eye. Horner's syndrome in a patient with brachial plexus suggests avulsion of C8 and T1 nerve roots.

Horton's test
Artificial erection test. Tests for chordee. *See* HYPOSPADIAS.

HOX
- The *HOX* are 38 genes, which encode proteins responsible for the establishment of cell identity along the AP axis in limb development.
- The position of gene on the chromosome correlates with the axial level of the limb bud where they are expressed.
- They determine timing and extent of local growth rates.

See EMBRYOLOGY.

Hueston's tabletop test
Test in patients with *Dupuytren's contracture*. Positive if the patient is unable to place fingers flat on the table. Usually surgery is indicated.

Hughe's tarsoconjuctival flap
- Used for *Lower eyelid reconstruction* of posterior lamella.
- A two-stage superiorly-based tarsoconjunctival flap taken from the central portion of the upper lid.
- Cut out defect in lower lid. Evert upper lid and cut out proximally based flap of conjuctiva and tarsal plate 5 mm from lid margin to preserve inferior upper tarsus. Advance down to fill defect. Close anterior lamella defect with FTSG or local flap.
- Divide pedicle after 3 weeks.

Human amniotic membrane
- Composed of inner membrane (amnion) and outer membrane (chorion).
- Used as temporary dressings for ulcers, burns and donor sites.
- Can get freeze-dried gamma sterilized amniotic membrane.
- It may reduce bacterial count and pain.
- Neovascularization does not occur and it does not promote healing and get hypertrophic scarring.

See BIOLOGICAL SKIN SUBSTITUTES.

Hutchinson's sign
May refer to a number of distinct clinical signs:
- Eponychial pigmentation on proximal nailfold in nail matrix melanoma.
- Vesicles on tip of nose preceding ophthalmic herpes zoster (because nasociliary branch of V1 innervates nasal tip and cornea).
- An enlarged unresponsive pupil ipsilateral to an intracranial mass.

Hyaluronic acid
Naturally occurring molecule in the body functioning to hydrate tissue, lubricate joints and form a tissue scaffold. 50% of hyaluronic acid (HA) found in skin. In ageing skin, HA depletes,

particularly in epidermis resulting in loss of skin moisture and contributing to loss of elasticity.

Preparations such as Restylane™ and Perlane™ are composed of synthetically manufactured hyaluronic acid. 20–50% are absorbed by 6 months. They are typically injected superficially to treat wrinkles and increase lip definition. *See* ALLOPLASTS.

Hydradenitis suppuritiva (HS)
- Chronic inflammatory skin disease with recurrent abscesses, sinus tracts and scarring occurring in areas of apocrine sweat glands.
- Incidence of 1:300. F:M 3:1, mainly 20s–30s. No racial difference.

Clinical features:
- Tender nodules usually start in puberty and in women flare premenstrually and may ease in pregnancy and after the menopause.
- Deep abscesses develop which may resolve or discharge. Adjacent abscesses may become linked by scar tissue. Perianal HS may mimic Crohn's disease.
- It is related to obesity, acne and hirsutism.

Three conditions, which are similar and are called the follicular occlusion triad are acne conglobata, dissecting cellulitis of the scalp and HS. Pus is usually initially sterile. Bacteria isolated are *Staph. aureus, Strep. milleri, Peptos-trepto-coccus* and *Chlamydia* (anogenital).

Sites: in order of frequency—axillary, inguinal, perianal, mammary, buttock, chest, scalp, retro-auricular, eyelid.

Aetiology:
- Likely combination of genetic and environmental factors leading to excessive inflammatory response.
- There is an autosomal dominant inheritance. Several genes have been implicated including *NCSTN, PSEN1* and *PSENEN*.
- There is a strong influence of sex hormones.
- Obesity exacerbates possibly by shear.
- Incidence of smoking is higher in HS.

Pathology:
- Apocrine glands are compound sweat glands, which extend into the subcutaneous tissues. Each has a deep coiled secretory component, which drains via a straight excretory duct into a hair follicle. Secretion is malodorous due to surface bacteria.
- Though the condition only occurs where there are apocrine glands the primary event seems to be follicular occlusion by keratinized stratified squamous epithelium. Apocrine glands which drain directly onto the skin are not affected.

- So it is a disorder of terminal follicular epithelium within apocrine gland-bearing skin. Follicular occlusion leads to rupture, spilling of contents including bacteria and keratin into the surrounding dermis. This leads to a vigorous chemotactic response; an abscess develops and this leads to destruction of the pilosebaceous unit. Epithelial strands generated from the ruptured follicular epithelium form sinus tracts.

Management:
Often complex and requires an individualized multimodal MDT approach based on distribution, severity and patient factors.

- *General:* weight loss, stop smoking, antiseptic soaps, tea tree oil, loose clothing to avoid friction, avoidance of skin trauma, analgesia.
- *Pharmacological:*
  - *Antibiotics:* evidence limited but topical or oral clindamycin can be effective if used early;
  - *Hormonal therapy:* the anti-androgen cyproterone acetate and ethinyloestradiol can be effective, but concerns are raised over the high doses required. *Finasteride* has been used to cause remission;
  - *Retinoids:* isotretinoin has been useful for acne and has been considered for HS, but it has not been shown to be effective probably because it has the maximal effect on sebaceous gland activity. Acetretin 25 mg bd. does, however, appear to be effective and acts more on keratinization. Cimetidine has been tried;
  - *Immunosuppression:* steroids may initially be effective, but relapse occurs when the dose is reduced. Intralesional triamcinolone can be effective. Immunomodulation with biologics (adalimumab followed by infliximab) has been recommended for severe HS.
- *Radiotherapy:* a German study had 38% complete relief of symptoms and 40% improved.

Surgical treatment:
- May be indicated in well circumscribed lesions:
  - The block of tissue needs to be adequately excised in depth to reduce risk of recurrence, as well as width as apocrine glands extend into the subcutaneous fat. Excise down to fascia or at least 5 mm of fat. The apocrine glands can be visualized by using the iodine/starch/oxytocin method.
- Defects can be left to heal by secondary intention or reconstruct with direct closure,

split skin grafts or local flaps. VAC can be used on SSGs;
- CO$_2$ laser with healing by secondary intention appears effective. It can be used for mild to moderate disease without any need for hospitalization.

Complications: Fibrosis and scarring can lead to contractures. Fistulae can occur. SCC in ano-genital HS has been described.

See SKIN.

Hydrocolloids

Hydrocolloid matrix backed with adhesive. It physically protects the wound, while absorbing fluid and maintaining a moist environment. Examples include Granuflex™ and Duoderm™.

See DRESSINGS.

Hydrofluoric acid

- One of the most dangerous and painful of chemical burns.
- Found in industrial and household settings, in photography laboratory products, glass etching, rust removers and petrochemical refining.
- Tissue damage caused in three ways:
  - Hydrogen ions cause superficial burns;
  - Fluoride penetrates to deeper tissue causing liquefactive necrosis (more like an alkali than an acid);
  - Free fluoride ions chelate calcium and magnesium leading to hypocalcaemia and hypomagnesaemia. Fluoride ion also inhibits NA-K ATPase which leads to an efflux of potassium. These electrolyte shifts cause the severe pain.
- >2.5% TBSA can be fatal via systemic hypocalcaemia and shock.

Treatment:
- *Hydrotherapy:* irrigate with water and clip or remove involved finger nails.
- *Topical:* inactivation of free fluoride ion by promoting formation of fluoride salt: Neutralize using topical calcium gluconate 10%—crush calcium gluconate tablets into an aqueous gel. Apply until pain free.
- *Infiltration:* subcutaneous injection is possible using calcium gluconate or magnesium sulphate in concentrations of 0.5 ml/cm^2 until pain free. Large volumes of fluoride ion can be neutralized via intra-arterial infusion. Systematic infusion of calcium and magnesium may be required.
- Monitor systemic response with serum calcium and ECG (watch for QT interval prolongation).

See CHEMICAL BURNS.

Hydrogels

Starch-polymer matrix, which swells to absorb moisture. They promote autolysis of necrotic material and are principally used to debride wounds.

See DRESSINGS.

Hydrogen cyanide

See INHALATION.

- Colourless gas form of cyanide. Exposure mainly from industrial situations.
- Binds to and inhibits cytochrome oxidase.
- Rapidly fatal in concentrations of >20 ppm and serum concentration of >1 mg/L.
- Smells of bitter almond.
- Treat with amyl nitrite, which traps cyanide, also sodium thiosulphate and hydroxy-cobalamin.

Hydroquinone

A skin lightening agent. Suppresses melanocytic activity and helps prevent hyperpigmentation.

Hydroxyapatite

- Ca10(PO$_4$)6(OH)2. Major inorganic component of bone.
- Coral of the genus *porites* has a calcium carbonate exoskeleton similar to bone. Exchange of carbonate for phosphate makes it identical to bone.
- This can bond to adjacent bone with no foreign body or inflammatory response.
- Comes as block and granules. Blocks are contoured and screwed.
- They are invaded by fibrovascular tissue with union in 2-3 months.
- HA implants are not resorbed. Blocks are brittle, but gain strength.
- Complication rates are 4-10% with low infection rate.
- BoneSource™ is a synthetic HA cement used for calvarial defects. HA can also be derived from bovine-deorganified bone.

See ALLOPLASTS.

Hynes pharyngoplasty

- A sphincter-type pharyngoplasty used for the treatment of *Velopharyngeal incompetence (VPI)*.
- Two superiorly based myomucosal flaps are raised from either side of the lateral pharyngeal wall. Flaps include a portion of salpingopharyngeus muscle and overlying mucosa. Probably a static pharyngoplasty.
- The flaps are transposed medially and sutured next to each other within a transverse incision on the posterior pharyngeal wall, above the level of the soft palate. A palatal split may be required to achieve this.

- Differs from the *Ortichochea pharyngoplasty* which uses flaps more laterally incorporating palatopharyngeus within the posterior tonsillar pillar, sits at the level of the palate and has the potential to be dynamic.

Hyperaesthesia
Increased sensitivity to a stimulus such as light touch.
See COMPLEX REGIONAL PAIN SYNDROME (CRPS).

Hyperalgesia
Increased sensitivity to pain or enhanced intensity of pain sensation.
See CRPS.

Hyperbaric oxygen
- Used for poor wound healing and radiation necrosis.
- In the normal wound a steep oxygen gradient exists between normal and damaged tissues.
- The mechanism by which hyperbaric oxygen can revascularize irradiated tissue is thought to occur through the creation of steep oxygen gradients naturally present in non-compromised wounds.
- These oxygen gradients allow the body to recognize irradiated tissue as being a true wound and the chemotactic and biochemical messenger response proceeds as in normal tissue angiogenesis.
- Clinically, hyperbaric oxygen may or may not be effective in complicated wounds.
  See RADIATION.

Hyperhidrosis
- Hyperhidrosis refers to excessive sweating on the palms of the hands, the soles of the feet and the axillae.
- The situation may be improved in cool conditions though it often remains a problem.
- Medical sympathetic block or surgical sympathectomy has been effective in carefully selected patients.
- Axillary hyperhidrosis can be treated by wide excision of the axilla to include most of the eccrine sweat glands, which are concentrated in the axillary vault.
- Raising bipedicled flaps and excising dermis will also denervate the sweat glands and reduce sweating.
- Subcutaneous curettage can be performed to superficial and deep surface after undermining the area of hydradenitis.
- Botox™ injections are effective for several months.

Hyperkeratosis
- An increase in the thickness of the stratum corneum and usually accompanied by an increase in the granular layer due to abnormal production of keratin.
- Can be caused by vitamin A deficiency or chronic exposure to arsenic.
- Manage with urea-containing topical preparations to promote desquamation.

Hyperpathia
Disagreeable or painful sensation in response to a normally innocuous stimulus (as touch). *See* RSD.

Hypertelorism
- A congenital increase in interorbital distance measured between the medial walls of the orbits at the junction of the maxillary, frontal and lacrimal bones (the dacryon).
- The intercanthal distance is measured between the medial canthal tendons and an increase in this dimension with a normal IOD is called pseudo-orbital hypertelorism (telecanthus) and can be caused by non-congenital causes.
- In adults the average IOD is 22–30 mm (in men 28 mm and women 25 mm).

Classification:
- *Tessier:* based on IOD.
  - IOD 30–34 mm;
  - IOD 34–40 mm;
  - IOD >40mm.
- *Munro:* according to shape.

Pathology:
- Hypertelorism is not a diagnosis in itself, but a description.
- Linked to failure of frontonasal process to move caudally.
- All have nasal deformity with widening of the ethmoidal sinuses.
- The nose is usually short and wide. Get turbinate hypertrophy with airway obstruction.
- May be underlying abnormalities of forebrain; 'the face predicts the brain'.

Aetiology:
- Associated with many congenital malformations.
- Seen in midline clefts (see *Tessier*) cranio-facial syndromes such as *Crouzon's* and *Apert's*, and sincipital (midline) encephalocoele. Also associated with dermoid cysts, teratomas.

Treatment:
Craniofacial MDT approach with ophthalmology involvement.

- Usually after the age of 2 years. 3-D CT scans are useful for planning.

- Tessier principles state whole orbit must be mobilized to allow translocation including the functional orbit posteriorly and a combined intracranial and extracranial approach.
- 2 main surgical options:
  - ○ *Box osteotomy:* good for normal facial width. Osteotomies around each orbit. Nasal bone and ethmoid sinus removed to allow medialization;
  - ○ *Facial bipartition:* good for inverted V deformity of maxillary occlusion. Osteotomies around orbit and midline allow medial rotation and transposition. Main difference to box osteotomy is the orbital floor is left in continuity with the maxilla.

  Both procedures require medial canthopexy.

Hypertrophic scar
- Excessive inflammatory response usually within 8 weeks of healing. Characterized by well-organized type III collagen bundles with nodules containing myofibroblasts.
- Remain within the borders of the scar, whereas *Keloid* scars extend beyond the borders.
- They may improve with time and may not recur if excised.
- M = F.

Management:
Multi-modal MDT management:

- *Prevention:* judicious acute care, splinting, positioning, mobilization and exercise.
- *Modulation:* pressure (bandage, splints, masks), silicone (gel, sheet), laser (non-ablative, ablative), immunomodulation (steroids).
- *Surgery* (last resort)*:* release contractures and resurface.

In burns:
- All wounds contract, but the degree of contracture and hypertrophy is related to the time taken to heal as the longer the time the longer the wound is in the inflammatory phase.
- Excess inflammation increases the amount of the fibrogenic TGF ß1 and TGF ß2.
- Hypertrophy is also increased by shortage of tissue.
- Laser is having an increasing role for hypertrophic scarring in burns. Non-ablative pulse dye laser can be used when scar is healed. Ablative CO_2 or ER-YAG can be used when evidence of hypertrophic scarring. Early evidence to show the use of laser reduces need for operative intervention.
  See SCAR.

Hypospadias
- Congenital anomaly of penis and urethra characterized by urethral meatus in ventral position.
- Associated with *Chordee*, hooded prepuce and torsion.
- May get clefting of the glans and scrotal bipartition.
- Patients/parents may report urinary stream dysfunction (misdirection, obstruction or post-void dribbling), sexual function (due to persistent chordee, scare or penile hypoplasia) and abnormal cosmesis.
- Distal hypospadias is likely to be an isolated anomaly. Proximal lesions more likely to have other anomalies including inguinal hernia, undescended testis, PUJ obstruction, renal agenesis, persistent Mullerian structures and intersex states.

History:
- Paul of Aegina (seventh-century Greek physician) advocated glandular amputation to position the meatus at the tip of the penis.
- Mettauer (1830) described a two-stage procedure without a graft, the first stage being left to heal by secondary intention.
- Nové-Josserand (1897) first used a graft.
- Thiersche and Duplay—2-stage procedure with first correction of chordee then tubularizing the urethra with lateral flaps.
- Cecil performed a 3-stage procedure with release of chordee followed by tubularizing ventral skin and burying in the scrotum. Later this skin is divided, but this means scrotal skin on the penis.

Incidence:
- Affects 1 in 300 males.
- Father-son 8%, sibling 14%, not all identical twins.

Aetiology and embryology:
- The ventral urethral groove normally fuses from proximal to distal and is complete at 5 months.
- Cessation of androgen stimulus (i.e. increased exogenous oestrogens, androgen receptor deficiency) causes meatus to form at distal point of fusion.
- Remnants of mesenchymal tissue form fibrous chordee.
- More common in IVF children.

Classification by pre-operative meatal location:
- Distal (glanular subcoronal, distal penile shaft) 65%.
- Mid-penile 15%.

- Proximal (penoscrotal, perineal) 20%—the most severe.

History: ask parents about erections, penile curve, urinary stream.

Examination: size of penis (testosterone cream may help), testicular descent (if not perform genetic analysis for intersex state), inguinal hernia (if present USS for upper urinary tract), watch urine flow and direction.

Investigation: formal investigation usually not required in distal hypospadias. Urinalysis, USS of urogenitary system and karyotype in proximal hypospadias.

Management: Glandular hypospadias may not require surgical intervention. Timing of surgery is debated but usually performed either 6–12 months of age or at 3–4 years of age. Aim to straighten (orthoplasty), even calibre of neourethra, reposition meatus (meatoplasty), reconstruct gland (glanuplasty) with good cosmesis and function.

- *One stage:* indicated in distal hypospadias when the urethral plate does not require transection:
  - Tubularized Incised Plate (TIP) described by Snodgrass. Involves a midline releasing incision of urethral plate followed by tubularization around a stent to form a neo-urethra;
  - 'Snod-graft' repair involves a skin graft to the releasing incision rather than leaving it to re-epithelialize. Particularly useful in salvage cases;
  - MAGPI described by Ducket. Involves meatal advancement and glanuloplasty via a vertical incision with horizontal closure;
  - Flip-flap.
- *Two stage:* indicated in more proximal hypospadias and offers the most reliable solution for patients who require transection of the urethral plate. Described by Bracka, the native urethral plate is transected and resurfaced with a full thickness skin graft

(prepuce, lip mucosa). The graft is tubularized at a second stage.
- *Addressing chordee:* deep fibres proximal to the meatus need to be incised. In the presence of ventral skin shortage, a V-Y advancement may be required using spare prepuce skin.

Complications:
- *Early:* bleeding, haematoma, infection, dehiscence, necrosis.
- *Late:* fistula, stricture, sacculation, residual chordee, spraying, urethral hair.
- *Fistula:* 90% detectable within 1 week of operation. In repairing, ensure that there is no distal obstruction. Wait for softening of tissues, close the hole and place a fascial flap over it. Test integrity of the repair.

See PENIS.

Hypotelorism Reduced interorbital distance seen in:

- Binder's syndrome.
- Down syndrome.
- Trigonocephaly (metopic synostosis).
- Holoprosencephaly.
- Arrhinocephaly.

Hypothenar hammer syndrome
- Thrombosis of the ulnar artery in Guyon's canal due to blunt trauma to the base of the hypothenar eminence.
- Get cold intolerance, pain and sometimes ulceration of the ring and little fingers.
- Treat by excision of thrombosed segment and vein graft.
- The localized sympathectomy caused by the resection may be important for recovery, allowing distal vascular dilatation or removal of a possible source of emboli.
- The effectiveness of resection may be due to resection of sympathetic fibres.

See VASCULAR INJURIES.

Iliac crest: free flap to Ito, naevus of

Iliac crest: free flap
- A source of vascularized bone on a long pedicle.
- Curved and useful for mandibular reconstruction.
- Skin and muscle can be included with minimal morbidity.
- There is a limited amount of bone to transfer resulting in a marked contour deficiency and may get abdominal herniation.
- Raised on the deep circumflex iliac artery but can also be raised on the superficial circumflex iliac artery or the dorsal branch of the fourth lumbar artery.

Anatomy:
- The deep circumflex iliac artery (DCIA) arises from the external iliac artery and passes on deep surface of inguinal ligament. It continues along the inside of iliac crest. It supplies bone through muscle so muscle must be raised as well. Artery diameter is 2 mm.
- The vessels send branches to skin and the first branch supplies the internal oblique and transverses abdominus. A muscle flap can be isolated as a separate pedicle.

Mandible reconstruction: for mandible the crest forms the lower border of the mandible, the ASIS the angle and the AIIS the condyle. So, use ipsilateral crest. Difficult to shape for angle to angle defects. The skin paddle is good for facial skin, but not so good for oral lining. Use for lateral segment defects.

Flap raise:
- The skin ellipse is centred over the upper border of anterior iliac crest. The medial incision is along the inguinal ligament.
- Divide external oblique. The conjoined fibres of internal oblique and transverses are incised just inside the iliac crest.
- The DCIA can be palpated adjacent to the ilium. Dissect distally. The descending branch is divided 1 cm anterior and medial to the ASIS.
- Isolate the bone. Preserve ASIS. Remove the flap.

- Take at least a 1-cm cuff of iliacus fascia below the course of the DCIA. If the full crest is taken, the TFL and gluteal muscles are detached from the anterior lip. A 2–3 cm fringe of externally attached muscle along the crest is taken if a skin paddle is used. Close in layers anchoring the muscle to the remaining iliac crest through drill holes.

Ilizarov technique
- Distraction osteogenesis was introduced in 1951 when a patient reversed the compression rods of a ring fixator.

See MANDIBULAR HYPOPLASIA. *See* BONE. *See* DISTRACTION OSTEOGENESIS.

Imiquimod
- Trade name: Aldara™.
- An immune response modifier. Binds to Toll-like receptor 7 on macrophages. Activates Langerhans cells.
- Used to treat actinic keratosis, basal cell carcinoma and Bowens disease.
- It has been used with success for *Keloids* following surgery with no systemic toxicity.
- It has also been used to treat molluscum contagiosum.

Implantation dermoid
See EPIDERMOID INCLUSION CYST.

Inadine
Non-adherent dressing made from a mesh impregnated with povidone-iodine for anti-microbial effect. Used in burns and chronic wounds such as ulcers.

See DRESSINGS.

Incisional herniation
- Associated with infection, dehiscence, age, obesity, malnutrition, steroids.
- Transverse abdominal incisions have the lowest rate of herniation. Lateral traction on the recti increases the protrusion.

See ABDOMINAL WALL RECONSTRUCTION.

Infection: upper limb

Infections caused by injury at home are most commonly *Staph. aureus*. Establish any underlying conditions such as diabetes.

See:

- *Felon*.
- *Paronychia*.
- *Tenosynovitis*.
- *Collar-button abscess*.
- *Herpes*.
- *Mycobacteria*.
- *Osteomyelitis*.
- *Flexor sheath*.
- *Palm infections*.
- *Dorsal infections*.
- *Animal bite: Pasteurella multicida*.
- *Human bites: Eikenella corrodens*.
- *Sporothrix schenkii*: in nurseryman.
- *Aeromonas hydrophilia*: gram-negative rod in freshwater lakes. Sensitive to tetracycline. Get rapid onset of cellulitis with abscess, myonecrosis and sepsis.

Infra-orbital nerve

- Terminal branch of V2 (maxillary) trigeminal nerve. Emerges from the infra-orbital foramen (10 mm below orbital rim) and divides into 4 branches:

  - Inferior palpebral;
  - External nasal;
  - Internal nasal;
  - Superior labial.

- Supplies the lower eyelid, upper lip, columella, lateral nose and ala, cheek, mucous membrane of cheek and lip.
- Block by palpating the infra-orbital foramen or notch which lies below the midline of the pupil with the eye looking straight. Intra-oral injection through the upper buccal sulcus in the line of the canine

Inheritance

- *Penetrance:* relates to the proportion of people with a genetic variant who exhibit signs and symptoms for a genetic disorder. For example, *BRCA1* and *BRCA2* have variable penetrance because not all carriers of the variant will go on to develop breast cancer. Complete penetrance is demonstrated by a specific point mutation in *FGFR3* which will always lead to achondroplasia.
- *Expression:* relates to the range of signs and symptoms that can occur with the same variant. For example, neurofibromatosis has variable expressivity of skeletal and neurological disorders.

- Van der Woude syndrome with a mutation in *IRF6* serves as an example of variable penetrance and expressivity.

Integra™

- Integra is an artificial skin composed of a 2-layer composite of dermis and epidermis.
- The dermal template is a porous bovine tendon collagen and shark glycosaminoglycan—condroitin-6 phosphate fibrous matrix arranged in a 3D pattern. It provides a biodegradable framework in which host fibroblasts migrate and lay down host collagen. The neodermis replaces artificial dermis and inherits a vasculature to become permanently incorporated as host.
- The epidermal portion consists of a temporary silicone layer, which acts as a mechanical barrier to bacterial invasion.
- Once the neodermis has developed, the silicone layer can be stripped away to accept a split skin graft. When using, excise the burn wound early. Graft with thin SSG. Donor site can be used many times.
- It has been used for post-burns excision and gives a better-quality scar, which is thicker and more supple than following SSG.
- The main problem relates to loss of integra due to haematoma and infection, and meticulous technique is required for success.

Integrins

- Matrix binding cell surface molecules.
- They are the main way that cells both bind to and respond to the extracellular matrix and are involved in a variety of cellular functions, such as wound healing, cell differentiation, homing of tumour cells and apoptosis.
- They are part of a large family of cell adhesion receptors, which are involved in cell–extracellular matrix and cell–cell interactions.

Interferon

Signalling proteins released by immune cells in response to a virus.

See CYTOKINES.

Interleukin

Signalling proteins released by CD4 lymphocytes, monocytes, macrophages and endothelial cells to promote the differentiation of lymphocytes and haematopoietic cells.

See CYTOKINES.

Interosseous muscles

- Four dorsal interossei abduct ('DAB') index, middle and ring (reference line is middle finger).
- Three palmar interossei adduct ('PAD') index, ring and little.

Palmar interossei:
- Single muscle belly arising from the anterior aspect of the respective metacarpal on the surface facing the middle finger.
- 1st inserts to ulnar side of index, 2nd to radial side of ring and 3rd to radial side of little.
- They cross palmar to the axis of the MCP joint dorsal to the deep transverse metacarpal ligament.

Dorsal interossei:
- Each arises from 2 metacarpals.
- 1st and 2nd insert into radial side of index and middle finger. 3rd and 4th insert into the ulnar side of middle and ring finger.
- The 1st, 2nd and 4th have superficial and deep muscles with medial and lateral tendons.
- The medial tendons travel under the sagittal band to insert into the lateral tubercle of the base of proximal phalanx. This abducts and weakly flexes.
- The lateral tendon runs superficial to sagittal band and continues as the lateral band. This flexes the proximal phalanx and extends the IPJs.

Nerve supply: deep branch of ulnar nerve.

Function:
- All assist MCP joint flexion and PIP and DIP joint extension.
- Also abduction and adduction, digital rotation and centralization of extensor tendon.
- Side-to-side movements of the index finger can be produced with EIP and EDC, but for the others it is solely by interossei. Rotation is important for fine control.
- They also stabilize the digit during pinch grip by preventing MCPJ hyperextension.

Interpolation flap

Similar in design to rotation and _Transposition flap_, but rotates into a nearby, but not immediately adjacent area so it must pass under or over intervening tissue. An example is a paramedian forehead flap used for nasal tip reconstruction.

Intersection syndrome
- Non-specific tenosynovitis of second dorsal _Extensor compartment_ containing ERCL and ECRB.
- Associated with repetitive trauma of the wrist.
- May mimic the more common _de Quervain's disease_: tenderness should be more proximal in intersection syndrome.
- It presents as a tender swelling localized to the region where the APL and EPB muscle bellies cross ECRB and ECRL 4 cm proximal to the wrist joint.

- Distinct crepitus can be felt in the swelling. _Finklestein's test_ is positive.
- Most are cured by injection and splintage.
- If symptoms persist the second dorsal compartment is released through longitudinal incision.

  See TENOSYNOVITIS.

Intracranial Pressure (ICP)
- Normally 7–15 mmHg.
- Changes in ICP are attributable to volume changes of the brain or cerebrospinal fluid within the cranium.
- Symptoms of raised ICP include headache, vomiting and altered levels of consciousness. Signs include papilledema.
- Raised ICP may be a feature of craniosynostosis. Multi-suture synostosis has a higher risk than single-suture synostosis
- ICP can be monitored indirectly via ocular monitoring for papilledema. Intracranial transducers are more accurate but are invasive.
- The management of raised ICP depends on the cause and may include medications (i.e. antihypertensive agents), cerebral shunts and decompressive craniotomies.

Intraluminal endothelial hyperplasia
See MASON'S HAEMANGIOMA.

Intravelar veloplasty
- Technique of velar muscle dissection and retropositioning during _Cleft palate_ reconstruction.
- Kriens described the abnormal orientation of the levator palatini muscles, and the need to detach them from their abnormally anterior insertion within the cleft palate margin and reorientate them in a more transverse direction.
- Sommerlad described radial muscle retropositioning and popularised use of operating microscope for intravelar veloplasty in landmark PRS papers in 2003.
- Surgical steps:
  - Mouth gag to provide access, vision and magnification (i.e. microscope);
  - _Marking:_ marginal incision between oral and nasal mucosa. LA infiltration;
  - _Raise oral mucosal layer:_ start on the hard palate to get the correct plane;
  - _Suture nasal muco-muscular layer:_ this provides tension for the muscles to be dissected;

○ Dissect muscles under tension and retro-position levator into a transverse muscular sling;
○ Close oral layer using lateral releasing incisions if required.

Intrinsic plus/minus

- The intrinsics flex the MCP joint and extend interphalangeal joints—the intrinsic plus position.
- Tight intrinsics will prevent interphalangeal joint flexion if the MCP joint is hyperextended.
- This can happen with tip amputations if the FDP retracts.
- Test for intrinsic tightness by testing passive PIP joint flexion with MCP joint extension—the *Bunnell test*.
- With extrinsic tightness IPJ flexion is possible on extension of MCP joint.
- Intrinsic minus refers to the absence of intrinsic function as seen in *Ulnar nerve palsy*, resulting in a *Claw hand*.

Inverting papilloma

- A papilloma which usually arises from the lateral wall of the nose.
- It is benign but can expand within the closed space and cause pressure necrosis of bone.
- SCC may arise from an inverting papilloma.

  See MAXILLA/MIDFACE.

Iron

- Essential cofactor for the replication of DNA.
- Also needed for proline hydroxylase used for converting proline to hydroxyproline.

Ischaemia-reperfusion injury

- Seen following re-establishment of blood flow in free tissue transfer or replant surgery.

- May get tissue injury beyond that caused by ischaemia.

Ischaemia: causes tissue and cellular hypoxia. Products of anaerobic metabolism, such as lactate, build up and disturb membrane transport systems resulting in influx of calcium into the cell. Inflammatory mediators are triggered.

Reperfusion: oxygen is returned and oxygen free radicals are produced by neutrophils—respiratory burst, neutrophils degranulation, and release of pro-inflammatory mediators.

  See NO REFLOW PHENOMENON.

Isolated limb perfusion

- Used in the treatment of *Melanoma* with multiple uncontrollable metastasis confined to the limb from where the primary was excised.
- May be effective for local control.
- The preferred chemotherapy regime is dacarbazine (DTIC), melphalan with platinum and carmustine.
- All agents have demonstrated a 15-30% response rate. The technique has been present since the 1960s.
- It involves perfusion with high dose chemotherapy under high oxygenation high pressure and high temperature (40°C). The limb is isolated with a tourniquet.
- The addition of tumour necrosis factor and interferon is also beneficial.

Ito, naevus of

Same features as the naevus of *Ota*, but in the distribution of the posterior supraclavicular and lateral cutaneous branches to the shoulder, neck and supraclavicular areas. *See* BLUE NAEVUS.

Jackson pharyngoplasty
- A dynamic sphincteric pharyngoplasty used for the treatment of velopharyngeal incompetence (*VPI*) described in 1985.
- A modification of the *Ortichochea pharyngoplasty* described in 1968, the pharyngoplasty involves two myomucosal flaps raised from the posterior tonsillar pillars (incorporating the palatopharyngeus), but the flaps are based higher, the tips of the flaps are sutured end to end, rather than interdigitated and the lateral donor sites are closed primarily.

Jackson's zones
Describe the zones of injury seen in acute *Burns*.
- *Zone of coagulation:* inner zone of irreversible coagulative necrosis.
- *Zone of stasis:* describes the adjacent at-risk tissue with marginal blood flow which without optimal conditions will progress to necrosis.
- *Zone of hyperaemia:* outer zone as a result of inflammatory mediators and vasodilation.

Jahss manoeuvre
- Technique for closed reduction of metacarpal neck fracture.
- Flexing MCP joint relaxes intrinsics and tightens ligaments.
- The proximal phalanx can thus be used to reduce the fracture with upward force on the flexed PIP joint and counterforce on the metacarpal shaft.

Jeanne's sign
- Clinical test in *Ulnar nerve palsy*.
- Loss of lateral or key pinch of thumb due to paralysis of adductor pollicis muscle, which adducts, flexes at the MCP joint and extends at the IPJ. Get hyperextension of MCP joint.

Jejunal flap
- Used as a free flap principally for oropharyngeal reconstruction.

- The jejunum constitutes the first 2/5s of the 7-m long small bowel from ligament of Treitz to the ileocaecal valve.
- The diameter is 4 cm and the root of the fan-shaped mesentery is 15 cm long.
- On average there are 12–15 branches to the jejunum and ileum.
- The blood supply of the jejunum is supplied by branches of the superior mesenteric artery. Each branch can support a segment of jejunum up to 24 cm long.
- Usually proximal jejunum is used.
- The first branch is not used because the pedicle length is short.
- Identify the jejunum and isolate the pedicle. Tie off other branches, divide the jejunum, divide the pedicle and transfer the flap. It can be opened out. Position it in an isoperistaltic fashion. Perform proximal bowel anastomosis then revascularize.
- A monitor segment can be fashioned from remaining jejunum and sutured to the neck.

See ORAL CAVITY RECONSTRUCTION.
See LARYNGOPHARYNGECTOMY. *See* PHARYNX.

Jewer classification of mandibular defects
HLC classification of mandibular defects following excision can have 8 potential permutations.
- H = lateral segment together with condyle—tend to swing to the contralateral side and reconstruction needs to give ramus height.
- L = lateral segments that exclude condyle—does not tend to get a big swing of mandible to the contralateral side. Can be reconstructed with a straight segment of bone.
- C = central defects including both canines. Require osteotomies in the bony reconstruction to achieve curvature.
- LCL—angle to angle and requires a more complex reconstruction than a simple L defect.

Joint contracture: hand
Pathology:
- The MCP joint tends to rest in extension following injury and swelling.
- The collateral ligaments then shorten. A flexion contracture is therefore caused by extrinsic forces.
- The PIP joint usually becomes stiff in flexion due to restriction of the volar plate and contracture of check rein ligaments.
- Restriction of DIP joint flexion is usually due to extensor adhesions.

PIP joint flexion contractures:
- Expose volar surface through Bruner incision which allows for a Y–V advancement, retract NVB and expose flexor sheath. C1 overlies PIP joint. Lift up C1 to expose flexor tendons.
- Perform tenolysis until FDS and FDP run freely. Retract tendon to expose volar plate with check rein ligaments, which extend from the proximal edge of the volar plate to the margin of the flexor sheath.
- Divide checkrein ligaments. Attempt to preserve the vincula which run between them. Gentle force is required to extend the joint.
- If there is still a contracture, gentle blunt dissection beneath the volar plate and/or sharp division of the volarmost fibres of the collateral ligament is undertaken. Enter joint through volar plate in midline and lift up volar plate off bone until joint freed. Hold joint out with K wire for short time before using dynamic splints.

PIPJ extension contractures:
- Require partial ligament resection. Approach dorsally.
- Divide transverse ligaments of Landsmeer. Retract lateral band dorsally.
- Resection part of collateral ligament to allow PIPJ flexion. Begin release dorsally. Assess the extensor hood and release adhesions before dividing collateral ligaments. Immobilize in partial flexion and start protected movement early.
- Occasionally PIP joint movement is restricted by chronic synovitis. Debridement may improve movement. Detach volar plate from one side to gain access to the joint. Debride.

MCP joint flexion contractures: almost always extrinsic and fully correctable by releasing extrinsic problem.

MCP joint extension contractures:
- Require selective release of the surrounding structures.
- Approach from the dorsal side using a longitudinal incision.
- Retract sagittal bands distally or divided on one side preferably the ulnar side, as it tends to prolapse ulnarly.
- Adhesions between the tendon and capsule are freed. Perform graded release of the collateral ligaments.
- Release dorsal fibres from their origin on the metacarpal head. Release should allow the proximal phalanx to track within the normal axis of joint motion.
- Volar structures can be freed by passing an instrument between volar plate and flexor.

Joint transfers: free
- Free non-vascularized joint transfers over time degenerate and collapse.
- Synovial fluid is required which requires an intact blood supply.
- There is, however, long-term bone and cartilage survival in vascularized joint transfers.
- The first free vascularized toe joint transfer was performed by Foucher in 1976. The alternative is arthrodesis or arthroplasty.
- The best indication for free joint transfers are in children and in young active adults with normal functioning flexor and extensor tendons. They are also useful when soft tissue is also required.

Anatomy:
- Toe blood supply is from the dorsal and plantar arch with the dominant supply to the 2nd toe from the dorsal arch by the first dorsal metatarsal artery (FDMA).
- The lateral digital artery to the big toe is sacrificed so a paddle of skin from the big toe can also be taken.
- As the growth plate for the metatarsal is distally and the phalanx is proximal if the MTP is taken both growth centres are included, which is important in children, but not in adults.

Joule heating
- Mechanism of tissue destruction seen in *Electrical injuries.*
- Passage of an electrical current through a solid body results in conversion of electrical energy to heat.

- Heat production (Q) is proportional to the square of the current (I), tissue resistance (R) and time of contact (t).
- $Q \propto I^2RT$.

Jumping man flap
- Five flap Y–V advancement and _Z-plasty_.
- Useful for releasing contractures on concave regions such as interdigital web space and medial canthal region.
- The central flap advances in a Y–V, while the two mirror image Z-plasties on either side are transposed.

Juncturae tendinae
- Tendinous bands connecting ring finger _Extensor digitorum communis_ (EDC) to EDC of middle and little fingers.
- They may also connect EDC of index and middle.
- Division of a tendon proximal to a junctura may result in only partial loss of extension.

- One of the earliest described elective tendon operations was the division of juncturae in harpists to improve independent finger movement.

Juri classification
For male pattern _Balding_.

- _Type 1:_ frontal.
- _Type 2:_ frontal and crown.
- _Type 3:_ vertex.

Juri flap
A local temporoparietal-occipital flap based on the superficial temporal artery. Used to reconstruct the anterior hairline in _Alopecia_. Flap is 4–5 cm in width and can be up to 26 cm long with the axial vessel incorporated. Elevation in sub-galeal plane.

Juvara: septa of
See LEGUEU AND JUVARA: SEPTA OF.

Kanavel's signs to Kutler V–Y flaps

Kanavel's signs
Seen in suppurative *Tenosynovitis* of the flexor tendon sheath (i.e. *Flexor sheath infection*).
- Tenderness over the flexor sheath.
- Pain on passive extension—the most sensitive sign as it reduces volume in the sheath.
- Flexed posture.
- Fusiform swelling of digit.

Kapetansky flaps
- Used in the correction of whistle tip deformity following bilateral cleft lip repair.
- Bilateral horizontally orientated V–Y flaps within vermilion tissue.
- Also a centrally-placed upside-down W creates a space into which the lateral flaps will advance. So they fill the central defect in all dimensions.

See SECONDARY LIP AND NASAL DEFORMITIES.

Kaplan's cardinal line
- A line drawn on the palm of the hand along the flexor surface of the radially abducted thumb, parallel to the proximal palmar crease.
- The bisection of this line with a line drawn from the scaphoid tubercle to the 3rd web space gives the point of origin of the motor branch of the median nerve. This is also the point where the flexed ring finger hits Kaplan's line.
- The bisection of Kaplan's line with a line drawn from the ulnar border of the abducted ring finger gives the position of the hook of the hamate and Kaplan's line overlies the deep palmar arch.

Kaposi's sarcoma
- A multicentric malignant disorder of vasoformative tissue. Initially presents with patches of purpura. Later, vascular polyps develop. Chronic lymphoedema occurs and ulceration secondary to RT.
- Described by Hungarian Moriz Kaposi in 1872.

- KS-associated herpes virus (human herpesvirus type 8 [HHV-8]) linked closely with all 4 types of KS.
- HHV-8 appears to interact with the HIV tat protein, excess levels of basic fibroblast growth factor, scatter factor and IL-6.
- Predispositions to KS include:
  ○ Older men of Mediterranean and Jewish lineage;
  ○ Africans from areas including Uganda, the Congo Republic, Congo (Brazzaville) and Zambia;
  ○ Persons who are iatrogenically immunosuppressed.
- Endemic African KS has accounted for 10% of cancers and has been seen in a male-to-female ratio of 15:1. In Uganda, KS has caused almost one half (48.9%) of cancer cases in men and 17.9% in women. It is rare in African Americans.
- For endemic M:F 1:1 in childhood, 15:1 by puberty.

Clinical:
- Multiple vascular nodules. Multifocal though can metastasize. Course may be indolent or fulminant. May occur on oral mucosa and lymph nodes only. Chronic lymphedema may precede KS.
- KS is described in 3 forms including localized nodular, locally aggressive, and generalized KS. KS typically occurs in these 3 forms and in 6 stages including patch, plaque, nodular, exophytic, infiltrative and lymphadenopathic. Often start in lower extremities.

Causes: HHV-8 linked, but other factors needed. Most important is immunosuppression.

Treatment:
- Treatment is based on the extent of disease and the patient's immune status.
- Management modalities for KS include non-intervention, surgical removal of skin nodules or severely affected areas (e.g. areas of the extremities, intussuscepted bowel), laser surgery, conventional and mega-voltage radiotherapy, chemotherapy,

immunotherapy, antiviral drugs and cessation of immunosuppressive therapy in iatrogenically immunosuppressed patients.
- Indolent skin tumours in elderly may not need treatment, but systemic vinblastine affects cutaneous and visceral lesions.
- Localized nodular disease responds well to surgery, radiotherapy, intralesional and systemic vinblastine. Vinblastine by both routes is preferable.
- *Taxanes:* e.g. paclitaxel have anti-angiogenic properties and is effective for HIV-KS.
- *Radiotherapy:* good for classic nodular. Conventional RT very effective for localized nodular. Electron beam RT with limited penetration good for superficial lesions. Usually response is complete and better on newer lesions.
- *Laser therapy:* argon laser, beneficial for classic KS.
- *Chemotherapy:* IV vinblastine titrated against white cell count. Also intralesional and intra-arterial. Can also use vincristine, vinblastine, dacarbazine, doxorubicin, and actinomycin D. Alkylating agents (e.g. cyclophosphamide, chlorambucil, bleomycin, doxorubicin, etoposide).

Kaposiform haemangioendothelioma
See KASABACH–MERRITT SYNDROME.
- A vascular tumour generally present at birth.
- Histologically distinct from haemangiomas. Marked by irregular sheets of spindle-shaped endothelial cells and slit-like vascular channels. Positive for D2-40, LYVE1 and Prox-1 but negative for GLUT-1 (marker for haemangioma).
- Mortality rate of 24% from coagulopathy and local infiltration.
- Treatment as for *Haemangiomas* with close monitoring of coagulopathy.

Karapandzic flap
- Used for *Lip reconstruction*.
- A modification of the *Gillies fan flap*, which maintains the neurovascular pedicle in the soft tissue, giving better functional results.
- Can be used for upper or lower lip defects.
- Semicircular incisions are used and facial nerve branches preserved. The commissure rotates.
- Does not import new lip tissue and may give microstomia. The vertical height of the defect determines the width of the flap.
- The incisions are full thickness medially, but at the commissure it is only down to subcutaneous tissue and neurovascular structures are preserved.

- If the defect is central, rotate flaps equally from either side. If more to one side bring more from the contralateral side so as not to distort the commissure.

Kasabach–Merritt syndrome
- A rare consumptive coagulopathy. Primary platelet trapping is a life-threatening complication of *Haemangioma*-like tumours, specifically *Kaposiform haemangioendothelioma*. Also seen rarely with tufted angioma and congenital haemangiopericytoma.
- Diagnosed by a rapidly enlarging tumour and a constellation of profound thrombocytopenia (typically <10,000/mm³) and consumptive coagulopathy (hypofibrinogenaemia).
- The prothrombin time (PT) and activated partial thromboplastin time (APTT) are variably elevated. D dimer and fibrinogen degradation products are elevated.
- An infant with Kasabach–Merritt thrombocytopenia is at risk for intracranial, pulmonary, intraperitoneal or gastrointestinal haemorrhage.
- Management:
  o Critical supportive care. Platelet transfusion should be avoided due to potential to exacerbate intratumoral bleeding and platelet trapping;
  o Pharmacological: steroids are often first line to help achieve haemostatic stability;
  o Surgical excision of the tumour, when physiologically safe to do so, offers potentially definitive cure.

Kazanjian and Converse classification: mandibular fractures
Based on presence of teeth in relation to the fracture line.
- *Class 1:* teeth on both sides of the fracture line.
- *Class 2:* teeth on one side of the fracture line.
- *Class 3:* patient is edentulous.

This relates to the ability to manage a mandibular fracture by intermaxillary fixation (IMF).

Keloid
- Pathological scarring characterized by proliferation of scar tissue outside the border of the scar, as opposed to *Hypertrophic scar*, which remains within the borders of the scar. Rarely spontaneously regresses and can cause itchy, pain and hyperesthesia.
- 'Chel' derived from the Greek for crab claw.
- Can develop over a year after injury.
- More common in dark-skinned people. Autosomal dominant or recessive pattern.

Associated with blood group A. Correlates with IgE and allergic symptoms.

- Most commonly located on earlobe, sternum and shoulders.
- Hormonally related as it appears in puberty and resolves after pregnancy.
- Histologically characterized by disorganized type I and III collagen. Fibroblast numbers not increased. Both keloids and hypertrophic scars have rich vasculature and thickened epidermal layer. Collagen is fragmented and shortened. Get collagen nodules. Collagen synthesis in both is elevated, but higher in keloids. There is less cross-linkage and more type III. The influence of growth factors is unclear.

Treatment:

- *Surgery:* high recurrence rate 45–100%. Helpful combined with other treatment.
- *Pressure:* 60–85% response rate. Wear garments for 18–24 hours/day for 6/12. May work by causing ischaemia, decreasing tissue metabolism and increasing collagenase.
- *Steroids:* give a variable response of 50–100%. Most effective on younger hypertrophic scars. No steroid has been shown to be more superior. May get skin atrophy, hypopigmentation, necrosis or ulceration. In conjunction with surgery use preoperatively, then immediately post-operatively followed by weekly injection for 2–5 weeks, then monthly for 3–6/12. Acts by decreasing collagen synthesis.
- *Radiotherapy:* use for scars resistant to other treatment. Need at least 900 Gy. Surgery then RT gives a 76% success rate. Irradiation destroys fibroblasts. Risk of later development of skin cancer which can be reduced by using iridium wires.
- *Silicone materials:* decrease scar volume and increase elasticity in 60–100% of patients. Get mild heat rash. These can be fluid, gel or rubber. Effective in 75–85% after surgery. Wear for 24 hours/day for at least 3/12. The effect is not due to pressure or the difference in O_2 or temperature. It may relate to static electricity and hydration, as keratinocytes need a moist environment to downregulate fibroblasts.
- *Laser:*
  ○ Non-ablative pulsed dye has the best response with scars being more pliable and less hypertrophic;
  ○ Ablative ER:YAG and CO2 laser.
- *Cryotherapy:* leads to cellular anoxia. Response rate of 50–70%. Younger scars have a better response.
- *Calcium antagonist:* verapamil has been shown to have some beneficial effect on the

control of cell growth and matrix accumulation in keloids. It has been shown to decrease IL-6 and VEGF production.
See SCAR.

Keratoacanthoma

- Benign self-limiting skin tumour.
- Occurs in sun-exposed areas and appearance closely resembles *Squamous cell carcinoma*.
- Derived from the hair follicle and usually a solitary firm keratinous 1–2 cm papule. Triphasic natural history:
  ○ Proliferative phase—rapid early over 2–8 weeks;
  ○ Stabilization;
  ○ Regression when the central plug is expelled and spontaneous resolution occurs.
- The central portion of the lesion is filled with a keratin plug. These lesions share similar dermoscopy features with SCC and differentiation with histology is subtle: typically, there is ground glass cytoplasm, cytological atypia, mitoses, margins rounded with no infiltration.
- *Management:* despite low potential for malignant transformation, surgical excision remains gold standard with approximately 5 mm peripheral margin, as difficult to distinguish from an SCC clinically.
See FERGUSON–SMITH SYNDROME.

Kernahan classification

Graphical classification of *Cleft lip and palate*.

- The deformity is likened to a letter Y with the two diagonal limbs representing anatomical structures belong to the primary palate anterior to the incisive foramen and the common limb representing structures belonging to the secondary palate posterior to the incisive foramen.
- Stippling indicates a cleft in an anatomical area whereas cross-hatching indicates a submucous area.
- Modifications to the Kernahan classification have been made to enable documentation of the cleft nasal deformity.

Kienbock's disease

- Kienbock described avascular necrosis of the lunate or lunatomalacia in 1910.
- May result from stress fracture. Negative ulnar variance is more common. Probably have a tenuous blood supply, which is disrupted by repetitive loads to the wrist.

Presentation: usually young adult male with a painful stiff weak wrist. Usually dominant wrist. Rarely a history of acute trauma. Find dorsal wrist swelling, limited wrist movement, but forearm rotation unaffected. Tenderness over lunate dorsally. Diminished grip strength.

Progression: wrist movement is decreased with progressive radiology, but function is fairly good and symptoms don't correlate with XRs.

Aetiology:
- Relates to vascularity, ulnar variance, lunate fossa inclination, and lunate geometry.
- Blood supply:
  - *Extra-osseous:* 3 types: 1. single vessel. 2. Several vessels 3. several vessels with anastomosis;
  - *Intra-osseous:* Y, I or X shape. Y and I are at risk of losing dorsal or palmar blood flow after trauma.

Ulnar variance: refers to the relationship of the distal articular surfaces of radius and ulna. Ulna minus is when the distal radius is longer than the distal ulna. 74% of wrists in Kienbock's are ulna minus, whereas only 23% of normal controls were. This may increase the load on the lunate. Check ulnar variance with a neutral rotation PA view. Shoulders abducted 90°, elbows flexed 90° and palm flat on the XR.

Geometry: triangular-shaped lunate concentrates shear forces.

Radiological classification: by *Stahl*.
- Normal radiograph.
- Increased radiodensity of lunate +/− decrease of lunate height on radial side.
- Lunate collapse with:
  - No scaphoid rotation;
  - Fixed scaphoid rotation.
- Degenerative changes around lunate.

Treatment:
- Early disease may benefit from intermittent casts or braces, but the wrist pain may be well tolerated for many years.
- Precollapse and negative ulnar variance may benefit from joint levelling, by radial shortening.
- Lunate bone grafts and revascularization is being investigated.
- Limited wrist arthrodesis (*Triscaphe*), aim to unload the lunate.
- Proximal row carpectomy provides functional range of pain-free motion, and is useful for stages II and III.
- Wrist arthrodesis for stage IV.

Kirner's anomaly
- Skeletal anomaly characterised by progressive palmar and radial curvature of the distal phalanx of the 5th digit.

- Not usually associated with functional impairment but if deemed necessary, epiphysiodesis or wedge osteotomy can be utilized. However, difficult to perform without damaging overlying nailbed or nearby extensor tendon insertion.

Kite flap
See FLAG FLAP.

Kleinmann shear test
- Test for *Carpal instability*.
- Place thumbs on dorsum of pisiform and lunate. The bones usually translate in opposite directions.

Klinefelter's syndrome
- 47, XXY.
- The most frequent abnormality of sexual differentiation.
- Occurs in 1:600 males but may remain undiagnosed.
- Get infertility, gynaecomastia, impaired sexual maturation and under-androgenization. Increased risk of diabetes, osteoporosis, breast cancer and non-Hodgkin's lymphoma.
- Multidisciplinary management involving speech therapy (for delayed speech), testosterone replacement and assisted reproduction techniques. May present for correction of gynaecomastia.

Klippel–Feil syndrome
- A congenital condition of at least 2 cervical vertebrae fusion characterized by a triad of short neck, low posterior hairline and limited neck movement.
- Most cases sporadic.

Cause:
- The process is failure of segmentation of the cervical spine. The cause of this has been postulated to be a lack of midline fusion with disruption of the notochord. A second theory is that the subclavian artery has been disrupted.
- Associated with cleft palate and Poland syndrome.

Treatment:
- This depends on the extent of the problem. MDT with neurology, neurosurgery and physiotherapy required. Anaesthesia may be a problem.
- Correction of neck webbing is difficult and consists of resection of excess skin with under-lying soft tissue with Z-plasty skin closure.
- The posterior hairline is corrected by expansion of the neck skin with subsequent

excision of the hair-bearing area with expanded skin advancement.

Klippel–Trenaunay syndrome
- Somatic mutation of *PIK3CA* gene. Cannot be inherited.
- May also be known as capillary-lympho-venous malformation (CVLM).
- Characterized by triad of low-flow vascular malformations (capillary, lymphatic and venous) in association with overgrowth of soft tissue and bone. Most common in the lower limb).
- Can be confused with Parkes-Weber syndrome (hallmarked by high-flow arterio-venous shunts).

Knight and North classification
For *Zygomatic fractures*, with frequency of occurrence.
- Undisplaced: 6%.
- Isolated arch: 10%.
- Unrotated body: 33%.
- Zygomatic body with medial rotation of ZF suture: 11%.
- Zygomatic body with lateral rotation of ZF suture: 22%.
- Complex: 18%.

Köbner's phenomenon
Skin trauma in *Psoriasis* resulting in new psoriatic lesions. Can occur with other skin conditions such as lichen planus.

Krukenberg operation
Converts the forearm into prehensile forceps. The flexors and extensors are converted to abductors and adductors. Main indication is for bilateral blind amputees. Also possibly bilateral congenital amputees.

Kuhnt–Szymanowski procedure
A procedure for paralytic or involutional *Ectropion* correction. It combines a blepharoplasty-type lower lid incision with a wedge resection of the lateral part of the posterior lamella of the lower eyelid and re-draping of the anterior lamella. The lateral placement of tissue excision helps to prevent cicatricial ecotopian, which could occur following central or medial tissue excision.

Kutler V–Y flaps
- For *Fingertip injuries*.
- Two laterally-based flaps. Use for transverse or volar oblique amputations at mid-nail level. Debride skin, trim bone. Tip of flap is at DIPJ. Gently spread to divide septa and advance flap. These flaps provide limited advancement.

Lacrimal system to Lymphoedema

Lacrimal system
- Lid lubrication is in three layers:
  - Inner mucin layer from goblet cells of conjunctiva;
  - Middle aqueous layer from lacrimal gland;
  - Outer lipid layer from meibomian glands in the tarsus and the glands of Zeiss and Moll at the root of the eyelashes.
- Lacrimal gland anatomy:
  - Located superotemporally in the orbit in the lacrimal fossa of the temporal bone;
  - Divided into two lobes by the levator aponeurosis;
  - Afferent sensory innervation from the lacrimal nerve from the ophthalmic trigeminal nerve;
  - Efferent parasympathetic innervation is via the greater petrosal nerve of the facial nerve, passing through the pterygopalatine ganglion before hitchhiking on the zygomatic branch of the maxillary trigeminal nerve.
- Lacrimal system anatomy:
  - Tears collect via the puncta of the upper and lower canaliculi at the medial aspect of the palpebral fissure. The canaliculi have a 2 mm vertical part and 8 mm horizontal part; they dilate to form ampulla at the junction of horizontal and vertical parts;
  - Canaliculi join to drain into the lacrimal sac which sits in the bony lacrimal fossa. The sac is surrounded by the lacrimal pump which are fibres of orbicularis oculi;
  - Lacrimal sac empties into the bony opening of the nasolacrimal duct which is composed of intra-osseous part 12 mm in length in the maxilla and membranous part in the nasal mucosa, which drains into the inferior meatus beneath the inferior turbinate.

Lacrimal duct damage following trauma (iatrogenic or nasoethmoidal fractures) can be visualised using CT-DCG (dacryocystography). Manage by repairing both upper and lower canaliculi over silicone splints (for 3 months) and ORIF fractures to correct the obstruction. Chronic obstruction will require a dacryocystorhinostomy which can be performed open or endoscopically.

Ladder
Reconstructive ladder principle is to perform the simplest effective procedure. More modern, however, is to consider the reconstructive elevator, i.e. the surgeon should jump straight to the most effective and appropriate reconstructive method. The range is:

- Secondary healing.
- Primary closure.
- Split skin graft.
- Full thickness skin graft.
- Skin substitute.
- Local flap.
- Tissue expansion.
- Distant pedicled flap.
- Free flap.
- Composite free flap.

Lagophthalmos
- The inability to close the eyelid.
- Causes of lagophthalmos include exophthalmos, an impairment of mechanical closure of the lids, e.g. burns of the eyelids, paralysis of orbicularis oculi or leprosy.

Lambdoid synostosis
- True isolated lambdoid synostosis is rare.
- <1% of synostosis.
- <1:10,000 births.
- Head shape is a posterior plagiocephaly.
- Get occipital flattening and marked mastoid bulging. The opposite occiput bulges.
  See CRANIOSYNOSTOSIS.

Landsmeer ligaments
Oblique retinacular ligament (ORL):
- The ORLs are attached proximally to the distal metaphysis of the proximal phalanx at the distal bony attachment of the A2 pulley.
- The ligaments run distally under the transverse retinacular ligament to join the lateral band.

- Each ORL lies volar to the axis of PIP joint motion and through the attachment to the conjoined tendon passes dorsally to the DIP joint. FDP initiates flexion at the DIP joint, which tightens the ORL, which increases flexion at the PIP joint giving synchronized flexion. It helps to prevent hyperextension of the PIP joint during extension.
- At the level of the PIPJ, ORL holds in place 7 tendinous structures—central slip of extensor tendon, 2 lateral bands, 2 slips from the central slip to the lateral bands and 2 slips from the lateral bands to the central slip.

Transverse retinacular ligament:
- Short wide fibres extend along the lateral side of the PIP joint superficial to the collateral ligament. They originate from the volar plate and the flexor tendon sheath in the area of the A1 pulley. They extend dorsally where they attach to the lateral margin of each lateral band.
- The transverse retinacular ligament pulls the lateral bands volarly during digital flexion. During extension they limit the dorsomedial displacement of the lateral bands. They play an important role in preventing swan neck deformity.

See RETINACULAR SYSTEM. *See* HAINES–ZANCOLLI TEST.

Langer's lines
- Lines of *Skin* tension originally demonstrated by Langer in 1861 by tapping holes in cadaveric skin with an ice pick-like instrument and noting direction of the resultant elliptical wounds.
- Useful for incision placement planning parallel to the Langer's line.
- Similar in many areas of the body to the relaxed skin tension lines (RSTLs), which are orientated perpendicular to underlying muscle fibres.

Langerhans cells
Located within stratum spinosum of the epidermis. Front line immune system. They process foreign antigens and present them to T lymphocytes.
See SKIN.

Laryngopharyngectomy
- Partial pharyngeal defects can be closed primarily or using pedicled myocutaneous flaps (such as pectoralis major) or free flaps.
- Circumferential defects where the lower anastomosis is above the clavicle are reconstructed with free flaps as a first-line. *Free jejunal, gastro-omental* or tubed fasciocutaneous flaps over a salivary tube

(RFFF or ALT) can be used depending on patient factors such as body habitus. The biggest problem remains fistula and stenosis, which occur in about 20% of patients. Excessive length may cause swallowing difficulties.
- Circumferential defects with resection below the clavicle may be reconstructed by gastric pull-up procedures, but these are associated with significant morbidity, with up to 40% fistula formation and operative mortality of up to 20%.
- *Voice restoration*.

Larynx carcinoma
The larynx is divided into 3 parts based on embryology which dictates vascular and lymphatic supply and therefore impacts spread of malignancies.

- *Supraglottic larynx:* extends from superior tip of epiglottis to apex of laryngeal ventricle. Lymphatics drain to thyrohyoid membrane.
- *Glottic larynx:* bounded superiorly by the apex of the laryngeal ventricle and inferiorly 1 cm below the ventricle apex or 5 mm below the free edge of vocal cord. A paucity of lymphatics in this region therefore isolated tumours associated with comparatively better prognosis.
- *Subglottis:* extends from inferior edge of glottis to inferior aspect of cricoid cartilage. Extensive lymphatics drain to cervical nodes.
- There are certain barriers to tumour spread, which may enable a less extensive resection. Metastasis to the neck varies depending on site with supraglottic being the highest risk.

Laser
- Based on Einstein's theory of Light Amplification by Stimulated Emission of Radiation (LASER). Developed by Maimon in 1960.
- Monochromatic collimated coherent light is produced. All light is part of the electromagnetic spectrum. Surgical lasers are between near infrared and ultraviolet, which includes visible light. Similar to a fluorescent light. The medium is a solid, liquid or gas, which when excited by absorbed energy causes the atom to be elevated to a higher energy state. Atoms in an excited state are a fixed energy level above ground state. As the atom returns to ground state the energy is released as an emission of radiation as photons.

Components:
- Active medium in a resonator. Parallel mirrors at each end. Energy supplied by an

energizer pump. Energy is absorbed causing population inversion. Energy is amplified by the reflecting mirrors. The radiation each atom emits is in phase with the radiation in the tube. The radiation is allowed to escape through a small unsilvered hole in the mirror. Monochromatic collimated coherent light escapes.

Light measurements:

- Used routinely in laser applications include energy, fluence, power and irradiance:

  o *Energy* is proportional to the number of photons and is measured in joules (J);
  o *Power* is the rate of delivery of the energy, measured in watts (W), where 1 W = 1 J/S;
  o *Irradiance* is the power per unit area, measured in W/cm^2;
  o *Fluence* is the energy delivered per unit area, measured in J/cm^2.

Electromagnetic spectrum: range from gamma rays to radio waves. Most clinical lasers are in the visible portion (400–700 nm).

Mode of delivery:

- Variety of delivery methods.
- *CW or continuous wave:* uninterrupted without pulses.
- *Pulsed mode:* light is delivered in single pulses or a train of pulses.
- *Superpulsed mode:* extremely high-peak powers with each pulse. Pulses are brief and repetition rate may be varied.
- *Q switching:* when one of the resonating mirrors is non-reflective for an interval of pumping. When this occurs the stored energy is emitted as a powerful pulse of light 10 billionths of a second in length.

Tissue action and interactions:

- On contact with tissue, laser light is scattered, reflected, transmitted, but mostly absorbed. Kinetic energy converts to heat which ablates tissue.
- The chromophore of the tissue determines which wavelength is absorbed.
- *Thermal:* the tissue effect is primarily thermal. The extent of the effect depends on the degree of absorption of light and diffusion to adjacent tissues. Key factors are the energy density, pulse duration and heat conduction.
- *Mechanical:* if pulse duration is shorter than thermal relaxation, then thermo-elastic expansion will occur. This change is sudden and generates acoustic waves.
- *Selective photothermolysis:* this theory has two components:

  o Wavelength determines absorption of energy;
  o Exposure time (pulse width) limits thermal diffusion if the pulse width is less than the thermal relaxation time of the tissues.

- *Thermal relaxation time:* the time required for a specific tissue to absorb and transmit thermal energy. To minimize thermal injury, the appropriate *pulse width* is chosen. Pulse width is the duration of pulse. Laser therapy has been refined by matching pulse widths to thermal relaxation time. Clinical result is maximized when laser passes through tissue and is absorbed by the target. The target substances are called chromophores.
- Primary chromophores are haemoglobin, melanin and water. They may also come from external sources such as tattoo pigments. Laser techniques have been limited by thermally-induced damage. Getting the wavelength right reduces this. Cooling with cryogen spray can protect epidermis when treating vascular lesions.

Laser systems:

- CO_2 (10,600 nm): the most frequently used. Chromophore = water. As the beam is invisible it is coupled with a visible beam of HeNe. Can be delivered as CW, or pulsed CW, which has less thermal injury.
- *Flashlamp-pumped pulsed dye (FLPD):* dye lasers contain fluorescent dyes, which are dissolved in solvents such as water or alcohol. These absorb light at one wavelength and emit at another. By changing the dye they can be tuned over a wide band (400–1,000 nm). Laser is delivered in short single pulses at high peak powers. So 585 nm wavelength is absorbed well by haemoglobin and a pulse duration of 450 ms matches the thermal relaxation time of blood vessels making it suitable for cutaneous vascular lesions. It penetrates to depth of 0.75 mm. In dark skin can lead to damage to melanocytes, leading to hypopigmentation.
- *Long-pulse dye laser:* for larger calibre vessels, a longer pulse width is required. 595–600 nm for 1.5 ms. Promising results with leg veins.
- *YAG lasers:* several types (neodymium Nd, erbium Er). The common denominator is a crystal of yttrium-aluminium-garnet. This is doped with an ion. Doping is the process where the crystal is grown with an impurity. Nd:YAG has a wavelength of 1064. There is no particular chromophore for this wavelength so its effect is coagulation and haemostasis. Effective for diffuse thermal injury such as deep vascular tumours. Q-switched Nd:YAG

used for tattoos. KTP:YAG has a wavelength of 532 nm. Good for oral mucosa. Er:YAG has a wavelength of 2940 nm close to that of water. Therefore, little heat transferred. Good for skin resurfacing.

- *Q-switched Alexandrite:* chromium-doped BeAl2O4. Tune from 701 nm to 826 nm. Good for tattoo greens and blues.
- *Argon:* one of the first used. Two wavelengths of 488 nm and 514 nm so it is absorbed by haemoglobin and melanin. Can give hypertrophic scars and depigmentation.
- *Copper vapour:* 578 and 511 nm wavelength. 578 nm is oxyhaemoglobin and 511 nm is melanin. Used for *Port wine stains* and telangiectasia.
- *Ruby:* first laser developed. Initially CW then Q-switched. 694 nm—melanin. Useful for pigmented lesions and tattoos. Long-pulse ruby penetrates deeper and has been used for hair removal. May get pigment changes.

Safety: CO_2 laser is in the invisible infrared spectrum. Protective plastic eyewear required. Glass may shatter. Patients require frosted metal scleral protectors with lubrication.

Clinical applications:

- *Vascular lesions:* the pulsed dye is most commonly used. Continuous wave lasers may be effective for large-diameter vascular lesions including nodular *Port wine stains*.
- Pigmented lesions: blue, green, red and near infrared wavelengths can be used. Q-switched ruby, Q-switched alexandrite and Q-switched Nd:YAG can be used to treat dermal lesions. Epidermal lesions respond to the green pulsed dye laser, frequency doubled Q-switched Nd:YAG, and the Q-switched ruby lasers.
- Benign naevi *Naevus of Ota/Ito*, *Café au lait macules*, *Naevus spilus*, *Becker's naevi*, *Melasma* have a variable response. Dysplastic naevi should not be treated and treatment of congenital naevi is controversial.
- *Tattoos:* the *Q-switched laser*, Nd:YAG, alexandrite and green pulsed dye lasers are all employed in tattoo removal. Each laser enables removal of specific colours of ink; however, none of these can remove all ink pigments. Multicoloured tattoos, especially fluorescent inks, are difficult to treat. Irreversible blackening of some inks has occurred with Q-switched lasers. CO_2 laser vaporizes the tattoo and the defect left to re-epithelialize resulting in a scar.
- *Laser resurfacing:* good for Fitzpatrick skin type 1 and 2. Type 3 can get pigment abnormalities. Continuous wave CO_2 lasers

were used, but resulted in significant scarring. Ultrapulsed laser limits damage with a high power for short duration. The ER:YAG lasers were the next to be used for resurfacing. Vaporization leads to re-epithelialization. Darker skin may hyperpigment. If so, treat with hydroquinone, hydrocortisone and tretinoin. Post-operatively the area can be dressed with an occlusive dressing or vaseline.

- *Laser depilation:* does not provide a permanent solution, but rather a hair-free interval. Use long pulsed alexandrite or Nd. YAG. Six treatments gives an 80% reduction in hair.
- *Others:* lasers have also been used in the treatment of warts, in incisional surgery and for actinic cheilitis.

Laser Doppler flowometry

Can be used to record blood flow in a small area or scan over a large area. It measures Doppler shift of light. These changes are produced by movement of macromolecules within vessels. The depth of penetration is limited to 1.5 mm.

Lateral arm flap

- Fasciocutaneous flap based on septal vessels. Initially described as a free flap, it can also be pedicled proximally or distally.
- The flap is supplied by the posterior radial collateral artery arising from the profunda brachii. Perforating vessels lie in the lateral intermuscular septum between triceps and brachialis/brachioradialis.
- Pedicle can be 8 cm long. The vessel diameter is 1.2 mm.
- The flap is supplied by the lower lateral cutaneous nerve of the arm which arises from the radial nerve and passes through triceps. The posterior cutaneous nerve runs through the flap.
- The flap can be sensate and can measure 14 × 30 cm.

Flap raise:

- Flap outlined on the distal 1/3 of lateral aspect of arm. Extend over lateral epicondyle. Flap axis and proximal incision is traced along a line between acromion and epicondyle. Incise deep fascia with skin and release posterior half from triceps until septum is seen. Septum separated anterior from posterior compartment and contains the vessel. Anteriorly separate fascia from brachialis, brachioradialis and extensors. Proximally separate deltoid from triceps to expose the pedicle and radial nerve. Ligate descending anterior branch. Identify two nerves—one to flap, the other going through it. Incise septum to release the flap. Ligate vessels distally.

See ORAL CAVITY RECONSTRUCTION.

Lateral femoral cutaneous nerve decompression

- T12.
- The lateral femoral cutaneous nerve runs along the inside of the iliac bone on iliacus and passes through transversus and through inguinal ligament at variable point 1–6 cm medial to the anterior superior iliac spine. Decompress through a transverse incision overlying the lateral 1/3 of the inguinal ligament and identify the nerve by dissecting through fascia inferior to ligament.
- Delineate nerve and split inguinal ligament and tendinous transversus tendon until completely released.

Lateral plantar flap

- Sensate flap below the lateral malleolar area along the lateral side of the foot.
- Pedicled on the lateral calcaneal artery, a terminal branch of the peroneal artery.
- Rotates to the Achilles tendon and lateral malleolar area.
- Can be raised as an adipofascial flap.

Lateral plantar nerve S1–2:

Terminal branch of tibial nerve. Supplies sensation to the lateral forefoot. Supplies motor to most of the deep muscles in the foot in a manner analogous to the ulnar nerve in the hand.

Lateral pterygoid

Origin: two heads. Upper from infratemporal crest, lower head from lateral surface of lateral pterygoid plate.

Insertion: upper head into capsule of joint and articular disc. Lower head into neck of condyle.

Action: upper portion pulls medially and forward. External portion pulls the condyle downward medially and forward.

Innervation: mandibular branch of the trigeminal nerve.

Latissimus dorsi flap

Origin: spinous processes T7–12, L1–5, posterior superior iliac crest, ribs 9–12.

Insertion: into humerus.

Blood supply: dominant pedicle, thoracodorsal artery, and segmental pedicles, posterior intercostals and lumbar artery perforating branches—type V muscle. The thoracodorsal artery comes off the subscapular artery. Mean length 9 cm, increase by 2 cm by following up subscapular artery. Usually a single artery and

vein. The vessels usually bifurcate into an upper transverse branch and a lateral vertical branch. It is possible to raise the muscle based on reverse flow from serratus anterior when the main pedicle has been cut.

Nerve supply: thoracodorsal nerve from the posterior cord of the brachial plexus.

Function: shoulder adduction, arm medial rotation and extension. Pulls the trunk forward. After raising flap there is no significant difference in shoulder power. Scar contracture causes up to 30% reduction in shoulder movement in 1/3 of patients (Laitung/Peck). No occupational problems.

Flap raise:
- *Position:* lateral decubitus. Prep ipsilateral arm so that it can be moved in the field.
- *Define landmarks:* Spine, Pelvic rim, Scapula, Posterior axillary fold.
- *Marking:* many options for raising skin as there are multiple perforators. More numerous in the proximal 2/3 of muscle. Start at posterior axillary fold and extend marking inferiorly and medially (obliquely) over the muscle. If no skin needed, mark a straight incision.
- *Raise:*
  - Easiest to identify correct plane in a muscle only flap raise if you start superiorly at the inferior edge of scapula as you can define the superior edge of the muscle. If a skin paddle is being taken—start at the anterior edge of the muscle—when you have identified the pedicle under the muscle the posterior skin incision can be made.
  - Extend dissection medially to midline and divide the attachments of the muscle to the midthoracic spine.
  - Raise the muscle towards the axilla, keeping pedicle on undersurface of muscle. Be careful not to raise serratus muscle with flap. Ligate branch to serratus and consider ligating circumflex scapular branch if more length is needed and pedicle needs to go to origin of subscapular branch. Decide wither to dennervate the flap or not.
  - Close in layers. Consider quilting stitches to reduce seroma. Consider drains.

See TRUNK RECONSTRUCTION. *See* BREAST RECONSTRUCTION. *See* CHEST WALL RECONSTRUCTION.

Le Fort fractures

René Le Fort was a French surgeon at the end of the nineteenth century. He looked at the fractures of skulls dropped from upper-storey windows. Fracture lines travel adjacent to thicker areas of bone, the buttresses. Maxillary fractures had the following patterns.

Alveolar fractures: fractured due to direct force or indirect force transmitted from the mandible. Usually reduce and fix with palatal splint.

Le Fort 1—transverse:
- Also called Guerin fracture.
- Get two segments—the lower floating palate contains the alveolus, palate and pterygoid plates.
- The fracture line passes transversely across:
  ○ Base of piriform aperture;
  ○ Base of maxillary sinus;
  ○ Pterygoid plates.

Le Fort 2 fracture—pyramidal:
- The fracture line passes:
  ○ Across the nasal bones;
  ○ Into the medial wall of the orbit;
  ○ Diagonally downwards and outwards through the maxilla;
  ○ Through the pterygoid plates.
- The bony fragment contains lacrimal crests, bulk of maxilla, piriform margin, alveolus, palate.

Le Fort 3 fracture—craniofacial dysjunction:
- The fracture line passes:
  ○ Through the nasofrontal suture;
  ○ Across the orbital floor to the NF suture;
  ○ Through the zygomatic arch and pterygoid plates.

This results in detachment of the entire midfacial skeleton from the cranial base. They are often asymmetrical. The midface is held to the skull only by soft tissues.

Vertical or sagittal fracture: the maxilla is split longitudinally along the junction of maxilla with vomer.

See MAXILLARY FRACTURES.

Le Fort osteotomy
Le Fort I: the most commonly used osteotomy. Perform 4–5 mm above the roots of the teeth. Go across maxilla below infra-orbital foramen. Through lateral and medial maxillary walls below nasolacrimal duct. Separate septum from vomer. Perform osteotomy between the maxillary tuberosity and the pterygoid plate of the sphenoid. Bone grafts may be used.

Le Fort II: this is the true total maxillary osteotomy. It is indicated in occasional cleft patients with severe maxillary hypoplasia involving the nose and infra-orbital rims and in Crouzon's disease without exorbitism, Binder's syndrome and patients with hemifacial microsomia, where

the naso-ethmoid complex is deviated to the affected side.

Le Fort III: this enlarges the orbital cavity and advances the maxilla. As the degree of exorbitism and retromaxillism may not correlate, the goal of this operation is to correct the bulging eye. A Le Fort I can also be performed to correct the malocclusion. *See* MAXILLA. *See* MAXILLARY OSTEOTOMY.

Le Mesurier–Hagedorn cleft lip reconstruction
Cleft lip reconstruction with a rectangular flap from the cleft side is inset into a releasing incision on the non-cleft side to create an artificial Cupid's bow.

Ledderhose's disease
Plantar fibromatosis associated with *Dupuytren's contracture*. Large tender nodules occur on the instep. Rarely get flexion contracture in the toes.

Leddy and Packer's classification of FDP avulsion
Classification for *Closed avulsion* of FDP. Based on the level at which the tendon lies.
- *Type I:* retracts to palm, vincula are disrupted.
- *Type II:* retracts to PIPJ after disruption of the short vincula. Tendon nutrition is preserved so it can be repaired up to 3/12 after injury. However, delay can convert it to a type I injury.
- *Type III:* bony fragment that doesn't pass the A4 pulley. Both vincula are preserved.

Leeches
Leeches are worms of the Annelid phylum, which feed on blood extracted from the host. The most common type used is *Hirudo medicinalis* from Southeast Asia and Europe. They were used 3,500 years ago in Egypt. Also in India. They were used in the Middle Ages and extensively in the nineteenth century for bloodletting. They have been used since 1960 in plastic surgery. In 1981 there was a reported success rate of 60% artery-only digit replants.

Indications: venous congestion may lead to oedema, reduced capillary and arterial flow, and venous and arterial thrombosis. Leeches may assist in flap salvage. They may be used to decongest replanted parts. If there is a good arterial inflow and poor venous outflow consider leech therapy. Venous competence is usually restored by day 4–5 for digits and 6–10 for free flaps.

Action:
- The front sucker conceals cartilaginous cutting plates that make a 2-mm incision. In 30 minutes a leech can ingest 10 times its own body weight or 5–15 ml of blood.

- Hirudin, an anticoagulant is injected. This inhibits the conversion of fibrinogen to fibrin. It also blocks platelet aggregation in response to thrombin. As thrombin is the final common pathway it is regarded as the most potent anticoagulant.
- Leech saliva also contains a local anaesthetic, hyaluronidase and a histamine-like vasodilator.

Complications:
- Infection with _Aeromonas hydrophila_, which is found in the gut of the leech. This is a Gram-negative rod and may infect up to 20% of patients. Give prophylaxis with third generation cephalosporin aminoglycoside.
- May cause significant blood loss.

Application: may prick the flap to encourage the leeches to feed. Direct the head (narrow end) to the flap. If they fail to feed it is a poor prognostic indicator for flap survival. They feed for about 30 minutes.

Leg ulcers
Aetiology: venous ulceration accounts for most cases of ulceration. 27% of adults have venous insufficiency, with 1.5% having ulceration. _See_ VENOUS HYPERTENSION. _See_ VENOUS ULCERS.

Differential diagnosis: VATIMAN:

- _Venous._
- _Arterial._
- _Trauma:_ insect bites, trophic, frostbite, radiation.
- _Infection:_ bacterial, fungal TB, syphilis.
- _Metabolic:_ DM, necrobiosis lipoidica, pyoderma gangrenosum, porphyria, gout.
- _Autoimmune:_ lupus, RA, polyarteritis nodosa.
- _Neoplasia:_ SCC, BCC, Kaposi's sarcoma, lymphoma.

Investigations: to determine the cause of the ulcer—wound swab limited benefit due to inevitable colonization with skin commensals, ABPI—normally 1.2. Venous duplex scanning and arterial studies. XR, biopsy.

Management: is tailored to the underlying cause of the ulceration. Arterial inflow deficiency will require arterial reconstruction, see _Venous ulcers_ for their management.

Non-operative treatment: elevate, hygiene, compression.

Surgery: subfascial ligation of perforating vessels, skin graft, flap reconstruction.

Plantar forefoot ulcers: usually over the metatarsal heads. Exposes bone and tendons and require digital amputations. Metatarsal head resection, conservative for big toe, resections for 2–4 and amputation for 5th. Plantar

V–Y advancement flaps, islanded toe flaps, or distally based muscle flaps.

Heel ulcer: wide osseous debridement. Local rotation/advancement flaps, medial plantar artery flap, turnover muscle flaps and free flaps.

Sickle cell ulcers: occur in 25–75% of homozygous sickle cell disease. They are chronic, recurrent, painful and disabling. Minor trauma causes sickling and thrombosis, ischaemia and further ulceration. Skin grafts are not helpful as they do not bring in any new blood supply. Free flaps are the procedure of choice. The ischaemia is not inevitably detrimental. Perform exchange transfusion, maintain haematocrit at 31–35%, washout flap with warm heparinized saline-dextran, give dextran and aspirin, warm, antibiotics, oxygen.

Legueu and Juvara: septa of
- The septa of Legueu and Juvara originate from the palmar fascia at the level of the proximal edge of the flexor tendon sheath and pass dorsally between the lateral surfaces of the A1 pulleys and the digital neurovascular bundles.
- They attach to the deep transverse metacarpal ligament at the point of insertion of the volar plate of the MCP joint.

   See RETINACULAR SYSTEM.

Leiomyomas
- Benign cutaneous tumours consisting of smooth muscle proliferation.
- Multiple cutaneous leiomyomas occur in widely varying numbers.
- Frequently they harden and become painful on pressure or application of cold. They may arise from arrectores pilorum muscles.
- Solitary angioleiomyomas are seen mainly on the legs. They may be sensitive to pressure and cold and may arise from venular smooth muscle.
- A third variety is found in the scrotum, labia majora, or nipple area.
- Treatment is by excision, but recurrence is frequent.

Lentigo
- Pigmented flat lesions that increase with age and are frequently found on the face and neck.
- They contain increased numbers of melanocytes. They persist in the absence of sunlight. This is in contrast to an ephelis (freckle) which contains a normal number of melanocytes and disappears in the absence of sunlight.
- Three types:

○ *Lentigo simplex:* not induced by the sun, may occur in young and middle aged and build in number with age;

○ *Lentigo senilis:* occur in the elderly;

○ *Solar lentigo:* occurs after sun exposure.

See NAEVUS.

Lentigo maligna

• It is a melanoma *in situ* confined to the epidermis. Also called Hutchinson's melanotic freckle.

• Elderly patients, sun-exposed areas of face and extremities. Patients usually present with an asymptomatic pigmented patch that has changed in size, shape or colour.

• Prolonged radial growth phase before entering into a vertical growth phase.

• Transformation to *Melanoma* occurs in 30–50%.

• Tissue diagnosis with incisional biopsy may miss subclinical microinvasion. Excision biopsy with 5 mm margin is ideal but may not be feasible because lesions are typically ill-defined, widespread and in cosmetically-sensitive areas. In these circumstances a peripheral margin technique, such as the *Linguine technique* may be considered.

Lentigo Maligna Melanoma

• A subtype of invasive malignant *Melanoma*, managed as per the melanoma guidelines.

LEOPARD syndrome

• An acronym: **L**entingines, **E**lectrocardiographic conduction abnormalities, **O**cular hypertelorism, **P**ulmonary stenosis, **A**bnormalities of genitalia, **R**etardation of growth, **D**eafness.

• Part of the RASopathies along with Noonan syndrome and *Neurofibromatosis* type 1. Result from germline mutations in the stem cell pool of the neural crest giving cutaneous and neurological defects. It is a rare condition.

• Lentigines are small dark macules.

Leprosy

Leprosy is a chronic infectious disease cause by *Mycobacterium leprae*. It primarily affects the skin and peripheral nerves, producing characteristic deformities. Reconstruction for leprosy includes:

• The commonest peripheral neuropathy is ulnar nerve palsy followed by median nerve palsy. Treatment may require tendon transfers.

• Common deformities that are typical of the face in leprosy:

○ Megalobule of the external ear;

○ Loss of eyebrows;

○ Nasal deformity;

○ Sagging and wrinkled redundant facial skin;

○ Lagophthalmos.

Lesion

When examining a lesion, remember S^3C^2M:

• Site.

• Size.

• Shape.

• Colour.

• Consistency.

• Mobility.

Leucoplakia

• White patch, found on oral, vulval, vaginal mucosa.

• In the mouth it is often seen in older men, linked to smoking, poor-fitting dentures and poor oral hygiene.

• Microscopically get hyperkeratosis and acanthosis. Get cellular atypia in epidermal layer and inflammatory infiltrate in dermal layer.

• 15–20% undergo malignant transformation. The *Squamous cell carcinoma* that develop are much more aggressive than those associated with *Solar keratosis*.

Levator palpebrae superioris

• Arises from lesser wing of sphenoid above superior rectus muscle. Passes forward for 40 mm to end just behind the septum as an aponeurosis.

• Close to the origin of the aponeurosis the muscle sheath is thickened above the muscle to form a band—Whitnall's ligament. This may be a definite structure or a more diffuse thickening. It inserts into the trochlea medially, and the capsule of the lacrimal gland and orbital wall laterally. It acts as a fulcrum for the action of the levator.

• The levator aponeurosis descends into the lid and the septum inserts onto its anterior surface as a thickened band 8 mm below Whitnall's ligament and 3 mm above tarsus. The angle formed contains the pre-aponeurotic fat pad. As the aponeurosis descends it becomes thinner and fans out. It inserts anteriorly into orbicularis muscle at the skin crease and below into the lower anterior surface of the tarsal plate.

• Innervated by CN3 oculomotor nerve

Levator veli palatini

Origin: inferior surface of petrous temporal bone and medial rim of Eustachian tube.

Insertion: palatine aponeurosis in middle third of the soft palate

Action: elevates, retracts and laterally deviates the soft palate. It may open the Eustachian tube on swallowing.

Nerve supply: pharyngeal branch of vagus nerve with motor fibres from the cranial accessory nerve.

See CLEFT PALATE.

Lhermitte sign

• Sudden painful or electrical sensation on flexing the neck.
• Spreads to the lower cervical or lumbosacral spine into the limbs.
• Seen in multiple sclerosis, cervical myopathy or after head injury.

Li-Fraumeni syndrome

• Autosomal dominant inheritance.
• *TP53* gene mutation.
• Primarily associated with sarcomas, breast cancer, brain tumours, leukaemia and adrenocortical carcinoma.
• Management may include high risk cancer-screening (i.e. MRI breast screening) and/or prophylactic operations.

Lichtman test

• To evaluate midcarpal instability.
• Examiner palpates triquetrum on dorso-ulnar aspect of wrist, 2 cm distal to ulnar head, with wrist positioned in pronation and palmar flexion. On radial deviation of wrist the triquetrum should become prominent whereas on ulnar deviation it disappears.
• If triquetrum initially becomes more prominent on ulnar deviation of wrist, suggests attrition of the triquetro-hamato-capitate ligament.

Lidocaine

• An amide *Local anaesthetic*.
• In comparison to bupivacaine, lidocaine has low toxicity, low lipid solubility, low potency, rapid onset and medium duration of 1–3 hours.
• Maximal dose plain is 3 mg/kg. With adrenaline is 7 mg/kg, e.g. 70 kg man and 2% lignocaine plain = $70 \times 3 \div 20 = 10.5$ ml; 80 kg man with 2% with adrenaline = $80 \times 7 \div 20 = 28$ ml.

Ligamentotaxis

• The principle of moulding fracture fragments into alignment via the maintenance of traction distal to an injured joint during a period of healing.
• This distal traction force on the peri-articular ligaments and palmar plate attachments results in reduction of some articular fracture fragments, and any associated joint dislocation with realignment of the joint surface.
• This principle is the basis for the use of external fixators in unstable long bone fractures.

Limberg flap *See* RHOMBIC FLAP.

Linburg-Comstock Anomaly

A tendinous communication between flexor pollicis longus (FPL) and flexor digitorum profundus (FDP) of the index finger. Causes simultaneous flexion of the IPJ of the thumb and DIPJ of the index finger (termed *Linburg's sign*). Present in 30% of people due to adhesions in the carpal tunnel between FPL and FDP index. Often unnoticed but may cause a problem in musicians.

Linburg's syndrome

Symptomatic restrictive thumb-index flexor tenosynovitis with hypertrophic tenosynovium between FPL and FDP. Forearm pain is aggravated when index DIP joint is blocked when the thumb is flexed.

Treatment: rest, NSAIDs, steroids. Surgery involved exploring the distal forearm and wrist and dividing any tendinous interconnections.

Lingual flap

Dorsal lingual flap:

• Must not cross the median raphe. Elevated at 8 mm thickness to include mucosa, sub-mucosa and superficial muscle.
• Posteriorly based can be used for retromolar triangle. Anteriorly based can repair cheek and commissure. Transverse flaps can repair floor of mouth (FOM) defects.

Lingual tip: perimeter flaps can be raised.

Ventral surface flaps: used for FOM with skin graft to donor.

See ORAL CAVITY RECONSTRUCTION.

Linguine technique

• Peripheral-margin controlled excision of skin cancer (indicated for lentingo maligna and non-melanoma skin cancer with non-distinct margins) in at least 2 operative stages.
• Anticipated pre-determined peripheral margin drawn. A 2 mm circumferential strip of tissue excised outside of margin and orientated for histology. Defect closed primarily with central lesion remaining *in situ*.
• Lesion excised at later stage when peripheral margin confirmed clear.

Linton flap

• Used in the treatment of *Venous ulcers*.
• Aims to divide the perforators between the superficial and deep system.

- Incision is parallel and 2 cm posterior to the medial tibial border from medial malleolus to midcalf.
- Deep fascia is divided and all perforating veins are ligated. It can be performed endoscopically.

Lip anatomy
Landmarks:
- Philtral columns:
  - Paired vertical linear protuberances—dermal thickenings, perhaps influenced by decussating fibres of orbicularis oris.
- Philtrum (aka philtral dimple or groove):
  - Central depression between the columns—perhaps due to fewer muscles fibres in this area.
- White roll:
  - Inferior cutaneous skin border with vermilion. Its anterior projection is due to pars marginalis of underlying orbicularis oris.
- Cupid's bow—described the curve of the vermilion-cutaneous border as it said to resemble the bow of the ancient roman god of love:
  - Peaks at the bases of the philtral columns;
  - Central trough (nadir).
- Vermilion (aka dry vermilion):
  - Keratinized mucous membrane of stratified squamous epithelium—on outer lip;
  - Median tubercle—central plumping of the dry vermillion.
- Red line:
  - Wet/dry mucosal border.
- Mucosa (aka wet vermilion):
  - Non-keratinized mucous membrane of stratified squamous epithelium—on inner lip.

Muscles:
- *Orbicularis oris:* provide oral competence. Originate lateral to the commissure (modiolus) and insert into the opposite philtral column:
  - horizontal muscle fibres compress the lips;
  - oblique fibres evert the lip; these fibres travel upward and medially from the modiolus to insert at the anterior nasal spine, nasal septum, and anterior nasal floor.
- *Levator labii superioris:* muscle originates from the inferior and medial orbital margin and curves around the alar base to insert into

the orbicularis oris fibres and the philtral column on the ipsilateral side.
- *Levator anguli oris:* muscle arises just below the lateral edge of the levator labii superioris.
- *Zygomaticus major:* muscle extends from the malar eminence and inserts into the modiolus.
- *Nasalis:* muscle has three components, which arise from bone below the piriform aperture.
- *Depressor septi:* muscle is the most medial muscle. This paired muscle arises from the periosteum over the central and lateral incisors to insert into the footplates of the medial crura. It depresses the tip of the nose and lifts the upper central lip.
- *Mentalis:* muscles elevate the lower lip. They originate from alveolar periosteum just below the vestibular sulcus and descend obliquely to insert into the skin of the chin.
- *Depressor labii inferioris:* (quadratus) arises from the lower border of the mandible. The fibres pass upward and medially, to join orbicularis oris. It depresses the lower lip.
- *Depressor anguli oris:* (triangularis) arises inferior to the quadratus muscle and continues upward to the modiolus. It draws the angle of the mouth downward and laterally.

Innervation:
- *Motor:* buccal and zygomatic branches of facial nerve for upper and mandibular for lower lip.
- *Sensory:* superior labial nerve from infra-orbital branch of trigeminal nerve for upper and inferior alveolar nerve from the mental nerve for lower lip.

Vascular: facial artery arises between mandible and anterior border of masseter, divides at commissure to form the superior and inferior labial artery.

Lymphatics: drain to submandibular and submental nodes.

Vermilion border: also white roll, transition between mucosa of the lip and skin. Alignment important.

Lip carcinoma
Diagnosis:
- Most tumours of the upper lip are BCCs and of the lower lip SCCs.
- 5% of SCCs occur on the upper lip. 2% affect the commissure, which is difficult to reconstruct and has a high metastatic potential.
- If nodes are present, disease survival drops from 90 to 50%.

Treatment: tumours involving the skin and dry vermilion of the lip only are treated as per the cutaneous skin cancer guidance whereas tumours involving the wet mucosa are treated as an oral carcinoma.

See HEAD AND NECK CANCER.

Lip reconstruction
Reconstructive principles:
• 1/4 to 1/3 of lip length can be excised and primarily sutured. Preserve sensation, and ensure anatomic alignment, particularly of white roll and cutaneous-vermilion border. Major problem is reduction of size of the mouth. The lower lip has a less complex shape and can be reduced without cosmetic compromise.

Vermilion reconstruction:
• Vermilion is a modified mucosal surface. It is the most visible portion of the lip. It is very sensitive.
• Lip shave procedure performed for widespread field change particularly of the lower lip. Primary closure may be possible. If there is too much tension perform a buccal advancement by releasing mucosa in the deep sulcus and elevated deep to salivary glands just superficial to muscle. This bipedicled flap is then advanced.
• *Vermilion switch flap* can be used.
• *Notch deformities* of vermilion: perform excision, Z-plasty, V-Y advancement.

Lower lip reconstruction:
• Anaesthesia with *Mental nerve block*. For the region below the labiomental fold also need local premandibular infiltration or bilateral inferior alveolar nerve blocks along the medial border of the mandibular ramus.
• *Wedge excision:* for tumour avoid simple V incision as this will not give adequate tumour clearance towards the apex of the V. Instead perform a W incision.
• *Step ladder technique (Johanson).*
• *Abbé flap:* for lower lip place flap at junction of mid and lateral thirds to spare the philtrum and commissure. If the incision is placed in the philtrum the scar will occur in a naturally occurring ridge.
• *Estlander flap:* a laterally based switch flap pedicled on the labial artery.
• *Karapandzic flap:* a modification of the *Gillies fan flap*, which maintains the neurovascular pedicle in the soft tissue giving better functional results.
• *Bernard operation:* advancement of full thickness flaps with triangular excision.

• *Webster modification:* of Bernard operation: excises skin only in the Burow's triangles.
• *Gillies fan flap:* fan-shaped rotational advancement flap based on the superior labial artery.
• *McGregor flap:* rectangular-shaped flap, based on superior labial artery, which is rotated around the commissure without reducing the size of the stoma.
• *Schuchardt flap:* the defect is excised as a rectangular defect and the incision is extended around the labiomental fold to the submental region on each side to allow lip to slide into the defect.

Defects over 65%:
• Depends on the availability of tissue. Bilateral cheek advancement or composite flaps, otherwise free flaps.
• *Free flap:* for very large defects. Radial forearm flap with palmaris longus tendon attached to the modiolus enables the flap to act as a dam. Ensure harvest of enough tissue to act as a sulcus. Antebrachial nerve can be coapted to mental nerve. Usually the lip remains immobile and insensate.

Upper lip reconstruction:
• More difficult to reconstruct because of the more complex shape:
  ○ Small defects can be closed directly.
• *Medium defects: Abbé flap.* Excision of periled crescents may enable a decrease in defect size to accommodate the Abbé flap.
• *Large defects:*
  ○ Reverse Karapandzic flap;
  ○ Bernard procedure for large defects;
  ○ Total reconstruction depends on the available tissue; bilateral cheek advancement, pericresenteric flaps, nasolabial flaps or innervated composite flaps can be used;
  ○ Composite radial forearm flaps with palmaris longus or bone may be used.
• *Vascularized scalp island flap:* to replace particularly burned upper lip with hair bearing skin in the male. An island of scalp centred over the posterior branch of the superficial temporal artery is designed high enough in the parietal area to allow for adequate rotation. The Dopplered vessels are dissected to anterior tragus and passed through a tunnel.

Lipodermatosclerosis
See VENOUS ULCERS. Brawny oedema seen in venous ulceration.

Liposuction

Liposuction is the aspiration of fat by cannulae attached to high vacuum. The skin shrinks, the stroma with vessels and nerves remains intact.

History:

- The beginnings of liposuction occurred in 1921 when Dujarrier attempted to reduce the fat from the knees of a ballerina. Injury to the femoral artery resulted in amputation.
- Curettage was commenced again in the 1960s by Schrudde, following which suction was added.

Assessment of patient:

History:

- Patient expectation and previous cosmetic treatment.
- PMH of abdominal surgery.

Examination:

- Skin quality, elasticity and scars.
- *Cellulite:* due to tethering of fibrous septa—not well treated by liposuction and may actually get worse.
- *Distribution and extent of fat:* is it intra-abdominal?—cannot be removed by liposuction.
- Examine for hernias.

Infiltration regimes:

- *Dry:* original method not now used due to substantial swelling, bruising and blood loss.
- *Wet:* 200-300 ml of infiltrate per areas—addition of adrenaline decreases blood loss by approx. 30%.
- *Superwet = 1:1 (1 mls of infiltrate for every 1 ml of fat removed):* developed in mid-1980s and results in similar blood loss to tumescent technique so tends to be favoured to the tumescent because you don't have the problems with such large volumes of fluid.
- *Tumescent = 3:1 (3 mls of infiltrate for every 1 ml of fat removed):* introduced by Klein in 1985.

Infiltration solutions:

- Standard infiltration involves adrenaline 1 mg/L of saline with or without the addition of lidocaine.
- Using local anaesthetic in the solution you can increase the normal safe dose from 7 mg/kg up to 35 mg/kg of lidocaine, although much smaller doses (500-1000 mg/L) are most commonly used—this is because lidocaine becomes sequestered within fat cells causing slow release over 12-24 hours and adipose tissue is minimally vascular so much of the infiltration is subsequently

aspirated. Plasma levels peak 10-12 hours later which can delay the onset of toxicity.

- Avoid using bupivacaine because of longer duration and higher risk of toxicity.

Liposuction technique:

- Mark patient standing:
  - Mark zones of adherence to avoid;
  - Mark topographic contour lines.
- Use multiple stab incisions to facilitate cross-tunnelling to get a smooth result.
- Remove deep fat first.
- End points:
  - Symmetry, shape and contour;
  - Skin pinch <1 inch;
  - Removal of equal volumes from each side.
- Large volume liposuction defined as aspirating more than 5L.
- Post-op:
  - Pressure garments;
  - Swelling for 6 months;
  - Return to work in one week, normal activity at 4 weeks.

Assistance:

- *Ultrasound assisted:* USS energy to liquefy fat cells—more effective in fibrous areas such as upper back and for gynaecomastia.
- *Power-assisted:* use motor for reciprocating motion.
- *Laser-assisted:* laser to subcutaneous tissue to target fat, collagen and blood.
- Radiofrequency assisted.

Complications:

- Early:
  - Seroma;
  - Infection—can be fatal (necrotizing fasciitis);
  - Contour irregularity;
  - Pulmonary embolism due to fat or venous thrombosis—can be fatal;
  - Lidocaine toxicity;
  - Perforation of organ—may require laparotomy or thoracotomy;
  - Bleeding;
  - Numbness—usually temporary.
- Late:
  - Contour irregularities—most common complication;
  - Pigment change.

  See FAT ANATOMY.

Littler neurovascular island flap

- For large volar thumb defects to bring sensation to thumb.
- Skin and subcutaneous tissue from the ulnar side of long or ring finger is transposed across the palm as a neurovascular island flap.

Digital nerve fascicles are dissected from common digital nerve in the palm. Preserve a cuff of tissue around the pedicle to preserve venous drainage. Perform a digital Allen's test.

Probably the middle finger should preferably be used as it is also median nerve.

See FINGERTIP INJURIES.

LOAF

Mnemonic for median nerve innervated small muscles of the hand:

- *L:* 2 radial lumbricals.
- *O:* opponens brevis.
- *A:* abductor pollicis brevis.
- *F:* superficial head of flexor pollicis brevis.

Local anaesthetics

History:

- *Cocaine* (an ester) was the first to be used but was addictive and dangerous.
- Procaine was used in 1905.
- Two groups, esters and amide. *Lidocaine* was discovered in 1948. True allergic reaction of amides is extremely rare.

Action:

- Reversibly prevent nerve conduction by blocking sodium channels.
- The rate of metabolism of local anaesthetics is related to the number of additional carbon atoms on the aromatic or the amine side of the molecule.
- Potency and toxicity are determined by the structure of the aromatic and the amine group.
- Anaesthetic potency is determined primarily by the degree of lipid solubility.
- The onset of action is primarily due to the pKa.
- They exist in anionic non-ionized and cationic ionized form. Preparations are acidic so have more cationic. The anionic form penetrates the nerve membrane. Adding sodium bicarbonate increases the anionic form and speeds onset. Also decreases discomfort.

Duration:

- Duration of action is related to the degree of binding to a protein receptor in the sodium channel and the vasodilatory effect. Metabolism is affected by age, liver failure and CCF.

Systemic toxicity:

- The CNS is more sensitive to toxicity and is made more sensitive by hypercarbia, hypoxia and acidosis.

- Patients may experience dizziness, tinnitus, circumoral numbness, loss of consciousness and fitting.
- After CNS excitation get depression and respiratory arrest.
- LAs prolong conduction time in the heart and produce a long PR interval. High concentrations will depress the sinus node and lead to sinus bradycardia and sinus arrest. They also exert a direct myocardial depressant affect.
- Bupivicaine can produce VF.
- The CVS toxic dose compared with the CNS toxic dose for lignocaine is $7\times$ and for bupivicaine is $3.5\times$.

Management of local anaesthetic toxicity:

- Stop LA injection.
- Call for help.
- ABC resuscitation principles with 100% O_2.
- Treat problems:
  - i.e. seizures;
  - *Arrest:* CPR (recovery from LA induced arrest may take over an hour so prolonged CPR may be required).
- *Intra-lipid infusion:* give 1,000 ml 20% lipid emulsion.

Long posterior flap below-knee amputation

- The rationale for this flap is that the anterior skin has the least good blood supply and the posterior skin is supplied by perforators through gastrocnemius/soleus.
- This muscle mass retains knee flexion.
- Tibia sectioned 10–12 cm below tibial plateau. Mark circumferential line at this level. Mark axial lines extending distally.
- The posterior flap should be rather more than 1/3 of the circumference of the limb—less will reduce vascularity, more will increase the dog ears. Anterior incision cuts to bone. Anterior compartment muscles divided at this level. Ligate anterior tibial vessels and divide nerve. Incise interosseus membrane. Divide peroneal muscles. Transect fibula high. Divide tibia 2 cm below anterior skin incision. Transect tibialis posterior. Extend skin incision distally cutting along gastrocnemius/soleus. Remove amputate. Cut muscle to give smooth slope. Resect muscle medially and laterally. Some suggest soleus should be completely resected. Ligate vessels. Fold over flaps and trim muscle and skin. Suction drain. Suture aponeurosis to anterior tibial periosteum or perform myodesis to tibial stump. Suture skin without tension.

- An alternative which may give a better stump shape is the *Skew flap*.

Longitudinal arrest: congenital hand

- Congenital hand anomaly with digital skeletal elements.
- Fit prosthesis activated by digits:
  - *Complete:* hand on trunk;
  - *Proximal:* forearm on trunk;
  - *Distal:* hand on humerus.

Lop ear

- Also cup ear or constricted ear.
- Encircling helix seems tight like a purse string with helical and scaphal hooding.
- 1:10 of prominent ears.

Treatment:

- Determined by the height of the lop ear in comparison to the normal side.
- Reshape existing tissues or supplement skin and cartilage.
- May need to excise overhanging cartilage and may require cartilage grafts or repair as for microtia.

See EAR RECONSTRUCTION.

Louis–Bar syndrome

Also called ataxia-telangiectasis.

- A neurovascular disorder.
- Autosomal recessive inheritance that appears at 3–6 years of life.
- Telangiectasis occur on the nasal and temporal area and then on the upper half of the body.
- Cerebellar ataxia also begins in early childhood, followed by progressive neuromotor degeneration.
- Also get endocrine dysfunction, chromosomal instability, immunologic deficiencies and growth retardation.
- Death usually occurs in the 20s from recurrent sinopulmonary infections and bronchiectasis or from lymphoreticular malignancy.
- Heterozygous carriers of the gene also may be at significantly increased risk for cancer.

Love's sign

- Clinical test seen with *Glomus tumour*.
- The presence of one very painful localized spot on palpation.

Lower limb anatomy
Thigh:

- *Femoral triangle:* bounded by: inguinal ligament, medial border of adductor longus, lateral border of sartorius. *Roof:* fascia lata. *Floor:* psoas, illiacus, pectineus, adductor longus. *Contents:* femoral nerve, artery and vein, deep inguinal nodes.
- *Anterior thigh muscles:* rectus femoris, vastus lateralis, medialis and intermedialis, sartorius.
- *Adductors:* adductor magnus, adductor longus, adductor brevis, gracilis.
- *Hamstrings:* biceps femoris, semimembranosus, semitendinosus.
- *Fascia lata:* deep fascia of the whole of the thigh. Tensor fascia lata (TFL) is inserted between its layers. Attachments are the sacrum and coccyx, inguinal ligament, iliac crest, superior ramus of the pubis, inferior ramus, tuberosity of the ischium and sacrotuberous ligament. Forms iliotibial band which attaches to the lateral condyle of the tibia.
- *Blood vessels:* femoral artery; profunda femoris, and its lateral and medial circumflex branches; muscular branches. Femoral vein, great (long) and short saphenous veins.
- *Nerve supply to muscles:*
  - *Obturator:* adductors (magnus, longus and brevis), gracilis;
  - *Femoral:* quadrates femoris, pectineus, sartorius, iliacus, superior gluteal, TFL;
  - *Sciatic:* semitendinosus, semimembranosus, biceps femoris, adductor magnus.
- *Cutaneous nerve supply:* cutaneous branches of femoral nerve (medial, intermediate, lateral and posterior), cutaneous branches of obturator nerve.

Lower leg:

- *Anterior compartment:* contains extensor muscles, tibialis anterior, extensor hallucis longus, extensor digitorum longus. Anterior tibial artery and deep peroneal nerve.
- *Lateral compartment:* peroneus longus, brevis and tertius. No artery, but a superficial peroneal nerve.
- *Posterior superficial compartment:* contains soleus and gastrocnemius.
- *Posterior deep compartment:* tibialis posterior, flexor digitorum longus, flexor hallucis longus. Contains posterior tibial artery, peroneal artery and posterior tibial nerve.
- *Nerves:*
  - Sensory supply:
    - *Sural:* lateral midfoot;
    - *Posterior tibial:* heel/plantar midfoot;
    - *Deep peroneal:* first web;
    - *Superficial peroneal:* dorsal midfoot;
    - *Saphenous:* medial ankle.

Lower limb reconstruction

Indications: required for open fractures, chronic wounds, unstable scars, sarcoma, diabetes, radiation, osteomyelitis, ischaemia.

Reconstruction may be required for the soft tissue coverage of bones, nerves, arteries and musculotendinous units, and/or to optimise amputation–for instance, pedicled or free flaps may allow preservation of the knee joint to optimise function.

Soft tissue coverage aims to provide robust vascularized cover for underlying structures such as exposed fractures, metalwork or neurovascular bundles. Can be achieved by locoregional flaps or free flaps depending on size and location of defect, donor site availability and fitness of patient.

Locoregional flap options by location:

Hip:

- TFL has little muscle bulk.
- Vastus lateralis has good muscle and a skin paddle with little functional loss.
- Rectus femoris can be used similarly, but with less bulk.
- Extended deep inferior epigastric flap is an alternative for large hip defects. This is essentially a VRAM with an adjacent random element. It may extend up to the knee (pennant flap).

Mid-thigh:

- Gracilis, but not much bulk.
- Vastus medialis is supplied by perforators along its length so it can not be rotated. It can be transposed medially.

Knee:

- Gastrocnemius, but may not cross to other side of knee or superiorly.
- Distally-based vastus lateralis is not reliable distally.
- Pedicled medial sural artery perforator (MSAP) or distally-based ALT may be useful.

Proximal tibia:

- Medial and lateral gastrocnemius (shorter than medial).

Mid-tibia:

- Turnover flap of tibialis anterior for small defects.
- Soleus muscle useful for larger defects.
- Fasciocutaneous transposition flaps.
- Fasciocutaneous keystone flap.

Ankle/distal tibia:

- Medial plantar artery flap—reliable and robust glabrous skin (to cover heel pad, medial ankle).

- Distally based peroneus brevis flap (to cover lateral ankle).
- Extensor digitorum brevis for small defects.
- Dorsalis pedis flap.
- Distally-based fasciocutaneous flaps including the reverse sural artery flap may be useful but may not be reliable if within the zone of injury.

Foot:

- *Classification: Hidalgo and Shaw.*

Achilles tendon and malleolar area:

- Medial plantar artery flap can provide sensate and robust cover.
- Local fasciocutaneous flaps.
- Lateral calcaneal flap can be sensate with a flap length of up to 14 cm if delayed.
- Dorsalis pedis flap can provide sensate coverage.
- The extensor digitorum brevis is the most useful local muscle flap, based on the lateral tarsal-dorsalis pedis pedicle.
- Temporoparietal flap and radial forearm free flap may provide thin coverage.

Heel and mid-plantar foot:

- Can use muscle flaps with skin grafts or fasciocutaneous flaps, but tissue needs to be able to withstand shear forces, ideally retain sensation, and be durable enough to allow patient to weight bear and wear shoes without compromising reconstruction.
- The flap should fit well, not be too thick and underlying bony problems should be corrected.
- For the neuropathic foot, ulcer may need to be debrided with the underlying bone.
- Medial plantar flaps can be raised with plantar nerves and can provide durable, sensate, specialized glabrous tissue.

Distal plantar and forefoot and dorsum:

- Most require free tissue transfer.

Free tissue transfer:

Free flaps are often the best reconstructive option for lower limb soft tissue coverage and have become commonplace, reliable and safe options. Choice of flap guided by:

- What is needed for cover:
  - Components;
  - Thickness;
  - Surface area;
  - Length of pedicle.
- Recipient vessels:
  - Ideally outside of zone of injury, although may be safely distal to this;

○ Can be either proximal or distal to defect—main factor is quality and patency of vessels, to be tested under direct vision under the microscope.

Benefits of muscle versus fasciocutaneous flap have been debated in the literature. Historically muscle flaps were thought to lead to better bony healing. This was demonstrated in some animal models but has not been born out in clinical studies.

• *Advantages of fasciocutaneous flaps:* replace like with like, skin is durable and can withstand footwear, limited donor site morbidity for many (FRFF notable exception), easier to re-raise down the line if needed, e.g. for deep infection.

• *Disadvantages of fasciocutaneous flaps:* may need thinning at a second stage to improve cosmesis and ability to don footwear, can be less reliable/slower to raise.

• *Advantages of muscle flaps:* will contour down, reducing need for thinning and improving cosmesis and ability to don footwear, often quick and reliable to raise.

• *Disadvantages of muscle flaps:* may be difficult to re-raise once healed, require a SSG to cover which creates second donor site and may not be as durable.

Approach to bone loss:
• Small:
  ○ Bone graft as an adjunct.
• Less than 5 cm:
  ○ *Primary bone shortening:* can be done for segments less than 5 cm. Care not to kink vessels;
  ○ *Masquelet technique:* (membrane induction) 2-stage approach which relies on an induced membrane that forms around a cement spacer (1st stage) and use of cancellous bone graft at a second stage which is revascularized by the induced membrane. Takes about 18 months in total to complete process and results can be unreliable;
  ○ *Bone distraction with frame:* at fracture site.
• 5 to 15 cm:
  ○ *Bone transport with frame:* lengthening with frame up to 15 cm as will take about 18 months (1 cm per month) and longer than that not realistic.
• Large (more than 12 cm):

○ Reconstruction with vascularized bone for defects over 12 cm, as under that other methods are probably better:
  ▪ *Fibula:* workhorse flap. Can do single or double strut, or reinforce with a (hemi) Capanna approach (reinforced with segment of cadaveric tibia). Takes 18 months for fibular to hypertrophy—in a protective frame for that time to allow tibialization of fibula;
  ▪ *DCIA:* more difficult, higher donor site morbidity;
  ▪ *Medial femoral condyle:* useful as you can take periosteum;
  ▪ *Scapula:* more common in head and neck recon.

Approach to arterial injury in lower limb:
• 'BOAST Standards for diagnosis and management of arterial injuries associated with extremity fractures and dislocations' describe up-to-date guidelines for MDT management of these injuries.
• Pulseless deformed limb should be re-aligned and vascular examination repeated—clinical signs are unreliable, an abnormal pulse oximeter waveform may be helpful to diagnose an arterial injury where there is uncertainty.
• Get CTA at time of trauma CT, but do not be falsely reassured by a normal CTA in context of abnormal clinical findings.
• Revascularize the limb within 4 hours.
• Consider arterial shunts whilst skeletal stabilization is placed.
• Repair artery directly or with interposition grafts—these are preferred to bypass graft.
• Make patient aware of possibility of amputation.
• Always consider fasciotomies—low threshold.

Reconstructive options in a vessel deplete leg (1 patent vessel):
• End-to-side for single vessel.
• Flow through flap.
• AV loops—can do in 2 stages (i.e. create the loop in the first stage then anastomose a flap in second stage).
• Cross leg flap.

Approach to nerve injury in lower limb:
• Sharp lacerations require immediate repair. If there is extensive contusion, wait 2–3 weeks. Prognosis varies and depends on distance.
• *Femoral nerve palsy:* unable to fully extend the knee giving a significant disability when walking uphill. Should be explored as some recovery should occur.

- *Sciatic nerve injuries:* get better recovery in the tibial than the peroneal distribution. Repair in the buttock may give some plantar flexion and some plantar sensation. High lesions often have severe vasomotor and trophic changes. Peroneal return does not usually occur.
- *Tibial nerve injuries:* are very disabling as the terminal branches supply plantar sensation and also sympathetic supply. Partial recovery of motor and sensation should occur following repair.
- *Common peroneal nerve:* the most frequently injured peripheral nerve as it is so superficial. Post-operative results are the poorest. Loss leads to foot drop and equinovarus (prevent equinovarus with fastidious use of foot drop splint and physiotherapy).

Amputation:
- Primary amputation for trauma if limb survival and function are unlikely. Sciatic/posterior tibial function important.
- Many scores exist to predict amputation including mangled extremity severity score (*MESS*) but all have problems.
- *Absolute indications:* unreconstructible NV, skeletal or soft tissue injury.
- *Relative indication:* when function or appearance of the limb will be inferior to a prosthesis.

Replantation:
- Frequently not performed as unable to restore neurology and good function from prosthetics.
- More favourable outcome in a child.
- Consider if a clean cut with short ischaemic time. If replantation is not going to be performed, consider using limb for spare part flaps and grafts.

Outcome measures for lower limb
Core outcomes for patients are:
- QoL.
- Return to life roles—work.
- Walking, gait and mobility.
- Pain and discomfort.

There are different types of outcome measures:
- Objective and clinical measures:
  o Time to fracture union;
  o Deep infection rates;
  o Flap failure rates;
- PROMs:
  o EuroQol-Five Dimensions Questionnaire;
  o Lower extremity Functional Scale.
- Physical performance measures:
  o Enneking.

Lower limb trauma
Open tibial fractures are limb threatening injuries. Must be managed in a Major Trauma Centre by appropriately specialist orthoplastic team. 'BOAST Standards for management of open fractures' provides up-to-date MDT guidelines for management of such injuries.

History:
- Establish mechanism of trauma to give an indication as to the amount of energy transferred and the urgency to initial wound excision and debridement.
- Timing.
- Treatment given at scene.

Examination:
- ATLS approach to identify concomitant life-threatening injuries.
- Focused lower limb examination:
  o Look:
    - Precise location of injury;
    - *Skin status:* evidence of degloving;
    - Bone status and periosteum.
  o Feel:
    - Neurovascular status.
  o Move:
    - *Active:* check motor supply of tibial and common peroneal nerve:
    - *Toes:* common peroneal;
    - *Ankle:* tibia;
    - Passive stretch for compartment syndrome.

Investigation:
- Clinical photos.
- Baseline bloods and crossmatch.
- Imaging:
  o XR;
  o CTA as part of Trauma CT (BOAST).

Immediate Management:
- Resuscitation and continued monitoring.
- Antibiotics within 1 hour of injury (now often given pre-hospital) and tetanus:
  o *Phase 1:* give until 24 hours post wound excision;
  o *Phase 2:* antibiotics is at definitive reconstruction.
- Analgesia—IV morphine.
- Remove gross contaminants and apply saline-soaked gauze covered with an occlusive dressing.
- Manage the fracture by reduction and splinting—XR and document NV status before and afterwards.

1st stage Wound Excision:
- *Personnel:* consultant orthoplastic team.
- Timing:
  - Immediate—agricultural/marine contamination, compartment syndrome, vascular injury, polytrauma;
  - *12 hours:* high energy injury;
  - *24 hours:* low energy injury.
- *Antibiotics:* give co-amoxiclav 1.2 kg and gentamicin 3mg/kg at start.
- Principles:
  - Wound extension along fasciotomy lines;
  - Tumour-like wound excision:
    - Peripheral to central;
    - Superficial to deep;
    - Deliver the bone ends;
    - 6L wash (not pulse lavage).
  - Wound classification (*Gustilo-Anderson classification*) and planning for definitive reconstruction.
  - If staged—temporize the skeleton and soft tissues.

Classifications:
- *Gustilo score.*
- *MESS.*
- *Hidalgo classification.*
- *Byrd and Spicer.*
- *Arnez and Tyler classification.*
- AO classification.

2nd stage definitive reconstruction:
- Within acute phase of 72 hours to reduce risk of deep infection as per NICE guidance and Godina paper.
- Some argue that this can be safely extended to 10 days.

Lumbosacral back flap
- Fasciocutaneous flap used for the coverage of *Pressure sores.*
- Based on contralateral lumbar perforators, L1–5.
- Covers medium-sized pressure sores of the sacrum, but only with skin.

Lumbrical muscles
- Worm like. Four lumbricals. Flex MCPJ and extend IPJs.
- The workhorse of the extensor apparatus.
- The only muscles with no bony attachment.

Origin:
- Arise from radial side of FDP tendons and pass volar to the intermetacarpal ligaments.
- 1st and 2nd are attached to index and middle FDP whereas 3rd and 4th are attached to

2 adjacent FDPs of middle and ring, and ring and little.
- They run on the radial side of the digits. A narrow flat tendon emerges from the muscle at the MCP joint to join the radial edge of the extensor aponeurosis at an angle of 40°.
- The radial 2 lumbricals join the dorsal interossei, whereas the ulnar two join the palmar interossei.

Insertion: the lateral slip of the extensor tendons.

Nerve supply: radial two are median and ulnar two are ulnar nerve.

Function: extension of IPJs in any position of MCP joint. They are important in balancing flexors and extensors. Relaxation of FDP decreases the antagonistic force and so decreases the resistance on the extensor apparatus.
See CLAW HAND.

Lunate: fracture
- Uncommon.
- Two patterns:
  - Impaction from axial load between capitate and radius;
  - Dorsal avulsion or impaction caused by impingement on the dorsal edge of the radius.
- Get mid-dorsal wrist pain. This may predispose to *Kienbock's disease.*
- Treat non-displaced fractures with immobilization.
- If displaced, perform open reduction through a dorsal approach.

Lund and Browder chart
Used to accurately assess the size of *Burns,* which allows for age group differences.

Lunotriquetral compression test
- Loads lunotriquetral joint along ulnoradial axis by palpating within the ulnar snuffbox.
- Direct pressure causes pain with lunotriquetral instability, synovitis, degenerative disease, partial synchondrosis.

Lunula
- White arc of *Nail* distal to eponychium. Due to persistence of nuclei in cells of germinal matrix.
- Nail becomes transparent as they disintegrate.

Lupus vulgaris
- Rare form of cutaneous tuberculosis.
- Destruction of soft tissues followed by atrophic scarring.
- Active areas of disease are studded with lupus nodules.

- It needs to be distinguished from cold abscess.

Treatment:
- Anti-tuberculosis chemotherapy.
- Scarring may require excision.
- Previous attempts to treat with radiotherapy led to SCCs within the lupus.

Lymph node levels in head and neck cancer
Level I:
- Divided into:

  A: *Submental:* between anterior belly of digastrics and above hyoid. Contains submental nodes and drains skin of the mental region, mid-lower lip, anterior portion of tongue, floor of mouth.

  B: *Submandibular:* between anterior and posterior belly of digastric and mandibular angle. Contains submandibular nodes and submandibular gland. Drains efferents from level 1, hard and soft palate and both alveolar ridges.

Level II:
- *Upper jugular:* from skull base to bifurcation of carotid (surgical) or hyoid (radiological). Posteriorly is the posterior edge of SCM, anteriorly is the sternohyoid. Contains upper jugular nodes and spinal accessory nerve.
  - A: above spinal accessory nerve;
  - B: below spinal accessory nerve.
- The lymphatics are adjacent to the upper third of the internal jugular vein. They are embedded in the carotid sheath and most lie anterolaterally to the vein.
- Level 2 drains efferent lymphatics from the face, parotid gland and level 1. There is direct drainage from nasal cavity, pharynx, larynx, external auditory canal and middle ear.
- It is the most commonly involved nodal level in head and neck cancer.

Level III:
- *Middle jugular:* from inferior border of level II to omohyoid crossing the IJV (surgical) or lower border of cricoid (radiological).
- Level III drains efferents from level II and V, retropharyngeal, pretracheal and recurrent pharyngeal nodes. Direct drainage from base of tongue, larynx, hypopharynx, base of tongue, tonsils and thyroid gland.

Level IV:
- *Lower jugular:* from omohyoid crossing IJV (Surgical) or lower border of cricoid (radiological) to clavicle.

- Level IV drains efferents from level III and V and directly from thyroid, larynx and hypopharynx.

Level V:
- *Posterior triangle:* around lower portion of spinal accessory nerve, along the transverse cervical vessels. Bounded by a triangle formed by the clavicle, posterior border of SCM and anterior border of trapezius.
- The nodes in the posterior triangle course along the spinal accessory nerve.
- Level V nodes drain lymphatics from occipital, retro-auricular and parietal scalp nodes. They are not often involved in oral cancers. Small nodes along the transverse cervical vessels are more frequently involved with chest primaries.

Level VI:
- *Anterior compartment:* from hyoid to suprasternal notch. Lateral border is medial border of carotid sheath. Includes parathyroidal and paratracheal lymph nodes and those along the recurrent laryngeal nerves.

See HEAD AND NECK CANCER. *See* NECK DISSECTION.

Lymphangioma circumscriptum
Cutaneous *Lymphatic malformations*, which can often be resected totally and the defect closed with a split-thickness skin graft.

Lymphangiosarcoma
- Rare consequence of long-standing *Lymphoedema.*
- Most are post-mastectomy with long-standing obstruction.
- Aggressive, metastasize early and non-responsive to chemo- and radiotherapy.
- Limb amputation is advised.
- Average survival 19 months. 5-year survival is <10%.
- When it is related to post-mastectomy oedema it is called Stewart–Treves syndrome. Occurs on average 10 years post-mastectomy.

Lymphatic malformations
- They can be described as either microcystic, macrocystic or combined forms.
- Previously microcystic was called lymphangioma and macrocystic was called cystic hygroma.
- They never involute, but expand and contract depending on the ebb and flow of lymphatic fluid.
- Most are seen at birth or within 2 years, but they can occur in the older child or the adult.

- Dilated lymphatics in the skin present as vesicles which form red nodules with bleeding.
- Those in the face are usually combined *Vascular malformations*, and cause facial asymmetry and possibly cause airway obstruction.
- It may be confused with a venous malformation or it may be a combined lymphovenous malformation.

Treatment:

- Sudden enlargement is usually due to bleeding or cellulitis. Treat with antibiotics and NSAIDs.
- Large cysts can be treated with aspiration of lymphatic fluid and instillation of sclerosant agents, for example, pure ethanol, sodium tetradecyl sulphate.
- Resection is the only way to remove a LM.
- Surgical guidelines are:
  - ○ Focus on a defined anatomic region;
  - ○ Define the duration of the procedure;
  - ○ Limit the acceptable blood loss;
  - ○ Perform as thorough a resection as possible, given anatomic restrictions.
- Transected lymphatic channels regenerate after subtotal excision leading to recurrence.

Complications: immediate post-operative complications include prolonged serous drainage, haematoma and cellulitis.

See LYMPHANGIOMA CIRCUMSCRIPTUM.

Lymphatics
Function:

- Endothelial-lined channels, which transport fluid, proteins and particles from the interstitial compartment to the vascular system.
- Also presents foreign matter to the immune system.
- In the intestines they also transport triglycerides and chylomicrons.

Anatomy:

- Embryologically the lymphatics develop from the venous system.
- They do not have well-defined basement membranes.
- Epidermal lymphatics have no valves, dermal lymphatics have small valves.
- A cutaneous network of valveless channels drain into valved vessels in the subdermal layer. These join to follow the major veins. These drain to nodal basins en route to the right and left subclavian veins.

- In the abdomen the lumbar lymphatic trunks join to form the cisterna chyli—a thin walled sac lying in front of the L1–2 vertebrae.
- This becomes the thoracic duct, which enters the left subclavian vein.
- The right lymphatic duct drains into the right subclavian from the arm, chest and head and neck.
- Lymphatics are not present in CNS, muscle, tendon, cartilage, bone.

Action: lymph is propelled by external muscle compression, helped by valves, pulsations from vessels, and intra-abdominal and intrathoracic pressures. Smooth muscle in the lymphatics regulates calibre.

See LYMPHOEDEMA.

Lymphoedema

- The accumulation of protein-rich fluid in the interstitial space leading to enlargement. The protein activates inflammation, but phagocytosis is impaired. Collagen deposition is increased in response to injury. Get thickened fibrosed channels which work ineffectively. In early disease stages, increased volume is related to fluid excess and partially resolves with elevation and compression. In later disease stages, abnormal fat is laid down and skin thickens and compression and elevation do not reduce volume excess. Stasis predisposes to infection, which can worsen the lymphoedema. Mainly *Strep.* and *Staph.* No medical or surgical cure exists.
- Goals of treatment are reduction of fluid accumulation, reduction of complications, and improved limb function. Typical history is of gradual oedema unilaterally.

Anatomy:

- If there is no particular insult, 77% of lymphatics are hypoplastic and 15% are aplastic. 8% are hyperplastic with tortuous lymphatics with valvular incompetence.

Malignant change: *Lymphangiosarcoma*.

Classification: primary (10%) vs. secondary (90%). Can also distinguish between low-volume disease (abnormal lymphatics with normal fluid volume) and high-volume disease (normal lymphatics with abnormally high fluid volume).

Primary lymphoedema:

- A diagnosis of exclusion. Classify into congenital, early and late.
- *Lymphoedema congenita* is 15% of primary lymphoedema and 15% are familial (Milroy's disease, F:M 2:1, lower extremities).
- *Lymphoedema praecox* (early primary lymphoedema) accounts for 75% of lymphoedema and onset is before 35 years.

More common in women and in the lower extremities. Left more commonly affected than right.

- *Lymphoedema tarda:* after 35 years.

Secondary lymphoedema:

- Results from damage to lymphatics. In developed countries mainly due to metastatic tumour and lymphadenectomies. In developing countries, filariasis by the organism *Wuchereria bancrofti* produces elephantiasis.
- Five I's:
  - ○ *Invasion:* primary lymphatic tumours, secondary tumours;
  - ○ *Infection:* filariasis, lymphogranuloma, TB;
  - ○ *Inflammation:* snake bites, insect bites;
  - ○ *Irradiation;*
  - ○ *Iatrogenic:* lymph node dissection, varicose vein stripping.

Grading:

- *Grade 0:* normal lymphatic channels with increased dermal backflow due to downstream blockage of flow (e.g. lymphadenectomy). Fluid excess.
- *Grade I:* ectasis of lymphatic channels. Fluid excess.
- *Grade II:* contraction and fibrosis of lymphatic channels. Fat excess.
- *Grade III:* sclerosis of lymphatic channels. Fat excess.

Imaging:

- On CT and MRI get honeycomb appearance. Lymphoscintigraphy with technetium-99 radiolabelled colloid gives 'transport index'. However, 2D image and poor anatomic resolution, uses radiation and is expensive.
- Indocyanine green (ICG) lymphography gives temporal and spatial information and can be performed by surgeons in outpatient setting. Useful for operative planning of lymphaticovenous anastomosis.
- Lymphangiograms are rarely performed as they are time-consuming, potentially dangerous and give little useful information.

Conservative treatment:

- First line for all patients is decongestive therapy.
- Initial intensive phase followed by maintenance.
- Intensive phase incorporates manual lymph drainage, multilayer compression bandaging, Therapeutic exercise.
- Maintenance phase—patients educated in self-management, skin hygiene, diet for obesity, custom-made compression garment.

- Early treatment of cellulitis is essential to limit progression of disease.
- Control cause if possible.

Restorative surgery:

- May be appropriate in the presence of patent lymph vessels
- Lymphaticovenous anastomosis—requires intact distal lymphatic vessels anastomosed to adjacent venules. Best when at least 2 or 3 anastomoses performed for grade 0 or grade I lymphoedema.
- Vascularized lymph node transfer (VLNT)— flap with superficial lymph nodes is harvested and anastomosed. Benefits include scar release, recruitment of healthy tissue and stimulated lymphangiogenesis by VEGF production. Indicated in stage I or early stage II lymphoedema. Newer techniques incorporate prophylactic VLNT into breast reconstruction surgery.
- Interposition lymph vessel transplantation (lymphaticolymphatic anastomosis)—using autologous lymphatic vessels to bypass an area of obstruction.

Excisional surgery:

- May be indicated when no patent lymphatic vessels (i.e. primary or chronic). Indicated in late grade II or grade III disease.
- *Suction-assisted lipectomy:* to remove excess fat associated with chronic lymphoedema. Requires post-op pressure garments permanently.
- *Charles operation radical excision:* excises all tissue down to muscle and applies skin grafts. Gives a poor result with insensate easily traumatized skin.
- *Homans technique:* longitudinal segment of skin and subcutaneous tissue is removed and the incision edges are sutured.
- *Staged subcutaneous excision:* remove subcutaneous tissue while keeping skin flaps. Less radical than Charles operation and is the most reasonable treatment for the symptoms of lymphoedema. 80% of the lymphatics fluid is carried in the superficial lymphatic system. The theory is to removed diseased lymphatics while preserving the dermal lymphatic plexus. Can give long-term improvement and minimize complications. Plan to remove as much skin and subcutaneous tissue while achieving primary closure. Perform in 2 stages separated by 3 months. Use a TQ. Raise medial flap 1.5 cm thick to mid-sagittal plane of calf. All subcutaneous tissue is removed. Sural nerve is preserved. Deep fascia is excised. Remain superficial to deep fascia at the knee

and ankle. Redundant skin is excised. Suction catheter. Laterally the same procedure is employed though deep fascia is preserved.

Genital lymphoedema: two systems of lymphatic drainage to the genitalia. Superficial lymphatics go to superficial inguinal nodes. A deeper network drains urethra and corpus spongiosum. Genital lymphoedema generally only involves the superficial system. Therefore, treatment involves excision of skin down to Buck's fascia from coronal sulcus to scrotum. Apply meshed graft to scrotum and non-meshed graft to penis.

See LYMPHATICS.

Macrodactyly to Myotomes

Macrodactyly
- Enlargement of all structures in the finger. Distinguish from *Haemangiomas, Vascular malformations, Ollier's disease.*
- In 70% an adjacent digit is affected. Index finger is the most commonly affected.
- The enlarged area often corresponds to specific nerve distribution.
- Associated with *PIK3CA* mutations.

Classification:
- Static or progressive:
  - *Static macrodactyly:* the enlarged finger grows in proportion to the rest of the child;
  - *Progressive macrodactyly:* the enlarged finger grows out of proportion to the rest of the child. More common than static.
- Syndromic or isolated:
  - Syndromes include *Ollier's disease, Maffucci syndrome, Klippel-Trenaunay-Weber syndrome.*
- *Type I-IV:*
  - *Type I:* gigantism and lipofibromatosis. Occur in the distribution of a peripheral nerve.
  - *Type II:* gigantism and neurofibromatosis.
  - *Type III:* gigantism and digital hyperostosis. Rare. Often bilateral. Nodular due to osteochondral masses.
  - *Type IV:* gigantism and hemihypertrophy. Rare. *Proteus syndrome.*

Management:
Extremely difficult—cannot make digit normal. Delay surgery until the digit is the same length as the parents' digit. Counsel parents and provide support. Beware relative ischaemia as the vessels may not be bigger than normal.

- Observation—when enlargement is not troublesome—some have minimal overgrowth that does not require intervention.
- Soft tissue debulking procedures:
  - Will never be normal—will always be stiff. Beware of stripping the nerves as may lead to dysaesthesia. Only address one side at a time;
  - Address bone;
  - Can remove growth plate—epiphysiodesis usually of proximal and middle phalanx only stops longitudinal group. Will still grow in width. Do at time when digit is size of same-sex parent;
  - Osteotomies for angulation.
- May need carpal tunnel release if median nerve.
- Can consider ray amputation of severely malformed digit—may be best option but difficult for a parent to accept. Can consider free toe transfer.

Macrophages
- Specialized cells arising from circulating blood monocytes that are involved in the detection and destruction of bacteria and other harmful organisms. They are a key element of the innate immunity.
- Important in *Wound healing* to remove debris and orchestrate the events of wound healing. They infiltrate the wound during the inflammatory phase and are the predominate cell type 3-5 days following injury. M1 macrophages are pro-inflammatory and predominate earlier whereas M2 macrophages are both anti-inflammatory and pro-angiogenic and predominate later.
- A primary source of *Growth factors.*

Macrostomia
- Congenital lateral opening of the oral commissure. Also known as *Tessier cleft* Number 7 or a transverse facial cleft.
- Most common of the atypical craniofacial clefts.
- Can be unilateral or bilateral.
- Associated with *Craniofacial microsomia* and *Treacher Collins syndrome.*

Reconstruction:
- Numerous techniques described.
- Principle to approximate the muscles at the modiolus (orbicularis oris and risorius) and align anatomical elements of the lips

including vermilion and white roll, whilst leaving an inconspicuous scar.
- Use of Z-plasty may be required if the facial cleft extends beyond the nasolabial crease.

Mafenide
- A sulpha medicine, particularly indicated for *Burns* involving cartilage.
- A broad antibacterial spectrum, though limited activity against MRSA *Staph. aureus*.
- It penetrates eschar well and also cartilage, so it is good for ears and noses. It is applied 12-hourly. It is painful to apply.

Maffuci's syndrome
- Multiple *Enchondromas* associated with soft tissue vascular malformations.
- Even higher frequency of malignant transformation to chondrosarcoma than *Ollier's disease* (which is 25% by aged 40 years).
- The vascular lesions are complex venous in type; they can occur in the subcutaneous tissue, bones (particularly the limbs), the leptomeninges, or the gastrointestinal tract. Patients may develop spindle cell haemangioendotheliomas.

See COMPLEX COMBINED VASCULAR MALFORMATIONS.

MAGPI (Meatal Advancement and Glansplasty)
- Used in true glanular *Hypospadias*.
- If used for subcoronal meatus get retrusive meatus.
- The meatus is opened vertically and closed transversely to advance the dorsal lip of the meatal mucosa out toward the tip of the glans.
- Glansplasty achieved by midline approximation of lateral glanular wings after freeing them from corporal tunica. Closure of the glans flaps in two layers moves the meatus towards the glans tip.
- It does not lengthen the urethra and does not correct chordee.

Malignant fibrous histiocytoma
- Historical term. Now referred to as pleomorphic undifferentiated sarcoma.
- Present as firm cutaneous or subcutaneous lesion in elderly patients.
- Pathological diagnosis can be difficult, but histochemical analysis for alpha-1-antitrypsin can be helpful.
- Consists of fibroblast like cells with pleomorphic giant cells.
- Two major types, myxoid and inflammatory, latter being the poorer prognosis.

- Associated with leukaemia, neurofibromatosis, Paget's and RT.
- Local recurrence rates are 70%. Propensity for lymph node metastasis.
- Give adjuvant RT.

See PSEUDOSARCOMATOUS LESIONS. *See* SARCOMA.

Mallet finger
Loss of continuity of extensor tendon with DIP joint with flexion of DIP joint. Left untreated the mallet can become a *Swan neck deformity*.

Classification:
- *I:* rupture of tendon insertion.
- *II:* tendon laceration.
- *III:* loss of skin and tendon.
- *IV:* avulsion fracture of distal phalanx.

Treatment:
- *I:* splint or closed reduction and consider fixation with a K-wire if unstable.
- *II:* tendon repair and splint.
- *III:* soft tissue repair with tendon repair or graft or DIP joint fusion.
- *IV:* controversial. XR and re-XR with splint. If well reduced continue splintage. If the joint is subluxed and the fragment displaced then ORIF.
- *Mallet thumb:* is rarer than mallet finger. If surgery indicated, the thicker EPL tendon holds sutures better than the EDC tendon.

Mammography
- UK national screening programme involves mammography every 3 years between 50 and 70 years.
- The American Cancer Society suggests annual screening from 40 years. The benefit of screening between 40–50 years is controversial.
- Perform younger if there is a family history, but the diagnostic accuracy is less.
- Mortality reduction between 20 and 45% has been reported.
- Suspicious lesions are fine microcalcifications, masses, architectural distortion. A mass with microcalcifications is the most suspicious.
- Suspicious lesions should be biopsied following needle localization.

See BREAST CANCER.

Mandible
The strongest bone in the facial skeleton. Thick bicortical structure. L-shaped with a horizontal portion (body and symphysis) and two vertical portions (rami). The angle, coronoid process, symphysis and condylar neck provide the sites of muscular attachment. The

alveolar supporting processes and condyle provide articulation.

Mandibular fractures
Symptoms and signs:
- Present with pain, trismus, malocclusion, crepitus, bruising.
- Palpation may reveal a step along the mandibular border or in dentition.
- Paraesthesia may be present in the distribution of the inferior alveolar nerve.

Location:
- Condyle 36%.
- Body 20%.
- Angle 20%.
- Symphysis 14%.
- Alveolus 4%.
- Ramus 3%.
- Coronoid process 3%.

Common patterns:
- Always exclude a second fracture as double fractures are common, particularly.
- Angle and contralateral body.
- Parasymphysis and contralateral subcondylar region.
- Symphysis and both condyles.

Classification:
- *Closed or compound:* compound through skin, buccal mucosa or tooth socket.
- *Kazanjian and Converse.*
- *Favourable and unfavourable fracture orientations:*
  - *Unfavourable:* tendency for instability with distraction of fragments at the fracture site due to pull of masseter, digastric and pterygoid muscles.
  - *Favourable:* tendency for stability with compression of fragments at the fracture site due to muscle action. Teeth in fracture segment may help to stabilize the fracture.

Radiology: perform OPG, PA, lateral oblique and reverse Towne's view to see condyles. CT.

Management:
- *Conservative:* for most condylar fractures and for stable undisplaced fractures with normal occlusion.
- *Intermaxillary fixation (IMF):* teeth of maxilla and mandible are wired together—called IMF as mandible can be termed the inferior maxilla. Fix with wires, arch bars or cap splints. Don't attach to incisor or canine as their single root makes them unstable. Leave for 3–6 weeks. It is not rigid, oral hygiene is difficult, eating is difficult and there is potential airway obstruction. If enough teeth

are present on either side of the fracture, a splint can be made without the need for bimaxillary fixation.
- *Open reduction and internal fixation:* the preferred method for most mandibular fractures. Use mono or bicortical fixation. Bicortical risks damaging tooth roots. Use Champy's principle of tension band plating. He noted that muscular forces distract upper and compress lower border, so a plate on the upper border acts as a tension band compressing the lower border—place between gum and nerve. Often used for fractures posterior to the mental foramen. Anterior fractures are treated with upper and lower bicortical plate fixation. Perform via an intra-oral approach where possible.
- *External fixation:* rarely used, but indicated with extensive bony defects and osteomyelitis.
- *Condylar fractures:* controversial. If immobilized, intracapsular fractures are prone to ankylosis. Options are:
  - Conservative with a soft diet;
  - Closed reduction and IMF;
  - ORIF—use:
    - When the condylar head is dislocated from the TMJ;
    - When the condyle is laterally displaced 30° or more from the axis of the ascending ramus;
    - In bilateral fractures associated with shortening of the ascending ramus and anterior open bite;
    - If adequate occlusion cannot be achieved by closed reduction;
    - If there is a foreign body in the TMJ.

See FACIAL FRACTURES.

Mandibular hypoplasia
- Micrognathia (undersized mandible).
- Can be congenital, developmental or acquired.
- Congenital mandibular hypoplasia commonly associated with *Pierre Robin sequence* and *Craniofacial microsomia.*

Classification: *Prozansky*; classification based on extent of hypoplasia.

Surgical management:
- *Distraction osteogenesis:* at operation, a corticotomy is performed at the angle. Screws are inserted in front and behind the corticotomy. These fit to the distraction device. Start distraction on the 5th day and continue for around 3–4 weeks. Leave for further 6–8 weeks until new bone is seen on XR.

- If the entire mandible is hypoplastic, a bidirectional distraction may be required. Two corticotomies are performed, one vertical in the mandibular body and the other horizontal in the ascending ramus. A bidirectional device is used on each side.

See ILIZAROV TECHNIQUE. *See* HEMIFACIAL MICROSOMIA.

Mandibular nerve
V3 of the trigeminal nerve exits the foramen ovale and branches to form the buccal, lingual, inferior alveolar and mental nerves. Block with a needle into the retromolar fossa parallel to the mandibular teeth at 45° angle. Provides anaesthesia for the lower face, mandible, teeth and anterior 2/3 tongue.

Mandibular osteotomy
- A procedure to move the position of the mandible if retruded or protruded.
- Sagittal splitting is the most versatile ramus osteotomy because it can be used for both mandibular prognathia and retrognathia.
- Main risk is neurosensory deficit to the lower lip and chin following temporary or permanent damage to the inferior alveolar nerve.

Mandibular reconstruction
Defects following tumour resection—*Jewer classification:*

Reconstruction options:
- Foreign implants—i.e. contoured recon plates. Technically less demanding and no donor site morbidity but require adequate soft tissues and most patients will need radiotherapy therefore risking implant extrusion.
- Non-vascularized bone (typically rib or iliac crest). Will need a good soft tissue cover and not robust against radiotherapy.
- Vascularized bone:
  - *Pedicled:* largely historical. Options include:
    - Sternocleidomastoid with clavicle although not possible if SCM devascularized following a neck dissection;
    - Trapezius with segment of spine of scapula;
    - Pec major with ribs (4–6—has most length).
  - Free:
    - *Fibular flap:* considered the gold standard reconstruction because positioning facilitates a 2 team approach of flap raise simultaneously with tumour resection, longest piece of vascularized

bone available, potential for multiple osteotomies and reliable skin paddle.
    - *DCIA flap:* good option as sufficient bone stock for hemi-mandible reconstruction.
    - *Scapular flap:* can take up to 14 cm of the lateral border of scapula based on the descending branch of the circumflex scapula artery. Can also harvest the tip of the scapula based on the angular branch of the thoracodorsal artery for reconstruction of the mandibular angle. Problematic because of patient positioning which does not facilitate 2 team approach.
    - *Radius flap taken with radial forearm skin:* risk of radial fractures afterwards and the small sliver of bone available is better suited for orbital rim reconstruction rather than mandibular reconstruction.
- Bone transport—if defect amenable.

Mandibular swing
- To gain access for oral tumour surgery.
- The lip is split in the midline. The straight line stops at the deepest part of the chin cleft then curves around the chin prominence to reach the midline below. The mandible is divided between the mental foramen and the insertion of anterior belly of digastric to increase exposure. A straight bony cut is performed. This approach divides the lingual mucosa and the mylohyoid muscle. The insertions of genioglossus, geniohyoid and anterior digastric muscles are preserved.

See HEAD AND NECK CANCER.

Mannerfelt syndrome
- Spontaneous rupture of FPL in *Rheumatoid arthritis*. Most common flexor to rupture. Due to carpal irregularities such as spurring of the volar surface of the scaphoid.
- Treat by tendon transfer, tendon graft or arthrodesis of the IPJ.
- Carpal spur should be excised and exposed bone covered with fascial flap.

Marcaine
- Brand name for the local anaesthetic agent *Bupivacaine*.
- Maximum safe dose 2 mg/kg.
- Marcaine plain or with adrenaline the same maximum dose, e.g. 60 kg woman with 0.5% marcaine = $60 \times 2 \div 5 = 15$ ml.

Marchac dorsal nasal flap
Good for closing defects 2.5 cm or less in diameter. Based on cutaneous perforating branches of the lateral nasal artery in the area of the medial canthus.

Design the flap at the medial canthal region of the opposite side, drawing a line to the glabella with a backcut.

See HATCHET FLAP. *See* RIEGER FLAP.

Marcus Gunn jaw-winking

- Rarely seen in some patients with upper eyelid *Ptosis* due to a congenital synkinesis between pterygoid muscles and levator palpebrae superioris.
- Ask patient to move jaw to the side opposite to the ptotic upper lid or open the mouth wide. The lid will lift if jaw-winking present.

Marcus Gunn pupil

- Get paradoxical pupillary dilatation when light is shone into the affected pupil.
- This occurs with injury to the optic nerve and suggests a partial lesion.
- First shine a light in the affected eye—get minimal or no response. Shining a light in the opposite eye causes constriction of both. Now shining in the affected eye causes dilatation.

Marfan's syndrome

- Disorder caused by genetic defect of connective tissue.
- Autosomal dominant inheritance.
- The defect itself has been isolated to *FBN1* gene on chromosome 15, which codes for the connective tissue protein, fibrillin.
- Develop *Arachnodactyly* with hyperextensibility.
- Also lens subluxation, aortic dilatation, mitral valve regurgitation, pes planus and protrusio acetabuli.

Marjolin's ulcer

- *Squamous cell carcinoma* arising in traumatized area such as burn scar, fistula tracts, osteomyelitis sinus.
- Described by Marjolin in 1828.
- Aggressive tumours with a poorer overall survival.
- There is a metastatic rate of 61%.
- The usual time to appearance is 25 years, but it can be as short as 3 years.

Martin–Gruber anastomosis

- Branches from the median nerve to the ulnar nerve in the forearm carrying all motor nerves to the ulnar nerve.
- Division of the ulnar nerve above the level of anastomosis will result in preservation of motor function whereas median nerve division causes a simian hand.
- Occurs in 23% of subjects. 5% send ulnar fibres to the median nerve.

See RICHE–CANNIEU ANASTOMOSIS.

Maruyama flap

- A retrograde dorsal metacarpal artery (DMCA) flap where the DMCA is ligated proximally and included in the flap as described by Maruyama in 1999.
- Considered a variation on the DMCA flap described by Quaba in 1990 and enhanced reach distally for digital cover. It can be used to cover defects up to the level of the PIPJ.
- Flap based on communicating web-space perforators that penetrate from the palmar arches through to the dorsal surface of the hand at the level of the metacarpal neck. These palmar perforators anastomose with the dorsal metacarpal arteries located on the dorsal interosseous muscles between each metacarpal.
- The skin paddles are designed over the intermetacarpal space. The skin paddle can measure 2–3 cm, but becomes unreliable proximal to the wrist.
- To raise the flap incise along the long axis of the flap deep to the fascia. The DMCA vessel is located under the fascia on the dorsal interosseous muscles. The DMCA is ligated proximally and the flap elevated from proximal to distally to the web space, taking care not to damage the interconnection between the dorsal metacarpal vessels and the communicating perforators emerging from the volar vessels. The donor site can be closed directly or with a skin graft.

See QUABA FLAP.

Mason's haemangioma

- Also called intraluminal endothelial hyperplasia.
- Less common than *Vascular leiomyoma*.
- It occurs on the fingers. It presents as a small dark subdermal lesion. It is a vascular lesion, but is clinically solid.
- It is benign though histologically resembles angiosarcoma.

Masquelet's test

- Ballottement test of lunotriquetral joint.
- Both hands used to apply shear force across articulation.
- Dorsal pressure applied to lunate and triquetrum with thumb and counter pressure with index finger.

See REAGAN'S TEST. *See* CARPAL INSTABILITY.

Masse's sign

- Clinical test in *Ulnar nerve palsy*.
- Loss of hypothenar elevation due to paralysis and wasting of *Opponens digiti quinti*.

Masseter muscle

Origin: zygomatic bone and zygomatic arch.

Insertion: lateral surface of ramus and inferior mandible at the angle.

Nerve supply: anterior division of mandibular nerve (V3).

Action: elevator, pulls mandible up and forward. *See* MUSCLE.

Mastocytoma

- May be present at birth, but can develop in early childhood.
- It initially starts as a recurring blistering patch with a persistent red-brown discolouration.
- In time, the patch becomes raised and may be 1 cm or more in diameter.
- When solitary they are generally benign and resolve spontaneously. Rarely they are generalized and very rarely malignant.

Mastopexy

An elevation +/− redistribution of breast parenchymal tissue and repositioning of the NAC in the setting of ptosis. Pure mastopexy (not in combination with breast reduction) has been defined as an excision of skin with minimal (<300 g) excision of breast parenchyma. Mastopexy techniques can be combined with breast augmentation or reduction.

Techniques: in a similar way to breast reduction, a combination of a skin pattern and NAC pedicle must be considered:

- Skin pattern options:
  - *Periareaolar:* not very effective at elevating the NAC alone but can be effective for minor ptosis in combination with an augmentation;
  - *Benelli mastopexy:* in addition to periareolar skin excision allows for parenchymal repositioning via coning of medial and lateral parenchymal flaps;
  - *Vertical:* the vertical limb added to the periareolar incision allows for a greater lift. Lassus described a vertical scar without undermining. Lejour described a vertical scar with undermining to create medial and lateral breast pillars in combination with liposuction.
  - *Inverted T:* facilitates reliable nipple elevation and parenchymal redistribution, especially in settings of severe skin excess, but has the biggest scar.
- NAC pedicle options:
  - If NAC moving small distance (<8 cm) then a vertical deepithelialized pedicle can be considered;
  - If more movement required, other pedicles commonly used in breast reduction (i.e. superomedial, inferior, central mound) should be considered.

Mathes classification of fasciocutaneous flaps

Classification of *Fasciocutaneous flaps* in 1981:

- *A:* direct cutaneous perforator, i.e. groin flap or dorsal metacarpal artery flap.
- *B:* direct septocutaneous perforator, i.e. scapular flap or posterior interosseous flap.
- *C:* indirect musculocutaneous perforator, i.e. paramedian forehead flap, nasolabial flap.

Mathes and Nahai classification of muscle flaps

Classification of muscle flaps in 1981 based on vascular supply:

- *Type 1:* single dominant pedicle enters muscle near its origin or insertion, i.e. gastrocnemius, TFL, abductor digiti minimi.
- *Type 2:* dominant pedicle and minor pedicles (circulation via minor pedicles is not reliable), i.e. gracillis, trapezius, soleus.
- *Type 3:* two dominant vascular pedicles each arising from a separate regional artery (flap can be based on either pedicle), i.e. rectus abdominis, pec minor, gluteus maximus.
- *Type 4:* multiple segmental pedicles (seldom compatible for transfer), i.e. sartorius, tibialis anterior, long flexors and extensors of the toes.
- *Type 5:* one dominant vascular pedicle and secondary smaller segmental pedicles, i.e. latissimus dorsi and pec major.

Matrix metalloproteins

These are responsible for the degradation of extracellular matrix. Imbalance between the active enzyme and their natural inhibitors may be seen in a number of diseases. They are zinc and calcium dependent.

Maxilla

Consists of a body and 4 processes—frontal, zygomatic, palatine and alveolar. The body contains the maxillary sinus. The bone thins to eggshell thickness. The alveolar process is thick as long as teeth are present.

Maxilla/midface tumours

- Maxillary sinus is an invagination of nasal mucosa into the maxillary bone. Ethmoid frontal and sphenoid sinuses do the same. They are air-bearing cavities.
- Disease within them is not recognized early. Most expand slowly giving nasal obstruction. Most tumours are large by the time they are discovered. The most common is the SCC.

Risk factors:
- Smoking, wood, nickel, chromium, radium.
- It may be associated with an _Inverting papilloma._
- Tumours below _Ohngren's line_ have a better prognosis, but are uncommon.
- Suprastructure tumours that involve the roof of the sinus are seen more commonly.
- Treatment usually involves maxillectomy and post-operative radiotherapy. Radiotherapy can give nerve problems, bone necrosis and trismus, and should be carefully planned.
- If there is lymph node involvement the mortality is 90%.

Tumour management:
- _Tumour grade:_ if low grade usually treat with surgery alone. Reconstruct with skin graft and dental appliance. Usually higher grade and may require orbital exenteration, craniotomy, RT and CT.
- _Stage:_ location as well as size is important.

Surgical approaches:
- _Lateral rhinotomy_ (Weber Ferguson), which can be extended into the lip.
- _Total rhinotomy_ provides access to the midline, cribriform plate and ethmoid.
- _Midface degloving,_ which avoids a facial incision by making a large gingivobuccal incision.

Surgical operations:
- _Medial maxillectomy:_ commonly used for benign tumours that involve the lateral wall of the nose. The main complication is stenosis of the nasolacrimal duct.
- _Suprastructure maxillectomy:_ addresses tumours in the sinus that involve the orbit and may have an intracranial extension.
- _Infrastructure maxillectomy:_ is the least common procedure. Used for tumours confined to the antrum, hard palate or superior alveolar ridge. It can be performed intra-orally and lined with a SSG.
- _Maxillectomy with preservation of the orbital contents:_ if tumour extends to orbital floor it is removed and the floor reconstructed with skin graft. If peri-orbital is involved the exenteration is performed.
- _Radical maxillectomy:_ for advanced tumours. Includes maxilla, ethmoid sinus, pterygoid plates and orbit.

Reconstruction:
- Many operations don't require reconstruction other than plating of osteotomies used to gain access.
- Reconstruction of radical maxillectomy is now performed using a free flap.

- If there is intracranial extension, muscle is transferred to seal the dura.
- Reconstructing the bony floor of the orbit requires vascularized bone. Scapula or fibula is useful. Two flaps may be required.

See ORAL CAVITY RECONSTRUCTION. _See_ LE FORT.

Maxillary fractures
- Maxillary fractures are less common than mandible, zygoma or nasal.
- The maxilla is reinforced by 3 vertical and 3 horizontal buttresses.
- The vertical buttresses include the:
  - Nasomaxillary buttress lying along the junction of cheek and nose;
  - Zygomatico-maxillary buttress, which passes through the body of the zygoma and upwards towards the zygomatic arch;
  - Pterygopalatine buttress, which passes posteriorly.
- The horizontal buttresses pass through the:
  - Infra-orbital rims;
  - Zygoma;
  - Alveolar arch.
- The maxilla is designed to absorb the forces of mastication and provide a vertical buttress for occluding teeth. Fractures are usually due to direct impact to the bone. The pattern and distribution depend on the magnitude and direction of the force. Upper _Le Fort fractures_ may injure the nasolacrimal canal. Higher fractures may involve the cranial fossa, with dural lacerations and fistulae. Fractures are caused by frontal or lateral impact.

Symptoms and signs include:

- _Bruising and swelling:_ usually superficial to the peri-orbital region and cheek and intra-orbital.
- _Battle's sign:_ bruising over the mastoid process.
- Changes in dental occlusion.
- Epistaxis.
- Enopthalmos.
- Diplopia.
- Paraesthesia in the distribution of the inferior alveolar nerve.
- Palpable step in bone with dish-face appearance from displacement downwards and posteriorly.
- _Mobility of the maxillary segment:_ pathognomonic of Le Fort fracture:
  - If alveolus alone suggests Le Fort 1 fracture;
  - Alveolus and nasofrontal suggests Le Fort 2;
  - Alveolus, nasofrontal and ZF suture suggests Le Fort 3.

Radiology: plain XR—Pa, Waters' views for sinus, CT and 3D CT.

Treatment:

- Establish an airway, control haemorrhage, close soft tissue wounds and fix fractures. ORIF is the preferred method. Gain access through:
  - Bicoronal incision for nasofrontal, orbital walls, ZF suture and zygomatic arch;
  - Lower eyelid incision for orbital floor and infra-orbital rim;
  - Upper buccal sulcus incision for lower part of maxilla.
- Reduce fragments with Rowe's distraction forceps. Apply IMF to stabilize maxilla. Apply plates across maxillary buttresses. Bone grafting may be required.

Complications: haemorrhage, airway compromise, CSF rhinorrhoea with infection, blindness (from nerve transection or haematoma), reduced nasal passage and rarely non-union.

See FACIAL FRACTURES.

Mayer–Rokitansky–Küster–Hauser syndrome
See VAGINAL AGENESIS.

McCune Albright's syndrome

- A congenital condition with variable expressivity. Sporadic mutation in GNAS1 gene.
- Characterized by triad of polyostotic (multiple site) *Fibrous dysplasia* of bone (commonly craniofacial), café-au-lait spots and multiple endocrinological dysfunction (leading to precocious puberty).
- Management is led by an MDT involving paediatrics, orthopaedics, endocrinologists and craniofacial. Treatment is tailored to individual symptoms. Bisphosphonates (pamidronate or alendronate) have been used to reduce bone turnover for fibrous dysplasia.
- Surgical management to prevent functional loss, treat primary deformity and reduce secondary deformity may be required. The vascularity of the skeletal lesions lends itself to a conservative and staged approach.

McGregor flap: cheek

- A lateral orbital transposition flap used for *Eyelid reconstruction*.
- For a lower lid defect of >60% of lid margin.
- The flap extends from the lateral canthal tendon upwards to the lateral temporal hairline. A Z-plasty is made laterally. A canthotomy is performed and the lid advanced medially.

McGregor flap: lip

- Used for lower *Lip reconstruction* to reconstruct the entire lower lip.
- Rectangular-shaped flap based on superior labial artery, which is rotated around the commissure without reducing the size of the stoma. Modification of *Gilles' fan flap* it is adynamic and insensate.
- The width of the flap equals the height of the defect, the length of the flap equals the width of the defect and the width of the flap. A mucosal advancement is required.

McKinney's point

6.5 cm inferior to the external auditory canal marks the greater auricular nerve crossing the sternocleidomastoid muscle. The greater auricular nerve is the most commonly injured nerve during a facelift.

Medial plantar artery flap

Axial pattern fasciocutaneous flap raised from the glabrous tissue on the medial plantar surface of the foot (the 'instep'). This area is not weight-bearing and therefore can be harvested with relatively little donor morbidity, although a proportion of the plantar fascia is harvested with the flap. The flap can be sensate as the *Medial plantar nerve* is usually taken with it.

Blood supply:

- Medial plantar artery, which is a terminal branch of the posterior tibial artery.
- *Innervation:* medial plantar nerve.

Flap raise:

- *Position:* supine.
- *Markings:* distal extent of skin paddle is the 1st MTPJ. Proximal extent is the edge of the heel pad. Avoiding extending the skin paddle onto the dorsum of the foot.
- *Raise:* can raise either from distal to proximal or vice versa. Safest is to expose the posterior tibial artery proximally first and chase this to adductor hallucis, which is the posterior edge of the flap. Then, raise the plantar edge of the skin flap with underlying plantar fascia followed by the dorsal edge of the flap. Finally, raise skin paddle from distal to proximal. FHL tendon will be exposed but adductor and FDB can be tacked over it and grafted. Abductor hallucis needs to be divided to continue to chase the pedicle proximally under the tarsal tunnel, and this should be repaired afterwards.
- *Closure:* donor site is split skin grafted.

Medial plantar nerve

- *L4–L5:* terminal division of the tibial nerve.
- Passes with the medial plantar artery deep to the abductor hallucis muscle.

- Mixed motor and sensory nerve supplying the medial forefoot. Muscular branches innervate abductor halluces, flexor digitorum brevis, flexor halluces brevis and the first lumbrical.

Medial pterygoid muscle
Origin: pterygoid fossa from lateral pterygoid process.

Insertion: medial surface of ramus and angle of the mandible.

Innervation: medial pterygoid nerve from the mandibular branch of trigeminal nerve (V3).

Action: upward, medial and forward traction on the mandible.
See MUSCLE.

Median nerve anatomy
- Arises from medial and lateral cords (C5-T1). Runs with brachial artery in arm, initially lateral then medial to brachial artery at elbow. In antecubital fossa, passes beneath bicipital aponeurosis and through two heads of pronator teres. In forearm runs between FDS and FDP. In wrist it passes under the transverse carpal ligament in the carpal tunnel.
- Terminal branches:
  - Forearm:
    - Anterior interosseous nerve (AIN) arises from the dorsal ulnar aspect of the median nerve at the distal end of the cubital fossa and travels along the interosseous membrane;
    - Palmar cutaneous branch arises 5–7 cm proximal to wrist crease.
  - Palm:
    - Recurrent branch;
    - Digital cutaneous branches to radial 3.5 rays.
- In the forearm it innervates PT, FCR, PL and FDS. The AIN innervates FDP and FPL and terminates in PQ.
- In hand *Median nerve motor branch* innervates lumbricals (radial two), opponens pollicis, abductor pollicis brevis, flexor pollicis brevis (superficial 1/2). *See* LOAF.
- The digital nerves supply sensation to thumb, index, middle and radial half of ring finger.

Median nerve compression sites
- From proximal to distal, the sites of compression are:
  - Distal 1/3 of humerus beneath projecting supracondylar process;
  - *Ligament of Struthers*;
  - Lacertus fibrosis;
  - Bicipital aponeurosis.

- In the forearm the potential sites are:
  - Between the humeral and ulnar heads of pronator teres;
  - The arch of FDS.
- In the wrist:
  - Carpal tunnel.

See CARPAL TUNNEL SYNDROME. *See* PRONATOR SYNDROME.

Median nerve motor branch
Three main variations, called Lanz variations:
- *1/2 of patients:* branches distal to the carpal tunnel with a recurrent course into the muscles.
- *1/3 of patients:* branches in the carpal tunnel, but follows the same course.
- *1/5 of patients:* branches inside the carpal tunnel and pierces ligament to supply the muscles.

Also:
- Accessory variations of the thenar branch at the distal carpal tunnel. Multiple branches may arise distally and travel parallel to the thenar muscles.
- *High division:* with the thenar branch dividing in the forearm, but running the same course with the median nerve separated by a persistent median artery.
- *Accessory variation of the thenar branch in the carpal tunnel:* these are branches that course superficial to the ligaments and supply the thenar muscles. These may be confused with a cutaneous branch. Sometimes they rejoin the main nerve distally.

Median nerve palsy
Presentation:
- Low lesions classified as occurring distal to the origin of the AIN. Results in sensory disturbance in the prehensile zone of the hand and paralysis of the thenar muscles (FPB frequently spared due to dual supply from ulnar) resulting in loss of thumb opposition.
- High lesions proximal to AIN origin involve paralysis of FPL, FDS and lateral half of FDP in addition to intrinsic hand muscles, therefore loss of thumb and index flexion in addition to thumb opposition. Pronator teres spared if lesion at or distal to elbow.
- Management depends on aetiology of palsy. Loss of sensation is arguably more devastating than loss of motor function.

Tendon transfer options:
- If a low palsy an opponensplasty addresses loss of thumb opposition. Options include FDS 4 (innervated by median nerve), EIP (radial nerve), ADM (ulnar nerve) or PL (median nerve).

- If a high palsy can consider:
  - Opponensplasty—EIP or PL;
  - Thumb flexion—BR to FPL;
  - Index finger flexion—ECRL to FDP (seldom performed)—can also buddy the FDP ulnar side FDPS—this will improve range of movement but decrease strength.

Medpor™
- High-density porous polyethylene.
- Used material for facial augmentation and ear reconstruction.
- Pore sizes allow stabilization of the implant through bone and soft tissue ingrowth with minimal foreign body reaction. It is strong, flexible and easy to shape.
- Risk of extrusion and exposure of implant.

See ALLOPLASTS.

Meibomian glands
Sebaceous glands, which drain directly onto the skin, found in the labia, penis and tarsus.

Meissner corpuscles
- *Sensory receptors* only found in the hand.
- Rapidly adapting myelinated A fibres, which mediate moving touch and vibration.
- They are encapsulated mechanoreceptors in the dermal papillary ridges of the skin. They range from 20 on the finger tip to $5/mm^2$ on the palm.

Melanin
- Source of pigment in skin and has a protective role from UV radiation.
- Melanin production is stimulated by sunlight and by the pituitary hormone melanocyte-stimulating hormone (MSH).
- Produced by Melanoctyes in the basal layer produce melanosomes containing melanin, which is synthesized from tyrosine. Melanin accumulates in melanosomes, which pass to surrounding cells via the dendritic processes where they fan around the nucleus superficially.

Melanocytes
- Spindle-shaped clear cells with a dark nucleus and dendritic processes. They synthesize melanin from tyrosine.
- Derived from neural crest and usually located in the stratum germinatum.
- The number of melanocytes is the same between races, but the amount of basal melanin production is greater in darker skin.
- Malignant transformation leads to melanoma.

Melanocytic naevi
- Benign pigmented skin lesion, containing either melanocytes or naevus cells.

- When melanocytes move from epidermis to dermis they become naevus cells. These are round, do not have dendritic processes and congregate in nests.
- Can be categorized as:
  - *Congenital melanocytic naevi*;
  - Epidermal:
    - Ephilis (freckle) containing normal number of melanocytes but increased melanin. Disappear in absence of sunlight;
    - *Lentigo* containing increased number of melanocytes and persists in absence of sunlight.
  - Dermal:
    - Intradermal—nest of naevus cells cluster in dermis;
    - Mongolian blue spot—over sacrum;
    - Naevus of Ota—bluish pigmentation on face in distribution of ophthalmic and maxillary divisions;
    - Naevus of Ito—bluish pigmentation in shoulder.
  - Mixed depth:
    - Junctional—nest at dermoepidermal junction. Associated with raised plaque.
    - Compound—nest at junction extending into dermis. Increase in thickness during late childhood and may be associated with coarse hairs.
  - Special:
    - Spitz—firm reddish-brown nodules that tend to present in childhood;
    - Atypical or dysplastic naevi—difficult to differentiate between melanoma. Excise with a clear margin;
    - Halo—melanocytic naevus surrounded by peripheral area of depigmentation due to regression.

Melanoma
A skin cancer involving malignant transformation of melanocytes.

Risk factors:
- Previous melanoma.
- *Sun exposure:* exposure to *Ultraviolet radiation (UV)*, mainly UVB, but also UVA.
- *Genetic:* 5–10% have family history. Alterations of *CDKN2*, a tumour suppressor gene for the protein p16 and in N-*ras* oncogene have been associated.
- Immunosuppression: renal transplants and cancers, such as lymphomas.
- Pigment traits: blue eyes, red hair, pale complexion have increased risk.

Clinical presentation:
- Very rare in children. Most cases occur in giant congenital naevi.
- *Major indicators* (ABCD): asymmetry and change in shape, colour and size.
- *Minor indicators* (DISC): diameter >6 mm, inflammation, sensory change (itch), crusting or bleeding.
- Diagnostic accuracy improved with use of dermatoscope. Can identify irregularities in borders, pigment network and globules. Presence of a blue veil from the Tyndall effect.

Types:
- All have horizontal growth phase and vertical growth phase. As no blood vessels in epidermis get no metastatic spread in horizontal phase.
- *Superficial spreading:* 70%. Upper back in men and women, legs in women. Growth is radial without the propensity to metastasize.
- *Nodular:* 20%. Legs and trunk. Get rapid growth without radial growth phase. Can get ulceration and bleeding. The most aggressive.
- *Lentigo maligna melanoma:* 4–10%, head, neck arms, elderly. Lentigo maligna present for 10–15 years before malignant change.
- *Acral lentiginous melanoma:* 2–8% in Caucasians, but most common type in dark skins. Palms or soles, or beneath nail plate. Not all melanomas in these sites are acral lentiginous except in dark skins.
- *Amelanotic melanoma.*
- *Desmoplastic melanoma:* found in the head and neck. They contain a malignant desmoplastic spindling stromal. May present as non-pigmented nodules or plaques. They recur locally and invade along nerves.

Diagnosis
Excisional biopsy with 2 mm peripheral margin and cuff of fat. Ask for full biopsy report:
- Breslow Thickness (BT).
- Ulceration.
- Mitoses.
- Subtype.
- Micro satellites.
- Invasion.
- Margins of excision.

AJCC 8th edition groupings based on TNM classification:
T based on Breslow Thickness:
- T1 <1 mm.
- T2 1.1–2.
- T3 2.1–4.
- T4 >4:
  - Without ulceration;
  - With ulceration.

N—involved lymph nodes:
- N1 0–1 nodes.
- N2 1–3 nodes.
- N3 >3 nodes.

M—distant metastases:
- M1 Skin or distant lymph nodes.
- M2 Lung.
- M3 Viscera.
- M4 Brain.

Clinical staging:

Stage 1A	T1aN0M0	10-year survival 98%
Stage 1B	T1bN0Mo T2aN0M0	94%
Stage 2A	T2bN0M0 T3aN0M0	88%
Stage 2B	T3bN0M0 T4aN0M0	82%
Stage 2C	T4bN0M0	75%
Stage 3	Any T, N>0. M0	24–88%
Stage 4	Any T, Any N, M1-4	Historically 10–15%

Management directed by skin MDT:
- Manage the local disease:

Wide local excision to deep fascia as per the 2015 NICE guidance:
  - 5 mm for Stage 0—melanoma *in situ*;
  - At least 1 cm for Stage 1, i.e. Pt2a;
  - At least 2 cm for Stage 2, i.e. PT2b (1-2 mm and ulcerated).

- Assess and manage lymph nodes if clinically node negative:

SLNB to analyse the first draining lymph node or nodes for Stage PT2a and above and (consider for Pt1b with aggressive features) as per the Melanoma Focus Guidance. PT4 get CT staging scan prior to SLNB:
  - If SLNB negative—it is stage 1 or 2 so can monitor clinically for 5 years;
  - If SLNB positive—it is at least stage 3:
    - CT staging and BRAF testing;
    - Refer to oncology for consideration of adjuvant treatment as 5 phase 3 clinical trials have shown improvement in relapse-free survival:
      1. Targeted therapy—BRAF inhibitor dabrafenib plus MEK inhibitor trametinib as per the Combi-ad trial (NICE approved);
      2. Immunotherapy (anti-PD1)—Nivolumab as per the Checkmate

trial (NICE approved for stage 3 melanoma for 1 year) 4 weekly IV cycles for a year then consider stopping.

- CLND not routinely indicted for positive SLNB following the consistent findings from MSLT 2 and DECOG in 2017. Can consider under certain conditions, i.e. heavy tumour burden (Extra-capsular spread, >3 nodes and multifocal or extensive disease (Dewar criteria) and people who cannot undergo adjuvant therapy);
- Follow up for 10 years with 6 monthly CT screening for 3 years.

- Manage macroscopic lymph node disease:
  ○ If clinically or radiologically suspicious nodes—FNAC or US guided core or open biopsy;
  ○ If palpable lymph node or macroscopic disease on CT—Lymph node dissection (axillary, superficial inguinal, pelvic or cervical) and refer for oncology for consideration of systemic treatment.

- Manage metastatic Stage 4 disease:
  ○ MDT decision about whether metastatic disease can be completely resected and intent of treatment—curative, palliative, best supportive care. Debulking does not improve survival but may have a role in palliation;
  ○ Refer to oncology for systemic therapy;
  ○ Consider role of radiotherapy in brain mets.

- Manage local recurrence. Consider:
  ○ Excision of local recurrence;
  ○ Electro Chemo Therapy (ECT) for extensive disease;
  ○ Isolated limb perfusion.

Melasma

- An acquired, hormonally influenced hyperpigmentation.
- Histologically the pigment may be located in either the epidermis or the dermis, or in both locations.
- *Lasers* may be effective in clearing pigments, including the Q-switched ruby, green pulsed dye, and Nd:YAG laser, but repigmentation is common.
- Additionally, hyperpigmentation following laser treatment may occur.

Meleney's gangrene

Streptococcal *Necrotizing fasciitis*.

Melolin

Gauze with polyethylene backing. *See* DRESSINGS.

Mental nerve block

- The mental nerve is the continuation of the inferior alveolar nerve, and it emerges from the mental foramen on the chin. located approximately 2.5 cm from the midline of the face in the midpupillary line, in line with the canine.
- It provides sensation to the chin, lower lip, mucosa, and gingiva of the lower lip.
- It is a branch of the mandibular division of the trigeminal nerve (V3).
- To block the nerve cutaneously, the foramen should be palpated and a wheal of anaesthesia placed. Then, the needle should be reinserted and advanced to the vicinity of the mental foramen but not into it. Approximately 1–3 ml of anaesthetic should be injected into the area.
- To block the nerve intra-orally, the foramen should be palpated with the middle finger of one hand and the lip lifted by the thumb and index finger of the same hand. The needle should be inserted at the inferior labial sulcus at the apex of the first bicuspid and 1–3 ml of anaesthetic injected. It may be located by rolling the lower lip outward and stretching the mucosa away from the canine root.

Merkel cell

- Present in the epidermis and thought to be a pressure receptor.
- Rare and only seen by electron microscopy.
- They are connected to keratinocytes by desmosomes.
- A slowly adapting mechanoreceptor which mediates constant touch and pressure through myelinated fibres.

See SKIN. *See* SENSORY RECEPTORS.

Merkel cell tumour

- Resemble *Basal cell carcinoma* histologically.
- Occurs as single tumour in older people.
- Tumour may be epidermal, dermal or subcutaneous.
- Microscopically get irregularly anastomosing trabeculae and rosette arrangement of basophilic uniform cells.
- They contain small granules similar to the neurosecretory granules of epidermal Merkel cell. Cytokeratin 20 stain.
- They resemble small cell carcinoma and a chest XR should be performed to exclude a secondary from a lung primary.
- They are aggressive and metastasize to nodes, viscera and bone.

Treatment:

- Cure is difficult.

• Excise with wide margin (3 cm) and consider adjuvant radiotherapy to the tumour bed and draining lymph nodes.

Mesh

Can be used in abdominal wall reconstruction, preferably as a scaffold to facilitate tissue ingrowth rather than a bridge to close a gap. Netherland Registry data shows the use of mesh repair is superior to suture repair when managing abdominal hernias.

• Types of Mesh:
  ○ *Synthetic:* stay around longer, better for strength. But not good for the infected setting, i.e. Prolene;
  ○ *Biologic:* better for infected setting as exhibit more of an inflammatory response, i.e. Strattice;
  ○ *Biosynthetic:* maintain tensile strength compared to biologic, i.e. Phasix™.
• Mesh location:
  ○ *Onlay:* on muscle;
  ○ *Inlay:* when defect not closed—mesh used to bridge, therefore not recommended;
  ○ *Sublay:* gold standard for reducing recurrence rate. Can be:
    ▪ Retromuscular;
    ▪ Pre-peritonea;
    ▪ Intra-peritoneal.

Mesodermal tumours

• *Acrochordon.*
• *Dermatofibroma.*
• *Dermatofibrosarcoma protuberans.*
• *Neurofibroma.*
• *Granula cell tumour.*

MESS Mangled Extremity Severity Score. Consider amputation with a MESS score of over 7.

• Skeletal/soft tissue injury:	low energy	1
	medium energy	2
	high energy	3
• Limb ischaemia: (double score if >6 hours)	near-normal	1
	pulseless, poor refill	2
	cold insensate	3
• Shock:	BP >90 mmHg	1
	transient hypotension	2
	persistent hypotension	3
• Age:	<30	1
	30–50	2
	>50	3

See LOWER LIMB RECONSTRUCTION. *See* LOWER LIMB TRAUMA.

Metacarpophalangeal joint dislocation

Finger:

• *Anatomy:* mobility is unique with lateral movement in extension, but stable in flexion. Looking laterally the shape is condylar and looking end on trapezoid being wider volarly. MCP joint contributes to finger convergence on flexion. Volar plate is firmly attached to proximal phalanx, but loosely to metacarpal allowing hyperextension. They are also stabilized by the deep transverse metacarpal ligament, which attaches to volar plates. Collateral ligaments originate dorsal to the axis of rotation on the metacarpal head and insert volarly on the proximal phalanx. ACLs insert into volar plate. The shape of the head and dorsal origin keeps them taut in flexion.
• *Dislocation:* rare and dorsal more common due to forced hyperextension. Most common in index finger. Hyperextension most commonly causes subluxation. Both entail proximal rupture of the volar plate, which is still in position in subluxation, but folded into the joint in dislocation. Dorsal dislocation is usually irreducible closed due to the noose formed around the neck by the flexor and lumbrical:
  ○ *Operation:* attempt closed reduction but if this fails, open reduction through a dorsal or volar incision for dorsal dislocation (where base of proximal phalanx is dorsal to metacarpal head). Clear the joint and repair ligaments;
  ○ *Subluxations are reduced closed:* don't apply longitudinal traction and hyperextension. Instead, flex the wrist, and apply pressure dorsally. Place in an extension-blocking splint for 3 weeks.
• *Collateral ligament injury:* uncommon, mainly in middle, ring and little. Caused by sudden deviation of the digit in flexion:
  ○ *Operation:* most are sprains. Treat conservatively. If unstable they will require repair through a dorsal incision. Reattach the ligament with a pull-out suture and hold in flexion.
• *Locked MCP joint:* get rigid loss of extension. Can be confused with triggering. It may be degenerative or spontaneous. Degenerative: >50, usually middle finger. Caused by osteophytes or changes around the joint capsule. Spontaneous: <50, usually index. No XR changes. Due to abnormal bands within the joint, loose bodies, capsular tears or irregular articular surfaces:

○ *Operation:* occasionally the joint can be freed under LA, but otherwise exploration is required.

Thumb

- *Anatomy:* stability important for power grip and precision grasp. ROM 5–100°. The metacarpal head is wider than the fingers and the sesamoid bones are incorporated into the volar plate. FPB and AP partial insert into these and provide additional support as do the other surrounding tendons.
- *Dislocation:* usually due to hyperextension. Much more common than the fingers as more exposed. Volar plate usually ruptures distal to sesamoid bones. There is no lumbrical so entrapment doesn't occur. Open reduction may be required:

  ○ *Operations:* closed reduction by flexing with traction. Open reduction is through a palmar incision. Some surgeons recommend volar plate repair. Sesamoid fracture can be held with a circular suture or removed. Volar dislocation is less common.

- *Collateral ligament injury.*

Metastatic bone carcinoma

- The most common malignant *Bone tumours* and the 3rd most common site for metastasis.
- Most affect the axial skeleton. 20% are in the upper limb but uncommon in the hand. Mimics infection.
- In the hand, most occur in the distal phalanx.
- *XR:* aggressive radiolucent lesion with periosteal reaction.

Treatment:

- Depends on many factors including life expectancy. Surgery is only indicated for impending fracture. Also use radiotherapy. These patients have a poor prognosis so treatment is usually palliative.
- In the hand, ray amputation is often the best treatment.

Methyl methacrylate

- Self-curing acrylic resin used for securing joint components to bone.
- Has minimal adhesive properties.
- Can be pre-formed or mouldable.
- Body response is minimal. Get exothermic reaction which may damage tissues. Cardiac arrest has been reported.
- Used in orthopaedics as a bone cement and neurosurgery for reconstructing cranial defects. Useful in thoracic surgery for *Chest wall reconstruction*, where it is placed between a Marlex mesh. It is used for dental prostheses.

- It does not biodegrade or become replaced by functional bone. It is associated with chronic inflammation.

See ALLOPLASTS.

Metopic synostosis

- The metopic suture is the first cranial suture to fuse, occurring variably at any time after 3 months.
- Lack of growth in the frontal bones, producing a keel-shape deformity—trigonocephaly. *See* HYPOTELORISM. *See* BITEMPORAL PINCHING. *See* BIPARIETAL WIDENING.
- Accounts for less than 10% of isolated suture, non-syndromic craniosynostoses.
- Isolated metopic synostosis not usually associated with raised ICP but may have higher risk of neurodevelopmental problems compared to other isolated synostoses.

Management:

- Non-operative.
- Open approach—bi-frontal orbital advancement (BFOA) via bi-coronal incision.
- Minimally invasive approach via endoscopic strip craniectomy.

See CRANIOSYNOSTOSIS.

MHC: major histocompatibility complex

- The most important antigens contributing to rejection.
- Found on chromosome 6 and are called different things in different species.
- Called HLA in humans. Two major classes:

  ○ Class I antigens have 3 loci in humans, HLA A, B and C, and are found on most nucleated cells;
  ○ Class II antigens in humans are HLA DR, DP and DQ, found on vascular endothelium and lymphocytes and macrophages; matching of HLA-A, B and DR are the most important.

- *Other antigens:* important for transplant are blood group, minor histocompatibility and skin specific antigens.

See TRANSPLANT IMMUNOLOGY.

Micropenis

Insufficient androgen stimulation. Usually caused by primary hypogonadism or hypothal-amic or pituitary dysfunction. It is 2.5 standard deviations below the mean length.

See EMBRYOLOGY.

Microsurgery

History:

- *1950s:* the first binocular microscope was developed by Carl-Zeiss.
- *1962:* Malt and McKhann, first limb replant.

- *1964:* Buncke performed the first successful ear replant.
- *1968:* Komatsu and Tamai first digit replant.
- *1968:* Cobbett first toe-to-hand transfer.
- *1969:* free omental flap to scalp.
- *1972:* temporal free flap in Japan by Harii and Ohmori.
- *1973:* Daniel and Taylor free groin flap.

Principles: calm disposition and patience. Surgeon must be able to concentrate without being hurried or interrupted. Trainees should begin in the laboratory. Reduce tremor by not drinking caffeine or exercising beforehand.

Positioning: position is key—movements will be easier and progress will proceed quicker. Surgeon should be seated with feet flat on the ground. The forearms should rest on drapes so that they are the same level as the anastomosis.

Choice of vessels: vessels need to be healthy with appropriate size and good outflow. Ideally away from zone of trauma and site of irradiation. A healthy vessel has a soft wall and a vascular sheath that can be dissected.

Preparation of vessels: inspect the lumens for irregularities such as intimal tears or separation from the media, thrombi, atherosclerotic plaques, friable walls. Wash away any debris.

Micro-sutures: the bite should incorporate all layers of the vessel—especially a good bite of the intima. Sutures are tied by sight (when the vessel ends meet and slightly evert)—not feel.

Patency: Acland described 5 important factors—surgical precision, size of the vessel, blood flow, tension, and the use of anticoagulant and anti-thrombotic medication.

See FREE FLAP.

Microtia

- Hypoplasia of the external ear, ranging from small to absent ear.
- Incidence: 1:7,000.
- M:F 2:1.
- Rt:lt:bilat 5:3:1.
- May have conductive hearing loss. Inner ear rarely involved.

May be associated hemifacial microsomia, and Treacher Collins syndrome.

Nagata classification:

- *Conchal type:* smaller ear but each part distinguished.
- *Small conchal type:* constricted ear—more difficult to distinguish each part.
- *Lobular type:* only lobule remains.
- *Anotia:* no ear.

Investigation:

- Audiometric testing for conductive or sensorineural hearing loss (Cochlea usually intact therefore expect conducting hearing loss—that is why patients usually benefit from BAHA).
- *Imaging:* CT to evaluate middle ear and inner ear anatomy.

Management:

Hearing is the primary concern and should be optimized bilaterally. Bone anchored hearing aids (BAHA) should be positioned at least 6–7 cm posterior to the external auditory meatus to allow for definitive pinna reconstruction at a later age.

Options for pinna reconstruction:

- Do nothing.
- Osseointegrated prosthesis.
- Alloplastic—single stage with porous polyethylene (Medpor™) implant covered with large temporoparietal flap.
- Autogenous with rib graft:
  - ○ *Brent:* four stages begun at 6 years;
  - ○ *Nagata:* two stages, begun at 10 years when more cartilage.

See EAR RECONSTRUCTION.

Milia

See EPITHELIAL CYSTS.

Millard cleft lip reconstruction

- A rotation advancement technique described by Ralph Millard in the 1950s which became globally popular.
- Involves a curvilinear incision on the medial lip element to provide rotation and a triangular flap on the lateral element to provide advancement.
- Modifications of the rotation-advancement included the Mohler which extends the incision into the columella to enhance the lip lengthening and Noordhof which adds a small triangle above the white roll and a laterally based vermillion triangle.

See CLEFT LIP.

Millesi classification of brachial plexus injury

Classification of *Brachial plexus injury*.

- *I:* supraganglionic.
- *II:* infraganglionic.
- *III:* trunk.
- *IV:* cord.

Milroy's disease Familial *Lymphoedema* congenita.

Minoxidil

- A powerful peripheral vasodilator that perhaps stimulates the passage of *Hair* from telogen to anagen phase.

- It causes hair growth or stops hair loss in 39% of men who use it for 1 year. It is more effective in men younger than 40 with recent hair loss limited to the crown area.
- It does not help the receding hair line. Efficacy plateaus at 1 year.

See HAIR TRANSPLANTATION.

Mirror hand
See ULNAR DIMELIA.

Moberg flap
- Volar advancement flap uses the entire volar surface of the digit. Mainly used for thumb defects.
- Flap will include both NVBs. Maximum length gain is 1 cm.
- Preserve branches to dorsal nerve and dorsal vessels otherwise can get dorsal skin loss.
- Proximal NVBs can be dissected to increase length and a large V–Y advancement created. Begin active extension by 10–14 days.

See FINGERTIP INJURIES.

Moberg pick-up test
- Stereognosis is the ability to recognize objects based on touch.
- Ten objects are picked up and identified first visually then blindfolded.
- Less useful for an isolated ulnar nerve lesion as the object can be identified using the intact median nerve.
- If median nerve is being tested, ring and little fingers are taped.

See SENSATION TESTING.

Mobile wad
Muscles of brachioradialis, ECRL and ECRB. Innervated by the radial nerve proximal to the bifurcation.

Möbius syndrome
- Developmental disorder with bilateral facial paralysis.
- Involves 6th and 7th cranial nerves and possibly the 3rd, 5th, 9th and 12th.
- 25% have limb abnormalities and 15% have abnormal pectoral muscles.
- The paralysis may occasionally be unilateral.

Reconstruction: aim for functioning nasolabial folds. Bring motor nerves—partial spinal accessory or trigeminal possibly with nerve grafts. Then provide muscle with a free transfer.

See FACIAL RE-ANIMATION.

Mohs surgery
- Margin control surgical excision of skin cancers—involves serial excisions which are examined microscopically until all the tumour has been removed.
- Pioneered by Frederick Mohs in 1940s—later refined to Mohs micrographic surgery. It combines staged resection with comprehensive surgical margin examination resulting in extremely high cure rates with maximal preservation of normal tissue.
- Generally reserved for high-risk facial lesions. 5-year cure rate of 99% in primary and 94% in recurrent BCCs.

Procedure:
- Entire lesion is excised at 45° with roughly 2 mm margin peripherally and deeply.
- Peripheral margins marked at 3, 6, 9 and 12 o'clock.
- Specimen squashed flat (potentially with releasing incisions) and rapidly frozen to allow sectioning parallel to surface of skin— this allows simultaneous assessment of the entire surgical margin.
- Residual tumour is mapped to the orientation markings and further excision targeted.
- Process repeated until clear margins obtained.

Mongolian spot
- Variably sized bluish-black patch over the lower back and buttocks in infants, occasionally over upper back and rarely in other sites.
- Usually present at birth, more common in Asians, rare in Caucasians.
- May be multiple. Usually regress in early childhood.

See NAEVUS.

Monocryl
Poliglecaprone 25. A monofilament synthetic suture. Similar absorption to *Vicryl*. Less prone to bacterial colonization.

Montgomery v. Lanarkshire Health Board (2015)
Redefined the standard for informed consent, previously governed by *Bolam*. In this case, a woman with diabetes delivered her son vaginally. He suffered shoulder dystocia and sustained hypoxic insult, resulting in cerebral palsy. She argued that had she known this risk, she would have requested an elective Caesarean section. This case established that patients should be told information that is relevant and material to them, even where the risk is rare, and informed consent should not be limited to what the doctor thinks is important to disclose.

Morley's compression test
- Test for *Thoracic outlet syndrome* producing tenderness at the root of the neck with pressure over the plexus in the interscalene groove causing neurological symptoms.

- Perform with patient sitting, feeling neck from behind. Feel the postero-lateral edge of the sternomastoid muscle. Slip fingers under the edge of the muscle at the root of the neck above the clavicle and feel the anterior scalene muscle. Roll fingers postero-laterally to feel the interscalene groove and then the scalenus medius.
- The plexus is felt on the interscalene groove, and reproduction of symptoms is diagnostic. Palpate for masses, listen for bruit. Fullness in the supraclavicular fossa is usually a cervical rib.

MRC grading of nerve function
Motor function:

- *M0:* no contraction.
- *M1:* flicker.
- *M2:* movement with gravity eliminated.
- *M3:* movement against gravity.
- *M4:* movement against gravity and resistance.
- *M5:* normal.

See SENSORY FUNCTION.

MRI

- Tissue is excited by a high-powered magnet. The energy emitted from the hydrogen ions in water and fat is measured.
- Upon the emission of energy, nuclei are said to relax, indicating that they assume a lower energy state by realigning with the applied magnetic field. The rate at which relaxation occurs is determined by two tissue properties, the T1 or longitudinal relaxation time and the T2 or transverse relaxation time.
- These relaxation times determine the amount of energy received from different tissues and are the basis for image contrast in MRI.
- *T1:* these images show anatomic detail and 'crisp' appearing anatomy. Fat-containing tissues will appear brighter (have higher signal) on T1-weighted images. These are sometimes referred to as FAT images. Structures with high H_2O content will appear darker (muscle, CSF).
- *T2:* These images appear slightly 'grainy' or 'pixely'. This sequence is designed to show fluid collections, can detect tumour infiltration of marrow, infection, acute fractures with haemorrhage or other pathological conditions that usually have with them associated oedema. CSF will be bright on this imaging sequence.
- STIR films are modified T2 images with the fat signal suppressed:
  - Gadolinium enhancement is taken up by pathological tissue and looks white, so it is best seen on a T1 image where the fluid is black;

  - *Positive points:* good for soft tissues, can view in any plane;
  - *Negative points:* poor for bone, takes a long time, expensive, metallic objects;
  - *NB* Fluid black and white—T1 and T2.

Mucous cyst
Subdermal cyst usually over the dorsum of the DIP joint. Cyst fluid arises from the joint and associated with *Heberden's nodes*. Excise if there is pain, enlarging cyst, infection or nail involvement. XR shows degenerative change with diminished joint space and osteophytes.

Treatment: if excision is indicated, perform through an H incision. Often overlying skin requires excision. Excise cyst down to joint. Remove any osteophytes, close the capsule, and perform a local flap to close the defect.

Muir and Barclay formula
For burns resuscitation using human albumin solution.

- TBSA% $\times$ 0.5 ml Wt (kg) = one ration:
  - Give one ration 4-hourly in first 12 hours;
  - Give one ration 6-hourly in next 12 hours;
  - Give remaining ration over 12 hours.

Muir-Torre syndrome
- Multiple internal malignancies.
- Cutaneous sebaceous proliferation.
- Keratoacanthomas.
- *Basal cell carcinoma* and SCC.

Muller's muscle
Smooth muscle with sympathetic innervation. Situated in the posterior lamellar of the upper lid and attaches to levator and tarsus.

Origin: posterior border of levator.

Insertion: superior border of tarsus. It is 10–12 mm long and 15 mm wide. It is adherent to conjunctiva.
See MUSCLES.

Mulliken and Glowacki classification
- Classification for vascular malformation (1982).
- Vascular abnormalities are classified as *Haemangiomas* or *Vascular malformations*.
- Vascular malformations are subcategorized based on predominant channel type and flow characteristics:
  - *Slow flow:* capillary (CM) and telangiectases, lymphatic (LM), venous (VM);
  - *Fast flow:* arterial and arteriovenous.

Munro classification of hypertelorism
Classifies *Hypertelorism* by shape of the orbit.
- *Type A:* parallel medial orbital walls.
- *Type B:* ballooning of anterior interorbital tissue.

- *Type C:* central portion of medial wall balloons.
- *Type D:* wide posterior ethmoidals. C and D are most difficult to correct.

Muscle

When injured, muscle can either form a scar or regenerate. Skeletal muscle usually regenerates, smooth and cardiac muscle do not.

Anatomy: each cell is circumscribed by its sarcolemma consisting of cell membrane, base-ment membrane, and endomysium. Bundles of fibres are fascicles, surrounded by perimysium and the whole muscle is covered with epimysium.

Injury: when cut the cell retracts leaving sarcolemma empty. This is filled with clot, which includes fibrin. Get inflammatory cell and fibroblast migration. By the 3rd day, the basal lamina are lined by macrophages. Fibro-blasts proliferate and collagen is laid down (type III then type I).

Regeneration:

- Occur from small satellite cells on the basal lamina of the sarcolemma. These satellite cells only occur in skeletal muscle. Only satellite cells can mitose.
- Satellite cells become myoblasts and fill the injured area. These fuse to produce multinucleated cells which then produce contractile proteins. These mature and finally become reinnervated. So fibroblasts produce the framework for muscle cells to regenerate. Excessive scar will block regeneration.

Treatment: mobilization accelerates revascu-larization but may cause more disruption. 5 days of immobilization is sufficient to prevent re-rupture of muscle in the rat model.

Muscles: upper limb
Extrinsic muscles:

- *Extensors—superficial:* 4 muscles, *EDC*, *EDM*, *ECU* and anconeus. They all share a common origin on the lateral epicondyle.
- *Extensors—deep:* 4 muscles, *APL*, *EPB*, *EPL*, *EIP*.
- *Extensors—lateral:* supinator, *Brachioradialis*, *ECRL*, *ECRB*. The latter 3 form the *Mobile wad* of Henry.
- *Flexors—superficial:* *PT*, *FCR*, *PL*, *FCU*. All from medial epicondyle.
- *Flexors—intermediate: FDS*.
- *Flexors—deep: FPL*, *FDP*.

Intrinsic muscles:

- *Interossei*, *Lumbricals*.
- *Of thumb:* *APB*, *FPB*, *OP*, *AP*.

Musculocutaneous/muscle flaps

- The motor nerve is always accompanied by a vascular pedicle, which is often the major source of circulation. There are often collaterals.
- A *dominant* pedicle can sustain an entire muscle.
- A *minor* pedicle can sustain only a portion of muscle. Some muscles have several *segmental* vessels each supplying a portion of muscle. Muscles with a single dominant pedicle are most useful as flaps.

Classification:

- *Taylor:* by nerve supply—for dynamic transfer.
- *Nahai and Mathes:* by vascular supply.
- Most are type II. Those with a dominant pedicle would be the most reliable.
- Skin in a musculocutaneous flap is supplied by perforators that are usually terminal branches of musculocutaneous perforators though there can be direct cutaneous perforators. Improve chances of survival of skin by having a broad-based skin paddle with bevelled edges, which is proximal to pedicle. Doppler or better colour duplex can assist in determining perforators.
- Neovascularization occurs particularly over the cutaneous area so a musculocutaneous flap will become pedicle independent much quicker than a muscular flap.

Function preservation: if a portion of muscle is left with intact origin, insertion and innervation. Examples would be a hemisoleus or part of a distally based latissimus.

Skin territory:

- The skin territory of each superficial muscle is defined anatomically as that segment of skin extending between the origin and insertion of the muscle and located between its edges along the course of the muscle. If fascia is included, the skin island may be extended beyond muscle dimensions in certain musculocutaneous flaps.
- Generally, the more narrow muscles (e.g. gracilis) have a greater limitation in skin territory because of the decreased number of perforating vessels to the overlying skin and the increased importance of septocutaneous vessels to the skin territory in proximity to the muscle.

Segmental flap: a type 3 muscle such as gluteus maximus can have part of the muscle raised so that some functioning muscle remains. Type IV muscles have to be raised segmentally as the rest of the muscle would not survive.

See FLAPS.

Mustardé flap
• A cheek rotation flap used for *Eyelid reconstruction*.
• In lower lid, can be used to reconstruct anterior lamella for defects of >2/3. Posterior lamella will require graft, i.e. palatal mucosa.
• The arc of rotation passes just below the lateral brow. Keep a wide base. It can be elevated subcutaneously or below SMAS.

See CHEEK ROTATION FLAP.

Mustardé lid switch
• A laterally based transverse flap of the lower eyelid is transposed to the upper lid.
• It may be possible to directly close the lower lid. If not, it can be reconstructed using one of the techniques described in *Eyelid reconstruction*.
• The transposition flap is divided at a second procedure.
• Also total lid switch.

Mycobacteria
Tuberculosis:
• 2% of infected patients have involvement of the upper limb.
• Get a cold abscess. XR show osteopenia with lack of bone destruction. Slight periosteal reaction and joint narrowing. Aspiration may be diagnostic. Biopsy may be necessary. Growth on Lowenstein–Jensen medium at 37°C. Some atypical mycobacteria grow at 30–32°C.
• Treat by aggressive debridement. Wound closure is acceptable.

Atypical mycobacteria:
• Incidence is increasing. Delay in diagnosis is common as they have an indolent course.
• *Mycobacterium marinum:* with aquatic exposure.
• *M. terrae:* with farm exposure.
• *M. avium:* particularly in immunocompromised patients.
• Treat with aggressive debridement and long-term antibiotics. Minocycline or combination therapy.

See INFECTION.

Mycosis fungoides
• Cutaneous T-cell lymphoma, or mycosis fungoides, is a cutaneous form of lymphoma.
• Presents with pruritic erythematous scaly patches, infiltrated plaques, and irregular skin nodules and ulcers.
• Diagnosed histologically.

• Extensive skin involvement precludes any definitive operative treatment.
• Topical nitrogen mustard or psoralen *Photochemotherapy* utilizing the photoactive psoralen drugs followed by long-wavelength ultraviolet irradiation (UVA) can be utilized.
• Patients who are unresponsive to these treatments can be treated with electron beam therapy. In most instances when irradiation ulcers have occurred, the extent of the disease and the extent of the previous electron beam therapy preclude the availability of adjacent tissues for pedicle flaps. Although mycosis fungoides is sometimes a fatal disease, in some cases the course is prolonged.
• New treatments include extracorporeal photophoresis.

Myeloma
See BONE TUMOURS.
• The most common primary bone malignancy.
• Occurs in >40s.
• Most produce monoclonal immunoglobulins.
• Bone involved contain red marrow, e.g. vertebral bodies, ilium, ribs.
• Long-term survival averages 4 years.
• *XR:* radiolucent punched out lesions.
• *Treatment:* very sensitive to chemo- and radiotherapy. Surgery is only indicated if there is a risk of fracture.

Myofascial dysfunction
See RSD.
• Myofascial dysfunction trigger points are often present in RSD.
• This is a clinical diagnosis.
• Specific proximal trigger points are found in muscle or fascia, which elicit immediate referred pain or numbness at distant sites.
• The trigger point is often a palpable lump. In the absence of treatment, trigger points become a chronic condition that does not spontaneously resolve.
• Treatment varies, but use muscle stretch and vasocoolant icing to inactivate trigger points.

Myofibroblast
Resembles a fibroblast but contains cytoplasmic filaments of α-smooth muscle actin. It is also found in smooth muscle. They are responsible for wound contraction. The number of fibroblasts in a wound is proportional to the contraction. Increased numbers are found in Dupuytren's disease.

Myoglobinuria
See ELECTRICAL INJURIES.

- Released from muscle following destruction.
- It is a monomer containing a haem molecule.
- Following electrical injury is indicative of rhabdomyolysis secondary to muscle destruction.
- If not treated, get intratubular deposition of pigments and acute renal failure.
- Treat with:
  - Forced diuresis with mannitol;
  - Alkalize the urine with 88–132 mEq/L sodium bicarbonate.

Myotomes
Upper limb:
- Shoulder:
  - *Abduct*: C5;
  - *Adduct*: C6–8.
- Elbow:
  - *Flex:* C5–6;
  - *Extend:* C 7,8.

- Forearm:
  - *Pronate:* C6;
  - *Supinate:* C6.
- Wrist:
  - *Flex:* C6–7;
  - *Extend:* C6–7.
- Fingers and thumb:
  - *Flex:* C7–8;
  - *Extend:* C7–8.
- Hand (intrinsics): T1.

Lower limb:
- Hip:
  - *Flex:* L2–3;
  - *Extend:* L4–5.
- Knee:
  - *Extend:* L3–4;
  - *Flex:* L5, S1.
- Ankle:
  - *Dorsi-flex:* L4–5;
  - *Plantar-flex:* S1–2.

m

Naevus to Nuss technique

Naevus
When a melanocyte leaves the epidermis and enters the dermis—becomes a naevus cell. They are distinctive:

- Round rather than spindle-shaped.
- No dendritic processes.
- Tend to congregate in nests.

Naevus flammeus neonatorum
See PORT-WINE STAIN.

Naevus simplex
Salmon patch.

- The common fading macular stain that occurs in 50% of neonates.
- Commonly located on the glabella, eyelids, nose, upper lip ('angel kiss'), and nuchal area ('stork bite').

  See PORT-WINE STAIN.

Naevus spilus
- Sharply demarcated brown patch speckled with smaller areas of black pigmentation.
- Get a background of *Café au lait macules* and multiple junctional nevi.
- Common. Found on the trunk and extremities.
- Treat by observation. Response to Q-switched pulsed *Lasers* is variable.

Nager's syndrome
- Autosomal dominant condition. Mutation in SF3B4 gene.
- Known as acrofacial (limbs and face) dysostosis.
- Craniofacial malformations are similar in appearance to *Treacher Collins* and include malar hypoplasia, downward slanting palpebral fissures, mandibular hypoplasia (leading to micrognathia), microtia and cleft palate.
- Limb abnormalities primarily involve the radial side of hand (i.e. thumb) and forearm.

Nail
Anatomy:
- *Entire nail unit:* perionychium consists of nail plate, proximal nail fold (eponychium), lateral nail fold (paronychium), distal edge of nail

(hyponychium) and germinal matrix. Nail plate is multi-layered of cornified cells derived from anuclear onychocytes from the germinal matrix of the nail bed.

- *Nail bed:* soft tissue below the nail plate. The germinal matrix (proximally) forms the early developing nail, the overlying fold contributes the smooth surface and the sterile matrix (distally) adds bulk. The entire nail bed including the overlying eponychial fold contributes material to the developing and growing nail lunula, which is a white arc of nail distal to eponychium due to persistence of nuclei in cells of germinal matrix. Nail becomes transparent as they disintegrate. The sterile matrix epithelium does not undergo *Parakeratosis*.
- *Keratinization:* there are three modes:
  - Germinal matrix forms the main substance of hardened nail plate with stratified layers of onychocytes;
  - Sterile matrix produces semi-rigid keratin, which also acts as an adhesive, sticking the nail to the nail bed;
  - External sheen is produced by epidermoid keratinization from the dorsal roof, nail bed is anchored to the periosteum.

- *Nail fold:* houses the proximal nail plate. The nail wall tapers distally to form the eponychium. Continuity of nail fold is required for nail growth. At the hyponychium the nail plate becomes non-adherent and extends over the tip of the finger. A build-up of cells occurs under the distal nail, which acts as a barrier. The nail bed has a rich vascular supply.

Growth: 1 mm per week or around 0.1 mm per day. Stress or illness can inhibit growth and trimming can increase growth.

Avulsion: nail avulsion will take surface epithelium and keratinous solehorn (keratin produced by the sterile matrix). Blood and plasma exudate creates a scab. Lateral nail folds and hyponychium provide reparative epidermis. This layer is hyperkeratotic but provides protection. New nail plate starts to regenerate in 2–3 weeks. Get a rolling front of advancing nail plate. Replacement of reparative epithelium with bed epithelium is synchronous with the progression of new nail plate. Both come from germinal matrix.

Traumatic nail deformities: it is easier to manage nail bed wounds acutely than perform secondary reconstruction. Anatomic alignment is crucial. If poorly aligned, nail will not adhere to the scar tissue. The nail should be removed and the nail bed examined and repaired following which the nail can be replaced if clean and adequate.

Subungual haematoma: caused by bleeding under the nail plate. How much bleeding requires exploration is not clear. Perhaps haematoma covering >50% of the nail bed should be explored. Pain requires release of the haematoma using a hand-held cautery (trephining), however this should be avoided with underlying tuft fractures unless nail bed repair is planned. Residual haematomas migrate distally with the nail.

Simple and stellate lacerations: usually due to a localized blow with compression. Requires debridement and accurate suture. Nail bed may need to be undermined to allow closure. Nail can be replaced as a splint if adequate and clean. If the nail is lost a splint can be put in place, although the multi-centre NINJA trial showed no benefit to splinting the repair (whether with nail plate or a splint). If the germinal matrix is involved the dorsal roof is lifted through lateral incisions.

Crush injuries: have a poorer prognosis. Repair what is possible. Avulsed nail bed can be removed and replaced with free grafts using split sterile matrix. Associated fractures may require a K-wire.

Avulsion injuries: with partial or total loss of nail bed. Nail bed adherent to the nail can be replaced as a graft. If the germinal matrix is avulsed it should be replaced under the eponychial fold. Split sterile matrix graft can be taken from the uninjured part of nail. Otherwise use big toe grafts. Take germinal matrix as well to prevent nail growth where there is no sterile matrix. A defect of germinal matrix requires a full thickness graft, but sterile matrix requires only a split graft. Harvest with a size 15 scalpel blade. Replacing a sterile matrix with SSG will not allow nail adherence.

Composite grafts: hyponychium and nail bed are unique structures. In children under 10 years composite grafts should be replaced. In older children and adults convert the composite graft into a full thickness skin graft. Defat the tissue and preserve nail bed.

Non-adherent nail: due to scarring of the nail bed. As the growing nail hits the scar tissue it becomes non-adherent. This catches and leads to trauma under the nail. Treatment involves trimming nail back to normal sterile matrix. Excise scar and close primarily or with split sterile matrix grafts. Non-adherence may be due to hyperkeratosis and requires scraping of the sterile matrix.

Split nail: often due to an axial scar, which divides the nail plate. It may also be caused by scarring of the dorsal roof or defect of the germinal matrix. Longitudinal scars may be excised or Z-plasty to change the direction of the scar. Larger scars require split grafts. Germinal matrix loss requires full thickness germinal matrix graft. Dorsal roof scarring may require a split sterile matrix graft. Cover grafts with a silicone sheet.

Hook nail: a nail that grows over the tip of the finger. Due to loss of structural support. The nail is sensitive and catches. Reconstruction involves recreating the injury and restoring bony and soft tissue support using Atasoy or Kutler flaps. Apply split nail bed graft. Bony support is more difficult and may require a composite toe flap.

Linear ridging: often associated with underlying bone or soft tissue abnormality. CT may be required to establish the cause. Treatment is the same as split nail.

Reconstruction of the eponychium: most commonly required after burns. Also friction injury. Get an irregular nail or a notched deformity. Can use a composite graft from toe. Dorsal skin may be rotated or transposed. A split sterile matrix graft is sutured to the undersurface to restore dorsal root bed.

Pincer nail deformity: normal nail shape is biconvex. The nail folds and the contour of the phalanx contribute to overall shape. With a pincer nail this shape is lost. It may be related to loss of lateral integrity of the distal phalanx. It is unsightly and may be ingrown and more prone to paronychia. Reconstruction involves dermal grafts laterally to restore contour. A tunnel is made laterally into which the dermal graft is inserted.

Nail lengthening

Can be used in fingertip reconstructions when nail sterile matrix has been destroyed. Eponychium is slid more proximally by de-epithelializing a strip of skin just proximal to the eponychial fold to allow it to move proximally. This gives more nail show. Described by Bakhach.

Nalebuff classifications

Thumb deformity in *RA*:

- *I:* Boutonnière deformity most common, MCP joint flexion, IPJ extended.
- *II:* Boutonnière deformity with adduction. Rare. Combined I and III—MCPJ flexion with IPJ hyperextension and subluxation of CMC.
- *III:* swan neck deformity with dislocated CMC, MCPJ extended and IPJ flexed.
- *IV:* UCL incompetence with CMCJ subluxation.
- *V:* like III, but not adducted. Due to stretching of the MCP joint volar plate.

Swan-neck deformity:

- *I:* flexible PIPJ deformity—generally responds to figure-of-eight splinting.
- *II:* limited PIPJ flexion with MCPJ extended due to intrinsic tightness—managed with splinting or intrinsic release.
- *III:* limited PIPJ flexion in all MCP joint positions due to fixed dorsal position of lateral bands—manage with translocation of lateral bands, PIPJ capsulectomy and collateral ligament release.
- *IV:* PIPJ destruction—manage with arthrodesis or arthroplasty

Boutonnière deformity:

- *I:* mild with extensor lag of 10–15°, passively correctable—manage with splinting, steroid injections or Dolphin or Fowler tenotomy.
- *II:* moderate with extensor lag of 30–40°, passively correctable—manage by shortening central slip or lateralizing lateral bands.
- *III:* severe with fixed flexion deformity— manage with arthrodesis or arthroplasty.

Narakas classification

Of *Obstetric brachial plexus* injury.

- *Group 1:* C5-6: paralysis of shoulder, absent elbow flexion—spontaneous recovery in >80%.
- *Group 2:* C5-7: As above with wrist drop—good hand, good shoulder and elbow in 60%.
- *Group 3:* All: complete paralysis—good hand in most, good shoulder and elbow in 30–50%.
- *Group 4:* All: complete paralysis, Horner sign, limb atonic—full recovery very rare.

Nasal fractures

Anatomy:

- The nose is comprised of 5 bones, the frontal process of maxilla, the nasal process of frontal bone, nasal bones, vomer and ethmoid.
- *Nerve supply:* trigeminal nerve—V1 (ophthalmic) infratrochlear and anterior

ethmoidal. V2 (maxillary)—infra-orbital and nasopalatine.

- *Rhinion:* the middle third of the nose which is the junction of the upper bony part and the lower cartilaginous part. At the rhinion the upper lateral cartilage overlaps the nasal bone and the lower lateral cartilage overlaps the upper lateral. Fracture of the rhinion may dislocate the upper lateral cartilages and cause a saddle deformity.
- *Blood supply:* from both internal and external carotids, but mainly from the external carotid via the maxillary artery and also the facial artery. The internal carotid contributes to the nose superior to the middle turbinate.

Fractures:

- Mainly occur in the thinner distal part of the paired nasal bones. Fractures may cause injury to the nasolacrimal system and epiphora. Severe blows may cause widening of the interorbital distance.
- Most commonly fractured facial bone. Lateral impact results in deviation of nasal bones and septum to the opposite side. Frontal impact results in splaying of the nasal bones, buckling or dislocation of the septum, collapse of the nasal dorsum.

Classification: *Stranc and Robertson*.

Symptoms and signs:

- Bruising and swelling.
- Obvious deformity.
- Look intranasally for septal haematoma, which should be drained at their most dependent portion to prevent pressure necrosis.

Treatment:

- Simple fractures may be treated by closed reduction.
- Ashe's forceps relocate the nasal septum.
- Walsham's forceps relocate nasal bones.
- The nose is packed and an external splint applied.
- Secondary rhinoplasty may be required.

See FACIAL FRACTURES.

Nasal reconstruction

The nose is a trilaminar structure comprising of external skin, a mid-layer of bone and cartilaginous support and an internal mucosal lining.

Nasal subunit described by Burget and Menick:

- *9 units:* dorsum, tip, columellar and paired sidewalls, alae and soft triangles. These subunits need to be respected during reconstruction.

- If a defect fills more than 50% of a convex subunit (i.e. tip, alae) then an entire subunit reconstruction may have superior aesthetic results, placing scars in subunit boundaries. The tissue filling the defect should be of the same thickness. Contour is important.

  See AESTHETIC UNITS.

Assessment for reconstruction:
- The goal of reconstruction is aesthetic and functional with a patent airway. Always analyse what is missing and what is available for reconstruction.
- All three elements of nose structure need to be assessed and replaced: skin cover, osseocartilaginous structural support and mucosal lining.
- Nose skin varies from thick stiff skin on the tip to thin smooth skin on the dorsum.
- If cheek, lip and nose are missing, first reconstruct cheek and lip and rebuild nose once the other is healed, thus allowing a stable foundation. Reconstruct according to the nasal subunits missing. Reconstruction can be prefabricated.

Skin cover:
- Upper 2/3 skin is thin and mobile, lower 1/3 is thick and adherent.
- Nasal dorsum options for skin cover:
  - FTSG;
  - <2 cm Reiger flap;
  - >2 cm forehead flap.
- Nasal alar options for skin cover:
  - <50% FTSG;
  - >50% reconstruct entire unit templated from contralateral. Can use nasolabial flap in a two stage or forehead flap.
- Nasal tip options for skin cover:
  - FTSG—superior to local flaps due to no pin-cushioning;
  - <1.5 cm bilobed but risk of pin-cushioning;
  - >2 cm forehead flap or nasolabial.

Structural support:
- The nasal skeleton is in thirds. The upper 1/3 is bony. These overlap the upper lateral cartilages and these overlap the lower lateral cartilages. Even though the alar rim does not have cartilage normally, any reconstruction in this area must involve cartilage support.
- The aim of support is to act against gravity and external forces, create nasal tip projection, form subcutaneous hard tissue, which acts against trapdoor contraction, recreate nasal subunit.

- Options for support include:
  - Septal cartilage (an 8-mm-wide L-shaped dorsum and caudal strut must be maintained to support the nose after harvesting a septal graft);
  - Conchal cartilage;
  - Rib cartilage;
  - Cantilever costochondral graft.

Mucosal lining:
- The lining of the nose is a thin mucosal layer except in the vestibule where it is keratinized. Reconstructions most often fail because of lack of lining. They must be vascular enough to support the cartilage grafts and supple enough to conform to the shape and thin enough not to obstruct the airway. It may be placed at the same time as external cover or the flap may be prelaminated.
- The options are:
  - Use residual nasal lining. It can be advanced 2-3 mm;
  - *Turn-in nasal flaps:* local hinge over flaps: turn over skin and scar adjacent to a healed nasal defect. The main disadvantage is an unreliable blood supply. These flaps should be kept short;
  - Nasolabial flaps have been used, but are always too thick. Vascularity is tenuous and cartilage grafts are risky;
  - *Septal hinge flap:* the technique involves removal of septal mucosa ipsilateral to the defect and dissection of an appropriately sized flap of septal cartilage. This septal 'door' is made to open on a dorsal hinge toward the reconstructive side, so that the septal mucosa on its far side bridges the wound and lines the airway. The technique promises more than it delivers;
  - *Prefabricated skin graft and lining:* cartilage and graft can be placed on the forehead flap and transferred once they have survived. However, the cartilage retains the shape of the concha or septum, and is fixed by scar so that it is difficult to alter the shape;
  - *Folding forehead or nasolabial flap:* this is not a good option. Doubling the flap increases donor site morbidity with a large flap and diminishes distal blood supply, increasing the risk of necrosis, and producing thick shapeless and unsupported alar margins;
  - *Intranasal lining flaps:* significant amounts of lining remain in the residual nose. Lining flaps from the vestibule, middle vault and septum are thin.

Columella:
- Difficult to reconstruct.
- Nasolabial flaps (unilateral or bilateral) on superior pedicles can be tunnelled under the alar base.
- Upper lip forked flaps may be useful in the elderly patient with a long lip.
- Forehead flaps and chondrocutaneous grafts are secondary options.

Total nasal reconstruction:
- A complex reconstruction requiring a staged approach.
- First described in 600 BC by Sushruta in the Hindu book of Revelation using forehead and cheek flaps. Tagliacozzi used lateral arm in the sixteenth century.
- May require distant tissue in the form of cartilaginous grafts and osseocutaneous free flaps.
- Prosthesis is a simple and effective option for those unable or unwilling to undergo surgical reconstruction.

Naso-ethmoidal fractures
Caused by trauma to the interorbital region. They often occur in conjunction with other fractures and involve the root of the nose, medial wall of orbit and ethmoidal air cells. Have high suspicion for brain trauma.

Symptoms and signs:
- Bruising and swelling.
- A palpable bony step.
- *Telecanthus*—if the medial canthal tendon is detached from its bony origin.
- Enophthalmos.
- Diplopia.
- CSF leak.

Treatment:
- Usually ORIF.
- Access is obtained via lacerations, bicoronal incision or medial orbital incision (Lynch incision). Nasal bones are elevated. A bone graft may be required to reconstruct the dorsum of the nose. The nasomaxillary buttress is reconstructed with plates and screws. The medial canthal tendon is reconstructed and secured.

See FACIAL FRACTURES.

Nasolabial flap
- Blood supply based on perforators from the facial and angular arteries passing through underlying levator labii and zygomatic muscles.
- Position flap just lateral to the nasolabial fold.

- Use inferiorly based flaps for buccal and FOM defects of 2.5–7 cm. The flaps including muscle may be transposed further. Small defects of the nasal ala can be reconstructed with a superiorly based flap. An inferiorly based flap can reconstruct lip above vermilion.
- Flaps can be pedicled and transposed, tunnelled, islanded, turned over for lining, V–Y advancement.

See ORAL CAVITY RECONSTRUCTION.

Natatory ligaments
Composed of transverse fibres, which run distal to the superficial transverse ligament at the palmar surface of the interdigital commissure. The proximal border extends from the ulnar border of the little finger to the radial border of the index finger. It occasionally extends to the thumb. Contracture results in limitation of abduction.

See RETINACULAR SYSTEM.

Neck dissection
Indications:
- *U.K. 2016 guidelines:*
  - Patients with a clinically N0 neck, with more than 15–20% risk of occult nodal metastases, should be offered prophylactic treatment of the neck–this includes almost all SCCs of upper aerodigestive tract except T1 and T2 cancers of the glottis and some T1 cancers of the oral cavity;
  - All patients with T1 and T2 oral cavity cancer and N0 neck should receive prophylactic neck treatment;
  - Selective neck dissection is as effective as modified radical neck dissection for controlling regional disease in N0 necks for all primary sites.

Types of neck dissection:
- *Comprehensive neck dissection:* Lymph nodes in levels 1–5 are removed. Indicated in macroscopic nodal disease. Radical neck dissections are fall under the umbrella of comprehensive neck dissections:
  - *Radical neck dissection:* level 1–5 lymph nodes plus the internal jugular vein, accessory nerve and sternocleidomastoid muscle are sacrificed;
  - *Extended radical neck dissection:* level 1–5 lymph nodes plus paratracheal and mediastinal nodes, and parotid gland;
  - *Modified radical neck dissection:* level 1–5 lymph nodes are removed but at least one of the non-lymphatic structures removed in the radical dissection are spared:
    - *Type 1:* accessory nerve preserved;
    - *Type 2:* accessory nerve and SCM preserved;

- *Type 3:* accessory nerve, SCM and IJV preserved.
- *Selective neck dissection:* fewer than level 1–5 lymph node dissection. Indicated in N0 neck:
  - *Anterolateral:* level 2–4; often for laryngeal and hypopharyngeal tumours;
  - *Anterior:* level 1–4 and tracheo-oesophageal nodes, for thyroid tumours;
  - *Posterior:* level 2–5, posterior scalp.

Principles:
- Sacrifice of spinal accessory nerve is debilitating. Get shoulder pain and droop with limited abduction. Modifications have been developed to preserve the spinal accessory nerve.
- Selective neck dissection aims to remove nodes which are likely to be involved in N0 necks. This concept is not applicable if there is clinical metastasis. Sentinel node mapping is less predictable in the head and neck, but may improve selection.

Operative steps:
1. Anaesthetic—GA.
2. Set up:
   a. Prophylactic antibiotics;
   b. Shoulder roll to elevate shoulders;
   c. Face pointing toward contralateral side;
   d. Surgeon at the ipsilateral side with assistant at the head.
3. Incision options—inverted wine glass, McFee, utility.
4. Raise the flaps in subplatysmal plane with preservation of great auricular nerve over SCM if possible.
5. Identify accessory nerve 1/3 down SCM and 1/3 up trapezius.
6. Mobilize the SCM.
7. Identify posterior belly of digastric and hypoglossal nerve superiorly in the dissection.
8. Dissect lymph nodes around the internal jugular vein with care to identify vagus in the carotid sheath. Thoracic duct will be found as it enters the junction of IJV and subclavian vein on the left. On the right you may see accessory thoracic duct.
9. Establish the deep limit of the dissection.
10. Post-op consideration of drains.

Structures that can be damaged in each level:
- *Level 1:* submandibular gland, facial vessels, marginal mandibular nerve, lingual nerve.
- *Level 2:* hypoglossal, vagus and accessory nerve. IJV (difficult to control if bleeds).
- *Level 3:* IJV, common carotid.

- *Level 4:* thoracic duct.
- *Level 5:* spinal accessory nerve, phrenic and brachial plexus.

Complications:
- *Intraoperative:* bleeding, <u>Air embolus</u>, pneumothorax, carotid artery injury, nerve injury—phrenic, CNX, brachial plexus, lingual, CNXII, CNIX, damage to lymphatics.
- *Intermediate:*
  - Skin flap necrosis;
  - *Carotid blow out:* often with salivary fistulas. Usually fatal. Can be proceeded by a sentinel bleed which must be explored surgically;
  - *Chyle leak:* due to thoracic duct injury, milky drainage, reduce by fat-free diet for a small leak, may need TPN for a large leak;
  - Salivary fistula.
- *Late:* scar contracture, neuroma, shoulder pain, facial oedema.

For intra-operative bleeding from IJV:
Pre-event:
- Pre-operative optimization with nutrition and good Hb.
- Ensure patient is cross matched.
- Defensive neck dissection to ensure proximal and distal control of IJV.
- Have an awareness of who is around that day and where they are.

Peri-event:
- Apply pressure immediately.
- Communicate with anaesthetist and theatre team.
- Trendelenburg—head down to prevent air embolus.
- Dissection to enable proximal and distal control.
- Repair vein or apply a patch of tissue—SCM.

Post-event:
- High care setting with close monitoring.

See HEAD AND NECK CANCER. *See* LYMPH NODE LEVELS IN HEAD AND NECK CANCER.

Neck reconstruction
Local flaps:
- Vertical scarring may be helped with Z-plasties. Elevate flaps in deep subcutaneous planes.
- Bilobed flaps and cervicohumeral flaps can be used, but can leave ugly scars.

Musculocutaneous flaps:
- Including trapezius, pectoralis major and latissimus dorsi can be used, but has a thick muscular pedicle.

- The cervicodorsal fasciocutaneous flap fed by cutaneous branches of the superficial cervical vessels and posterior intercostal perforators arises in the posterior neck and can be raised as large as 30 × 7 cm.
- The cervicoscapular flap may include a vascular network of the circumflex scapular artery which can be as large as 32 × 12 cm.

SSG and splinting:
- The most frequently used reconstruction.
- Release the contractures deep and along aesthetic subunit lines where possible.
- Orientated seams horizontally.
- Splint for at least 6 months, which gives less than 17% recurrence rate.

Tissue expansion:
- Placement in the unscarred supraclavicular region.
- Difficult to expand in the soft neck.

Microsurgical restoration of the neck unit:
- Radial forearm flap has been used, giving thin pliable skin but may be small, hairy with a poor donor site.
- The free scapular flap blends well. It may require debulking in fat patients. It may be pre-expanded.
- Other sources are the groin flap, thoracodorsal and TRAM/DIEP.

Necrobiosis lipoidica
- Commonly associated with diabetes mellitus, but may occur in patients without diabetes and it may precede the clinical onset of diabetes mellitus.
- The lesion begins as a dusky red plaque, which progresses to atrophy of the skin followed by central ulceration.
- It is more common in the pretibial area.
- The lesion is progressive, despite control of the diabetes.
- Some patients present with the cosmetic problem of unsightly legs.
- Resection of the involved area and resurfacing with split-thickness skin grafts have been successful.

Necrotizing fasciitis
- A rapid, aggressive and life-threatening infection of soft tissues characterized by the spread of infection and necrosis through the fascia and subcutaneous fat.
- Subtypes:
  - *Type 1:* polymicrobial;
  - *Type 2:* Gram positive from strep A infection. Aggressive and associated with high risk of mortality;
  - *Type 3:* Gram negative from marine species such as vibrio;
  - *Type 4:* fungal species such as candida—associated with immunocompromised state.
- Necrotizing fasciitis includes Fournier's gangrene, suppurative fasciitis and haemolytic streptococcal gangrene—Meleney's ulcer.
- Risk factors include advanced age, diabetes, peripheral vascular disease, immunosuppression, smoking, alcoholism and NSAID use.
- Necrotizing fasciitis is a clinical diagnosis, but LRINEC score may contribute if diagnostic uncertainty. Use with caution, as it has not performed well in external validation. Points based on CRP, WCC, Hb, Na$^+$, creatinine, and glucose.

Investigation:
- Bloods:
  - ABG for lactate;
  - FBC, U&E, LFT, calcium (low due to calcium precipitation with fat necrosis) CRP, glucose, clotting, crossmatch.
- Tissue cultures and Gram staining.
- Imaging as an adjunct if patient stable enough and should not delay surgical intervention—*see* SUBCUTANEOUS GAS.

Management:
- Aggressive resuscitation with oxygen and fluids.
- Analgesia.
- Broad-spectrum antibiotics that can subsequently be tailored by gram stain and cultures.
- Aggressive surgical debridement. Reconstruction once patient has recovered from the insult.

  Hyperbaric oxygen: may be a useful adjunct via induction of phagocytosis by neutrophils.

Negligence
A breach of duty of care by falling below a reasonable standard and causing harm. In the context of informed consent, this was previously governed by the *Bolam test* (1954), now superseded by *Montgomery v. Lanarkshire Health Board (2015)*.

Neoplasm
Abnormal mass of tissue, the growth of which exceeds and is uncoordinated with that of normal tissue and which persists after the initial stimulus which provoked the change. A malignant neoplasm invades normal tissue and may metastasize.

Characterized by:

- *Initiation:* change in genome of cell.
- *Promotion:* change made permanent by cell division.
- *Progression:* further division to form an invasive tumour.

Neovascularization

- Free transfer of arteriovenous pedicles to another site can lead to neovascularization allowing the surrounding tissue to be raised on the new pedicle.
- For example, the radial arteriovenous pedicle of the radial forearm flap has been transferred to the neck and buried under the supraclavicular area and subsequently used to resurface a severely burned face.
- After 6 weeks the surrounding tissue can be raised.
- The Crane principle has been used to implant the same pedicle in a second donor site.

Nerve compression

- Nerve compression can be occur spontaneously at predictable anatomical points or result from traumatic, metabolic, metaplastic or iatrogenic events.
- Pathophysiology: acutely, increased pressure from nerve compression leads to decreased perfusion from neural microvasculature. Chronically see irreversible inflammatory changes in the form of fibrosis, demyelination and axonal loss.
- Classical clinical triad:
  - ○ Neurological pain;
  - ○ Sensory disturbance;
  - ○ Motor dysfunction.
- Assessment:
  - ○ History to determine onset and progression, aggravating and alleviating factors and risk factors;
  - ○ Examination to determine site of compression by eliciting provocative tests. Signs of chronicity including muscle atrophy.
- Investigation:
  - ○ Consider electrodiagnostic studies—nerve conduction studies (NCS) and electromyography (EMG);
  - ○ Consider imaging.
- Management options:
  - ○ Non-operative:
    - ▪ Activity modification;
    - ▪ Exercise and physiotherapy;
    - ▪ Splints;

- ▪ Analgesia;
- ▪ Steroid injection.
  - ○ Operative decompression which may be open or endoscopic.

Nerve conduction studies

Nerve conduction study involve two electrodes placed on the skin along the course of the nerve. The first electrode stimulates an electric response, the second electrode records the characteristics of the action potential.

Measures:

- *Amplitude:* size of response which is roughly proportional to the number of depolarizing axons in the nerve.
- *Latency:* the time taken for the response to travel.
- *Conduction velocity:* divide inter-electrode distance by the latency.

In early chronic nerve compression there is an increase in latency and decrease in conduction velocity.

Differentiate from electromyography which assesses the integrity of muscle function to help determine whether axonal damage has occurred. Electrode is inserted into the muscle. Needle is moved to different locations in the muscle to test for fibrillation potentials then kept in the same position to check for fasciculations. As more severe axonal loss occurs in chronic nerve compression, EMG will exhibit increased fibrillation potentials and fasciculations.

Nerve graft

- The *Sural nerve* can provide 30–40 cm of nerve graft. It is identified approximately 2 cm posterior and 1–2 cm proximal to the lateral malleolus and is posterior to the short saphenous vein. Courses towards midline of popliteal fossa. Harvest gives a numb lateral calf and dorsum of foot.
- When a limited amount of graft material is required the medial or lateral antebrachial cutaneous nerve can be harvested from the injured upper extremity.
  - ○ The lateral antebrachial cutaneous nerve is found adjacent to the cephalic vein. 8 cm of nerve graft can be obtained and the loss of sensation is slight;
  - ○ The medial antebrachial cutaneous (MABC) nerve, found in the groove between the triceps and biceps muscles adjacent to the basilic vein, has a posterior and an anterior division. Harvesting of the anterior branch is preferred because the posterior branch causes numbness over the elbow. 20 cm of graft can be obtained.

- In patients with median nerve sensory loss the third web space nerve can be harvested to reconstruct the median nerve defect, providing up to 24 cm of nerve graft.
- The dorsal branch of the ulnar nerve can be harvested to reconstruct the ulnar nerve.
- The terminal branch of the *Posterior interosseous nerve* is useful for bridging small defects in small diameter nerves. It is located on the radial side of the base of the 4th extensor compartment at the wrist.

Nerve injury
Anatomy:
- Axons are surrounded by *Endoneurium*. Large axons are individually myelinated, smaller axons are grouped together and wrapped by Schwann cells. The greater the myelination the faster the conduction.
- Groups of axons are bundled together and surrounded by *Perineurium*.
- Fascicles are arranged in groups which are surrounded by the inner epineurium.
- The periphery is encased in outer epineurium.
- Peripheral nerves originate where the dorsal and ventral roots of spinal cord coalesce. Afferent (sensory) fibres originate in the dorsal spinal cord with cell bodies outside the spinal cord as the dorsal root ganglia. So brachial plexus lesions can be diagnosed as supraganglionic if there is sensory loss, but no Wallerian degeneration.
- The axon extends from spinal cord to the motor end plates and sensory receptors. Proteins are produced in the cell body and transported to where they are needed. If the cell body dies the entire cell dies.

Injury:
- Get Wallerian degeneration distally. Without the nucleus the axon degenerates along with the myelin sheath. Adjacent Schwann cells become phagocytic. Get a hollow endoneurial sheath, which collapses. Proximally get limited degeneration.
- Various cytokines such as NGF are released by Schwann cells stimulating axonal regeneration.
- The cell body produces structural proteins.
- Axons sprout both from the cut end and from the nodes of Ranvier, producing a growth cone. Tendrils called filopodia reach out from the growth cone until they find a favourable substrate. Then the axon grows into it within several days of injury. Once this is found the other sprouts degenerate.

- All the structures need to come from the cell body and this is the rate limiting step in nerve production.
- Nerves by preference grow towards other nerves, but this is dependent on a critical gap distance.
- Models using neuroprotective substances, such as acetyl-L-carnitine.

See SEDDON AND SUNDERLAND CLASSIFICATIONS OF NERVE INJURY.

Nerve repair
- Can be performed as epineural, perineural (fascicular) or group fascicular repair. No technique has been shown to be superior.
- If end-to-end repair is not possible, then non-vascularized nerve grafting, vascularized grafting and nerve conduits can be used.
- No evidence that vascularized is better than non-vascularized, but it makes sense if the bed is poor.
- Conduits have been made out of vein or synthetic material.
- To ensure correct alignment, topographical maps can be referred to. Muscle can be stimulated directly for the first 72 hours. Histochemical techniques have been described to allow differentiation of motor from sensory nerves.

Prognosis:
- Better in young patient and distal lesion. Regeneration occurs at 1 mm per day with a 1 month lag before recovery starts.
- Muscles can regain function up to 1 year after denervation. Get loss of up to 40% of sensory neuron population after nerve division. Neuron rescue has been attempted in animals.

Nerve stimulator
Can be used to stimulate a nerve and observe muscle contraction. Useful in identifying the facial nerve and its branches. In a laceration, a motor nerve may continue to conduct impulses distal to the division resulting in muscle contraction up to 72 hours after division. When using the disposable stimulator, attach the earth to the muscle being stimulated otherwise the current may not be strong enough to detect a response.

Neurilemmoma
- A benign tumour of nerve sheath.
- Also called schwannoma as they originate from Schwann cells. The tumour appears as a slightly elongated swelling along the course of a nerve, which may cause some pain or sensory change. Tapping may cause paraesthesia. They present when they are

small. The tumour should be separated from normal fascicles. Recurrence is uncommon.

Neurocutaneous flap

Suprafascial paraneural vessels supply not only the nerve, but the skin that the nerve supplies via the formation of choke vessels or true anastomoses between networks of fascial perforators. The major superficial venous channels serve as the outflow from the paraneural plexus, e.g. the sural flap includes the short saphenous vein. See FASCIOCUTANEOUS FLAPS.

Neurocutaneous melanosis

- The association of a large CMN with multiple small CMN ('satellites') with CNS involvement.
- CNS manifestations include hydrocephalus, seizures, focal deficits, or partial paresis usually occurring before 2 years of age.
- If neurological symptoms occur most patients will die from progression of melanosis or malignancy.

See CONGENITAL NAEVUS.

Neurofibroma

- Solitary tumour or multiple as part of *Neurofibromatosis* type 1 (von Recklinghausen's disease).
- Plexiform neurofibromas are large with thickened nerves.
- Treatment may be required for cosmetic reasons or functional disturbance.
- Neurofibromas are difficult to resect from the nerve.
- Malignant degeneration can occur when the neurofibroma is associated with neurofibromatosis type 1.
- Solitary lesions are seen in the first decade, multiple lesions after 30 years.

See MESODERMAL TUMOURS.

Neurofibromatosis

Autosomal dominant inherited syndrome with variable penetrance and high rate of spontaneous mutations.

Type I: most common type

- Also known as von Recklinghausen's disease.
- Multiple neurofibromas, café au lait spots, axillary freckling, Lisch nodules on the iris (ocular neurofibromatosis) and other findings.
- Incidence 1:3,000. Manifests in infancy with the café au lait spots. Also have freckling in the axilla. It progresses to affect skin, soft tissue, nerve and bone. Tumour progression is most aggressive at the time of puberty.
- The commonest presentation is with facial masses.

Type II: rarer

- Presents with less skin lesions, but more meningiomas and acoustic neuromas (bilateral). Plexiform neurofibromas are large infiltrative lesions usually found in the head and neck region.

Head and neck neurofibromas can occur in 5 types:

- *Localized/plexiform:* originate from nerve sheath cells and can be superficial or deep. Have potential to grow and be highly vascular.
- *Cranio-orbital:* can be minor (involving lateral orbital wall) or major (with dysplastic sphenoid bone and orbital enlargement). Characterized by hypoplastic zygoma and abnormal ipsilateral sinuses.
- *Facial:* involving branches of the trigeminal nerve.
- Parotid, auricular or occipital.
- Neck.

Surgical management: Debulking of problematic or larger lesions is challenging due to the vascularity and high risk of recurrence. Structures such as the globe may need support with alloplastic or autologous implants. Psychological input advised for this challenging lifelong condition.

Neuroma

Present with pain and localized tenderness and dysaesthesia in the distribution of the nerve.

Types:

- *Neuroma-in-continuity:*
  - ○ *Spindle:* with chronic irritation in an intact nerve;
  - ○ *Lateral:* at site of partial nerve division;
  - ○ Following nerve repair.
- *End-neuroma:* following traumatic division and amputation.

Common upper limb neuromas:

- Palmar cutaneous branch of median nerve.
- Superficial branch of radial nerve.
- Radial digital nerves.
- Dorsal branch of ulnar nerve.

Palliation: desensitization, TENS, drugs such as carbamazepine.

Surgery:

- Resection and coagulation.
- Ligation, crushing or capping (with vein or histocryl glue).
- Multiple sectioning (may form multiple neuromas).
- Epineural repair over cut end.
- Bury nerve end in bone or muscle.
- Implantation into a nerve—another or the same nerve.

Neurapraxia
See SEDDON AND SUNDERLAND CLASSIFICATIONS OF NERVE INJURY.

Neurotmesis
See SEDDON AND SUNDERLAND CLASSIFICATIONS OF NERVE INJURY.

Nexobrid™
See BROMELAIN-BASED ENZYMATIC DEBRIDEMENT.

Ninhydrin printing test
To test for sweating. The hand is cleaned with soap and alcohol. Place hand under a lamp and obtain an imprint. Spray with ninhydrin. Get a purple pattern with normal sweating.
See SYMPATHETIC FUNCTION TESTING.

Nipple
Nerve supply: *p*rincipally from the anterior branch of the 4th lateral intercostals nerve. It enters the breast at the chest wall 1.5 cm from the lateral edge of the breast.

Nipple inversion
Classification:
- *I:* inverted, but everts easily and stays out. Try suction with nipplet or home-made nipplet using cut-off syringe.
- *II:* inverted. Able to evert, but retracts.
- *III:* inverted and will not evert.

Surgery: for II and III treat operatively. Evert nipple with skin hook. Using scalpel or nipple cut fibrous bands at the base of the nipple until it remains everted. Use purse string suture with clear non-absorbable monofilament suture to maintain eversion.

Nipple reconstruction
- Perform as second stage after breast reconstruction to get accurate positioning. Banking is usually not safe oncologically and gives a poor cosmetic result.

Nipple sharing: can be used if there is an adequate size contralateral nipple, but will usually result in small nipples and a scar on the previously unaffected breast.

Local flap: the best way to produce nipple projection. Determine position of nipple by comparing with the opposite breast and/or asking patient to choose position. Measure nipple to sternal notch and nipple to midline distance. Make small adjustments to fit nipple correctly on to the reconstructed breast mound. Nipple diameter should be the same as the opposite nipple, but projection should be at least twice as much. Can improve projection using cartilage graft. For nipple projection use one of a variety of flaps, e.g. skate flap, C–V flap, mushroom flap, Maltese cross (de-epithelialized areas), also arrow flap, star technique.

Areola: use tattooing—4 months after the reconstruction, a tattoo should be darker as it fades within the first few weeks or FTSG from inner thigh.

No man's land
Flexor tendon zones (zone II) from distal palmar crease to middle of middle phalanx. Coined by Bunnell due to the historically poor results after attempted repair.

No-reflow phenomenon
- Different tissues can tolerate different amounts of ischaemia. Skin and bone tolerate ischaemia well—up to 6 hours of warm ischaemia. Muscle shows irreversible damage after 4 hours.
- No-reflow describes the state of failure of perfusion once flow is re-established.
- The theories of no-reflow are:
  - Capillary leak increases haematocrit causing sludging;
  - Endothelial swelling increases resistance;
  - Capillaries are plugged by leucocytes;
  - Interstitial oedema causes external compression on capillaries.
- Small capillary beds are occluded causing AV shunting. Treat with fibronolytic drugs, NSAIDs.

See MICROSURGERY.

Nodular fasciitis
An uncommon lesion that must be distinguished from palmar fasciitis—part of Dupuytren's disease. It occurs more commonly in the forearm sometimes after a traumatic event. It presents as a small (<3 cm), tender, growing mass. It can be confused with a fibrosarcoma.

Noma
- Noma, also known as cancrum oris or necrotizing ulcerative stomatitis, is an orofacial gangrene which occurs in young children and untreated has a high mortality. WHO classified NOMA as a neglected tropical disease in 2023.
- The pathogenesis is non-specific polymicrobial organisms.
- Mainly affects children aged 2-6 years old. Most prevalent in sub-Saharan Africa but also cases reported in Asia.
- Noma comes from the Greek 'nome' meaning to devour. Starts as a soft tissues lesion of the alveolus then develops into an acute necrotising gingivitis. Rapid progression often leads to extensive unilateral loss of the lips, oral commissure, nose, cheek and occasionally the lower eyelid. The bones of the maxilla, nose, zygoma, and mandible may

be eroded and masticatory muscle involvement often causes trismus.
- If patients survive, they often have severe facial disfigurement characterized by tissue loss, scarring and trismus.

WHO classification into 5 clinical stages:
- *Stage 0:* simple gingivitis
- *Stage 1:* acute necrotising gingivitis
- *Stage 2:* oedema
- *Stage 3:* gangrene
- *Stage 4:* scarring
- *Stage 5:* sequelae

Management:
- *Medical:* early reversible stages of the disease can be successfully managed by antibiotics, oral hygiene and nutritional supplements.
- *Surgical:* reconstruction of noma sequelae is challenging and requires wide release of scarred tissue and importation of well-vascularized tissue to reconstruct the layers of the face.

Non-ossifying fibroma
- Localized defects in the cortex of long bones.
- Seen in first decade of life.
- They form eccentric metaphyseal lesions.
- *Histology:* abundant immature fibroblasts.

Treatment: Observe. Most ossify at skeletal maturity.

See BONE TUMOURS.

Notta's node
Nodule palpable in *Trigger finger*.

Nuss technique
Used for the treatment of *Pectus excavatum*. A preformed hooped bar inserted via thoracoscopic guidance through incisions in the 4th intercostal space.

Obesity
WHO weight classifications are based on the _Body Mass Index (BMI)_.

Underweight	<18.5.
Normal range	18.5–24.9.
Class I overweight	25–29.9.
Class II obese	30–34.9.
Class IIa obese	35–39.9.
Class III obese	≥40.

Oblique retinacular ligament (ORL) of Landsmeer
See LANDSMEER LIGAMENTS.

Oedema
Impairs wound healing. In normal tissue, each cell lies close to a capillary and receives oxygen and nutrients by diffusion. Increase of extracellular fluid increases this distance. Also leads to protein deposition which can act as a barrier to diffusion. Growth factors and nutrients are also diluted.

Ohngren's line
Theoretic plane that joins the medial canthus of the eye with the angle of the mandible. Divides the maxillary sinus into two. Head and neck tumours below the line are considered to be associated with a better prognosis than those above.

See MAXILLA/MIDFACE.

Ollier's disease
- Multiple _Enchondromas_.
- Up to 25% of patients may get malignant degeneration of enchondroma to chondrosarcoma by the age of 40 years.
- Not associated with the cutaneous lesions seen in the setting of multiple enchondromas in _Maffucci syndrome_.

OMENS classification
For _Craniofacial microsomia_. Classifying the condition by the major affected structures:

- Orbit.
- Mandible.
- Ear.
- Nerve (facial).
- Soft tissue.

'OMENS plus' is used to include the expanded spectrum: cardiac, skeletal, pulmonary, renal, gastrointestinal, and limb anomalies.

Omentum flap
- Can be used pedicled, particularly for _Sternotomy wounds_ and free, e.g. to provide soft tissue bulk in _Hemifacial atrophy_.
- Type 3 flap: 2 dominant pedicles are right and left gastroepiploic vessels. Right vessel is usually larger in diameter.
- Entire or part of the omentum can be isolated on right or left gastroepiploic vessels (branches of the gastroduodenal and splenic artery respectively).
- Flap elevation can be performed open or endoscopically.
- Upper midline incision. Lift omentum from colon. Free any adhesions. Isolate filmy attachments and divide. Clamp small vessels. Divide the short vessels between the gastroepiploic arcade and the greater curvature of the stomach. Now the omentum is attached by the left gastroepiploic (branch of splenic) and the right gastroepiploic.
- Using a lengthening technique, the tunnelled omentum can usually reach the head and neck. It should fit loosely into the defect. Close the abdomen. Leave the upper wound open for 3–4 cm. Close skin and uncover chest. Either tunnel or lay open and skin graft. Potential complications include hernia, wound infection and bowel injury.

Omohyoid: anatomy
Origin: inferior belly, tendon and superior belly. Inferior is from scapula and suprascapular ligament. It passes upward and forward across posterior triangle. Passes under sternocleido-mastoid to tendon held by loop of deep fascia slung to clavicle. Superior belly goes up in anterior triangle.

Insertion: hyoid.

Nerve supply: ansa cervicalis.

Action: acts to depress hyoid.

Omphalocoele
- Developmental anomaly occurring in 1 in 3,200–10,000 births.
- Often have sternal and diaphragmatic abnormalities, heart defects and bladder

extrophy. Large defects have a high mortality rate.
- Results from failure of fusion at the umbilical ring.
- The sac of amnion and chorion commonly contains liver and midgut.
- The defect develops during the 6–12th week of gestation when the midgut passes out of the abdomen. Defects range from those around the umbilicus to those extending to the xiphoid and pubis. It is not a hernia.

See ABDOMINAL WALL RECONSTRUCTION. *See* GASTROSCHISIS.

Oncogene
A gene that normally directs cell growth. If altered, an oncogene can promote or allow the uncontrolled growth of cancer. Alterations can be inherited or caused by an environmental exposure to carcinogens.

Onychomycosis
- 50% of patients with dystrophic nails have a nail bed fungal infection.
- Diagnosis is confirmed by microscopic visualization of hyphae on nail scrapings using a 20% KOH preparation.
- Other causes are psoriasis, lichen planus and trauma.
- More common in the foot.
- Treatment was previously problematic.
- Lamisil (terbinafine) is an effective antifungal. The dose is 250 mg per day for 6 weeks. LFTs are not required unless there is a history of liver disease. The dose is different for feet. 30% of patients will have a recurrence. An alternative is itraconazole.

Oppenheimer effect
Most implants in animals can induce tumours regardless of the material. Maximal tumorigenesis occurs with smooth surface. In rats the minimal size was 0.5 cm^2 and minimal time was 6 months with latent time of 300 days. There is not a strong association in humans.

See ALLOPLASTS.

Opponensplasty tendon transfers
All insert at the APB insertion, i.e. dorsoradial to the 1st metacarpal head.

- *Bunnell/Royle-Thomson:* FDS ring through pulley of FCU. Good for young, fit patients.
- *Camitz:* PL with strip of palmar fascia to APB. More commonly used in elderly, frail patients.
- *Burkhalter:* EIP. Useful in ulnar nerve palsy or high median nerve palsy as supplied by the PIN (radial nerve).
- *Huber:* ADM. Most often used for children with hypoplastic thumb, but vector is not as

good at recreating opposition as a FDSIV transfer and ADM may not be long enough to also reconstruct the UCL.

Opponens pollicis
Origin: TCL deep to APB, ridge of trapezium and capsule of 1st CMC.

Insertion: radial border of 1st MC.

Nerve supply: motor branch of the median nerve.

See MUSCLES.

Opposition
- Thumb opposition is a composite motion through 3 joints to position the thumb pad opposite the distal phalanx of the middle finger.
- Abduction, pronation and flexion occur at the CMC joint, abduction and flexion at the MCP joint and flexion or extension at the IPJ.
- Get 40° abduction at the CMCJ and 20° at the MCP joint.
- Get 90° pronation.
- IP extension gives pulp-to-pulp grip and flexion for pinch.

Oral cancer
Risk factors:
- Tobacco products, alcohol. Also poor oral hygiene, mechanical from dental appliances, mouthwash, syphilis, Plummer–Wilson syndrome, candida, toxic irritants.
- *Leucoplakia* and erythroplakia are premalignant—white and red lesions.

Features:
- Account for 30% of head and neck cancer.
- Tongue the most common—30% of cases, most being in the anterior part, next is floor of mouth.
- 90% are SCC, next adenocarcinoma. SCCs can be differentiated, undifferentiated, adenoid squamous and verrucous.

Outcome: determined by tumour size, thickness and nodes. Treatment based on TNM. Surgery mainstay of treatment, but also radiotherapy.

See HEAD AND NECK CANCER.

Oral cavity reconstruction
Extend from vermilion to junction of hard and soft palate. Aim to maintain oral continuity, aid swallowing, prevent aspiration, preserve speech, promote wound healing.

Anatomy:
- *Lips:* extend from skin vermilion to mucosa in contact with opposite lip.
- *Buccal mucosa:* all the mucosa on the inner surface of cheek and lip up to alveolar ridge.

- *Lower alveolar ridge:* formed by the alveolar process of the mandible and gingival mucosa.
- *The retromolar trigone:* is the mucosa overlying the ascending ramus of the mandible up to the maxillary tuberosity.
- *The upper alveolar ridge:* is the counterpart on the maxilla.
- *Hard palate:* extends over the palatine shelves.
- *Floor of mouth* (FOM)*:* extends from the gingiva of mandible to ventral tongue. The anterior tongue is from the tip to the V-shaped circumvallate papillae.

Specific sites:
- *Hard palate:* rare and should be biopsied first.
- *Alveolar ridge:* may get poorly fitting dentures. Metastasis unusual, but mandibular invasion is common.
- *Retromolar trigone:* easily invade adjacent structures up to skull base.
- *FOM:* become large before presenting. Often get occult bilateral neck metastasis.
- *Buccal mucosa:* aggressive metastatic potential.
- *Tongue:* invades easily and reaches a large size before presentation.
- *Lip:* tend to present early.

Surgical approach:
- Preserve tongue mobility.
- Small defects can be grafted or closed with local flaps or nasolabial flaps. Tongue flaps may be used.
- Radial forearm flap is the most commonly used flap for larger defects. Can be sensate with lateral antebrachial nerve to lingual nerve.

Oral cavity:
- *Small defects:* FOM defects may be able to be closed directly, but this may interfere with speaking and swallowing. Tongue and buccal mucosa can be closed directly. Tongue flaps can be useful and a posteriorly based lateral flap can fill a tongue defect but the tongue should not be tethered.
- *Large defects:* tongue, FOM and buccal mucosa defects can be reconstructed with a SSG using the quilting method. With anterior FOM defects coverage is important to prevent tongue tethering. It can be covered with nasolabial flaps. The pedicle is divided at 2 weeks. Bite blocks are required if there are teeth. Distant pedicle flaps have been used: forehead flaps, cervical apron flap, deltopectoral, pectoralis major, trapezius, latissimus dorsi, platysma and sternocleidomastoid flaps. The most frequently used flaps are the deltopectoral

and pectoralis major. Bone can be carried with trapezius, latissimus dorsi, serratus anterior, pectoralis major and sternocleidomastoid. Trapezius carrying spine of scapula is the most reliable.
- *Free tissue transfer—mucosa:* the best mucosa replacements are the radial forearm flap, ulnar forearm flap, scapular flap, lateral arm flap and dorsalis pedis flap. The radial and ulnar forearm flaps and the scapular flap are the most commonly used. Jejunal patches have been used but jejunal mucosa may be somewhat exuberant and may continue to produce mucus. Small doses of radiotherapy have been given to flatten the mucosa and reduce secretions.

Tongue:
- Hemi-glossectomy commonly reconstructed with radial forearm flap.
- Total glossectomy needs a bulkier reconstruction such as free rectus abdominus or ALT. Laryngeal suspension in a cephalad and anterior vector is important.

Complications:
- Salivary fistula may occur and be difficult to deal with in the irradiated patient.
- The incidence of complications is increased when a simultaneous neck dissection is performed.
- *Carotid blowout:* particularly associated with a fistula and radiotherapy. Immediate cover with a muscle flap is advocated and may be performed prophylactically at the time of neck dissection.
- *Chyle leak:* may be repaired immediately if noticed, but usually become apparent once the patient is fed. Rarely require reoperation. Treat with fat free diet or TPN.
- Long-term complications include problems with the scar, shoulder pain and cosmesis.

See HEAD AND NECK CANCER.

Orbicularis oculi
- Innervated by facial nerve.
- There are two portions, the orbital and palpebral.
- Orbital overlies orbital rims. It facilitates forceful eye closure.
- The palpebral portion is subdivided into pretarsal and preseptal. Continuous with SMAS in upper face:
  - Pretarsal orbicularis oculi is divided into superficial and deep components and is primarily responsible for involuntary eyelid blink;

o Preseptal orbicularis oculi also has a superficial and deep component. Lacrimal pump intimately associated with muscle. Contraction of the pretarsal muscle shortens and closes the canaliculi, preseptal muscles pull on the diaphragm giving negative pressure in the sac. On relaxation tears are driven into the nasolacrimal duct. Also involved with voluntary eye closure. The orbital orbicularis acts as a medial brow depressor and performs forced eyelid closure. The muscle of Riolan is the smallest striated muscle in the body and is situated on the lid border.

See EYELID RECONSTRUCTION. *See* EYELID ANATOMY.

Orbit

Anatomy:

• The orbit is comprised of 7 bones—frontal, zygoma, lesser and greater wing of sphenoid, ethmoid, lacrimal, palatine and maxilla.
• The optic foramen is situated medial to the superior orbital fissure.
• The anteromedial portion of orbital roof is the extension of frontal sinus. The rest is made of thin orbital plate of frontal bone and lesser wing of sphenoid. The roof is triangular in shape.
• The lacrimal gland sits in a concavity behind the rim. The optic canal is 8–12 mm in length. The floor is triangular. Most is made of the orbital plate of the maxilla. The palatine bone lies in the posterior aspect of the floor. Medially is the ethmoid.
• The infraorbital nerve traverses the floor of the orbit in a groove.
• The sphenoid bone is the bone through which all neurovascular structures pass.
• Tenon's capsule is a fascial structure that divides the orbital cavity in two. The anterior half is filled with the globe and the posterior half with fat, muscles and neurovascular structures.

Orbital dystopia

Vertical or horizontal. With vertical dystopia the orbits do not lie on the same horizontal plane. In horizontal or transverse dystopia, the orbits are displaced laterally (orbital *Hypertelorism*) or medially (*Hypotelorism*). Orbital dystopia must be distinguished from ocular dystopia where the position of the globe is altered.

Causes: vertical include craniosynostosis, torticollis, craniofacial microsomia and facial clefting. The most common cause of vertical orbital dystopia is a congenital condition. Surgery is beneficial.

Surgery: the box osteotomy moves the entire orbit. Frontal craniotomy allows movement of the orbital roof. The medial and lateral walls, floor of the orbit, zygoma, and maxillary osteotomies are performed. The procedure is performed through coronal, eyelid and gingivo-buccal sulcus incisions. Diplopia may occur post-operatively, and more commonly with vertical repositioning.

See EXORBITISM. *See* EXOPHTHALMOS. *See* ENOPHTHALMOS.

Orbital fractures

• Occur in conjunction with zygomatic fractures, nasoethmoid fractures, high Le Fort fractures.
• Isolated orbital fractures result from pressure applied to the globe. The orbit fractures at its weakest point, the inferomedial floor known as the lamina papyracea (paper layer).
• The orbits can be divided into thirds. The orbital rim consists of thick bone, the middle third is thin then thickens in the posterior third. So the middle frequently breaks first followed by the anterior portions of the rim. This protects the important neurovascular structures posteriorly from severe displacement.

Symptoms and signs:

• Bruising and swelling.
• Subconjunctival haematoma with no posterior limit.
• Palpable steps in the orbital margin.
• *Enopthalmos:* caused by increased volume of the orbit due to fracture, decreased volume of contents due to herniation, tethering at the fracture line. May occur late due to fat atrophy.

Diplopia:

• Caused by entrapment of fat, fascia or muscle within fracture, or contusion of recti or oblique muscles. Usually on upward gaze due to fractures being tethered inferiorly.
• Visual field, globe pressure, fundoscopy. Assess lacrimal system. Examine for trapped muscle by the forced duction test. The insertion of a rectus muscle is grasped and the globe is moved.

Radiology: plain XR—PA, Water's views—teardrop sign may be present resulting from herniation of orbital contents through fracture line into maxillary sinus. CT and 3D CT.

Indications for surgery: perform if there is diplopia, enophthalmos, evidence of orbital entrapment radiologically, large bony defects, or other fractures requiring fixation.

Fracture pathology:
- The commonest orbital fractures are zygomatico-orbital and malar fractures. The commonest infraorbital fracture is the orbital floor. A blow-out fracture is due to a blow usually on the orbital rim causing an increased intraorbital pressure resulting in a fracture to the thin inferior and medial wall. Orbital contents herniated through the fracture.
- Frequently get hypoaesthesia in the distribution of the infraorbital nerve. The inferior oblique arises from the medial aspect of the orbital floor adjacent to the lacrimal groove behind the rim. Objects greater than 5 cm will increase intraorbital pressure resulting in a pure blow-out fracture. Objects <5 cm diameter will cause globe rupture.

Fracture treatment:
- Aim to release trapped structures and restore muscular function, replace orbital contents into the orbit and restore orbital size.
- The orbital floor can be approached through a bicoronal incision, subciliary lower eyelid incision, midlid incision, transconjunctival incision, lateral brow incision, medial canthal and intraoral incision.
- Fractures are fixed with interosseous wires or miniplates. The orbital floor is reconstructed with bone grafts or implants—rib, iliac crest anterior maxilla or split calvarial bone graft, titanium mesh, Gore-tex™, silicone or Medpor™.

See FACIAL FRACTURES.

Oropharyngeal tumours
Commonest sites in oropharynx are tonsils, tongue base, soft palate and pharyngeal wall.

Glottic and subglottic cancer:
- The glottis is surrounded by ligamentous structures, which act as a barrier, and it is poorly supplied with blood vessels and lymphatics. Therefore the risk of cervical metastasis is low for T1 and T2 tumours: <10%.
- Supraglottic region is richly supplied with vessels and therefore the risk of cervical spread is much higher with 50% of T1 and T2 tumours having cervical metastasis.

Elective neck dissection: supraomohyoid neck dissection is recommended for stage I and II tongue cancers as there is a high chance of occult metastasis: 30% for stage I and 50% for stage II. If two or more nodes present then also perform radiotherapy.

Surgery vs. radiotherapy:
- Stage I and II disease of the oropharynx is relatively uncommon, and often present with a neck mass. Either modality is effective for early disease.
- *Surgical complications:* dysarthria, dysphagia, aspiration.
- *Radiotherapy complications:* xerostomia, dysgeusia (distortion or absence of sense of taste), dysphagia, but symptoms after radiotherapy less than after surgery.

Surgery:
- Oncological resection most commonly performed via transoral robotic surgery.

See VOICE RESTORATION. *See* HEAD AND NECK CANCER. *See* ORAL CANCER.

Orthodontics
Appliances to move alveolar ridges and teeth. For *Cleft* and *Craniofacial* disorders. Dental development is usually slower than normal. Teeth are not removed unless they are causing problems. Maxillary central incisors are usually rotated.

Passive prosthetics (neonate):
- To fill the cleft palate.
- It is made from *Methyl methacrylate*.
- It aids breathing and feeding and placing the tongue in the correct position.
- It prevents medial collapse and promotes maxillary transverse growth.
- It must be adjusted every 6 weeks.

Presurgical orthopaedic (PSO) (neonatal):
- To mould the maxillary and alveolar tissues to correct abnormal bony relationship and provide a better platform for repair. It can be passive or active device.
- Naso-alveolar moulding (NAM) has an extra-oral nasal element attached to the oral plate to mould the nasal tissues.
- Passive devices are difficult to maintain, they are unpredictable and take a long time. Dutch cleft trials disproved efficacy.
- Pinned retention using devices such as designed by Latham are more invasive, but quicker. A screw is turned regularly to realign segments which is usually complete within 3 months. POC may cause reduced maxillary growth.

Mixed dentition (age 7–11 years):
- By maxillary expansion, orthodontics, extractions and tooth straightening.
- Alveolar bone grafting occurs in this period.

Adolescent and adult dentition (age 12–17 years and over):
- 50% patient with UCLP will be missing the lateral incisor on the cleft side—orthodontics

need to make space for this missing tooth. The missing lateral incisor is replaced with a prosthetic tooth or by moving other teeth into position.

- Class 3 malocclusion prevalent in 26% cleft population. Maxillary retrusion may be in multiple planes (vertically, lateral and AP). Maxillary expansion may be used.
- Retention is important at the end of orthodontic treatment to overcome tendency to relapse from scarring.

Orthognathic surgery

Addresses malposition of the dentofacial skeleton. Two most common conditions treated are mandibular and maxillary retrusion. Also maxillary vertical excess and mandibular prognathism. Most are developmental. Some are associated with congenital problems such as cleft lip and palate.

Evaluation:

- Assess form and shape of face. Use aids such as the classic canon of vertical facial thirds. Also look at the AP relationship. The nose is the key to the central face and the lip-tooth-chin for the lower third.
- Look at occlusion: _Angle classification_, assess overbite and overjet. _See_ TEETH. Assess the temporomandibular joints, looking for any dysfunction which may first require treatment. _Cephalometric analysis_ is used.
- _Radiological analysis with CT:_ 3D virtual planning is advantageous for yaw and midline adjustments according to skull base and bony collision—especially with asymmetry. The CAD/CAM approach is rapidly replacing traditional cephalometric analysis and mock surgery on models. Surgeon can plan incisions fixation, need for bone grafts and removal of overlapping bone segments.

Treatment plan:

- Based on severity of deformity. MDT planning with orthodontist, dentist, speech and language therapist and psychologist. Orthognathic surgery may precipitate velopharyngeal dysfunction. Aim to obtain a Class 1 occlusion after jaw repositioning. _See_ LE FORT.
- _Maxillary vertical excess:_ dissect subperiosteally to piriform rim and infra-orbital nerve. Osteotomy made at least 5 mm above the root apexes. Resect bone.
- _Vertical maxillary deficiency:_ only one osteotomy cut is needed placed 5 mm above the apex of the roots. Intermaxillary fixation is performed with an acrylic wafer inserted to get correct position. Bone graft is inserted, cranial strips. Rigid internal fixation.

- _Maxillary retrusion:_ often idiopathic. Also associated with cleft lip and palate. Get flattened midfacial region. Get Class III malocclusion. Get reduced SNA angle and normal SNB angle. Perform a Le Fort I osteotomy and rigidly fix. Relapse is high so some perform an overcorrection.
- _Mandibular retrusion:_ most evident in the profile view. Get Class II malocclusion. Get a decreased SNB angle. Prior to surgery, orthodontics corrects any flaring that will limit the amount of advancement. 3 types of osteotomies are performed:
  - ○ Vertical and oblique ramus;
  - ○ Inverted L;
  - ○ _Sagittal split osteotomy:_ may relapse, but less with rigid fixation, the most common problem is mental nerve dysfunction; this is common, but usually resolves, may get limited mandibular opening.
- _Mandibular prognathism:_ often get mild midface flattening. Need set back. Use sagittal split for less than 1 cm and inverted L for larger osteotomies.
- _Bimaxillary osteotomies:_ osteotomies of both maxilla and mandible for larger repositioning >10–14 mm.

Chin deformities: can occur independent or together with other facial deformities. 7 types of deformity—macrogenia, microgenia, combination macro and microgenia, asymmetric chin, pseudomacro- and pseudomicrogenia, witches' chin deformity (soft tissue ptosis).

Ortichochea flap

- Used for _Scalp reconstruction_ with large scalp defects.
- Axial flaps, which allow the entire remaining scalp to be elevated.
- The 3-flap technique (banana peel) uses an anterior pedicle based on supratrochlear and supraorbital vessels, a lateral flap on superficial temporal artery vessels, and a posterior flap incorporating occipital vessels. Good for frontal and occipital defects. Galeal scoring may allow as much as 20% increase to flap area.

Ortichochea sphincter pharyngoplasty

- A type of sphincteric pharyngoplasty for the treatment of _Velopharyngeal dysfunction_.
- Originally described by Ortichochea and modified by others, such as Jackson.
- Involves the construction of palatopharyngeus myomucosal flaps from the posterior tonsillar pillars, which are sutured to the posterior pharyngeal wall.

Osborne's ligament
A tendinous arch formed by the two heads of *Flexor carpi ulnaris* under which the ulnar nerve passes.

Osseointegration
- Direct anchorage of an implant by the formation of bony tissue around the implant without the growth of fibrous tissue at the bone-implant interface.
- Developed in the 1970s in edentulous patients for the anchorage of dental prosthesis. Also used for fixation of hearing aids to the temporal bone and for small joint reconstruction in the hand and for the fitting of prosthesis in the hand and other sites. Osseointegration for proximal limb prostheses has become increasingly commonplace and increasingly successful.
- Titanium fixtures are used and the titanium oxide layer formed at the surface of the implant is probably important in this phenomenon.
- In thumb prosthesis there is a capacity for tactile stimulation—osseoperception. This may be based on the transfer of tactile stimuli from the thumb to the intra-osseous nerves via the osseointegrated implant.

Ossification of hand
Age of appearance of ossification centres:

- Capitate and hamate: 2/12.
- Thumb metacarpal: 1.6 year.
- Triquetral: 1.7 year.
- Thumb proximal phalanx: 1.7 year.
- MCP joint of fingers: 1.5 year.
- Distal phalanges: all by 2.5 year.
- Lunate: 2.6 year.
- Middle phalanges: all by 2 year.
- Scaphoid, trapezium, trapezoid: 4.1 year.

Ossifying fasciitis
- Rare benign tumour similar histologically to nodular fasciitis, composed of metaplastic bone with calcification.
- Rapidly growing lesion which may be mistaken for a malignancy. Usually found in the trunk and upper and lower limbs.
- Most common in women 20-30 years, may be associated with trauma (10%).
- Treatment is local excision.

Osteoarthritis
Epidemiology: commonest cause of disability in the UK. In the hand, IPJs and base of 1st CMCJ are most often affected. IPJ arthritis has a good prognosis, 1st CMCJ arthritis is progressive and a major cause of disability.

Pathogenesis: destruction of hyaline articular cartilage. Most osteoarthritis is primary (idiopathic). Can be secondary to *Gout*, Wilson's disease, haemochromatosis, trauma, *Kienbock's*, infection, *Ehler's–Danlos syndrome*, haemophilia.

Radiological findings:
- Loss of joint space.
- Osteophyte formation.
- Subchondral sclerosis.
- Subchondral cysts.

Classification of 1st CMCJ arthritis: *Eaton-Littler*.

Treatment:
- Non-operative:
  - Analgesia: topical or systemic NSAIDs, selective COX-2 inhibitors, opioids. (NICE 2014: no good evidence for management of chronic pain with paracetamol, intra-articular hyaluronic acid, glucosamine or chondroitin, or rubefacients);
  - Physiotherapy, occupational therapy and splintage;
  - Behaviour and lifestyle modifications;
  - Injection of intra-articular steroids.
- Operative:
  - Aim to treat pain and improve function;
  - In general:
    - Arthroplasty (joint replacement, excision arthroplasty, interposition arthroplasty);
    - Arthrodesis;
    - Osteotomy.
  - DIPJs are fused at 0–20° of flexion.
  - PIPJs can be arthrodesed (increasing from 40° at the index finger to 55° at the little) or replaced, e.g. with Swanson silicon joint replacements.
  - MCPJs are usually replaced. Fusion is a salvage procedure.
  - 1st CMCJ: *see* CMC JOINT ARTHRITIS THUMB.

Osteoblastoma
See BONE TUMOURS.

- Similar histologically to osteoid osteoma, but a different XR appearance and clinical course.
- They are larger—usually over 2 cm.
- They occur in the cancellous bone of the posterior column of the spine.
- They are slightly more aggressive.
- They have plumper osteoblasts.
- Some are stage 3 with a high recurrence rate.

Osteochondroma
- The most common benign *Bone tumour*.
- Cartilage-capped bony exostosis near the epiphyseal cartilage plate.

- Usually painless.
- Growth often stops within 2 years of skeletal maturity.
- Most occur in the 20s.
- May get local pressure on adjacent structures.
- May be solitary or multiple.
- Multiple may be hereditary as autosomal dominant (20% have a negative family history).
- Most commonly in the radius and ulna and in the hand in the metacarpal and phalanges.
- Treat if becomes large and causing cosmetic or functional problem.
- Malignant transformation may occur though very rare—more likely with multiple osteochondromas.

Osteogenic sarcoma

- >80% occur in patients <30 years old.
- Present with pain unrelated to activity.
- Most common in the distal femur then the proximal tibia.
- In the upper limb, the proximal humerus is the most common site followed by the distal radius. In the hand, usually found in the metacarpals or phalanges.
- 90% are stage IIB on presentation.
- Secondary osteosarcomas with Paget's or after radiotherapy is very aggressive.

Histology: consists of malignant proliferating spindle cell stroma producing osteoid bone.

XR: *see* SCLEROTIC EXPANSILE DESTRUCTIVE LESION. MRI shows widespread marrow involvement. With soft tissue extension with sunburst pattern.

Treatment: aggressive radical excision with neoadjuvant and adjunctive chemotherapy. >90% can have limb salvage surgery. Survival is 50–70% 5-year without lung metastasis.
 See BONE TUMOURS.

Osteoid osteoma

- Benign osteoblastic lesion consisting of a well demarcated core (nidus) with surrounding zone of reactive bone.
- *XR:* get area of sclerosis with central radiolucency. CT will differentiate from a Brodie abscess.
- 3 types are cortical, medullary and subperiosteal.
- They are reported in all bones, mainly in the lower limb. In the hand they are most common in the proximal phalanx.
- They present in the 20s and 30s.
- Patients complain of a dull aching pain with point tenderness.
- Treat with observation and NSAIDs until the disease burns out in 2–3 years.

- *Surgery for pain:* complete excision of the nidus. Also radiotherapy has been used.
 See BONE TUMOURS.

Osteomyelitis

Inflammation of bone caused by an infecting organism.

Osteomyelitis in children:

- Bimodal distribution <2 years and 8–12 years.
- Typically, metaphysis of long bones via haematogenous spread of staphylococcal or streptococcal organisms.
- If untreated progresses to sequestrum formation and chronic osteomyelitis.
- IV antibiotics are mainstay with surgical draining if required for sequestrum.

Osteomyelitis in adults

- Can be acute (<2 weeks) or chronic.
- Most caused by penetrating trauma and predisposing conditions such as DM. Direct trauma will most often lead to *S. aureus* or streptococcal infection. Infections following ORIF are often *Staph. epidermidis*.
- Classification: *Cierny and Mader classification*.
- See BOAST Standards for Fracture Related Infection.
- Manage with MDT to include microbiology and infectious disease in a specialist centre.
- Principles of management:
  - Confirm diagnosis and isolate pathogen: if patient is well, allow an antibiotic holiday prior to deep bone biopsy to isolate organism and guide treatment. Use a bone sampling kit to avoid cross-contamination between specimens. Take 5 samples for microbiology and one for histology;
  - Tumour-like excision of dead and infected tissue;
  - Fill dead space and achieve bony stability.
- Single-stage debridement and reconstruction is ideal in appropriate patients. Chronic osteomyelitis treated with combination of surgical debridement and long-term antibiotics. OVIVA study shows equivalent outcomes with long term oral antibiotics compared to long term intravenous antibiotics.

Ota: naevus of

- A blue naevus seen at birth or in adolescence.
- Mainly in women of eastern Asian descent.
- Flat, irregular, grey-blue patch on the face in the distribution of 1st and 2nd trigeminal nerve may involve the eye. 5% are bilateral.

Do not disappear spontaneously, and may hyperpigment.
- Benign, but associated melanoma has been reported.
- Q-switched ruby and argon lasers may be effective.

See BLUE NAEVUS. *See* NAEVUS.

Oxandrolone
Synthetic derivative of testosterone that may be used in severe burn injuries to reduce protein catabolism.

Oxyhaemoglobin dissociation curve
A plot of saturated haemoglobin on y axis and oxygen tension on x axis. The sigmoid curve is determined by the haemoglobin's affinity for oxygen and can be reshaped and shifted to the right (decreased affinity for oxygen) or left (increased affinity for oxygen).

Factors leading to a rightward shift of the oxy-haemoglobin curve in situations where tissues need oxygen to be released (i.e. exercise or shock) include:

- Increased temperature.
- Increased carbon dioxide.
- Increased acidity.

Factors leading to a leftward shift are the opposite to the factors above and also:

- Carbon monoxide.
- Cyanide poisoning.
- Fetal circulation.

Ozone
- O_3, which occurs in the stratosphere due to the splitting of O_2 to O by *Ultraviolet radiation (UV)*, which then combines with O_2 to form O_3.
- Ozone is more effective in blocking UVA than UVB.
- 95% of radiation, which reaches the human skin is UVA. However, the minimal UVB causes the acute sunburn and malignant skin changes.
- Since 1969 there has been a 3–7% decrease in ozone. With each percentage decrease there is a 1% increase of melanoma.

p53
Tumour suppressor gene, mutated in the majority of cancers. UV-related mutations have been linked to mutations of this gene.

Pacinian corpuscles
- Only found in the hand.
- Rapidly adapting myelinated A fibres mediating fine touch and vibration. They respond to the onset of mechanical stimulus.
- They are situated in connective tissue along nerve trunks. They are served by a single myelinated fibre.
- There are up to 120 on the palmar surface of each finger.

  See SENSORY RECEPTORS.

Paget's disease
- Eczematous lesion of the nipple and areola, which is also found in extramammary areas.
- Extramammary Paget's occurs in both sexes, more common in older women.
- Found primarily in the anogenital region, mainly the vulva.
- Biopsy is required. Microscopically large round Paget cells lie within the epidermis. These have large nuclei and lots of pale staining cytoplasm. Mucin stains differentiate these cells from melanoma.
- Paget's disease of the breast without an underlying mass requires excision and has a good prognosis. If a lump is present this will require treatment and prognosis will depend on the nature of the lump.
- Extramammary Paget's requires wide and deep excision with a careful search for an underlying carcinoma. Paget's cells may be found outside the clinical limits of excision and wide excision will reduce chance of recurrence. Prognosis is poor if an underlying carcinoma is present.

Pairolero classification
For *Sternotomy wound* infections. *See* CHEST WALL RECONSTRUCTION.

Palatal flap
Total palatal mucoperiosteal tissue can be raised on a single greater palatine artery. This can be transposed to cover defects in buccal mucosa, retromolar triangle, tonsillar and soft palate. Donor area left to granulate. Not pliable, contraindicated with previous RT.

See ORAL CAVITY RECONSTRUCTION.

Palate carcinoma
- More commonly in older men. Rare in the West.
- Associated with tobacco and alcohol.
- Presentation may be with swelling, bleeding or pain. Bone invasion occurs late. Nodal involvement is seen in 16% of hard palate cancers and 37% of soft palate lesions.

Treatment:
- Resection through the mouth with underlying bone.
- Radiotherapy may cause bone exposure and necrosis.
- With more extensive lesions, a partial hemimaxillectomy is performed through a Weber-Fergusson incision, and reconstructed with a skin graft and a prosthesis.
- More extensive lesions require total hemimaxillectomy.
- As long as the inferior peri-orbitum is not breached, there is no change in position of the eye and no double vision. If the orbit is involved, the orbital contents must be removed; if the tumour extends into the ethmoid sinus, an intracranial approach is advised.
- Cervical node involvement requires neck dissection, which includes the parotid region.
- Radiotherapy is given for large tumours, for incompletely excised tumours, and after neck dissection.

Results: the 5-year survival rate is 31%.

See HEAD AND NECK CANCER.

Palm infections
3 potential spaces deep to flexor tendons.

- *Thenar space:* radial to oblique septum, which extends from palmar fascia to 3rd metacarpal. Flexor sheath infection of the index finger may rupture here. Incise in thenar crease.

- *Mid-palmar space:* ulnar to oblique septum. Middle and ring sheath infections may rupture here.
- *Hypothenar space:* rarely involved. Incise on radial side to avoid a tender scar.

These are only potential spaces. Distinguish from the radial and ulnar bursae which are synovial sheaths enclosing the flexor tendons of the thumb and little finger, which communicate with the space of *Parona*. Infection can lead to a horseshoe abscess.

See INFECTIONS.

Palmar branch of the median nerve
Arises 5–6 cm proximal to the distal wrist crease between palmaris longus and flexor carpi radialis. It passes superficial to the radial margin of the flexor retinaculum to supply the skin of the palm. It is frequently injured during carpal tunnel release though it never runs ulnar to a line drawn from the ulnar side of the middle finger.

Palmar fascia
See RETINACULAR SYSTEM.

Palmaris longus
Origin: flexor pronator origin. Muscle belly is small with a long thin tendon which runs superficial to TCL.

Insertion: apex of palmar aponeurosis. Absent in 10–15% people.

Nerve supply: median nerve.

Action: weak flexor of wrist. Good donor for tendon grafts or transfers.

See MUSCLES.

Papillomatosis
An increase in depth of corrugations at the junction between the epidermis and dermis.

See SKIN.

Papineau technique
Staged bone grafting for infected non-union of a tibial fracture:

- *Stage 1:* excision of infected bone, external fixation, pack with antibiotic swabs.
- *Stage 2:* cancellous bone grafting with antibiotic swabs.
- *Stage 3:* flaps and skin grafts to achieve soft tissue cover.

See LOWER LIMB RECONSTRUCTION.

Parakeratosis
The presence of nucleated cells at the skin surface.

See SKIN.

Parascapular flap
See SCAPULAR/PARASCAPULAR FLAP.

Parkes–Weber syndrome
- Autosomal dominant condition. *RASA1* gene mutation.

- May be categorized as part of the *Complex combined vascular malformations*.
- Characterized by capillary malformations on the skin, hypertrophy of bone and soft tissue and multiple high-flow arteriovenous fistulas (AVFs). AVFs can be associated with bleeding and heart failure.
- Can be confused with Klippel-Trenaunay syndrome (characterized by low-flow vascular malformations).

Parkland formula
- Fluid regimen used in *Burns* resuscitation.
- Uses crystalloid fluid (Hartmann's/Ringer's lactate).
- Fluid for first 24 hours = $4\,ml \times kg \times TBSA\%$ burn.
- Half given in first 8 hours, second half in next 16 hours.
- For children, also give maintenance fluid calculated by body weight. Beware hypoglycaemia.
- Tends to overestimate fluid needs in adults with moderate-sized burns. Monitor urine output and other parameters closely, and adjust based on the patient's response.

Parona: space of
Retrotendinous potential space in the distal forearm between FPL tendon, FDP tendon and pronator quadratus. The synovial sheath enclosing FPL can connect with that of the little finger through this space. This can give rise to a horseshoe-shaped abscess if all three spaces are involved in septic tenosynovitis.

Paronychia
- An infection in the nail fold along the perionychium. Cellulitis can be treated with antibiotics. Pus under the nail requires removal of whole or part of the nail. If chronic, it may require marsupialization of the nail fold.
- Chronic paronychia may point to an underlying disease such as diabetes or scleroderma. Most commonly seen in middle-aged women. Many have *Candida albicans*. Treatment is difficult. Marsupialize eponychium. Remove nail and apply anti-fungals to nail bed.

Parotid duct: trauma
The duct travels from the anteromedial border of the parotid gland to the anterior border of masseter on a line between the tragus to the middle of the upper lip and exits in the mouth opposite the second maxillary molar (bicuspid). A vertical line drawn from the lateral canthus indicates where it divides intra-orally. Lacerations in this area may divide the duct. It lies very close to the buccal branch of the facial nerve so the two are likely to be injured at the same time. The

duct can be cannulated and if divided should be repaired over a stent.

Parotid tumours
See SALIVARY TUMOURS.

Parotidectomy
• Avoid muscle relaxant to aid identification of the facial nerve branches.
• *Blair incision:* upper anterior ear, down along pre-auricular crease and back over mastoid process then anteriorly towards the hyoid bone.
• Elevate skin flaps, preserving great auricular nerve.
• Separate the tail of the parotid from the sternocleidomastoid and digastric muscles.
• *Facial nerve:* approach proximally or distally:
• *Antegrade:* visualize cartilaginous tragal pointer; facial nerve 1 cm deep to this point; use nerve stimulator; separate superficial lobe from the nerve.
• *Retrograde:* identify distal branches at the following sites:
  o Cervical branch alongside retromandibular vein;
  o Marginal branch below lower border of mandible as it runs over the facial artery;
  o Buccal branches alongside parotid duct which can be cannulated to identify it.

Parry–Romberg's syndrome
See HEMIFACIAL ATROPHY.

Parsonage–Turner syndrome
Also known as brachial plexitis. Pain around shoulder and upper arm is followed in a few hours by atrophic paralysis of anterior interosseous nerve. Pain can be bilateral though paralysis is unilateral. May have recent flu-like illness. Recovery occurs after 15–36 months. Treat conservatively.
See ANTERIOR INTEROSSEOUS SYNDROME.

Passavant's ridge
This is the bulge on the posterior pharynx caused by the contraction of superior constrictors. May be seen in *Velopharyngeal dysfunction* in an attempt to assist velopharyngeal closure.
See CLEFT PALATE.

PDS
Polydiaxanone. Monofilament suture. Absorbed more slowly than other absorbable sutures. It loses its strength at 3 months, absorbed by 6 months. Used as a dermal suture in areas prone to stretched scars.

Pectoralis major
Origin:
• *Clavicular head:* anterior surface of medial half of clavicle.
• *Sternocostal head:* sternum, upper 6 ribs, external oblique aponeurosis.

Insertion: intertubercular groove of humerus.

Action: adducts and medially rotates humerus. Clavicular head flexes and sternocostal head extends humerus.

Nerve supply: lateral and medial pectoral nerves. Clavicular head C5 and C6, sternoclavicular head C7-8, T1.

Arterial supply: pectoral branch of thoracoacromial trunk.
See MUSCLE.

Pectoralis major flap
• Described by Ariyan in 1979.
• Often considered the mirror image of the latissimus dorsi flap. Used to be a work horse for the head and neck but largely surpassed by free flaps now. Still used for infected median sternotomy wounds.
• *Origin:* sternocostal and clavicular heads.
• *Insertion:* bicipital groove of humerus.
• Type 5 muscle. Dominant vessel is the thoracoacromial artery, pectoral branch. Minor segmental supply from the internal mammary perforators or branches from 5-7 intercostals. Thoracoacromial branch can be found just beneath the junction of middle and lateral third of clavicle—anterior to the medial border of the pectoralis minor muscle.
• *Venous drainage:* venae commitantes.
• *Motor innervation:* medial and lateral pectoral nerve.
• Raise different for men and women.

Raise for male patients:
• Position supine, sandbag under the shoulder.
• Landmarks:
  o Mark likely position of pedicle: junction of middle and lateral third of clavicle to xiphoid process.
• Markings:
  o Mark deltopectoral flap as a lifeboat—do not violate;
  o First line to draw is a curvilinear from superior anterior axillary crease, medial to nipple and down to upper rectus sheath—this is line of the pedicle;
  o Skin paddle medial and inferior to nipple—maximum dimension of 8 cm to close directly want the skin paddle to be completely over the pec major muscle to improve vascularity.
• Raise:
  o Incise on the curvilinear line down to superficial fascia of pectoralis major;
  o Identify inferior border of pectoralis major;
  o Adjust proposed skin paddle accordingly;
  o Place interrupted silk sutures between skin and muscle to stop it avulsing the vessels;

p

○ Bluntly dissect plane between pectoralis major and minor;

○ Pectoral branch of thoracoacromial can be seen on the deep aspect of pectoralis major;

○ Then release the medial aspect (keep the humeral attachment at this stage or the flap will spring away from you);

○ Then release the humeral attachment;

○ Medial and lateral pectoral nerves are divided for ease of rotation and additional flap length.

• Close in layers.

Raise for female patients:

• Based on breast size.

• Small breasts: inframammary skin paddle—slightly superior to IMF.

• Large breasts: the IMF can be pulled inferiorly below the pectoralis major muscle—therefore to get a reliable skin paddle it is better to design the skin paddle in the same place as men (even though less cosmetically acceptable).

Methods to increase reach:

• Design skin paddle more distally (and only partially overlying pectoralis muscle although this risks vascularity of the skin).

• Detach muscle from clavicle.

• Pass pedicle under the clavicle or cut portion of clavicle.

Pectus carinatum

• *Pigeon breast:* protrusion deformity of anterior chest wall.

• The opposite of *Pectus excavatum.*

• Much less common.

• Can be chondrogladiolar (most prominent at xiphisternum) or chondromanubrial (most prominent at sternomanubrium).

Management: can be non-operative with a brace, or operative management similar to pectus excavatum. Resect abnormal costal cartilage. Reposition sternum. Support sternum with a sub-sternal metallic strut. Secure strut with wires. Shave sternum and use shavings as on-lay for the hollows.

See CHEST WALL RECONSTRUCTION.

Pectus excavatum

• Chest deformities occur in 1 in 300 births. M:F 2:1, may be familial.

• May be associated with Marfan's syndrome.

• Pectus excavatum (funnel chest) is the most common.

• The depression begins at the sternal angle and reaches the deepest point at the xiphoid. It may be so severe that the sternum contact

the vertebral bodies. This results in cardiac displacement, rotation of the heart and reduction in lung space.

• The Haller index is calculated by transverse chest diameter / anteroposterior chest diameter. The normal value is 2.5, pectus excavatum has values of >3.25.

• Due to overgrowth of costal cartilages forcing it posteriorly or anteriorly (pectus carinatum). In a 5-year-old child a sternovertebral distance of <5 cm is severe, 5–7 cm is moderate and >7 cm is mild.

Reconstruction:

• Prosthesis can be inserted into the defect.

• *Ravitch technique.*

• *Sternum turnover procedure:* transection of ribs and intercostal muscles at costal arches. Transect sternum above deformity. Remove and turn over. Suture sternum with wires and heavy silk.

• *Nuss technique.*

See CHEST WALL RECONSTRUCTION.

Pelvic wall reconstruction
Anatomy:

• Defined as the region above lower extremities and below abdomen. Bony landmarks are iliac crest, pubic symphysis, sacrum and greater trochanter.

• Major arteries are the common iliac, deep circumflex iliac and inferior epigastric artery. Internal iliac artery enters the true pelvis, and divides into anterior and posterior. Anterior divides into inferior gluteal, obturator, internal pudendal, umbilical, inferior vesical, middle rectal, uterine and vaginal arteries. The posterior divides into superior gluteal, iliolumbar and lateral sacral.

Operations: local muscle flaps are often the first choice for small defects. Include gluteus maximus, *Rectus abdominus,* rectus femoris, vastus lateralis.

Anterior defects: abdominoperineal hernias can be a problem and reconstruction should include fascia. Also mesh can be used covered with muscle flaps. TFL and rectus femoris can be used for inside and outside mesh cover.

Lateral defects:

• Local muscle flaps for smaller defects, including rectus abdominus, external oblique and rectus femoris.

• *Hemipelvectomy:* involves removal of the entire lower extremity and hemipelvis. If radical the bone is divided proximal to the sacroiliac joint. For a groin tumour choose a posterior flap. For a posterior tumour choose an anterior flap.

- *Posterior flap:* anteriorly start 5 cm proximal and 2 cm medial to ASIS. Follow inguinal ligament. Laterally from ASIS over anterior greater trochanter then distal to the gluteal groove. Divide iliac vessels, preserve sacral roots to bladder and rectum. Elevate myocutaneous flap.
- *Anterior flap:* uses a myocutaneous flap supplied by perforators of the external iliac and superficial femoral arteries.

Penile prosthesis
2 types available. A permanently stiff rod which keeps the penis firm, the other is inflated with a saline pump.

See PEYRONIE'S DISEASE.

Penis: anatomy
Root:
- Attached to perineal membrane.
- Bulb is the posterior end of corpora spongiosum.
- Lateral crura are the posterior ends of corpora cavernosa.
- Ischiocavernosus muscle moves the erect penis.
- Bulbospongiosus muscles empty the urethra of semen and urine.

Body: 3 erectile bodies, 2 corpora cavernosa and corpus spongiosum surrounding the urethra. The NVB contains the deep dorsal vein, dorsal artery, paired dorsal nerves.

Fascia:
- Tunica albuginea surrounds corpus cavernosa and spongiosum.
- This is surrounded by Buck's fascia (deep) and Dartos fascia (superficial).
- Between tunica albuginea and Buck's fascia lie the dorsal artery of penis, dorsal nerve of penis and deep dorsal vein of penis.
- The suspensory ligament attaches the penis to the symphysis pubis.

Urethra:
- *Posterior:* prostatic and membranous.
- *Anterior:* penile.
- The urethra is lined by transitional epithelia just proximal to the external urethral meatus and distally is lined by squamous epithelium.
- The cross-section is a horizontal slit changing to a vertical slit at the meatus causing urine to spiral.

Blood supply:
- The common penile artery comes from the internal pudendal artery.
- Its branches are the bulbourethral, dorsal and cavernosal artery.

- Venous drainage is by venae comitantes draining into the internal pudendal veins and the deep dorsal vein, which drains into the prostatic plexus. Superficial veins drain skin.

Lymphatic drainage:
- Lymphatics running with the superficial dorsal vein drain to superficial inguinal nodes.
- Lymphatics of the glans drain to deep inguinal nodes and internal iliac nodes.

Nerve supply: the dorsal nerve carries afferent sensory stimulation to the pudendal nerve. Erotic or tactile stimulation stimulates the cavernous nerve, which relaxes the cavernosal smooth muscle. Relaxation causes a decrease in arterial resistance and expansion in the lacunar spaces leading to an erection.

- *Erection:* parasympathetic, pelvic splanchnic nerves from the sacral plexus (S2–4).
- *Ejaculation:* sympathetic nerves (L1 root from sacral ganglia).
- *Skin:* posterior scrotal and dorsal branches of the internal pudendal nerves (S2–4).
- *Muscles:* the perineal branch of the pudendal nerves.

Development: *see* EMBRYOLOGY.
See HYPOSPADIAS.

Penis reconstruction
Indications: ambiguous genitalia, female to male gender reassignments and a number of acquired conditions of penile loss, such as trauma, cancer, burns, infection.

Goals:
- Normal appearance and adequate length for intercourse.
- Should contain the urethra and allow voiding while standing.
- Protective sensation to contain erectile prosthesis.
- Tactile and erogenous sensation.
- One stage. These are only possible with newer microvascular techniques.

Total penile reconstruction: radial forearm flap is most commonly used.

- *Chinese method:* using radial forearm flap. centre over radial artery. Include two sensory nerves. 15 × 15 cm flap. Bone can be harvested or rib graft inserted as prosthesis. Ulnar skin which is less hairy is used to create the neourethra. 3 cm width of urethra and 10 cm to tube around it. For gender-affirming surgery, the urethra will need to be longer.
- *Modified Chinese:* centre neourethra over radial artery to give best possible perfusion. Shaft either side of this. Cricket bat design places urethra over radius and shaft in

tandem but with significant loss of penile length. As the ulnar border is less hirsute, it can be raised on the ulnar artery.

Disadvantages of forearm flap:

○ Hair causes problems in neourethra;
○ Not much bulk;
○ Extrusion of the prosthesis;
○ Large graft;
○ Cold intolerance.

• *Lateral arm flap:* extends from deltoid insertion to proximal 1/3 forearm. Proximal forearm becomes glans and is innervated by posterior brachial and antebrachial nerves. The urethra is centred over the pedicle and a flap 18–20 cm wide is required. In a thin arm the urethra is prefabricated with a FTSG centred over the pedicle and sutured around a catheter. This is left 3–6 months. This ensures a good urethra is formed prior to lifting the flap and allows all available skin to be used for the phallus.

• *Others:* free sensate osseocutaneous flap. This requires a FTSG for urethra. Second toe dorsalis pedis flap has been used with jointed skeleton allowing rigidity and yet folding.

• *Recipient site:* T incision. Dissect out left and right erogenous branches of internal pudendal nerve from clitoris or penile remnant, also ilioinguinal or genitofemoral nerve. Use inferior epigastric vessels, gaining 15 cm of length. For a prosthesis a pocket is made beneath the rectus abdominus.

• *Transfer:* for gender-affirming surgery, a neourethra is made from labia minora flaps. Perform neurorrhaphy first then anastomose vessels.

Subtotal reconstruction: release any existing scar. Deglove corporal bodies down to base. Skin graft. Z-plasty to break up longitudinal scars. W flaps. Division of suspensory ligaments in the midline (avoid neurovascular structures). Silicone spacer can be inserted. Girth can be augmented by fat-dermal composite graft. Take from abdomen and include 5-10 mm of fat. Excise suprapubic fat. Penoscrotal webbing may need Z-plasty. New coronal sulcus can be created by undermining. Tattooing can be performed for colour mismatch.

Complications: fistulae and strictures secondary to ischaemia. Making it stiff enough is the biggest problem. An inflatable prosthesis inside a sensate phallus gives the best chance of success.

Perforator flaps
Developed from *Fasciocutaneous flap* and *Musculocutaneous/muscle flaps* when it was realized

that the muscle itself didn't need to be raised as long as the perforating vessels were preserved.

Performance status
World Health Organization.

Grade	Explanation of activity
0	Fully active, able to carry on all pre-disease performance without restriction.
1	Restricted in physically strenuous activity but ambulatory and able to carry out work of a light or sedentary nature, e.g. light house work, office work.
2	Ambulatory and capable of all selfcare but unable to carry out any work activities. Up and about more than 50% of waking hours.
3	Capable of only limited selfcare, confined to bed or chair more than 50% of waking hours.
4	Bedbound. Completely disabled. Cannot carry on any selfcare. Totally confined to bed or chair.
5	Dead.

Perifolliculitis capitis abscedens et suffodiens
Also called dissecting cellulitis of the scalp.

• Occurs most often in men of African descent.
• Disease of the scalp similar to *Hidradenitis suppurativa*.
• The scalp is involved with a perifolliculitis that results in burrowing, encysted epithelium-lined tracts with associated chronic infection and granulation tissue. Abscess and fistula formation and keloid scarring can occur.
• Non-operative treatment includes oral antibiotics, oral isotretinoin, oral or intralesional corticosteroids, analgesia, topical antiseptics and biologics such as TNF-α inhibitors (adalimumab).
• Surgical treatment includes CO_2 laser ablation and excision of the scarred, infected areas and resurfacing with split-thickness skin grafts or skin flaps from the adjacent scalp if the disease is limited.
• Treatment is challenging and often results in recurrent relapses, patchy scarring and alopecia.

Periodontium
Also known as gums. Specialized dense fibrous tissue covered with mucous

membrane that attaches to the cervical margin of the roots of the teeth and the alveolus of the jaws. Long-term survival of the tooth is dependent on this periodontal attachment.

Peri-orbital ecchymoses

Also known as raccoon eyes, which if bilateral are highly suggestive of basal skull fracture. May also be a sign of disseminated neuroblastoma or amyloidosis.

Permacol™

A cross-linked, acellular porcine collagen/elastin matrix. Permanent, non-allergenic, cell-friendly, biocompatible, supports revascularization. Comes in sheets.

Peyronie's disease

- Peyronie was a French barber surgeon who commanded the surgical corps of Louis XIV. He described scar tissue causing upward curvature of the penis.
- Connective tissue disorder affecting 1% of males.
- Get painful erections, curve, nodules.
- The plaque may be an inflammatory response to traumas to the penis.
- Associated with beta-blockers.
- Dupuytren's disease is seen in 10–30% of patients with Peyronie's disease.
- Curve is usually up and to the right.
- Condition usually progresses over 2 years and then stabilizes or improves.

Goals of treatment: preserve or restore sexual function. Consider erectile dysfunction, penile pain.

Investigations: penile ultrasound for vascular anatomy.

Medical: vitamin E until plaque matures or curve stable.

Surgical:
- Various implants have been tried.
- Plication (Nesbit plication) or excision of plaque and dermal graft (from non-hair-bearing groin skin).
- Dermal graft gives straight erections in 85% of patients.
- Consider a penile prosthesis at the same time as surgery for plaque if there is erectile dysfunction.

See PENILE PROSTHESIS.

Pfeiffer's syndrome

See CRANIOSYNOSTOSIS.

- Autosomal dominant and caused by mutations in *FGFR-1* or *2*.
- Similar craniofacial features to Apert's syndrome.
- Craniosynostosis—turribrachycephaly secondary to a bicoronal and occasional sagittal synostosis.

- Midface hypoplasia with shallow orbits and exorbitism.
- Hypertelorism and down slanting palpebral fissures.
- Nose is often downturned with a low nasal bridge.
- Enlarged broad thumbs and toes and may have partial syndactyly of 2nd and 3rd digits.

Clinical subtypes:
- *Type 1:* mild consisting of brachycephaly, midface hypoplasia and digit abnormalities: associated with normal intelligence.
- *Type 2:* features of type 1 with the addition of clover-leaf skull, proptosis; associated with developmental delay.
- *Type 3:* similar to type 2 but without the clover leaf skull.

Phalen's test

- A clinical test for *Carpal tunnel syndrome.*
- Hold the wrist in maximal palmar flexion. Test is positive when symptoms occur within 60 seconds.
- Reverse Phalen's test is similar with the hands and fingers dorsiflexed.

Pharyngeal structures

Also called branchial structures (branchia meaning 'gill').

Pharyngeal arches: from migrating neural crest cells. 6 in total but the 5th diminishes.

- *1st arch:* trigeminal nerve (CN V). Maxillary artery. Bones: Maxilla, Mandible, greater wing of sphenoid, incus malleus, temporal (squamous). Muscles: muscles of mastication, anterior digastric, mylohyoid, tensor tympani, tensor veli palatini.
- *2nd arch:* facial nerve (CN VII). Stapedial artery. Bones: Stapes, styloid process, lesser horn and upper body of hyoid. Muscles: muscles of facial expression, posterior digastric, stylohyoid, stapedius.
- *3rd arch:* glossopharyngeal nerve (CN IX). Common carotid artery. Bones: greater horns and lower body of hyoid. Muscle: stylopharyngeus.
- *4th and 6th arch:* vagus nerve (CN X, superior laryngeal and recurrent laryngeal nerves). Aortic arch. Cartilage: laryngeal cartilages. Muscles: pharyngeal constrictors, levator veli palatini, palatoglossus, striated upper oesophageal muscles, laryngeal muscles.

Pharyngeal grooves: also called clefts. These are on the external surfaces of the arches.

- *Groove 1:* external auditory canal.
- *Grooves 2–4:* Cervical sinus. Usually obliterated by 6 weeks of gestation.

Pharyngeal pouches: these are on the internal surfaces of the arches.

- *Pouch 1:* internal auditory canal.
- *Pouch 2:* palatine tonsil.
- *Pouch 3:* inferior parathyroid and thymus.
- *Pouch 4:* superior parathyroid.
- *Pouch 5:* thyroid C cells.

Pharynx

- A muscle-lined, tubular continuation of the oral cavity. It regulates food entry into the oesophagus and is a modulator for speech.
- *Nasopharynx:* rigid mucosa-lined, box-shaped structure with the posterior openings of the nasal cavity (choanae) anteriorly.
- *Oropharynx:* includes tonsils and tonsillar pillars, base of tongue and cephalad portion of middle constrictor.
- *Hypopharynx:* lies lateral and posterior to the larynx and is surrounded by cricopharyngeus.
- The oral cavity prepares food for swallowing. When ready, the tongue pushes it up and back, the middle constrictor relaxes, the larynx elevates and closes and the food moves into the oropharynx and hypopharynx. The bolus moves down into the oesophagus. As it passes, the larynx descends and airway is reopened.
- *Nerve supply:* sensation is primarily the internal laryngeal branch of the superior laryngeal nerve, from vagus. Also glossopharyngeal nerve. Motor supply to upper pharynx is from the external laryngeal branch of the vagus and the lower pharynx is from the recurrent laryngeal branch. High injury to the vagus gives severe functional disruption to the pharynx and larynx. Lower injury gives only motor problems.

Malignancy:

- Paediatric tumours such as rhabdomyosarcoma can be treated with chemotherapy and RT without surgery.
- SCC of the larynx and pharynx is treated with resection +/– neck dissection and RT.
- Oropharynx and hypopharynx carcinoma frequently spread to the nasopharynx with lateral spread to lymph nodes. Intrinsic larynx carcinoma is less likely to spread. Cancer of cervical oesophagus spreads to thoracic oesophagus and may require total oesophagectomy. Removal of tumour with a 2 cm margin frequently results in a circumferential defect.

Reconstruction:

- *Total oesophagectomy:* for malignancy, stricture and motility disorders.

Reconstruction is performed with a right, left or transverse colon as a pharyngogastric conduit in a subcutaneous or substernal position. To gain extra length an arcade can also be anastomosed in the neck.

- *Gastric pull-up:* occasionally used.
- *Local flaps:* for small defects. Tongue flap and islands of buccal mucosa and muscle can be transposed.
- *Deltopectoral flap:* in two stages.
- *Pectoralis major flap:* can carry a skin island, so it can be a one-stage operation. More challenging in women and the skin is thick. It can be used as an onlay patch for defects which are not circumferential.
- *Sternocleidomastoid flap:* with skin can be used for small defects.
- *Jejunum free flap:* good choice of vessel is the transverse cervical vessels. Usually perform the pharyngoenteric anastomosis first followed by the microvascular anastomosis followed by the distal anastomosis.
- *Other free flaps:* radial forearm, lateral arm, tubed ALT and scapula flaps can be used. These have potential for sensory reinnervation. They are anastomosed to the lingual, alveolar or cervical lexus sensory nerves. It is not clear whether this improves swallowing.
- *Gastro-omental free flap:* useful when a long vascular pedicle is needed. The gastroepiploic vessels that supply the greater curvature of the stomach can reach the axillary vessels and can replace gullet with omentum to cover neck structures.

See VOICE RESTORATION.

Phenol peels

- Use as a *Chemical peel* produces profound long-lived results.
- It induces a controlled predictable partial thickness chemical burn.
- This results in a smoother more youthful-looking skin.
- Penetrates to the upper reticular dermis causing a new stratified collagen layer.
- Effective for fine and coarse wrinkling and irregular pigmentation.
- Prolonged recovery period and significant bleaching with demarcation line.

Mechanism of action:

- Chemical injury that extends to the superficial dermis.
- This is reconstructed with neocollagen.
- Healing proceeds from epithelial appendages.
- Initial marked inflammatory reaction with epidermal regeneration at 48 hours.

- Most of the healing is complete within 3 weeks.
- The new collagen is more rigid and compact.
- The changes can last as long as 20 years.
- After a peel the melanocytes remain, but they do not produce as much melanin.

Toxicology:
- Phenol ingestion causes injury to kidneys and liver.
- Only small volumes of phenol are absorbed topically.
- If applied in less than 30 minutes there is a higher incidence of cardiac arrhythmias which can be avoided by applying over an hour. All patients should be monitored.

Patient selection:
- Not beneficial for acne scarring, capillary haemangioma, facial telangiectasia or hyperpigmentation after skin grafting.
- It is good for fine and coarse wrinkles, and blotchy skin pigmentation.
- Severe epithelial dysplasia after actinic keratosis responds well to deep facial peel.
- Regional peeling works in fair-skinned patients, whereas in darker complexions and red-haired freckled patients a full peel should be performed.
- Use on the neck, thorax and limbs can lead to hypertrophic scarring.

Technique:
- Sedation is needed for full facial peels.
- *Baker formula*: 3 ml phenol (88%), 2 ml water, 8 drops of soap, 3 drops of croton oil. The croton oil is a vesicant.
- It is applied with an applicator over at least an hour.
- After each region of the face is completed it is covered with an occlusive dressing to increase the depth of phenol penetration.
- Burning sensation occurs 30 minutes after the tape is applied.
- Sedatives are required for the first 6 hours after which the burning subsides.
- The mask is removed after 24–48 hours. The wounds are washed.
- Re-epithelialization occurs 7–10 days after phenol application.
- Lubricate the skin. Sun exposure should be avoided after.

Phocomelia
Intercalated deficiency of the upper limb.
  See TRANSVERSE ARREST.

Photodynamic therapy
- Used for treating BCCs, actinic keratosis and Bowen's disease.
- An inactive photosensitizer is administered and accumulates in the tissue.
- Light is delivered to the tumour, which photoactivates the sensitizer, which in turn converts molecular oxygen to free radicals that are tumoricidal.
- It may have a role for treating widespread disease.
- 5-aminolevulonic acid is highly selective for tumour cells. It is a prodrug which is metabolized by the haem biosynthetic pathway. The active metabolite is protoporphyrin IX. This is activated by illumination at 635 nm.
- Cream is applied for 3 hours then illuminated for 9 minutes.

Phyllodes tumour
Large benign tumour of the breast that typically occur in the perimenopausal patient.

Piano key sign
Seen with *Caput ulna*.

Pierre Robin sequence
- Pierre Robin (1867–1950) was a French dental surgeon.
- The sequence consists of airway obstruction in a child with micrognathia and glossoptosis. Most also have a cleft palate (60–90%). Infants also often have feeding difficulties. It is a sequence rather than a syndrome as the primary developmental difference is micrognathia, which causes glossoptosis and cleft palate.
- It may be associated with syndromes, notably *Stickler syndrome* and 22Q11.2 deletion syndrome.
- The neonate may require intervention to assist the airway obstruction. The measures which can be taken are:
  o Non-operative:
    ▪ Nurse side-to-side;
    ▪ Jaw thrust;
    ▪ Oxygen via nasal specs;
    ▪ Nasopharyngeal airway.
  o Surgical:
    ▪ Mandibular distraction;
    ▪ Tongue lip adhesion;
    ▪ Tracheostomy.
- Neuromuscular control and airway diameter usually improves in the first 6 months of life. Optimal early management of PRS airway is debated and surgery is controversial.
- PRS associated with feeding problems due to exhaustion associated with upper airway

obstruction and inability to feed and breath simultaneously. NG tubes often required to supplement feeding.

- Timing of cleft palate reconstruction may occur later than usual due to airway concerns.

See CLEFT PALATE.

Piezogenic pedal papules

- First described in 1991.
- Painful or asymptomatic papules of the feet and wrists, which result from herniation of fat through the dermis.
- They are common, non-hereditary and not related to a connective tissue defect. They are apparent when weight is applied to the heels and resolve when weight is removed. Usually bilateral.
- Histology reveals fragmentation of the dermal elastic tissue.
- There is no recommended medical or surgical treatment.

Pigmented villonodular synovitis

See GIANT CELL TUMOUR (PVNS).

Pilar cyst

Also called *Tricholemmal cyst*. *See* EPITHELIAL CYSTS.

Pilomatrixoma

Also known as calcifying epithelioma of Malherbe.

- A superficial benign solitary skin tumour arising from hair follicle cells usually on the face and neck or upper extremities mainly in children or young adults but can occur at any age.
- Presents as asymptomatic firm bluish dermal nodule 0.5 cm in diameter, rarely greater than 2 cm. Get foci of calcification or ossification.
- They are firmly fixed to the overlying skin.
- Histologically there are sheets of epithelial cells with basophilic shadow (ghost) cells arranged in irregular bands. Masses of keratin are found interspersed between cells with calcification.
- Lesions do not tend to regress. Definitive treatment is surgical excision with clear margins.

Pincer deformity

Nail deformity. *See* NAIL.

Pisiform

Fracture:

- Uncommon, often overlooked as difficult to see and half associated with severe injuries. Most common mechanism of injury is a direct blow. Also repetitive trauma. Difficult to see on XR. May need supination, oblique and carpal tunnel views.
- May get avascular necrosis. May get non-union or pisotriquetral arthritis.
- Examine by loading the subpisiform joint laterally as with the thumb CMC joint.

- If symptomatic treat by excision, which doesn't appear to affect wrist flexion.

Dislocation:

- For dislocation to occur there must be massive disruption of the FCU tendinous complex. Rarely reported.
- Due to violent contraction of the muscle with a flexed wrist. If the rupture is proximal to pisiform get distal dislocation. If the rupture is distal to the pisohamate and pisometacarpal ligaments get proximal dislocation. May be associated with avulsion of the hook of hamate.
- Treat either by tendon reattachment or excise pisiform and restore tendon continuity.

Pisotriquetral arthritis

- Characterized by pain over the palmar ulnar aspect of the wrist. Palpation elicits tenderness over the ulnar aspect of the pisotriquetral joint (PTJ).
- The pisiform is a sesamoid bone. Flexion of FCU relaxes the pisiform and allows side to side or radioulnar sliding. With compression this causes pain. It should be distinguished from lunotriquetral synovitis (*see* CARPUS, and FLEXOR CARPI ULNARIS TENOSYNOVITIS).
- *XR:* obtain a 30° supinated oblique view tangential to the pisiform. A standard carpal tunnel view further defines the joint. XR may reveal an osteochondral loose body emanating from the joint.
- Injection may help to localize the point of the pain. Osteophytes may cause ulnar nerve symptoms.

Operation: pisiform excision is carried out through a longitudinal palmar incision that crosses the wrist joint obliquely. The incision is radial to the pisiform. Incise the periosteum and peel off the FCU tendon. Excise the pisiform. Mobilize after a week.

Pitanguy's line

Identifies surface landmark of frontal branch of facial nerve which runs from 0.5 cm below the tragus to 1.5 cm above the lateral eyebrow.

See FACIAL NERVE.

Pitres–Testut sign

In *Ulnar nerve palsy*. Two signs. Inability to abduct in radial or ulna direction the middle finger. Also inability to cone the extended fingers.

Plantaris: anatomy and harvest

- Located anterior and medial to Achilles tendon.
- Absent in 7%–20% of limbs. Can be detected with CT scan or USS. Also unusable at times due to its insertions.

- Harvest with transverse incision just anterior to medial aspect of Achilles tendon. Divide and pass suture then stripper.

See TENDON RECONSTRUCTION.

Platelet-derived growth factor
See CYTOKINES AND GROWTH FACTORS (Growth factors).

Platysma flap
Based on the submental branch of the facial artery and raised on a superior muscle pedicle. The skin island is designed on a transverse axis distally. Innervated so can be used to give motor function to the lip and provide sensation. It can be transposed to reconstruct defects of the floor of mouth and tongue. Can be used as a free flap to reconstruct orbicularis oculi function in facial palsy.

See ORAL CAVITY RECONSTRUCTION.

Poirier: space of A fenestration in the capitolunate articulation where a capsular tear occurs with a lunate dislocation.

See CARPUS.

Poland's syndrome
- Described by Alfred Poland 1841 when he was an anatomy demonstrator at Guy's hospital.
- Aetiology may be hypoplasia of the subclavian artery.
- Usually sporadic, occasionally genetic.
- 1:30,000, right > left. M > F.

Chest wall: congenital, partial or complete absence of pectoralis major and pectoralis minor: absence of sternocostal head of pectoralis major is a key finding. Hypoplastic musculoskeletal components. Get partial rib and sternal agenesis, mammary aplasia, absence of latissimus dorsi, serratus anterior and pectoralis major. Also hypoplastic scapula. If mild get breast hypoplasia and nipple displacement. There may be extensive deformities of the costochondral cartilages and sternum and absence of portions of the 2–4th ribs.

Upper limb deformities: symbrachydactyly—short fused fingers. Usually central 3 digits. Short arm.

Other disorders: scoliosis and renal disorders.

Reconstruction: in females need to address the breast asymmetry. Both male and female patients may require latissimus dorsi transfer to reconstruct the anterior axillary fold. Sternal prominence may need correction.

See CHEST WALL RECONSTRUCTION.

Pollicization
- A surgical technique to create a thumb from an existing finger. First described by Gosset and Hilgenfeldt then refined by Little and Buck-Gramcko.

- With *Thumb hypoplasia* pollicization is required for Blauth type IIIB, IV and V. Pollicization using index finger is preferred for congenital absence.
- Pollicization is the only procedure that can restore the CMC joint. Damaged fingers may make useful pollicization as they only really need to function well at the CMC joint.

Principles:
- Incisions:
  - Need to get access to vessels to maintain flap circulation;
  - Dorsal veins;
  - Palmar arteries;
  - Need to access digital nerves;
  - Need to access skeleton, intrinsic and extrinsic tendons;
  - Need to be left with excess skin to be able to create the first web.
- Take the metacarpal out. Use MC head to make CMCJ, which sits into a pocket that you create at the base of thumb.
- Make an opposable digit.
- Make a first web space.
- Re-position so that it faces the right way—do tendon rebalancing with EDM, ADM.
- Make a CMCJ.

Technique for index finger pollicization
- GA, arm abducted on hand table, antibiotic prophylaxis.
- Incision.
- Raise dorsal flap preserving dorsal veins to index.
- Vessels:
  - Raise volar flap and dissect neurovascular bundles to thumb, index and long finger;
  - Divide radial digital artery to long finger and transverse metacarpal ligament.
- Nerves:
  - Radial is already separate;
  - Ulnar digital nerve needs intra-neural dissection from long finger.
- Bones:
  - Distal osteotomy at 2nd metacarpal physis and remove
  - growth plate—this will become the neo-trapezium;
  - Rotate finger down 135° into new position.
- Tendons:
  - Index finger extensors are shortened;
  - Index flexors are not shortened.
- Interossei:
  - Re-routed into lateral bands to act as adductor and abductor pollicis.

- Skin:
  - Flaps used to create generous first web space.

See THUMB RECONSTRUCTION.

Pollock's sign
- Clinical test in *Ulnar nerve palsy*.
- Loss of FDP to ring and little with inability to flex distal phalanges.

Polydactyly
- Extra digits. May be pre-axial, central or postaxial.
- Post-axial or ulnar sided most common. Worldwide it is the most common congenital malformation of extremities. May be associated with syndactyly (termed polysyndactyly).

Surgery:
- If joints are involved, preserve collateral ligament. If at the MCP level take care to preserve the physis. A closing wedge osteotomy may be required.
- Revisional surgery may be required if there is recurrence of clinodactyly.

Ulnar polydactyly:
- Also called post-axial polydactyly.
- The most common single hand malformation. 8 × greater than other fingers. Often bilateral.

Classification: *Stelling*. Treat by simple excision.

Central polydactyly:
- Usually with syndactyly, often bilateral.
- Treat by releasing the syndactyly, excising the excess tissue and soft tissue reconstruction.

Radial polydactyly:
- Also called pre-axial polydactyly.
- *See* THUMB DUPLICATION.

See CONGENITAL HAND ANOMALIES.

Polyethylene
- Polyethylene refers to plastics from polymerization of ethylene gas.
- Ultra-high molecular weight polyethylene has a very low frictional coefficient against metal and ceramics and is used as a bearing surface for joint replacement prosthesis. Also wear resistance is low.
- *Medpor™* is a high-density porous polyethylene.

See ALLOPLASTS.

Polymethylmethacrylate
See METHYL METHACRYLATE.

Polypropylene
Similar structure to *Polyethylene*. They differ by a methyl group instead of hydrogen in each unit

of the chain. Marlex™ mesh has a high tensile strength and allows tissue ingrowth.

See ALLOPLASTS.

Polytetrafluoroethylene
Examples are Proplast, Gore-tex™ and Teflon™. Proplast HA contains hydroxyapatite. Can be used for onlay without biofunctional loading. It supports fibrovascular ingrowth. Gore-tex comes in sheets and can be used for *Guided bone regeneration*.

See POLYETHYLENE.

Porokeratosis
- Autosomal dominant disorder of abnormal keratinization with malignant degeneration into *Basal cell carcinoma* and SCCs.
- The most common type is porokeratosis of Mibelli.

Port-wine stain
Also called Capillary malformation or naevus flammeus neonatorum.

- Combined capillary *Vascular malformations*.
- Incidence 0.3%.
- An intradermal vascular malformation present at birth and persists through life with no regression.
- Developmental weakness of vessel wall.
- It can be localized or extensive.
- Differentiate from the fading macular stain (*Naevus simplex*).
- In distribution of trigeminal nerve.
- Deep red-purple.
- Grows with child.
- Later become nodular (cobblestoning).
- Some fade others darken.
- Associated with *Sturge–Weber*, *Klippel–Trenaunay*, *Parks–Weber*.
- *Treatment:* cosmetic camouflage, argon pulsed dye laser. Significant lightening occurs in 70–80% of patients.

Position of safe immobilisation (POSI)
- Refers to the 'safe' position of hand splintage, i.e. the position from which it is easiest to regain mobility after a period of splinting.
- *Metacarpalphalangeal joint* flexed, PIP joint extended, thumb abducted, wrist mild extension.
- MCP joint has variable tightness of collateral ligaments in flexion and extension. The head is ovoid in the sagittal plane with a palmar flare in the transverse plane so the collateral ligaments are stretched to their longest when the MCPJ is held in flexion. Lax ligaments tend to shorten leading to extension contracture.
- The interphalangeal joints are the same in flexion and extension, but the volar plate

overlies cartilage, where it will readily become adherent. The extensors are stable in extension and stressed in flexion. In flexion they will easily become attenuated with disruption of the transverse retinacular ligaments, leading to volar slip of the lateral bands and a boutonniere deformity.

Positron emission tomography (PET)
- First developed and used in 1953.
- Used for the detection of micrometastasis based on abnormal cellular metabolic activity, rather than relying on structural changes.
- Non-invasive high-resolution imaging.
- Used in oncology because malignant cells have a higher rate of utilization of glucose. Glucose accumulates in malignant cells as does 2-deoxyglucose. This can be labelled with ^{18}F (^{18}F-FDG), which is a glucose analogue that is taken up by glucose-using cells and phosphorylated by hexokinase.
- As this decays it emits a positron, which collides with an electron. These annihilate each other leading to formation of two photons emitted at 180° to each other. The PET scanner detects these and where they came from.

Posterior interosseous artery flap
Anatomy:
- The posterior interosseous artery arises from the common interosseous artery or ulnar artery just distal to the antecubital fossa.
- It passes through the interosseous membrane under supinator and above the APL close to the PIN.
- At distal end of supinator it divides into descending and ascending recurrent branches. The ascending branch courses retrogradely to anastomose with the posterior radial collateral artery just distal to the elbow.
- The descending branch travels on the dorsal aspect of the forearm on APL within the intermuscular septum between ECU and EDM.
- It terminates at the wrist where it anastomoses with the dorsal branch of the carpus and perforating anterior interosseous artery.
- Multiple septocutaneous perforators supply the overlying skin. The largest arises just distal to supinator.

Flap raise:
- Draw a line from lateral epicondyle to DRUJ.
- A large perforator which should be included is found distal to the junction of posterior 1/3 and distal 2/3, usually between 5–11 cm from

the radial humeral condyle. Centre the skin island over the artery. It can be a width of 6–8 cm. Incise the radial side of the flap through fascia.
- Extend incision to wrist. At the wrist the anastomosis between the posterior interosseous artery and communicating perforators of anterior interosseous artery can be seen. Retract EDC and EDM to expose supinator. The artery is seen emerging from the distal edge of supinator with nerve. Perforating vessels to skin can be seen. Divide artery proximally. Dissect ulnar side of flap. Elevate proximal to distal. Inset flap into defect. It can be elevated as an osseocutaneous flap.

Posterior interosseous nerve
- Supplies all wrist extensors except ECRL. ECRB and supinator are supplied before entering the arcade of Frohse.
- Just proximal to the elbow, the radial nerve divides into superficial and deep. The superficial branch is sensory and the deep branch (PIN) is motor. It supplies ECRB then passes to the forearm entering the supinator muscle. After emerging from supinator, it supplies EDC, ECU, and EDM. Long motor branches supply APL, EPL, EPB and EIP. ECRL is innervated proximal to the PIN so some wrist extension is preserved with loss of PIN.

Posterior interosseous syndrome
Compression can be caused by:
- *Trauma:* dislocation of elbow, fracture of the radial head.
- *Inflammation:* RA of radiohumeral joint.
- *Swellings:* ganglia, lipoma.
- *Iatrogenic:* after tennis elbow injection.

Contusion of the dorsal proximal forearm can injure the PIN. In this situation, triceps and ECRL will be spared. Supinator is tested in extension. Thumb adduction is weakened due to the loss of EPL.

Posterior Thigh Flap
- Fasciocutaneous flap based on descending branch of inferior gluteal artery.
- Skin innervated by the posterior femoral cutaneous nerve.
- Can reconstruct pelvic and perineal defects.

Preiser's disease
Idiopathic avascular necrosis of the proximal pole of the *Scaphoid*.

Prelamination/prefabrication
- Involves creating a multilayered flap prior to transfer. Thus, the surgeon is not limited by natural flaps.

- Especially for head and neck reconstruction. For example, forehead flaps can be lined with cartilage and skin grafts before transferring for a total nasal reconstruction.
- It also includes *Neovascularization*.

Premaxilla

The alveolar segment of the maxilla which includes the nasal spine and 4 incisor teeth. It is located centrally anteriorly to the incisive foramen.

See CLEFT LIP.

Pressure sores

Definition: an ulcer resulting from unrelieved pressure. All of the other factors are secondary to the effects of pressure.

History:
- Charcot (1879) thought that nerve injury released a neurotrophic factor.
- Brown-Sequard (1853) believed that moisture and pressure were key.

Aetiology: as well as unrelieved pressure, other factors are altered sensory perception, incontinence, immobility, shear and friction, poor nutrition.

Pathophysiology:
- *Pressure:* is the single most important factor. Capillary pressure ranges from 12 mmHg at the venous end to 32 mmHg at the arterial end. External force exceeding these pressures will cause a reduced capillary perfusion. There is an inverse relationship between the amount of pressure and the length of time to ulceration. Studies confirming this also demonstrated that the initial changes occur in the muscle overlying the bone. Low pressure for long periods is more destructive than higher pressures for short periods and a rest of just 5 minutes can reverse damage.
- *Denervation:* neurologically injured patients are more susceptible to ulceration than patients with cerebral palsy. Denervated flaps have a higher bacterial count than innervated flaps.
- *Infection:* bacteria accumulate in areas of increased pressure. Proposed mechanisms include impaired lymphatic function, ischaemia, denervation and impaired immune function.
- *Oedema:* once external pressures are greater than 12 mmHg, veins become engorged, and tissue pressure increases. Plasma extravasation occurs leading to oedema. Denervated tissues also lead to loss of sympathetic tone, vasodilatation and oedema. Lymphatic pump requires active skeletal muscle so denervation also exacerbates

oedema by this indirect way. Also secondary to release of inflammatory mediators.
- *Shear:* vertical shear occurs when patients are pulled up the bed. Shear is eliminated with an air mattress.

Preoperative care: all components of care must be optimized before surgery.

- *Nutrition:* 25–35 cal/kg should be delivered daily. 1.5–3 g/kg of protein is required daily. *Vitamin C* and Vitamin A. *Zinc*, *Iron* and *Copper*. Supplemental feeds may be required. Consider TPN.
- *Infection:* patients prone to pressure ulcers may be prone to urinary sepsis, leading to bacteraemia. Pulmonary infections more common with high spinal lesions. Osteomyelitis may be present within the pressure sore and may require a bone biopsy.
- *Relief of pressure:* turning associated with *Mattress* systems.
- *Treatment of spasms:* spasms develop in spinal cord injury due to the separation of spinal reflex arcs from higher control. Efferent fibres from muscles end directly on afferent fibres. Treatment includes drugs, e.g. diazepam (10–40 mg/day) and baclofen (15–100 mg/day). Also intrathecal phenol or alcohol. Severe case may require cordotomy or rhizotomy (sectioning of some of the sensory nerve fibres entering the spinal cord).

Risk factors: immobility, incontinence, nutrition, altered level of consciousness. Braden, Norton and *Waterlow* scales are risk assessments for pressure sores.

Staging system: National Pressure Advisory Panel (1–4), also Shea and Yakony-Kirk.

- *Stage 1:* non-blanchable erythema of skin.
- *Stage 2:* partial thickness skin loss involving epidermis and dermis, superficial ulcer.
- *Stage 3:* full thickness skin loss extending down to fascia. Deep crater.
- *Stage 4:* full thickness skin loss with damage to muscle, bone and other structures.

Osteomyelitis: may need to perform bone biopsies, CRP, CT scan and treat with antibiotics for 6–8 weeks prior to reconstruction.

Surgical principles: surgery may be required for grade 3 and 4, drain collections, debridement, excision of pseudobursa, ostectomy, haemostasis and suction, closure without tension using well-vascularized tissue. *Vastus lateralis flap*, *Rectus femoris flap*, gluteal thigh flap.

Ischial pressure sores:

- Plan a flap that will cover the ulcer, but allow the use of secondary flaps.

- The inferior gluteal musculocutaneous rotation flap uses the lower half of the gluteus maximus muscle.
- Also a superiorly based gluteal flap.
- The biceps femoris V–Y flap.
- The TFL flap.

Sacral pressure sore:
- Mostly musculocutaneous and fasciocutaneous flaps.
- Mainly based on the *Gluteus maximus*, based superiorly or inferiorly, rotated, advanced or turned over.
- Also *Lumbosacral back flap*.
- Attempts have been made to place sensate skin in the back, but with limited success.

Trochanteric sores:
- Develop in patients who lay laterally for long.
- *TFL* is most commonly used.
- Sensation is from L1–3 so this is potentially a sensate flap in patients with a spinal cord lesion lower than L3.

Proflavine
Proflavine hemisulphate (proflavine 3,6- dia-mino-acridine sulphate dihydrate) is a quin-olone antimicrobial. It is bacteriostatic against many Gram-positive bacteria, but less useful against Gram-negative organisms and ineffect-ive against spores. Can get hypersensitivity. Used as it forms a malleable dressing.

Progeria
- Rare autosomal recessive disorder.
- Characterized by growth retardation, craniofacial disproportion, baldness, prominent ears, heart disease.
- Premature ageing in children.

  See WERNER'S SYNDROME.

Prominent ear correction
- 5% of Caucasians, 2/3 having a family history.
- The commonest deformity is absence of anti-helical fold. True conchal hypertrophy is rare. Also may have lobular hypertrophy.
- Helix to mastoid distance >2 cm. Pinna to mastoid angle > 25°. Conchoscaphal angle > 90°.

Non-surgical treatment: splinting (such as EarBuddies™) can be performed in the neonatal period and for up to 18 months, although younger age child is associated with shorter period of splinting. Maternal oestrogens circu-late from 3 days to 3 weeks after birth. Long-term outcome is not known (Matsuo 1984).

Surgery:
- Alter concha by:
  - *Furnas setback:* suturing concha to mastoid fascia;
  - Conchal excision (rarely required);
  - Cartilage scoring—anterior or posterior. May have unpredictable results.
- Alter anti-helical fold by:
  - Suturing techniques, e.g. Mustardè stitch between scaphoid and conchal fossae. Can stitch over a graft of soft tissue to create a softer fold;
  - Cartilage scoring techniques relying on Gibson's 'release of interlocked stresses', e.g. Chongchet anterior cartilage scoring.
- Alteration of soft tissues:
  - *Earlobe:* the fibrofatty core can be sutured to the concha or skin can be excised posteriorly;
  - *Excision of auricularis posterior muscle and soft tissues:* this provides a space for the concha to sit in for the Furnas setback.

Complications:
- *Early:* haemorrhage, haematoma, infection, pressure necrosis, wound dehiscence, suture failure.
- *Late:* under- or over-correction, asymmetry, irregular anti-helix, telephone ear, shallow sulcus, keloid, suture extrusion, recurrence.

Pronator syndrome
- Compression neuropathy of the median nerve proximally in the forearm (4 sites), the most common being bands within pronator.
- Compression points:
  - *Ligament of Struthers:* arises from lateral supracondylar process on lower 1/3 of humerus. Test by resisted elbow flexion;
  - *Lacertus fibrosus:* arises from biceps. Test by resisted supination with flexed elbow;
  - *Pronator teres:* test by resisted forearm pronation with the elbow extended. Pronator teres can be tender, firm or enlarged;
  - *Arch of FDS:* test by resisted flexion of PIPJ of middle finger.
- Get forearm pain, as well as paraesthesia in the distribution of the median nerve. Palmar paraesthesia will be present from involvement in the palmar branch of the median nerve.
- May get weakness secondary to pain. Patients often perform repetitive tasks. Get pain on palpation of the median nerve. No weakness of muscles. Tinel's sign positive in the forearm. Muscle cramps can occur.

Treatment:
- Try immobilization with elbow at 90°. 50% respond to non-operative treatment.
- *Operative technique:* lazy-S incision over the elbow. Find median nerve proximal to elbow.

p

Excise ligament of Struthers if present. Incise bicipital aponeurosis, follow to superficial head of pronator teres. Incise fibrous band of pronator teres. If there is a variation in passage through pronator, the deep head can be detached to expose the nerve. Next look at superficialis arcade. Incise superficialis arch. Relieve any site of compression. Pronator is reattached.

See ANTERIOR INTEROSSEOUS SYNDROME.

Pronator teres

Origin: from medial epicondyle. It passes distally and radially.

Insertion: through a flat tendon into radial aspect of mid-radius. It pronates the forearm, wrist and hand in extension. Valuable for wrist extension in radial nerve palsy.

Nerve supply: median nerve.

Blood supply: ulnar artery, anterior recurrent ulnar artery.

See MUSCLES.

Prosthetics: myoelectric

Utilize EMG potentials from residual neuromuscular systems to control the terminal device. The EMG potentials are obtained from skin surface electrodes over agonist/antagonist muscle groups. The main advantage is durability, reliability and function.

Prosthetic joint infection

Limb-threatening condition. Manage in MDT. Can consider DAIR (debridement, antibiotics, implant retention) in appropriate cases. Most require management in stages including deep sampling off antibiotics, removal of implant or components, debridement and wound excision, soft tissue reconstruction, long term antibiotics, and revision arthroplasty. For soft tissue reconstruction options around the knee, *see* LOWER LIMB RECONSTRUCTION.

Proteus syndrome

• A sporadic vascular, skeletal, and soft tissue disorder.
• Asymmetric growth.
• Tumour-like lesions consist of connective tissue, adipose tissue, Schwann cell structures and vascular tissue.
• More often in thorax and upper abdomen.
• The vascular anomalies are of the CM, LM, CVM, and CLVM type.
• Get macrocephaly (calvarial hyperostoses); asymmetry of the limbs; partial gigantism of the hands or feet, or both; plantar thickening ('moccasin' feet) can be present. Verrucous (linear) nevus also occurs.
• Proteus syndrome may be on a spectrum with *Epidermal naevus (Solomon) syndrome.*

• May result from a dominant lethal gene that survives by somatic mosaicism.

See COMPLEX COMBINED VASCULAR MALFORMATIONS.

Proximal interphalangeal joint (PIPJ)

Anatomy:

• Normal ROM 0–110°, lateral motion 8°. Hinge (ginglymus) joint.
• Two condyles on the proximal phalanx articulate with facets on the middle. A median ridge creates a tongue in groove preventing lateral movement. Get convergence of the fingertips on flexion due to the slight asymmetry of the finger joints. The condyles of each joint are of differing heights. In the coronal plane they angle away from the second web space. There is also some rotation occurring during flexion.
• *Ligaments:* form a 3-sided box. The sides are the collaterals, the floor is the volar plate. Collaterals are proper (PCL) and accessory (ACL). PCL is thicker and provides most joint stability. It fans out from proximal to distal. It blends with volar plate at the critical corner. ACL is a suspensory ligament for *Volar plate* and flexor tendon sheath. ACL prevents tendon sheath from moving away from PIPJ in flexion.
• Dorsal stability is provided by central slip.

Hyperextension injuries:

• Injuries can occur dorsally, volarly or laterally, but are most common as hyperextension. Assess stability under a ring block.

Classification: *Dray and Eaton.*

Operations:

• If stable, provide extension block splint for 1–2/52. Buddy strap for 1/12. Treatment of unstable type III is more difficult and varied. 3 main treatments are open reduction, skeletal traction or volar plate arthroplasty.
• *Open reduction:* most successful with a single fragment. Approach through volar Bruner incision. Elevate flexor sheath between A2 and A4. Reduce joint. Apply dorsal blocking K-wire (flex PIPJ and pass wire through head of proximal phalanx). Hold fragment with a small screw or K wire from volar side. Remove dorsal block at 4/52. Cerclage wire fixation can also be performed.
• *Volar plate arthroplasty:* if the fragments are multiple, they can be excised with the collateral ligaments. The volar plate is freed from collateral ligaments. The volar plate is attached to bone through a pull-out suture avoiding the lateral bands. Collateral ligaments are then reattached.
• *Dynamic traction:* traction with movement for 6 weeks.

Chronic fracture dislocation of PIPJ: difficult problem with pain and stiffness. Can perform capsulotomy and reduction. Also K-wire in 30° of flexion and perform osteotomy to base of middle phalanx to tilt the volar lip. Bone graft may be required. Chronic hyperextension may require *FDS tenodesis*.

Collateral ligament injuries: most can be treated with splinting. Instability is usually due to proximal rupture or avulsion fracture. Repair with suture, bone anchor or interosseous wire. Only a small group require operative treatment.

Volar dislocations: much less common. May get rupture of the central slip with some collateral ligament involvement. With some rotation one of the collateral ligaments may tear. The ipsilateral proximal phalanx condyle slips through the extensor mechanism making it irreducible. Attempt closed reduction but may need open. If irreducible the prognosis is better as the extensor mechanism is intact.

Arthritis: the PIPJ is not commonly involved in OA. Treat conservatively. Occasionally, an osteophyte requires excision. Implants are more indicated for ring and little finger as they are used to grasp. If conservative treatment fails, patients will require an *Arthroplasty* or *Arthrodesis*.
    See JOINTS.

Proximal row carpectomy
- Motion-preserving wrist *Arthrodesis* procedure.
- Excision of scaphoid, lunate and triquetrum, allowing the capitate to articulate with the radius.

Indication: radiocarpal or intercarpal arthrosis, spastic wrist contractures, malalignment of proximal carpus—Kienböck's disease, SLAC, scaphoid non-union.

Requirement:
- Undamaged articular surface of the lunate fossa of distal radius and proximal pole of capitate.
- Also perform radial styloidectomy to prevent impingement against the trapezium.

Prozansky classification
(Murry and Mulliken) *Mandibular hypoplasia* in *Hemifacial microsomia*.
- *Type I:* all parts present though hypoplastic.
- *Type IIa:* condyle articulates as a hinge.
- *Type IIb:* no condyle.
- *Type III:* the mandibular ramus is absent.

Prune belly syndrome
Also called Eagle–Barrett syndrome.
- Seen in newborn boys.

- Get absent abdominal wall muscles, cryptorchism, and dilated urinary tract.
- The muscle deficiency may be limited to one area.
- The abdomen is wrinkled and with growth looks more like a pear.
- Surgery is required to correct urogenital problems and muscle deficiency may require muscle flaps.
    See ABDOMINAL RECONSTRUCTION.

Pseudo-epitheliomatous hyperplasia
Seen in long-standing chronic ulcers, often in pressure sores. Epidermal thickening may look like malignant change. Get downward proliferation of epidermal cells and micro abscesses. It may be difficult to differentiate from malignancy.
    See SQUAMOUS CELL CARCINOMA.

Pseudogout
- Calcium pyrophosphate dihydrate deposition.
- Calcification through the triangular fibrocartilage of the wrist is diagnostic.
    See GOUT.

Pseudohypertelorism
A normal interorbital distance but an increased intercanthal distance—measured between the medial canthal tendons.
    See HYPERTELORISM.

Pseudosarcomatous lesions
- Several clinically benign localized fibromatous proliferative lesions may show cellular changes and numerous mitoses that easily lead to a mistaken diagnosis of fibrosarcoma.
- *Infantile digital fibromatosis:* is a rare pseudosarcomatosis characterized by asymptomatic, firm, red, smooth nodules up to 1 cm in size on the dorsal and lateral aspects of the distal phalanges of the toes and fingers during infancy and childhood. Surgical excision is the recommended treatment, but recurrences are reported to be frequent.
- *Atypical fibroxanthoma.*
- *Nodular pseudosarcomatous fasciitis.*

Pseudoxanthoma elasticum
- Degenerative disorder of elastic fibres.
- Mainly affecting skin eyes and arteries.
- Autosomal recessive and dominant types.
- Get premature skin laxity looks like plucked chicken skin.
- Redundant skin around the neck, axilla, trunk and limbs.

- May benefit from plastic surgery, but severe arteriosclerosis commonly develops as early as the third decade of life.

Psoriasis

- Common, benign, chronic, erythematous, scaling skin disease.
- Surgery should be avoided when the disease is worsening:
  - May induce *Köbner's phenomenon;*
  - High skin colonization bacterial count may increase infection.
- Treatments range from topical therapy to phototherapy and systemic therapy.

Psoriatic arthritis

- Negative RhF.
- 5% of patients with psoriasis develop arthritis.
- 1/3 have a family history of psoriasis.
- 20% of patients can develop skin changes after the arthritis.
- Asymmetric.
- Classically affects DIPJ.
- Arthritis mutilans or telescoping occurs in psoriatic arthritis and severe seropositive arthritis.
- *Nails:* get pitting, leukonychia and crumbling.
- *XR:* osteolysis with bone destruction and widening of the joint spaces. Get pencil in cup changes.
- *Treatment:* usually osteotomy, arthrodesis or arthroplasty.

PTFE

See POLYTETRAFLUOROETHYLENE.

Ptosis: breast

See REGNAULT'S CLASSIFICATION.

Ptosis: eyelid

- Drooping of the upper lid.
- Differentiate from *Blepharophimosis.*
- Aim of surgery is to correct ptosis by increasing the power of the lid.
- The 3 sources of power are levator palpebrae superioris, Müller's muscle and frontalis muscle. Müller's muscle is sympathetically innervated with slow lifting effect. It adjusts lid level. Paralysis of Müller's muscle drops the lid by 2-3 mm. Paralysis of frontalis causes brow ptosis. Levator is not strongly fixed to the tarsal plate. Fixation is through fibrous bands. So in correcting ptosis, aponeurosis can be lifted off the tarsus and fixed more firmly. This is effective as the attachment is now firmer than the rather elastic attachment prior to fixation.

Aetiology:

- *Myogenic:*
  - Congenital levator dystrophy;
  - Blepharophimosis syndrome;
  - Progressive external ophthalmoplegia;
  - Myaesthenia gravis.
- *Neurogenic:*
  - 3rd nerve palsy;
  - Horner's syndrome;
  - Marcus Gunn jaw-winking, aberrant 3rd nerve regeneration.
  - *Aponeurotic:* defects in levator aponeurosis.
- *Mechanical:*
  - Dermatochalasis;
  - Tumour;
  - Scar;
  - Anophthalmos.

Clinical tests:

- Determine the lid margin level and the amount of levator function. Normal lid covers 1-2 mm of the upper limbus.
- *Margin-reflex distance:* patient looks at torch held 1/2 m away. Measure distance of lid from corneal reflex.
- *Levator function:* fix brow with thumb and measure excursion of upper lid between upgaze and downgaze. Normal levator function is 12-15 mm.
- *Bell's phenomenon.*
- *Jaw-winking:* ask patient to move jaw to the side opposite to the ptotic upper lid or open the mouth wide. The lid will lift if jaw-winking present.
- Also measure aperture and distance from upper margin of iris to lid. Check visual acuity, extraocular muscle movements.

Classification of ptosis:

- Ptosis severity:
  - *Mild:* 1-2 mm;
  - *Moderate:* 3 mm;
  - *Severe:* 4+ mm.
- Levator function:
  - *Good:* >10 mm;
  - *Fair:* 4-10 mm;
  - *Poor:* <4 mm.

Summary of surgical treatment:

- *Good levator function with mild ptosis: Fasanella–Servat* procedure i.e. Müller's muscle shortening.
- *Good levator function with severe ptosis:* repair levator aponeurosis.
- *Fair levator function with any degree of ptosis:* resect levator aponeurosis.
- *Poor levator function:* perform brow suspension.

Surgical treatment based on aetiology:

- *Congenital:*
  - *Severe:* frontalis sling;
  - *Less severe:* levator advancement/ tarsectomy.
- *Senile ptosis:* disinsertion and reattachment of levator.
- *Post-traumatic:*
  - *Neurogenic:* use frontalis sling;
  - *Trauma:* reinsert.
- *Myogenic:* treat disease then reinsert or plicate.
- *Neurogenic:*
  - *Stroke:* use a sling;
  - *Horner's:* Müllerectomy, reinsertion of aponeurosis or Fasanella–Servat procedure.
- *Mechanical:* remove the weight.

Surgical techniques:

- *Fasanella–Servat:* Müller's muscle shortening with additional resection of part of conjunctiva and superior third of tarsal plate
- *Excision of segment of levator aponeurosis:* through posterior or anterior approach. Excise transverse segment of levator and resuture the incised edges to correct the ptosis.
- *Excision of segment of levator palpebrae superiosis:* through an anterior or posterior approach. The amount resected depends on the levator function and the degree of ptosis.
- *Frontalis sling:* harvest fascia lata. Place sling in U or W shape. Place stab incisions in the brow and upper eyelid. Pass a needle, pass a wire and snare the fascia. The placement of fascia on the lid should be as close to the tarsus as possible and as distally as possible. This fibrous tissue will hold whereas a sling placed in orbicularis will relax with time.
- *Frontalis myofascial flap from eyebrow:* the frontalis originates from galea and ends in the skin at the eyebrow region. Some fibres interlace with orbicularis. A superiorly based flap can be isolated and advanced downwards and attached to the tarsal plate. Frontalis power is measured by marking the inferior margin of the eyebrow arch and measuring the elevation. The flap is elevated through an incision where the superior palpebral fold should be. The flap is fixed to the midtarsal level with silk.

Complications: the commonest technical error is in suturing the edge of Whitnall's ligament to the tarsal plate. Also under- and over- correction, dry eyes, bleeding.

Pulleys

- Thickened areas within the <u>Flexor sheath</u> which enclose the Flexor tendons. In finger there is the palmar aponeurosis (PA), 5 annular pulleys and 3 cruciform pulleys. PA pulley is the transverse fibres of palmar fascia. Annular pulleys—odd numbers are over joints (A1 over MCPJ, A3 over PIPJ, A5 over DIPJ).
- The pulleys keep the tendon close to the bone, preventing bowstringing without restricting joint movement. They also help to distribute the flexor tendon excursion across the digital joints.

Annular pulleys:

- *A2 and A4:* are the most critical pulleys to prevent bowstringing.
- *A1:* is 10 mm long. It is attached to the volar plate and distally to the proximal phalanx.
- *A2:* is the strongest and longest at 17 mm. It is attached to the proximal half of the proximal phalanx.
- *A3:* thin band 3 mm long over the PIPJ, attached to volar plate.
- *A4*: mid-portion of middle phalanx, 8 mm long.
- *A5:* very thin over DIPJ volar plate, often absent.

Cruciate pulleys:

- Enable the sheath to conform to the position of flexion.
- C1 and C3 are most frequently found. In the thumb there is one oblique pulley at the level of the shaft of the proximal phalanx. It is 11 mm in length. It extends obliquely in a distal radial direction.

Thumb: have an A1 pulley overlying MCP joint and an A2 pulley overlying IPJ and an oblique pulley. The latter is considered the most important.

Pulvertaft weave

See FLEXOR TENDON. *See* LATE RECONSTRUCTION.

Pyoderma gangrenosum

- An autoinflammatory disorder characterized by rapidly enlarging, painful skin ulcers with purple/blue edges and pathergy (the development of ulcers following minor trauma).
- It is often associated with ulcerative colitis (50% of patients).
- Also other gastrointestinal disorders, such as diverticulosis, regional enteritis, peptic ulcer disease, hepatitis and carcinoid tumour.

- Associated with rheumatoid arthritis, pulmonary diseases and haematological disorders.
- No associations with 20% of the patients with pyoderma gangrenosum.
- No specific organism associated.
- The basic lesion may be a necrotizing cutaneous vasculitis.
- The course is protracted and, in some instances, fulminant.

Treatment:

- Diagnosis is confirmed on histology which shows a neutrophilic infiltrate. Samples should also be taken for microbiology to exclude infection.
- Local and systemic steroid therapy, other immunosuppressives (e.g. azathioprine, methotrexate) and biologics (e.g. infliximab) have been helpful. Local injections may cause local skin trauma, which may induce new pyoderma gangrenosum lesions.
- Systemic and topical antibiotic therapy can be used as supportive treatments but do not form the mainstay.
- Surgery reserved as a last resort due to potential exacerbation. Conservative debridement may be required for grossly necrotic tissues. Do not incise the adjacent intact tissues, to avoid extension of the disease beyond the operative debridement. Reconstruction should be delayed until the active disease stage has resolved.

Pyogenic granuloma

- A proliferation of capillaries often at a site of trauma.
- There may be an associated infection, but the condition is not an infective process.
- They rarely appear before the age of 6 months, frequently occur in children, but may occur at any age.
- They are rapidly growing in the early stages, later remaining unchanged. They have a pliable surface and bleed easily.
- Red or blue-black, haemorrhagic.
- Most commonly found on the face and distal extremities.
- They may be excised or destroyed with diathermy, laser or silver nitrate. They may recur. Vascular proliferation may be deep and therefore may require excision.

Q-switched laser to Quantitative microbiology

Q-switched laser

- Q-switching is when one of the resonating mirrors is non-reflective for an interval of pumping, which produces a pulsed output beam and allows for a very high peak power.
- Stored energy is emitted as a pulse of light 10 billionths of a second in length.
- 3 available—ruby (694 nm), YAG (1064 nm or 532 nm) and alexandrite (760 nm).

See TATTOO. *See* LASER.

Quaba flap

- A distally-based dorsal metacarpal artery (DCMA) flap described by Quaba and Davison in 1990. Most commonly used to resurface dorsal surface of proximal digits (index or middle finger).
- Based on a skin perforator from the dorsal metacarpal artery present at the level of the neck of the metacarpal approximately 0.5–1 cm proximal to the metacarpophalangeal joint (MCPJ) and just distal to the juncturae tendinum. The anatomy is most reliable on the radial side of the hand from the 2nd or 3rd DCMA.
- *Flap raise:* a Doppler can locate the perforator in the second or third intermetacarpal space. The skin paddle is designed using reverse planning as an ellipse between the metacarpals and can extend proximally to the wrist crease. Incise a longitudinal edge of the flap down to paratenon then raise proximally to distally. The pedicle is identified distal to the intertendinous connection. The flap is islanded, avoiding skeletonization of the pedicle in order to preserve the small veins in the connective tissue. The flap can be rotated up to 180° into the defect.

See MARUYAMA FLAP.

Quadrangular (quadrilateral) space

Defined by the long head of triceps medially, teres major inferiorly, teres minor superiorly, humerus laterally. The posterior circumflex artery and axillary nerve pass through it.

Quadriga syndrome

Diminished grip strength caused by tethering or tightening of one flexor tendon thus creating laxity and reducing power in remaining flexors. Derived from the Roman chariots with 4 horses on one rein and coined by Verdan.

See AMPUTATION.

Quickert's procedure

Preferred procedure to treat involutional entropion by correcting horizontal lid laxity, attenuation of lid retractors and overriding orbicularis oculi.

Radial artery
- Radial artery runs superficially in the forearm from the division with the brachial artery to its exit under APL.
- It first lies on pronator teres beneath brachioradialis then on the radial head of FDS and FPL. Gives branches to the fascial plexus and on to the skin, radius and muscles. Accompanied by 2 or more venae comitantes.
- Runs medial to APL and EPB.
- Passes deep to these to cross the anatomic snuff box.
- It enters the palm between two heads of the 1st dorsal interosseous muscle and is covered by AP.
- It gives off princeps pollicis which gives the two thumb digital arteries.
- It runs medially between interosseus and AP to become the main component of the deep palmar arch.
- A dorsal branch joins a branch from ulnar artery to become the dorsal carpal arch.

Radial dysplasia
- Formerly known as radial club hand.
- Congenital longitudinal radial ray deficiency.
- May affect all preaxial structures from shoulder to hand. May involve thumb and/or index finger
- Wrist unstable and hand radially deviated, flexed and pronated. ROM of fingers reduced.
- Often other syndromes.
- No known aetiology.
- 50% bilateral.

Classification: *Bayne and Klug*. Type IV most common: 50-90% of cases.

Prevalence:
- 1:55,000. 0.5-10% of congenital hands.
- Bilateral > unilateral. M:F 3:2. Absence > partial absence.

Aetiology: may be sporadic, syndromic, or associated with thalidomide or valproic acid.

Associations: *see* FANCONI'S ANAEMIA. *See* TAR SYNDROME. *See* HOLT-ORAM SYNDROME. *See* VACTERL ASSOCIATION.

Clinical features:
- Short forearm, bowed radially, hypoplastic or absent radius with anlage (fibrous band).
- Hand radially deviated. Skin deficient radially.
- Elbow stiff and extended (may be due to synostosis) but improves with age and determines when to operate.
- Hypoplasia of radial structures such as radial nerve.
- Reduced wrist movement. Check mobility. Carpus is deviated radially and displaced palmarly. The scaphoid and trapezium are usually absent in type III and IV.
- Muscles abnormal (both extensors and flexors) and relate to severity of the radial ray deficiency. Muscles most commonly affected are pectoralis major, brachioradialis, supinator, extensor carpi radialis, flexor carpi radialis, muscles of thumb. FDS is usually present but abnormally fused to FDP with absence of index tendon. EDC is usually present but fused with ECRL or EDM. Thumb extrinsics are usually absent.
- *Nerves:* ulnar nerve normal, musculocutaneous nerve is missing. Median nerve supplies anterior compartment, radial nerve often terminates at elbow after supplying triceps. Sensation radially is supplied by median nerve with an anastomosis to ulnar nerve.
- *Arteries:* radial artery often absent or small. Interosseous arteries are well developed.

Treatment principles:
- *I:* do nothing or lengthen.
- *II:* lengthen.
- *III and IV:* centralize or radialize.

  Treatment: regular manipulation and splinting. Operate between 6-18 months of age.

- *Centralize:* carpus on ulna by carpal excision and transfer radial wrist muscles to ulna side, closing wedge osteotomy. Stabilize with a pin through the 3rd metacarpal.
- *Radialize:* requires full passive correction. Place the scaphoid over the ulna and secure with a pin through 2nd metacarpal. Transfer

FCR to ulnar side of carpus to reduce radial deviating force.
- *Pollicization:* release constricting radial soft tissue.
- Later may require ulnar osteotomy, distraction lengthening or fusion.

Operative technique:
- Bilobed flap to make use of redundant ulnar skin. Preserve dorsal veins and sensory nerves. Beware the radial-median nerve just under the skin on the radial side.
- Incise extensor retinaculum and identify radial extensors and flexors. They may be fused. If present detach BR, FCR, ECRL, ECRB. Protect and retract finger extensors, and find ECU, FCU and ulnar nerve and artery.
- Incise dorsal and palmar wrist capsule transversely to release ulno-carpal joint, but preserve ulnar collateral ligament. Dissect distal ulnar head avoiding damage to cartilage and epiphysis.
- Excise residual fibrotic tissue until hand is easy to move, attached only by skin, tendons and NVBs.
- Transpose with carpal bones over ulnar head and fix with pin passed retrograde through ulna then into 2nd metacarpal.
- If ulna is markedly bowed or there is marked soft tissue contracture, perform wedge osteotomy of ulna.
- Suture back capsule. Radial tendons may be transposed, but may be atrophic. Shorten and tighten ECU. Close bilobed flap.
- Long arm plaster for 6–8 weeks, then removable splint until 6 year.

Complications: recurrent deformity, premature distal ulnar epiphyseal closure.

Outcome: determined by presence of thumb, wrist motion, digital motion and ulnar length.
See CONGENITAL HAND ANOMALIES.

Radial forearm flap
- First described in 1978 as a proximally based free flap. Distally based pedicled flap described in 1981.
- One of the thinnest fasciocutaneous flaps in the body. Can also be osseocutaneous or fascia only.
- *Arterial supply:* radial artery—lies underneath BR proximally then between FCR and BR in the distal third; it gives off most of its perforators here: 9–17 branches.
- *Veins:* both the deep and superficial systems play a part—the deep radial venae commitantes have collateral branches that allow circumvention of the valves to permit retrograde

venous flow for a reverse-based flap. The superficial system (i.e. cephalic vein) provides a reliable source for the anterograde flap.
- Flap can be taken with the lateral antebrachial nerve (extension of musculocutaneous) to provide sensory supply.
- *Complications:*
  ○ *Circulation:* sacrifice of the radial artery can jeopardize hand circulation—this can be avoided with perforator-based flaps;
  ○ Venous congestion is a risk in reverse flaps. There is an option to super charge a retained superficial vein to a dorsal hand vein;
  ○ *Donor site:* often needs a skin graft unless the flap is very narrow;
  ○ *Nerve injury:* the superficial radial nerve and lateral antebrachial cutaneous nerves are at risk.

Operative steps in raising the flap:
- Mark the arm pre-operatively to ensure anaesthetist does not place any lines in the ipsilateral arm.
- Allen's test pre-operatively to test arterial dominance in hand.
- Arm out on arm board, padded arm tourniquet.
- Landmarks:
  ○ FCR, BR, PL.
- Feel radial pulse and mark likely course. Mark cephalic vein.
- Mark skin paddle to incorporate vessels—beware that the more radial skin will be hair-bearing.
- Raise starts distally deep to fascia but leaving paratenon. Locate the radial artery between FCR and BR—needs ligation to proceed with raise. Going proximally, BR will need to be retracted as the artery goes beneath it. Will need to ligate multiple branches going deeply—but be careful to leave perforators going into flap. Be careful not to injure SBRN.
- Small defects can be closed primarily. Most require skin graft.

Radial nerve
- Radial nerve from posterior cord—C5–T1.
- Passes along the spiral groove beneath the lateral head of triceps.
- Through the lateral intermuscular septum 10–15 cm proximal to the lateral epicondyle.
- Continues between brachialis and biceps with brachioradialis and ECRL laterally. Motor branches to 3 muscles come off before the elbow. It divides at the elbow into superficial and deep (posterior interosseous.). PIN goes deep to supinator (arcade of Frohse).

Superficial radial nerve: passes between tendons of brachioradialis and ECRL near the midforearm, and pierces the deep fascia to become subcutaneous. It runs towards the snuff box superficial to APL and EPB. It gives sensory branches to the dorsum of thumb to radial half of ring finger and hand.

Radial tunnel syndrome

- The most frequent site for radial tunnel compression is the arcade of Frohse.
- Sites of compression:
  - A fibrous band tethering nerve to the radiohumeral joint;
  - *The leash of Henry:* radial recurrent vessels, which pass across the radial nerve;
  - The tendinous margin of ECRB;
  - *The arcade of Frohse:* a fibrous band on the surface of supinator.

Symptoms:
- Pain is the predominant symptom. It can be confused with tennis elbow. Motor and sensory disturbance is uncommon.
- Pain on extension of middle finger is positive in radial tunnel syndrome. Nerve conduction studies are unreliable.

Treatment: surgical decompression from posterior muscle splitting or anterior approach.

See RADIAL TUNNEL SYNDROME. *See* POSTERIOR INTEROSSEOUS SYNDROME. *See* WARTENBERG'S SYNDROME.

Radiation

See HEALING. *Acute effects* include erythema, inflammation, oedema, ulceration. *Late effects*: depigmentation, atrophy, fibrosis, necrosis, neoplasia.

Radiation injury: caused by:
- DNA disruption that can cause a lethal injury or cell death from disruption of division.
- O_2 free radicals that are directly toxic.

Early and late effects:
- *Early:* inflammatory response with erythema and hyperpigmentation.
- *Late:* fibrosis, pigment changes:
  - Endothelial cell, capillary and arteriole damage with loss of blood vessels in the affected area and hypoperfusion;
  - Fibroblasts proliferate less and collagen is deficient;
  - Lymphatics are damaged causing oedema and infection;
  - Keratinocytes are injured; dry desquamation if there are enough cells to replace the dead ones; moist desquamation if the dermis is exposed in places and an

ulcer if all epidermis and adnexal structures are destroyed.

Treatment: local wound care, flaps from outside the radiated field, and hyperbaric oxygen.

Technique: absorbed radiation is measured in grays (Gy). 1 joule/kg = 1 Gy = 100 rads. The therapeutic dose for carcinoma is tissue dependent, but range from 45 to 80 Gy.

- *Fractionating irradiation:* allows treatment of the cancer, while not exceeding tolerance of the surrounding normal tissue. The dose for tumour irradiation is indexed to tumour volume. Also only dividing cells will be killed so that fractionating will target more cells.
- *Altered fractionation:* is external beam radiation outside the conventional treatment.
- *Hyperfractionation:* is used for rapidly growing tumours—smaller doses every 6 hours.
- *Accelerated fractionation:* is the same total dose over a shorter period.
- *Hypofractionation:* is used as palliation of advanced tumours.

Principles: ionizing radiation occurs as either electromagnetic waves or particulate forms. Electromagnetic radiation used therapeutically is as short wavelengths, such as X-rays and gamma rays. Also discrete energy packets called photons. Particulate irradiation consists of small energized particles such as electrons, neutrons, protons, alpha particles and others.

Delivery: by external beam e.g. linear accelerators or by *Brachytherapy*. External beam is applied in daily fraction of 200 cGy/day over a 5–6 weeks course. Brachytherapy allows continuous radiation. Photons are short pulses of high energy. Absorption depends on their energy level. High-energy megavoltage treatments are used for deep-seated tumours as they pass through the skin and are therefore skin sparing. Low-energy photons are used for superficial lesions.

Carcinogen: ionizing radiation including electromagnetic (X-rays and gamma rays) and particulate radiation (electrons, protons, neutrons, α-particles) cause change by ionizing cell constituents. A single exposure may produce a tumour after a long latent period.

Tolerance dose: of different tissues and organs has been established as the likelihood of treatment-related complications in 5 years using conventional fractionation. So if complications will occur in 50%, it is expressed as TD 50/5. The dose likely to eradicate a tumour is for example TD5 = 5% of tumours will be eradicated. The sensitivity of normal tissues is the LD (lethal dose). So LD50 is the dose which will kill 50% of normal cells.

See HYPERBARIC OXYGEN.

Radiation treatment of head and neck cancer: *see* HEAD AND NECK CANCER.

Indications: for small lesions RT may be as effective as surgery. For larger lesions both are required. When combined, survival is not particularly improved. Pre-operative RT is thought to eradicate subclinical disease and prevent tumour implantation and possibly make more tumours operable. However, it interferes with healing. Post-operative RT is indicated for large tumours, nodes with extracapsular involvement and for vascular and perineural invasion. As healing has already occurred, higher doses can be given.

Outcome: T1 or T2 tumours do well with either surgery or RT with 80% disease-free for 3 years. 30% survival for T3–4.

Complications:
- *Acute:* mucositis, loss of taste, xerostomia with dryness, which is permanent and progressive.
- *Chronic:* progressive. Dry uncomfortable mucous membranes. Atrophic skin with poor healing. Oral hygiene should be good to prevent loss of teeth. Osteoradionecrosis can be a serious problem requiring hemimandibulectomy. Carcinogenesis. Spontaneous fistulization, carotid blow out.

Radiotherapy for sarcomas:
Most *Sarcomas* are radiosensitive to varying degrees. Ewing's sarcomas are very radio-sensitive. Liposarcomas are reasonably radiosensitive. Post-operative radiotherapy reduces the risk of local recurrence. Radiotherapy typically consists of 50 Gy delivered in 25 fractions over 5 weeks. Indications for post-operative radiotherapy include high-grade tumours, incompletely excised tumours, tumours >5 cm in diameter, deep head and neck sarcomas.

Radio-ulnar synostosis
Proximal forearm, 60% bilateral.

- *Primary:* no radial head and extensive synostosis.
- *Secondary:* radial head normal, but dislocated.
- Get fixed pronation, but hypermobile wrist.
- XR shows heavy bowed radius.
- Restoring rotation is unsuccessful:
  - Mild or unilateral, no treatment;
  - Severe, do rotational osteotomy, synostosis may occur in metacarpal.

Ramsay–Hunt syndrome
Post-infective facial nerve palsy. *See* FACIAL NERVE RE-ANIMATION.

Random pattern flaps
See FLAPS. No directional blood supply. Not based on any known vessel. Include local flaps to the face. Length breadth ratio is 1:1 in the lower extremity, but up to 1:6 in the face.

Ravitch technique
- Operative technique for the correction of *Pectus excavatum*.
- Elevate perichondrial flaps and resect involved costal cartilage (4–5 on each side, preserve costochondral junction).
- Divide xiphoid process to allow sternal elevation.
- Posterior transverse osteotomy of superior sternum and fracture sternum forwards.
- Bone wedge used to stabilize the sternum.
- Stabilize sternum with wires to ribs.
- Bilateral pectoralis flaps to cover sternum.

Raynaud's disease
- Vasospastic disease of small vessels of unknown aetiology with intermittent episodes of skin colour and temperature change.
- Raynaud's phenomenon has an underlying disorder such as scleroderma, RA or cryoglobulinaemia.

Investigations:
- Bone scan:
  - *Phase 1:* within 2 minutes of injection shows nucleotide in the vascular system;
  - *Phase 2:* 5–10 min, shows nucleotide diffusing into soft tissue;
  - *Phase 3:* 2–3 hours, binding to skeletal structures;
  - In Raynaud's get decreased perfusion in phase 1 and 2, sympathetic block may help to establish the sympathetic contribution.

Conservative treatment:
- Stop smoking.
- Prevent cold exposure.
- *Drugs:* calcium channel blockers, serotonin receptor blocker (Ketanserin) topical nitroglycerin, and alpha-adrenergic blockers such as reserpine. Reserpine has been the most valuable.

Surgery:
- Principally sympathectomy.
- Cervicothoracic sympathectomy only provides short-term improvement.
- Distal sympathectomy provides longer-term relief. The radial artery receives sympathetic nerves from the radial nerve and lateral cutaneous nerve. The ulnar artery receives 3 branches from the ulnar nerve and one from the medial cutaneous nerve of the forearm.

r

- *Digital sympathectomy:* the sympathetic fibres to the digital vessels ramify in the adventitia so adventitia stripping will provide effective sympathectomy. Results are best with pure vasospasm.

  See VASOSPASTIC DISORDERS.

Reagan's test
- Test for lunotriquestral instability.
- Press the thumb on the lunate dorsally and the index finger on triquestrum volarly.
- Compare with *Masquelet's test*.

  See CARPAL INSTABILITY.

Recall phenomenon
- Seen in *Extravasation injuries*.
- An inflammatory reaction at the site of a previous extravasation injury following recommencement of administration of the toxic substance (mostly seen with doxorubicin).

Rectus abdominus flap
- Vertical muscle from xiphoid to pubic symphysis. Type 3 muscle with dual dominant vascular pedicle. All of the overlying skin can be based on the musculocutaneous perforators.
- The muscle is contained beneath the anterior rectus sheath throughout its entirety. Above the arcuate line (midway between umbilicus and pubis) it has the posterior rectus sheath behind it.
- Superior pedicle is the superior epigastric artery from the internal mammary—it pierces the posterior rectus sheath behind the 7th costal cartilage to enter the medial posterior surface of the muscle. The inferior pedicle is the deep inferior epigastric artery from the external iliac and is larger calibre. It enters the muscle 3–4 cm below the arcuate line giving off 1–3 substantial musculocutaneous perforators.
- Innervation—ventral rami of lower 6–7 segmental thoracic spine.
- The two anastomose within the rectus muscle bulk at around the level of the umbilicus.

Flap raise:
- Position—supine.
- Landmarks: xiphoid, public symphysis, umbilicus.
- Markings:
  - *Muscle flap:* vertical paramedian incision over muscle;
  - *Musculocutaneous flap:* skin paddle can be vertical or transverse.

- Raise (for muscle flap):
  - Dissection down to rectus sheath;
  - Split anterior rectus sheath vertically;
  - Retract the lateral border of the muscle medially to expose the pedicle—can trace down to the origin near the pubis—can then divide the muscle inferiorly under direct vision;
  - The superior portion of the muscle can be encircled and divided—must securely ligate the SEA;
  - The muscle is now islanded on the DIEA.
- Close the defect by closing the anterior rectus sheath.

Rectus femoris flap
Anatomy:
- One of the quadriceps.
- Originates at the ASIS, inserts into patellar tendon.

Blood supply:
- The lateral femoral circumflex vessels, running from medial to lateral.
- 2–3 branches enter the muscle in the proximal third, 10 cm below ASIS.
- A secondary supply is located 2 cm below the primary supply.

Reconstruction:
- Elevate through a lateral thigh incision.
- After transposition, approximate vastus lateralis and medialis.
- Good for reconstructing the lower abdominal wall. The tip reaches between the xiphoid and umbilicus.
- The mutton chop flap is an extended rectus femoris myocutaneous flap.
- Get slight weakness of knee extension.

  See ABDOMINAL WALL RECONSTRUCTION. *See* PRESSURE SORES.

Reflex sympathetic dystrophy
See COMPLEX REGIONAL PAIN SYNDROME (CRPS).

Regnault's classification
Classification for the grading of breast ptosis:
- *1st degree (minor):* nipple-areolar complex (NAC) at or slightly above inframammary fold.
- *2nd degree (moderate):* NAC below the inframammary fold, but on the anterior projection of the breast mound.
- *3rd degree (major):* NAC is in the dependent position. If very severe the nipple points downwards.
- *Pseudoptosis:* the NAC remains above the inframammary fold, but the breast mound descends below the inframammary fold with glandular hypoplasia.

- *Glandular ptosis:* the breast is normal except that the breast mound has descended below the inframammary fold.

  See MASTOPEXY.

Rendu–Osler–Weber disease
Hereditary haemorrhagic telangiectasia (HHT).

- Occurs in 1–2 per 100,000 births.
- A group of autosomal disorders of similar phenotype caused by several genes. The homozygous form is lethal.
- Get multisystem vascular dysplasia and recurrent haemorrhage.
- Spider-like bright-red maculopapules, 1–4 mm in diameter occur on the face, mucous membranes, fingers and nail beds. Also on internal mucosal surfaces.
- They usually present after puberty and increase in number with age.
- Epistaxis is the most common presenting symptom.
- Arteriovenous malformations may develop in the brain, spinal cord, liver and lungs.
- Septic emboli from pulmonary AVMs may cause brain abscesses.

  See TELANGIECTASES.

Replantation
- Single digit replants distal to FDS insertion give good results. Zone 2 replants may have poorer functional results and require extensive hand therapy. Replants distal to the DIPJ/beyond the trifurcation of the NVBs are technically difficult and not often attempted in the U.K. Important to counsel any patient carefully about recovery time and likely functional outcomes and discuss alternative options.
- *Multiple digit:* thumb has highest priority followed by middle or ring finger to give grasp and pinch. Little finger important for power grip. Index finger is most dispensible.
- *Storage:* place part in damp normal saline gauze and place in sealed bag surrounded by ice-saline bath to maintain at 4°C. Never place directly on ice.
- *Absolute indications:* for replantation. Thumb, multiple digits, paediatric, mid-carpal wrist or distal forearm.
- *Relative indications:* single digit distal to FDS, proximal limb in child.
- *Ischaemic time:* measure from time of amputation to replantation. Warm ischaemic time should be <6 hours if proximal to the wrist or <12 hours for fingers though survival after 42 hours of warm ischaemia has been reported. Cold ischaemic time should be <24 hours for fingers.

Operation:
- Start by operating on the amputated part. Use 2 midlateral incisions and tag structures. Tag tendons and veins as well as the NVB. Insert choice of bony fixation. Low threshold to shorten bone on amputated part to facilitate ease of vessel anastomosis.
- Bony fixation can occur by a range of methods including K-wires, dental intraosseous wires, plates and intramedullary nails.
- Veins grafts may be required if there is significant trauma to the vessels and superficial veins can be harvested from the volar wrist (mark pre-operatively with tourniquet up). Digital arteries can be transposed or a digital artery from an adjacent healthy finger can be used.
- If there is flow across the anastomosis but no perfusion then there may be spasm distally. Keep digit warm. Try topical papaverine. Heparin or 50,000–100,000 units of streptokinase or urokinase can be used.

Treatment of the failing replant:
- *Poor inflow:* reduce dressing and ensure there is no constriction. A marcaine block can be given at the wrist. Papaverine can be injected through the skin incision. If there is no improvement proceed to surgical exploration. Thrombosis should be resected and vein grafted. Heparinize.
- *Poor outflow:* leech therapy or chemical leeching using heparin-soaked swabs on de-epithelialized patch or directly onto sterile matrix after removing the nail plate.

Retinacular system
There are 4 layers of fascia in the palm. The retinacular system has several important functions. The attachment of retaining ligaments to the skin enhances stability. It also provides fascial compartments for hand structures.

Palmar fascia:
- *Midpalmar fascia:* triangular in shape. Proximally it is attached to palmaris longus or transverse carpal ligament. It extends to the base of the fingers and has longitudinal, transverse and vertical fibres. Longitudinal fibres can be superficial or deep.
- *Longitudinal fibres:* superficial fibres are the pretendinous bands palmar to the flexor tendons and sheaths. They diverge as they approach the MCP joints. The central fibres run parallel to the flexor tendons. The band to index angles radially to the radial side of the MCPJ and the band to the little finger does the opposite. The bands are attached to skin. Most end at the palmar skin crease. Some

bifurcate at the MCP level and extend into fingers to contribute to the spiral bands of Gosset. The deep longitudinal fibres pass distally beneath the natatory ligament to insert into the lateral digital sheet.

- *Vertical fibres:* a deep system divides the midpalmar space into several compartments. The superficial vertical fibres pierce the palmar fat pad to anchor skin to the palmar aponeurosis. The septa of Legueu and Juvara originate from the palmar fascia at the level of the proximal edge of the flexor tendon sheath and pass dorsally between the lateral surfaces of the A1 pulleys and the digital neurovascular bundles. They attach to the deep transverse metacarpal ligament at the point of insertion of the volar plate of the MCPJ. There are fewer vertical fibres over the thenar and hypothenar eminence giving a relative laxity here.
- *Transverse fibres:* thin strong shiny fibres which run transversely deep to the pretendinous bands in the distal palm just proximal to the A1 pulley. The vertical fibres pass between the transverse fibres forming the A0 pulley. The transverse fibres are not involved in Dupuytren's contracture.
- *Natatory ligaments* (in web spaces).

Retaining ligaments of the digits:

- These stabilize the skin and the extensor mechanism and support the neurovascular bundles.
- *Grayson's ligament* (dorsal). Extend to the middle phalanges.
- *Cleland's ligaments* (volar). Extend to the middle phalanges.
- *Landsmeer ligaments* (oblique retinacular and transverse retinacular).
- *The spiral band:* a fibrous condensation formed by the pretendinous band, natatory ligament, and vertical septa. Distal to the natatory ligament it progresses to the digit as the lateral digital sheet.

See DUPUYTREN'S CONTRACTURE.

Retromolar trigone carcinoma

- The retromolar trigone is a poorly defined area covered under the terms 'posterior floor of the mouth', 'posterior alveolus' and 'anterior tonsillar pillar'.
- The main points of significance about this region are that diagnosis may be delayed, the region is less accessible, and reconstruction is more difficult.

See HEAD AND NECK CANCER.

Rhabdomyosarcoma

- Sarcoma that tends to occur in younger children.
- Often involves the orbit and usually doesn't metastasize.
- Surgery, irradiation and chemotherapy has improved the 5-year survival to 55%.
- Most failures are due to local recurrence, so wider excision will improve local control and obviate the need for RT.

Rheumatoid arthritis

- Affects 2% of the population. F:M 3:1. 90% have hand involvement, 10% have significant hand involvement. 15% get severe disease.
- *Aetiology:* autoimmune reaction to an unknown agent in synovial tissue. Antigen interacts with IgG and IgM antibodies to produce synovial inflammation. 70% RhF +ve (IgG or IgM abs in serum). 50–80% of RA patients are positive for RhF or anti-citrullinated protein antibody (ACPA) or both. ACPA is more sensitive and specific.
- American College of Rheumatology 2010 *Criteria for diagnosis* replaces the previously widely used 1987 criteria: Based on a points system, with a score of 6 or above diagnostic for RA:
  - Number and size of joints involved (0–5 points);
  - RhF or ACPA serology (0–3 points);
  - CRP or ESR abnormal (0–1 points);
  - Duration of symptoms >6 weeks (0–1 points);

  Typical XR findings can also lead to diagnosis.

Classification:

- *Monoarthropathy:* 1 joint, pauciarthropathy 2–4 joints, polyarthropathy >4.
- *Clinical course:* monocyclic (one attack) or polycyclic. Progressive if worsening.
- *3 phases:* proliferative, destructive and reparative.

Pathology: 5 stages

- Macrophages in synovium ingest and present foreign antigens to T cells, which initiates B cells to produce antibodies.
- B cells proliferate. Angiogenesis occurs and synovial cells proliferate. Chronic inflammation is perpetuated. Expansive hyperplasia within synovium forms a pannus.
- Patient becomes symptomatic with warm swollen joints.
- Synovial pannus invades cartilage, bone, ligaments and tendons.
- Damage produces joint destruction, contractures and tendon ruptures. Cartilage is

destroyed. Subchondral bone is eroded. Synovium expands and joint capsule is stretched with ligament destruction. Joint instability and subluxation.

Non-articular manifestation:

- *Eyes:* iritis, scleritis, uveitis. Sjögren's syndrome (dry eyes, dry mouth, RA).
- *Nervous system:* polyneuropathy, carpal tunnel syndrome.
- *Blood:* anaemia, Felty's syndrome (RA with splenomegaly and neutropenia).
- *Heart:* pericarditis, myocarditis, pericardial effusions.
- *Lungs:* pleural effusions, rheumatoid nodules, Caplan's syndrome (nodular pulmonary fibrosis in RA exposed to industrial dusts).
- *Kidneys:* amyloidosis.
- *Skin:* vasculitic ulcers, rheumatoid nodules are present in 20% of patients.

Investigations:

- RhF and ACPA serology.
- CRP and ESR. Also useful to monitor disease progression once diagnosis established.
- *XR:* soft tissue swelling, peri-articular osteoporosis, erosions, and loss of joint space.

Non-surgical treatment:

- Mainstay of treatment for RA. The advent of effective medical treatment has largely obviated the need for surgery for many patients.
- Disease modifying antirheumatic drugs (DMARDs) are first line: methotrexate, sulfasalazine, leflunomide, hydroxychloroquine, gold. Side effects can be limiting.
- Biologic agents including TNF-α inhibitors (e.g. adalimumab, etanercept, infliximab), IL-1 inhibitors, IL-6 inhibitors, T cell inhibitors and B cell inhibitors reduce inflammation.
- Diet, rest, exercise, splint and medication.

Surgery:

- *Rheumatoid nodules.*
- *Tenosynovitis.*
- *Tendon rupture.*

Indications: for pain, function, prophylactic (to prevent further deformity) and for cosmetic improvement.

Surgical options: synovectomy, arthroplasty, tendon repair/replacement/repositioning, and arthrodesis.

Wrist RA: Pannus occurs in the volar radiocarpal ligaments. Scaphoid becomes unstable. Get volar flexion of scaphoid, carpal collapse and distal ulna subluxation. Carpus supinates on radius with ulna translation.

- Synovectomy.
- *Darrach procedure.*
- Arthroplasty (not commonly performed).
- *Arthrodesis:* gives stability, but sacrifices wrist movement.
- *Limited carpal fusion:* may be possible as the midcarpal joint may be spared.

Dorsal tenosynovitis:

- Proliferative tenosynovitis leads to a swelling that may cause tendon rupture due to synovial infiltration, abrasion (*Vaughn–Jackson syndrome*).
- Perform dorsal synovectomy and place extensor retinaculum under the tendons.

Extensor tendon rupture:

- Starts from ulnar to radial.
- Repair by adjacent suturing, EIP transfer or FDS-4 transfer.

Flexor tenosynovitis:

- Present with pain on flexion and decreased movement with crepitus. Tendon rupture may occur.
- Treatment is by flexor synovectomy.

Flexor tendon rupture:

- FPL is the commonest to rupture (*Mannerfelt lesion*).
- Treat with direct repair, graft, and FDS transfer. FDP rupture in the palm—attach stump to adjacent tendon.
- For FDP rupture in the finger perform DIPJ stabilization.

MCP joint:

- Get ligament disruption by pannus. Cartilage and bone destruction remove stability. Wrist radial deviation alters balance of finger deviators. Radial sagittal band attenuation. Tightened ulnar intrinsics.
- *Treatment:* synovectomy. Soft tissue alignment with intrinsic release, crossed intrinsic transfer and extensor tendon stabilization, *Arthroplasty*.

See SWAN NECK DEFORMITY. See BOUTONNIÈRE DEFORMITY.

Thumb deformities:

- *Classification: Nalebuff.*
- *Aetiology:*
  - Boutonnières occurs when the pannus affects the dorsal MCP joint structures leading to flexion and subluxation;
  - Hyperextension of IPJ caused by EPL;

○ Swan neck occurs when the CMC joint ligaments are destabilized with dorsal subluxation, adduction contracture and compensatory hyperextension of the MCP joint.
• *Treatment:* depends on the stage of disease.
   ○ For flexible Boutonnières treat by synovectomy and extensor reconstruction;
   ○ MCP joint arthrodesis;
   ○ Swan necks are treated with CMC arthroplasty.

Rheumatoid factor

IgM autoantibody to IgG immunoglobulin. Not specific to RA. Patients with RA who are negative tend to have a milder disease.

Rheumatoid nodules

• Collagenous matrix over bony prominence. Commonly over olecranon. Can appear on the dorsum of the fingers.
• Probably over areas of attrition with microvascular damage and complement cascade and chronic inflammation.
• Histologically get central fibrous tissue surrounded by macrophages which show pallisading. As it expands get central necrosis.
• More common in males.
• They occur in 25% of patients with RA and are associated with aggressive disease.
• Surgery is indicated for relief of symptoms and cosmesis. Recurrence is common.

Rhinophyma

A severe form of acne *Rosacea* affecting the nose. There are 4 stages of rosacea, the 4th being rhinophyma.

Pathology: possibly the vascular instability leads to fluid in dermis with inflammation and fibrosis. Sebaceous ducts become plugged. Get a lymphocytic infiltrate.

Epidemiology:

• Rosacea is common with a higher incidence in women though rhinophyma is more common in men possibly due to the androgenic influence.
• More common in English and Irish descent with a familial component.
• Rosacea begins in the 30s, acne rosacea in the 40s and rhinophyma in the 50s.
• Triggers may include UV radiation, temperature change, alcohol use, spicy foods and exercise. Skin tumours can easily be missed within rhinophyma or mimic rhinophyma.

Treatment:

• *Non-surgical:* rosacea is treated with topical and oral antibiotics and retinoids. None has

been shown to halt progression to rhinophyma. Irradiation has been reported to be successful for rhinophyma.
• *Surgical:* the mainstay of treatment is surgical. There are many treatments such as dermabrasion, cryosurgery, shave excision and CO_2 laser therapy. No one method has been shown to give superior results. All skin should be sent for histology. Only graft for severe nodular rhinophyma or underlying malignancy.

Rhinoplasty

Challenging as the anatomy is variable, form and function must be corrected and it is highly visible.

Anatomy:

• The external nose consists of an osseocartilaginous framework which can be divided into upper, middle and lower thirds.
• The upper third, or bony vault, consists of nasal bones and frontal process of maxilla, which overlaps the cartilage—upper lateral and dorsal septum.
• The middle third, or upper cartilaginous vault, consists of paired upper lateral cartilages which meet at the dorsal cartilaginous septum. The internal angle between these two is the internal nasal valve, and should be 10-15°.
• The lower third, or lower cartilaginous vault, consists of paired lower lateral cartilages (also called alar cartilages) which meet to form the nasal tip. Each alar cartilage has a medial, middle and lateral crus. The external nasal valve is in this third and is formed from the lower edge of the lateral crus, the soft tissue alae, the nostril sill and the membranous septum.
• The lobule is the entire area covering cartilage, but the tip is just the area in the tip defining points.
• *Lower lateral cartilages:* 3 crura—medial, middle and lateral with 2 junctions—columellar breakpoint and dome-defining point. Excising lateral crura will reduce tip volume and modifying the domal segment of middle crura will increase tip definition.
• *Base:* alar base, nostrils and columella.
• Septum, anterior nasal spine and pyriform maxilla.

Function:

• The five functions of the nose are respiration, filtration, humidification, temperature regulation and protection.
• 50% of airways resistance occurs in the nose. Resistance is determined by the internal valve as described above. If this area is affected by

septal deviation, mucosal disease etc., respiratory obstruction can occur.
- If lateral cheek traction will reduce obstruction (positive Cottle sign) then spreader grafts may be of benefit.
- The turbinates also increase resistance. Inferior turbinate hypertrophy may require reduction.

Assessment:
- External:
  - Frontal view: skin quality:
    - *Upper third:* bony vault;
    - *Middle third:* dorsal aesthetic lines—should be regular from medial brow to the nasal tip;
    - *Lower third:*
      a. Broad tip;
      b. Position of alar rims and base.
  - Lateral view: labiocolumellar angle and chin-nose-lip proportions:
    - *Upper third:* position of root—nasofrontal angle;
    - *Middle third:* dorsal hump;
    - *Lower third:*
      a. Supratip point;
      b. Tip projection.
  - Basal (worm's eye) view:
    - Alar flaring.
- Internal:
  - Septum: position and perforation;
  - Turbinate hypertrophy.
- Functional:
  - Smile to see what happens to nose: depressor septi nasi may cause an animation deformity to depress tip;
  - *Internal valve:* Cottle's manoeuvre;
  - *External valve:* do they collapse on deep inspiration.

Surgery:
Open approach:
- Anaesthesia:
  - GA with oral tube south facing;
  - IV antibiotics, dexamtheasone, tranexamic acid;
  - LA with adrenaline infiltration in columella and along infracartilaginous incision;
  - Trim nasal hair.
- Incisions—transcolumellar and infracartilaginous:
  - Transcolumellar at the narrowest point of columella—lots of designs including step and V incisions;

- Infracartilaginous—joined to the transcolumellar incision along caudal margin of lower lateral cartilages.
- Skin elevation (submuscular) with dissection of the lower and upper lateral cartilages:
  - Cut and push technique with sharp curved iris scissors to lift skin off columella and avoid injury to the medial crus cartilage which can be easily damaged;
  - When you reach the soft tissue triangles, stop and approach through the infracartilaginous incision—it is safer to approach lateral to medial;
  - Maintain dissection close to the cartilages as the dorsal skin is raised;
  - When the keystone area is reached, a periosteal elevator is used to dissect periosteum off the bone—important to keep the periosteum with the skin flap to protect the thin skin here.
- Intraoperative diagnosis and assessment of tip projection.
- Treatment includes:
  - Dorsal hump reduction or augmentation:
    - Separation of upper lateral cartilages from septum;
    - Incremental reduction of the septum proper;
    - Incremental dorsal bony reductions;
    - Verification by palpation;
    - Final modifications if required can include spreader grafts, suturing techniques, osteotomies.
    - Potential grafts can include dorsal onlay, dorsal sidewall onlay, radix graft—provides appearance of lengthened nose.
  - Midvault and septal reconstruction:
    - Full exposure;
    - Release of mucoperichondrial attachments;
    - Straightening of septum;
    - Restoring support—with struts, batten grafts or spreader grafts;
    - May need submucous resection of hypertrophied inferior turbinates;
    - Precisely planned percutaneous osteotomies;
    - Potential grafts:
      1. *Spreader:* between dorsal septum and upper lateral cartilages in submucoperichondrial pocket. Can also do auto-spreader grafts if excess upper lateral cartilage;
      2. Septal extension to control rotation and support the shape of nasal tip:

a. *Type 1:* a spreader graft that extends anteriorly into interdomal space;
b. *Type 2:* paired batten grafts that extend diagonally across septal L-strut.

○ Alar rims—can be changed with sutures or grafts:

■ Potential grafts:

1. *Alar batten:* a pocket from piriform aperture in alar sidewall to improve valve collapse;
2. *Alar rim:* subcutaneous pocket parallel to rim to prevent alar retraction or collapse;
3. *Alar spreader graft:* a bar that bridges the intercrural space under the lower lateral cartilages—to correct pinched nasal tip.

○ Tip projection.
• Wound closures.
• Splints and dressings.

Closed approach:

• It is simple, quick and without external incisions. Limitations: Most patients on whom it is used have single identified issue such as a dorsal hump, wide nose or minor tip problems.
• *Transcartilaginous:* involves a single intracartilaginous incision which penetrates the lateral crura 4–5 mm above the caudal margin which allows removal of excess cephalic lateral crura. The incision should mirror the external tip defining line.
• *Delivery method:* two incisions, a marginal incision at the caudal border of lateral crura and an intercartilaginous incision at the cephalic border of the lateral crura, where it meets the upper lateral cartilage. The lateral crura is exteriorized. This method may be better if some tip modification is required. Dorsal exposure is performed in close contact with the upper lateral cartilages. Extramucosal tunnels are formed. Septal surgery is performed and dorsal hump reduction. Osteotomies are made. Small tip grafts may be required.

Consequences of surgery:

Expected consequences of surgery include oozing for 2-3 days, bruising, swelling, nasal congestion for 2-6 weeks, temporary loss of smell, tip numbness and tip swelling.

Complications of surgery:

Immediate complications include airway obstruction due to haematoma, mucoperichondrial tears and fracture of the nasal L strut. Other complications include epistaxis, septal haematoma and perforatoin, infection, wound dehiscence, CSF leak, skin necrosis, nasal airway obstruction, deformities including inverted V deformity, rocker deformity and Polly beak deformity), over- or undercorrection and need for revision surgery.

Rhomboid flap

Also called Limberg flap.

• A transposition flap that borrows adjacent loose skin for covering a rhombic defect.
• A rhombus is an equilateral parallelogram with 60° acute angles and 120° obtuse angles.
• The short diagonal equals the length of each side. Extend the short diagonal by an equal length and draw a line of equal length at 60° which will be parallel to side of rhombus.
• Consider relaxed skin tension lines when planning orientation of rhomboid defect and flap donor site.
• A large defect can be converted into a hexagon to facilitate closure using 6 rhomboid flaps.

See DUFOURMENTAL FLAP.

Rib graft

• Split rib grafts can be used for *Cranium reconstruction*.
• Ribs can regenerate as long as the periosteum is left intact.
• Don't take more than two ribs in continuity.
• Manage pleural puncture by lung expansion. The defect is then closed. Cut the ribs as long as possible and split with a fine chisel.
• They can be embedded in various ways.

Ribbon sign

• Curled up arteries lying proximally.
• May get faint red streaks on amputated digit.
• Suggest the arteries have been avulsed distally and are a poor prognostic sign.

Riche–Cannieu anastomosis

Anastomosis of motor fibres between the median nerve and ulnar nerve at the level of the palm causing ulnar muscles to be supplied by the median nerve.

Ricketts' aesthetic plane

• A line drawn from nose tip to chin.
• The lower lip lies on this plane, the upper lip 2 mm behind.

See CEPHALOMETRICS.

Rieger flap

• A rotation advancement flap of dorsal nasal skin.
• Initially described as a random pattern flap with a wide pedicle encompassing the whole side of the nose, it can be based on a branch of the angular artery that enters the skin of the

nasal radix just below the medial canthal tendon.

- Elevating the flap on a narrow vascular pedicle gives greater mobility.
- The dorsal nasal flap provides good coverage for <2 cm defects in the nasal dorsum up to the tip defining points.
- If used for infratip defects, it pulls the nasal tip cephalad and causes alar notching.
- It provides a single unit of closely matching tissue while leaving scars that coincide with 'aesthetic unit' junctions.

See NASAL RECONSTRUCTION. *See* MARCHAC DORSAL NASAL FLAP.

Riley–Smith syndrome
Microcephaly, multiple vascular malformations and pseudopapilloedema, but no lipomas unlike *Bannayan syndrome*.

Ring avulsion injuries
Originally classified by Urbaniak 1981:

- *Type 1:* circulation adequate—treat with standard bone and soft tissue care.
- *Type 2:* circulation inadequate—treat with vessel repair.
- *Type 3:* complete degloving or complete amputation—amputation.

Modified by Kay, Werntz and Wolff 1989:

- *Type 1:* circulation adequate—standard bone and soft tissue care.
- *Type 2:* arterial compromise only—vessel repair.
- *Type 3:* inadequate circulation with bone, tendon or nerve injury—amputation.
- *Type 4:* complete degloving or complete amputation—amputation.

See DEGLOVING INJURIES.

Rintala flap
For nasal tip and columella, rectangular dorsal nasal flap based on nasion with Burow's triangles cut at canthal level.

See NASAL RECONSTRUCTION.

Rolando's fracture
Same place as a *Bennett's fracture*, but comminuted, with a Y- or T-shaped intra-articular component.

Romberg's disease
See HEMIFACIAL ATROPHY.

Roos test
- Clinical test in *Thoracic outlet syndrome*.
- 'I surrender position'.
- Patient seated. Arms abducted to 90°, elbows flexed to 90°.
- Hands closed into a fist and opened repetitively for 3 minutes. Each cycle lasts 2 seconds.
- May get colour change or neurological symptoms. Rarely carried out for 3 minutes.

Rosacea
4 stages of rosacea—a cutaneous vascular disorder.

- Facial flushing.
- Thickened skin and facial erythema.
- Some progress to acne rosacea with erythematous papules and pustules.
- *Rhinophyma* in some patients. The nose is usually the only structure affected. The nasal skin is erythematous with pits. Skin becomes chronically infected. May get nasal airway obstruction. The framework is unaffected.

Rotation flap
- Semicircular flap raised from the edge of a triangular defect which rotates about a pivot point into an adjacent area.
- The line of greatest tension is from the pivot point of the flap to the edge of the defect bordering on the leading edge of the flap. If the tension is great, a backcut may be made or a Burow's triangle excised at the base of the flap.
- Most commonly used for scalp and sacral defects.
- Another type of rotation flap is the bilobed flap.

See TRANSPOSITION FLAP.

Rubens flap
- Flap raised from the peri-iliac fat pad, which is portrayed in subjects of the artist Peter Paul Rubens.
- Based on the deep circumflex iliac vessels.
- Can be used for *Breast reconstruction*.

Saethre–Chotzen syndrome
- Autosomal dominant syndromic *Craniosynostosis*.
- Caused by a mutation in the *TWIST* gene, which codes for a transcription factor.
- Characterized by bicoronal synostosis, facial dysmorphology, brachydactyly and cutaneous syndactyly.
- Can be confused with Crouzon's if no limb abnormalities.
- Get a low-set frontal hairline.
- Facial asymmetry.
- Ptosis of the eyelids.
- Maxillary hypoplasia with a narrow palate.
- Intelligence is usually normal.
- A partial syndactyly or brachydactyly involving the second and third digits.

Sagittal band
- A passive stabilizer for the *Extensor tendons* over the MCP joint.
- The distal part is covered by transverse fibres of the interosseous hood.
- It attaches to volar plate.
- It also limits the proximal excursion of the extensor and it is the primary extensor of the MCPJ. As the extensor contracts, the sagittal band is pulled, which lifts the base of the proximal phalanx.

Subluxing tendons:
- Loss of integrity of sagittal band by trauma or attrition results in subluxation usually into the ulnar gutters.
- The tendons may centralize in extension but slip in flexion. Eventually active extension is lost though it can be maintained if positioned passively.
- Most commonly affects the ulnar 3 digits.

Tear:
- Get swelling over the MCP joint, pain on extension, extensor lag and deviation of the finger (to intact side).

- Treatment controversial. Splint initially, but if this fails perform primary repair with centralization and stabilization of the extensor tendon.

Sagittal synostosis
- The most common form of *Craniosynostosis*.
- Scaphocephaly (boat-like) due to premature fusion of the sagittal suture. Characterised by frontal bossing, parietal narrowing, anterior positioned vertex and occipital bullet.
- Mostly non-syndromic and sporadic, 2% genetic or familial predisposition.
- Get compensatory growth at the coronal lambdoid and metopic sutures.
- The entire sagittal suture may not be involved so that deformity may be predominantly anterior, predominantly posterior or both.
- Raised intracranial pressure in isolated sagittal synostosis is rare but reported.

Operative procedure: there is no consensus as to the best surgical option which range from:

- Sagittal strip synostectomy plus helmeting— effective if performed less than 6 months of age. Shorter operation than total vault remodelling but associated with a higher relapse rate.
- Sagittal strip with springs.
- Calvarial remodelling. Ranges from subtotal to total. Pi procedure is one example which involves a coronal osteotomy and two parasagittal osteotomies, with the frontal bone being drawn back onto the central sagittal section. Total vault remodelling aims to correct all of the phenotypic head shape changes associated with sagittal synostosis and gain intracranial volume.

Salivary gland tumours
- 3% of head and neck malignancies.
- 80% in parotid.
- 80% parotid masses are benign.
- 80% of malignant salivary tumours are in the parotid.
- 50% salivary masses are benign.

Factors indicating malignancy: pain, obstruction, nerve involvement, invasion, bleeding, rapid progression.

Classification:
- Benign or malignant.
- Primary or secondary.
- Long list of possible tumours.

  See WHO CLASSIFICATION.

Benign parotid tumours:
- *Pleomorphic adenoma:* benign mixed tumour. The commonest benign tumour of the parotid. Classified by some as a low-grade malignant tumour. Presents as a slowly growing mass. Invasion of facial nerve is rare. Simple enucleation leads to a high rate of recurrence. Treatment is by superficial parotidectomy.
- *Adenolymphoma:* Warthin's tumour. Located in the tail of the parotid in elderly males. 5–10% are bilateral. Most are treated by superficial parotidectomy.
- *Others:* oncocytoma, sebaceous adenoma, cystadenoma.

Malignant parotid tumours: most arise in the body of the gland. Occasionally in the tail and rarely in the deep lobe. They can be primary or secondary. All malignant parotid tumours require adjuvant radiotherapy.
- *Mucoepidermoid carcinoma:* most common malignancy, 30% of malignant parotid tumours. 3 histological grades.
  - Well differentiated with limited local invasiveness;
  - Intermediate, which behave like well differentiated SCCs;
  - Poorly differentiated—local invasion and regional spread, treat high grade with total parotidectomy, but preserve nerve if functioning and if possible; give radiotherapy to all.
- *Adenoid cystic carcinoma:* most common non-parotid malignancy. 20% of malignant tumours. 3 grades—cribiform, tubular and solid. Skip lesions along the facial nerve are common and perineural invasion common. It may recur many years after presentation. If the follow-up is long enough few patients are cured.
- *Carcinoma ex pleomorphic adenoma:* malignant transformation may occur after 10 years.
- *Others:* adenocarcinoma, acinic cell carcinoma, sebaceous carcinoma, lymphoma.

FNA:
- FNA biopsy can be useful particularly if the patient is at a high risk or if it is thought to be a metastasis.
- Some controversy as to the value of tissue diagnosis, but it is argued that tissue diagnosis should always be obtained first with FNA and if this is negative, with ultrasound assisted core biopsy. This is to exclude a tumour, which doesn't require surgery, principally a lymphoma.

Facial nerve: resect facial nerve if it is invaded with tumour or the tumour cannot otherwise be removed.

Neck dissection: the role in N0 tumours is unclear, usually perform RT.

Salmon patch
See NAEVUS SIMPLEX.

Salter–Harris classification
For epiphyseal injuries in children. Mnemonic SALTR, describing fracture position in relation to physis (I: Slipped, II: Above, III: Lower, IV: Through, V: 'Rammed').

- *Salter-Harris I:* fracture through growth plate. Epiphysis separates from metaphysis with shear force. Good prognosis.
- *Salter-Harris II:* after age of 10, fracture through plate and metaphysis.
- *Salter-Harris III:* after age of 10, fracture in epiphysis.
- *Salter-Harris IV:* any age, rare in hand, fracture in epiphysis and metaphysic.
- *Salter-Harris V:* compression fracture of epiphyseal plate—rare in hand.

Saphenous flap
A *Venous flap*, based on the short saphenous vein and used to reconstruct defects around the knee.

Sarcoidosis
- May present with cutaneous lesions as reddish translucent, smooth papules on the eyelid and nasal margins or as plaques and nodules.
- Steroid treatment for generalized disease often improves cutaneous lesions.
- Large masses may be excised after failure of medical therapy.

Sarcoma
Incidence:
- 1% of malignant disease.
- 50% of deep sarcomas are in the lower limb and most are in the thigh.
- Metastasis is largely via haematogenous route, so metastases are most commonly seen in the lungs. Less commonly to soft tissue,

liver and brain. Lymph node involvement is rare but ominous.
- U.K. guidelines published in 2016.
- Most common types are:
  - Liposarcoma;
  - Malignant fibrohistiocytoma;
  - Fibrosarcoma;
  - Synovial sarcoma;
  - Rhabdomyosarcoma.

Aetiology:
- Previous radiation. Most likely to develop on the edge of the radiation field where less devitalized tissue exists. It can happen even with low-dose treatments such as for keloid scars but there is a long latency period. With higher dose treatments the latency is 10–15 years. The most common sarcoma secondary to RT is osteogenic sarcoma and fibrosarcoma. Radiation-associated angiosarcoma (RAAS) of the chest wall can occur after radiotherapy for breast cancer (rare).
- Retinoblastoma and Wilms tumours are associated with subsequent sarcoma formation, with a chromosomal anomaly on 13q responsible.
- Association with some benign conditions such as neurofibromatosis, fibrous dysplasia and Paget's disease.
- Some chemicals, such as polyvinyl chloride, arsenic and dioxin are sarcomagenic.
- AIDS is linked to Kaposi's sarcoma.

Classification:
- *Tissue of origin:*
  - *Smooth muscle:* leiomyosarcoma;
  - *Striated muscle:* Rhabdomyosarcoma;
  - *Fat:* liposarcoma;
  - *Blood vessels:* Angiosarcoma, Kaposi's sarcoma;
  - *Lymph channels:* lymphangiosarcoma;
  - *Fibrous tissue:* fibrosarcoma;
  - *Nerve:* malignant Schwannoma;
  - *Synovial tissue:* synovial sarcoma;
  - *Skin:* Dermatofibrosarcoma protuberans, Atypical fibroxanthoma, Malignant fibrous histiocytoma.

Staging AJCC
T:
- T1 <5 cm.
- T2 >5 cm.
- T3 >10 cm.
- T4 >15 cm.
- A—superficial.
- B—deep.

N:
- 0 = no regional lymph nodes.
- 1 = regional lymph node.

M:
- 0 = no metastases.
- 1—distant mets.

Grading: Trojani grade
- *Grade 1:* Well differentiated: no necrosis and mitotic count <10.
- *Grade 2:* Moderately differentiated: <50% necrosis and mitotic count 10–19.
- *Grade 3:* Poorly differentiated: >50% necrosis and mitotic count >20.

  Prognosis is linked to Trojani grade.

Clinical presentation: Typically presents as a mass, maybe with pressure effects and systemic symptoms. U.K. guidelines suggest if any of the below features are present, then a referral for urgent ultrasound and/or review at a specialist sarcoma service is warranted:
- Size >5cm.
- Increasing size.
- Painful.

Investigations:
- *Ultrasound.*
- *MRI:* gadolinum-enhanced to improve resolution.
- *CT:* for metastasis and/or bony involvement.
- *Angiography.*
- *Radionuclide imaging:* arterial, venous and osseous phase.
- *Biopsy:* after imaging. With FNA, Tru-cut or open—site of incision planned to enable excision of the scar and tract.

Management: Always manage within an MDT within a specialist sarcoma service.
  Goals:
- Maximize long-term survival and function.
- Minimize local recurrence and morbidity:
  - Surgery: mainstay for patients with resectable disease, aim to completely excise by wide local excision with a margin of 1 cm, aiming for a histological margin of R0 >1 mm (histological margins R0 = no tumour at inked edge, R1 = tumour extends to inked edge, R2 = macroscopic residual tumour). Amputation may be required. Structures needing to be removed in the resection would drive the need for primary reconstruction:
    - *Arteries:* vein grafts from greater saphenous nerve;
    - *Veins:* may be able to rely on superficial system;

- *Nerves:* nerve cable grafts;
- *Muscle:* need for regional or free muscle;
- *Skin:* need for free flap.
- *Radiotherapy:* recommended along with surgery for most high-grade tumours and for some large or marginally excised low-grade tumours:
  - *Adjuvant:* because of Toronto study Lancet 2002 showing equivalent efficacy to neo-adjuvant at 5 years and less short-term side effects. 60–66Gy (pronounced grey) in 1.8-2Gy fractions;
  - *Neo-adjuvant:* uses lower dose of 50Gy. Advantage: you radiate a smaller area with a smaller dose. Disadvantage: higher wound complications.
  - *Chemotherapy:* paediatric rhabdomysarcoma, soft tissue Ewing's sarcoma and synovial sarcoma are chemosensitive sarcomas. Usually given as both neoadjuvant and adjuvant treatment in combination surgery and/or radiotherapy. Chemotherapy may also be considered in other scenarios but not routinely recommended.

Sauvé–Kapandji procedure

Fusion of distal ulna to radial sigmoid notch with removal of a section of ulna proximal to fusion.

See DRUJ.

Scalenus muscles

Scalenus anterior:
- *Origin:* transverse process of 3-6 cervical vertebra.
- *Insertion:* tubercle of first rib.
- *Nerve:* anterior rami of C5 and C6.
- *Action:* stabilizes the first rib or rotates and flexes the neck if the first rib is fixed.

Scalenus medius:
- *Origin:* posterior tubercle of transverse process of C2-7.
- *Insertion:* superior aspect of neck of first rib.
- *Nerve:* posterior branches of anterior ramus of C3-8.
- *Action:* flexes and rotates cervical vertebra, raises first rib. When acting bilaterally flexes the neck.

Scalp anatomy

S: skin.
C: subcutaneous fat.
A: aponeurosis (galea) connects frontalis with occipitalis.
L: loose connective tissue.
P: pericranium.
- *Skin:* the thickest in the body, up to 8 mm thick. It is attached by fibrous septa.

- *Subcutaneous layer:* of dense connective tissue and fat binds the skin to the underlying galea. It contains the principal arteries and veins of the scalp, as well as the sensory nerves and lymphatics.
- *Galea aponeurotica:* the tough fibrous layer of the scalp. It is extensive in its attachments and is a part of the subcutaneous musculo-aponeurotic system (SMAS) of the face. It connects the occipitalis muscle posteriorly with the frontalis muscle anteriorly and the temporoparietal fascia (superficial temporal fascia) in one temporal region with the same layer on the contralateral side. The frontalis muscles originate from the galea aponeurotica and insert into the dermis at the level of the supraciliary arches.
- *Loose areolar plane:* beneath the galea, composed of thin, avascular connective tissue. It is the layer most often involved in avulsion injuries. The laxity within this layer provides for the mobility of the scalp. Haematoma and infection spread easily through it, and thrombosis of the emissary veins may extend to the dural sinuses.
- *Pericranium:* densely adherent to the outer table of the skull, it has a good blood supply.
- *Arterial supply:* supra-orbital, supratrochlear, superficial temporal, occipital and postauricular. The main supply is from the occipital and superficial temporal arteries with the latter being the longest and largest.
- *Nerve supply:* CNV—supra-orbital and supratrochlear. The lesser occipital nerve supplies the posterior scalp.
- *Lymphatics:* forehead and frontoparietal drain to the superficial parotid gland and retromandibular node, posterior drainage is to the occipital and posterior triangle nodes.

Scalp reconstruction

Indications:
- *Congenital: Aplasia cutis congenita,* haemangiomas, AVM, extravasation injuries, *Craniopagus.*
- *Acquired:* trauma, burns, tumours.

Goals of reconstruction:
- Reconstruct with hair-bearing skin if possible, debridement should be limited as there is an excellent blood supply.
- Prevent desiccation of bone with bone necrosis. If bone exposed need immediate cover.
- Galea can be scored. Skin graft can be used on a vascularized surface—bone can be drilled or decorticated.
- Management of scalp wounds with radiotherapy may require a flap.

Surgery:

- *Local flaps.*
- *Regional flaps* or free flaps will be required if >30% of the scalp is involved. Examples include *Ortichochea flap*, Juri flap, *Trapezius flap*.
- *Replantation:* avulsed scalp can be replanted—use vessels outside zone of injury, which may require vein grafts. *See* CRANIUM RECONSTRUCTION.
- *Free flaps:* free flaps allow a one-stage procedure to cover exposed bone or brain. The most commonly used flaps are omentum, latissimus dorsi with or without serratus anterior and radial forearm. The radial forearm gives good cover with pliable tissue though it may need pre-expansion. Free flaps however are often bulky and non-hair-bearing. Superficial temporal vessels can be used or preferably use vessels in the neck—occipital or facial vessels.
- *Tissue expansion:* the preferred method for secondary scalp reconstruction as it enables hair-bearing skin to be used to cover the defect. The main disadvantage is the long duration of treatment. May develop skull deformation following prolonged expansion in children. Up to 50% of scalp can be replaced with expansion. Place multiple crescentic expanders adjacent to the defect. The risks are infection, extrusion and device failure.

Scalping flap

- The most reliable way to deliver a large amount of skin from the forehead to the nose.
- Originally described by Converse in 1942. Useful particularly in the older patient.
- Elevate through a coronal incision behind the superficial temporal artery, extending to a skin paddle on the contralateral forehead.
- The frontalis muscle is not carried in the distal end of the flap, but the remainder of the pedicle is dissected in the subgaleal plane.
- The donor site on the forehead is closed with a FTSG.
- The temporary defect on the scalp is covered with a non-desiccating dressing.
- After the skin paddle is completely revascularized on the nose, the pedicle is divided and the anterior scalp is replaced.
- The advantages of the scalping flap technique are the rich vascular supply of the broad skin paddle and the lack of incisions on the central forehead.

See NASAL RECONSTRUCTION.

Scaphoid fracture

- The commonest carpal bone to be fractured.
- Most fractures are either transverse or horizontal oblique, which tend to be stable. Vertical oblique are more prone to displacement and non-union.
- Earlier treatment with fixation leads to earlier bony union though no long-term difference.

Blood supply:

- From branches of radial artery through ligamentous and capsular attachments to the dorsal ridge. Orientation of blood flow is predominantly distal to proximal.
- The superficial palmar branch of the radial artery gives a volar supply to the distal scaphoid.
- The dorsal carpal branch gives a dorsal supply to the distal scaphoid. The proximal pole is therefore poorly supplied.
- Minimal intraosseous anastomosis so the blood supply to the proximal fragment may be disrupted following fracture leading to avascular necrosis (*Preiser's disease*).
- The scaphoid functions as a link between the distal and proximal carpal rows. 80% of fractures occur at the waist. Proximal 1/3 fractures don't heal well.

Treatment:

- If undisplaced, manage with cast. A long arm cast may reduce time of healing, so have a long arm cast for 6 weeks and a short cast until radiological healing.
- Displaced fractures require fixation.
- K-wires are simple with high union rates but no compression.
- Herbert screws and Herbert–Whipple screws provide compression by differential pitch concept.

Non-union: occurs in 30% of waist fractures and 100% of proximal pole fractures. Ligamentous injury leading to a *DISI* will increase instability.

Classification: of non-unions can be simplified to stable and unstable.

- *Stable non-unions:* have a firm fibrous non-union, which prevent deformity of the length and shape of the scaphoid. OA is minimal. Stable may become unstable with time.
- *Unstable pseudoarthrosis:* are nearly always associated with some degree of carpal collapse deformity. Get sclerosis, cysts and synovial erosion. May develop scaphoid non-union advanced collapse (SNAC).

Treatment:
- *Internal fixation:* compression screw provides the best fixation for routine non-unions. Approach volar or dorsal. Volar disrupts ligaments, dorsal may disrupt blood supply. Vascularity is assessed but most will also require bone grafting.
- *Bone grafting:* dorsal inlay, volar inlay and peg grafts have been used. Russe describes a bicortical bone graft through a volar incision. If collapsed then perform a volar wedge graft.
- *Vascularized bone grafting:* avascular necrosis is a serious late complication of scaphoid fractures. Patients develop increasing pain and stiffness. Reconstruction is by vascularized bone graft with or without bone stimulation. This produces faster incorporation and increased viability. The dorsal aspect of the distal radius is supplied by four vessels, two superficial to the retinaculum and two deep. Distally these anastomose with the dorsal intercarpal arch. A bone graft harvested here may be pedicled to reach the scaphoid. Zaidenberg graft relies on a septal pedicle between the 1st and 2nd dorsal extensor compartments. The benefit is the vascular reliability and the simplicity with a single incision. Volar grafting is based on the palmar carpal artery, the anterior interosseous and a branch of the ulnar. The pronator quadratus is usually transferred to maintain the blood supply. The flap has a limited reach.
- *Bone stimulation:* with electrical stimulation by external devices. Electromagnetic fields may upregulate mRNA of TGF-ß and BMP. One study showed 69% of non-unions healed with casting and electrodes. There is controversy regarding efficacy.

Salvage procedures: may be required for persistent non-union with carpal collapse.
- *Conservative treatment:* wrist support and change of activity. Neurectomy for pain, usually of the posterior interosseous nerve. Also the anterior interosseous nerve can be cut. Limited radial styloid incision can relieve impingement. Partial scaphoid excision can be helpful if the distal scapholunate ligament is preserved. The retaining palmar ligaments must be preserved.
- *Limited intercarpal and midcarpal fusion:* the most used are the capitolunate, scapho-capitolunate and scaphotrapeziotrapezoid arthrodeses. The various midcarpal fusions allow correction of midcarpal joint subluxation while preserving radiolunate joint motion.

- *Proximal row carpectomy versus scaphoid excision:* proximal row carpectomy is standard procedure for SLAC, involving removal of scaphoid, lunate and triquetrum. Scaphoid excision and four corner arthrodesis is more demanding with longer immobilization. They seem to have similar outcomes.
- *Total wrist fusion:* this gives pain relief at the expense of motion. The AO plate fixation uses bone graft and a plate to align 3rd metacarpal with radius with dorsal angulation of 0–20°.

See CARPAL INSTABILITY.

Scapholunate instability
See CARPAL INSTABILITY.

Scapular/parascapular flap
Blood supply:
- Based on cutaneous branch of circumflex scapular artery.
- Arises from subscapular artery and passes between teres major and teres minor on axillary border of scapula.
- Divides into scapular artery (horizontal) and parascapular (longitudinal).
- The position of the pedicle can be found by $D = (L - 2) \div 2$, where D is distance between the spine of scapula and pedicle, and L is distance from spine of scapula to inferior angle of bone.

Anatomic landmarks:
- Scapular flap is based on a horizontal line from *Triangular space* (2 cm above posterior axillary crease) to vertebra. The medial end lies midway between the medial border of scapula and the midline.
- The parascapular flap is centred on a vertical line from triangular space to posterior iliac crest. The distal line lies midway between the tip of the scapula and the iliac crest.

Uses: useful in lower limb reconstruction. Can be raised as a scapular-parascapular flap to achieve a large L-shaped skin paddle. Can be raised as chimeric flap with a bone from the lateral scapula. Disadvantage is positioning makes simultaneous orthopaedic fixation and flap raise difficult. Also good for cheek and hemifacial restoration. The thickness allows for sculpting and the colour match is reasonable. It does not atrophy and is good for Romberg's disease.

Technique: raise medial to lateral just above the deep fascia. As the lateral border of scapula is approached, carry the dissection beneath deep fascia. Identify the triangular space. Up to 10 cm of bone can be obtained from the lateral margin by identifying the distal branch of the circumflex scapular artery. Separate skin and bone paddles can be obtained.

See TRUNK RECONSTRUCTION.

Scar

- Scarring is the body's natural response to injury in an attempt to restore strength and integrity—demonstrates a trade of organisation for debridement and sterilization.
- If the signalling processes are abnormal can result in excess scar. Hypertrophic and keloid scarring are both fibroproliferative disorders of wound repair. In both, the fibroblasts have an upregulation of collagen synthesis, deposition and accumulation.
- *Hypertrophic scars:* well-organised type III collagen and upregulation of myofibroblasts. They stay within the boundaries of the original scar.
- *Keloid scars:* poorly organised types I and III collagen, with an upregulation of PCNA and p53 and normal to reduced numbers of myofibroblasts. They can extend outside the boundaries of the original scar.
- Scarring can be assessed using the Vancouver scar scale, which assesses height, pliability, vascularity and pigmentation.

Prevention:

- Surgical technique:
  - ○ Atraumatic technique;
  - ○ *Minimize tension:* wound tension causes edge separation and scar widening;
  - ○ *Skin eversion:* the exaggerated application of the principle of tension free closure;
  - ○ *Perfect apposition:* with unequal thickness of tissue—take a deeper bite of the thinner tissue and more superficial bite of the thicker tissue for proper alignment;
  - ○ *Use of natural skin tension:* Langer's lines have two advantages:
    - ▪ Place scar in natural creases;
    - ▪ Least amount of tension on the wound.
- Optimize patient factors—nutrition, diabetes, obesity, radiation exposure, steroid use.
- Manage infections and foreign bodies because they increase proinflammatory cytokines which trigger abnormal fibroblast response. Leave the dressing on for 48-72 hours—then you get epidermal closure and reduce infection risk.
- Adjuncts—taping, binding the wounds to release tension. Moisturise and massage scar. Protect from sun. Silicone to improve hydration. Pressure to induce relative tissue ischaemia thereby reducing collagen synthesis and increasing extracellular matrix remodelling.

Treatment:

- Early treatment as for prevention: avoid sun, reduce tension across wound by e.g. taping, silicone gel or sheets, pressure if applicable.
- Treatment options at 6 weeks to 3 months:
  - ○ *Intralesional corticosteroid:* reduces intracellular transcription of pro-inflammatory cytokines. Repeat every 2-4 weeks;
  - ○ Bleomycin, 5FU, verapamil.
- Treatment options after one year:
  - ○ *For hypertrophic scars:* surgery or laser;
  - ○ *For keloid:* no uniformly successful treatment. All have risk of recurrence:
    - ▪ Excision 'always' results in recurrence and is therefore 'always' combined with adjuvant therapy including intralesional steroid or radiotherapy;
    - ▪ Intralesional cryotherapy.

See KELOID. *See* HYPERTROPHIC SCAR.

Schirmer's test

- To assess the function of the greater petrosal nerve by measuring tear secretion.
- *Schirmer 1:* place a strip of filter paper in the lower conjunctiva for 5 minutes <10 m of wetting is abnormal.
- *Schirmer 2:* LA can be added to block reflex tear secretion (Schirmer's test 2).

See FACIAL RE-ANIMATION.

Schuchardt flap

- Used in *Lip reconstruction*.
- The defect is excised as a rectangular defect and the incision is extended around the labiomental fold to the submental region on each side to allow lip to slide into the defect.
- It requires the excision of triangles in the submental region unless a compensating crescentic excision along the fold can be made instead.

Schwannoma

See NEURILEMMOMA.

Schweckendiek technique

- Protocol for the repair of *Cleft lip and palate*.
- Lip and soft palate are repaired before the child is 1 year of age.
- Hard palate is repaired at 8 years of age.
- Reportedly excellent midfacial growth due to reduced disturbance of the important growth centres around the palate, but poor speech.

Scleroderma Hard skin.

- Chronic autoimmune disease mainly affecting women aged 30-60.
- Get thickening of skin, but also affects arteries, joints, lungs and kidneys.

- Sclerodactyly designates the characteristic hand changes, consisting of atrophic skin of the fingers held in partial flexion with limitation of motion in both flexion and extension.
- Wound healing is poor and ulcers should be treated like ischaemic ulcers.

See CREST.

Scleroderma circumscriptum

- Band-like lesions.
- They often follow a dermatome pattern on the trunk or an extremity.
- They may appear in the paramedian region of the forehead—scleroderma en coup de sabre—associated with *Hemifacial atrophy*.
- Severely deforming atrophy of skin, subcutaneous tissues, muscle, and bone may result from scleroderma.
- The eventual extent of the disease is unpredictable in its early stages and spontaneous resolution occurs in some cases.
- The treatment is conservative so long as active disease is present. When activity has ceased soft tissue may require augmentation possibly by microvascular transfer.

Scurvy

See VITAMIN C.

Sebaceous adenoma

- Non-descript solitary lesion.
- Histologically the lesion is an incompletely differentiated sebaceous lobule with irregular shape and size.
- Adenoma sebaceum, associated with *Tuberous sclerosis* is an angiofibromatous proliferation and not a true sebaceous adenoma.
- Multiple sebaceous tumours of the face, scalp and trunk with keratoacanthomas may be associated with internal malignancies in *Torre's syndrome.*

Sebaceous cell carcinoma

- A rare tumour, but accounts for 2% of *Eyelid tumours*.
- They arise from meibomian glands or pilosebaceous glands.
- Usually slow-growing and arise in the upper eyelid in patients over 60 years old.
- Delay in treatment significantly increases mortality.
- There is a 5-year survival of 60–70%.
- Diagnose by excision biopsy.
- Management is by wide local excision and orbital extension will require exenteration. Neck dissection may be required. Radiotherapy is controversial and is reserved for palliative therapy.

Sebaceous cyst

See EPITHELIAL CYSTS.

Sebaceous epitheliomas

- Resemble basal cell epitheliomas as pale or yellow papules with central ulceration.
- Usually a solitary lesion on the face or scalp.
- Treatment is by either excision, electrocoagulation and curettage, or carbon dioxide laser vaporization, depending on their size and location.
- Biopsy may be required to differentiate it from sebaceous carcinoma.

Sebaceous glands

- Holocrine glands that drain into the pilosebaceous unit.
- They are called meibomian glands when they drain directly onto skin.
- More frequent on the forehead, nose and cheek.
- They are not the (sole) cause of sebaceous cysts which are of epidermal origin.

Sebaceous hyperplasia

- 2–4 mm papules on the face of middle-aged adults.
- Pale yellow with central umbilication and telangiectasia.
- Histologically the lesions are collections of sebaceous glands with enlarged lobules located around a central enlarged sebaceous duct.

See FORDYCE'S SPOTS.

Sebaceous naevus of Jadassohn

- Superficial skin lesion, present at birth in head and neck and more rarely trunk and limbs.
- Well-circumscribed, irregularly raised plaque, usually solitary.
- Yellowish waxy appearance with no hair.
- In puberty it thickens and becomes verrucous.
- It is a hamartomatous conglomerate of sebaceous glands and defective hair follicles.
- Large lesions are associated with epilepsy.
- Naevus sebaceous syndrome includes naevus sebaceous, ocular dermoids, cognitive impairment, epilepsy and skeletal abnormalities.
- 15–20% rate of transformation into another tumour, eg *Syringocystadenoma papilliferum*, trichoblastoma, trichilemmoma. Rarely malignant transformation to *Basal cell carcinoma* or SCC. Rarely occurs before early adulthood.
- May observe or excise, including serial excision.
- Extensive lesions may require tissue expansion.

S

Sebaceous tumours

See SEBACEOUS NAEVUS OF JADASSOHN. *See* SENILE SEBACEOUS HYPERPLASIA. *See* SEBACEOUS EPITHELIOMAS.

Seborrhoeic keratosis

Also seborrhoeic wart, senile keratosis, basal cell papilloma.

- Occurs in males and females from 5th decade onwards.
- Related to sun exposure.
- 'Stuck on' appearance. May be pigmented or non-pigmented. Covered with greasy scale.
- Familial variant autosomal dominant.
- A variant called *Dermatosis papulosa nigra* is seen in people with Fitzpatrick skin types 4, 5 and 6.
- Get accumulation of immature keratinocytes between the basal and keratinizing layers.
- Treatment is for cosmetic reasons or for lesions in inconvenient locations and is by curettage, excision or cryotherapy.

Seddon and Sunderland classifications of nerve injury

Seddon described three grades of nerve injury in 1943. Sunderland expanded this in 1951 to five grades:

- *I – Neurapraxia:* local conduction block, no Wallerian degeneration. Spontaneous recovery.
- *II – Axonotmesis:* axonal damage with intact endoneurium, no Wallerian degeneration. Spontaneous recovery.
- *III – Axonotmesis:* axonal damage with damaged endoneurium but intact perineurium. Some Wallerian degeneration. Spontaneous recovery unlikely.
- *IV – Axonotmesis:* axonal damage with damaged endoneurium and perineurium, but intact epineurium. Wallerian degeneration. Spontaneous recovery very unlikely.
- *V – Neurotmesis:* complete nerve transection. No spontaneous recovery.

Semmes–Weinstein monofilament testing

- Technique of *Sensation testing* to evaluate light touch and deep pressure.
- Uses 20 nylon monofilaments with a constant length, but increasing diameter.
- They are applied perpendicular and the patient responds when feeling sensation.
- The figures range from 1.56 to 6.65 with 2.44–2.83 being normal for a finger.

Senile keratosis

See ACTINIC KERATOSIS.

Sensation testing

- *Four main types of testing:* threshold, functional, objective and sudomotor:
  - *Threshold:* temperature, pressure, touch, vibration, sharp stimulus;
  - *Functional:* 2PD, stereognosis;
  - *Objective:* object manipulation.
- *Light touch and pressure: Semmes-Weinstein* monofilament testing. *2PD* is a reliable way to test the quality of sensibility in the fingers.
- *Pain:* with a pin prick.
- *Vibration:* tuning forks of varying cycles.
- *Temperature:* tested with temperature specific probes.
- *Moberg pick-up test.*

Classification: *Highet's.*

Sensory receptors

- 3 types in the hands, thermoreceptors, mechanoreceptors and nociceptors.
- They are either encapsulated or present as free nerve endings.
- Free nerve endings are either myelinated or non-myelinated and lie between epidermal cells. Free endings are usually nociceptors or thermoreceptors.

Mechanoreceptors:

- Rapidly and slowly adapting fibres.
- Rapidly adapting are myelinated A fibres. They include *Pacinian* and *Meissner corpuscles,* which mediate moving, touch and vibration.
- Slowly adapting: *Merkel cell.*
- Corpuscles of Ruffini and Krause are poorly understood mechanoreceptors found in the deep dermis. Ruffini are slowly adapting and Krause rapidly adapting mechanoreceptors.

Sentinel lymph node biopsy

- First described in 1991 by Wong.
- The sentinel lymph node is that which first receives the lymphatic drainage from the involved area. It is therefore the first to receive tumour cells. If this node is tumour-free then the others in the chain will also be. So sentinel node biopsy will spare patients with tumour negative nodes the morbidity of lymphadenectomy. The sentinel node can be examined more extensively.
- SLNB is a staging procedure in *Head and neck cancer* and in *Melanoma.*
- The node is identified using vital blue dye and also a radioactive tracer. A scan pre-operatively can help to identify where the sentinel node is.
- Routine histology identifies 1 positive cell in 10,000. Serial sectioning and staining increases this to 100,000.
- Sentinel node biopsy is thought to be useful as a staging tool to predict prognosis and guide treatment rather than to improve prognosis.

Serratus anterior

Origin: outer surface of upper 8–9 ribs.

Insertion: costal surface of vertebral border of scapula.

Nerve supply: long thoracic nerve.

Vascular supply: lateral thoracic artery.

Action: abducts scapula at the scapulothoracic joint, raises ribs when scapula is fixed.

As a free flap: to avoid winging of the scapula use the middle and lower 4–5 digitations of the muscle.

Sex differentiation defects

- *Klinefelter's syndrome.*
- *Turner syndrome.*
- *Ambiguous genitalia.*

  See AMBIGUOUS GENITALIA. *See* EMBRYOLOGY.

SGAP and IGAP (Superior and Inferior Gluteal Artery Perforator Flap)

- Can be a muscle flap (type 3) or a fasciocutaneous flap.
- Arterial supply—superior and inferior gluteal arteries (terminal branches of internal iliac artery). Pass out of pelvis by passing above and below the piriformis muscle.
- Used as a free flap in breast reconstruction or as a pedicled flap in sacral sore reconstruction.

Flap raise:

- Position—prone.
- Landmarks:
  - PSIS;
  - Ischial tuberosity;
  - Greater trochanter;
  - Coccyx.
- Perforators—confirm with Doppler:
  - *SGAP:* junction of medial/middle third of line between PSIS and greater trochanter;
  - *IGAP:* junction of middle/inferior third of line between PSIS and ischial tuberosity.
- Flap raise:
  - Incise down to muscle;
  - *Undermine flap:* keep at least one of SGAP or IGAP.

Shprintzen's syndrome

See VELOCARDIOFACIAL SYNDROME.

Sick cell syndrome

Carbon monoxide binds to cytochromes, as well as haemoglobin. Cytochrome-bound CO is washed out after 24 hours causing a secondary rise in serum COHb and possibly post-intoxication encephalopathy.

Sickle cell disease

- Caused by substitution of glutamic acid by valine on the haemoglobin β chain.

- Inherited as an autosomal gene. Heterozygotes have both normal and abnormal haemoglobin.
- Sickle cell trait gives a relative resistance against malaria.
- Most common in West Africa, central India and also in Mediterranean populations.
- Distorted red blood cells increase blood viscosity with capillary and venous thrombosis, and organ infarction.
- Patients at risk should be screened by electrophoresis.
- For surgery, patient should be well hydrated. Keep well oxygenated with O_2 concentrations of 40–50%. Keep warm. Tourniquets should be avoided if possible but can be safe if other factors optimal.

Sickle flap

See HATCHET FLAP.

Silicone

- Silicon is an element. Silica is silicone oxide. Silicone is interlinked silicon and oxygen with methyl, vinyl or phenol side groups. Polydimethylsiloxane (PDMS) has a repeating chain of -Si-O- units with methyl groups attached to the silicone atoms.
- Consistency can be changed by varying the length and cross-linking of the PDMS chains. Fluids are short straight chains, gels are lightly cross-linked and elastomers are longer chains with cross-links.
- Silicone is highly biocompatible, non-toxic, non-allogenic and non-biodegradable.
- Get a mild foreign body reaction. Capsule formation is universal. Capsular contracture is the most common complication. Get synovitis in joint arthroplasty.
- *Disadvantage as implant:* rubbers tear or fail when stressed (Swanson finger joints). Gel foam is difficult to remove following rupture. Bone resorption can occur. Smooth implants are more prone to extrusion and capsular contracture. Textured (breast) implants appear to be linked to *BIA-ALCL*. Rubbers are permeable so proteins and lipids may be absorbed altering the physical property.
- *Uses:* in plastic surgery silicone is used for breast reconstruction, facial reconstruction, orbital floor, tissue expanders, penile devices and finger joint replacements.

  See ALLOPLASTS.

Silicone controversy

- *1962:* first implant inserted.
- *1982:* Van Nunen linked implants to connective tissue disease (CTD).
- *1992:* cosmetic implants were banned in USA, France and Spain.

- *1994:* a class action settlement of $4.25 billion for any of 10 CTD developed within 30 years.

Findings of UK independent review group: controversy over whether implants cause some autoimmune diseases or an increased risk of cancer. In 1998 the report concluded that:

- They are not associated with greater risk than other implants.
- No evidence of abnormal immune response.
- No association with connective tissue diseases.
- Local complications occur.
- National registry advised.

Findings of IMNAS in USA: Institute of Medicine of the National Academy of Science reported in 1999 that:

- No evidence that silicone implants are responsible for any major diseases.
- No evidence that recurrent breast cancer is more prevalent with implants.
- Silicone augmentation is not a contraindication to breast feeding and milk formulas have a higher level of silica than breast milk with implants.

See BREAST IMPLANTS. *See* BREAST AUGMENTATION. *See* BIA-ALCL

Silver nitrate

- Used in *Burns* dressings.
- 0.5% concentration.
- It is broad spectrum and resistance to the silver ion is rare. There is minimal absorption so toxicity is rare.
- It is very hypotonic so its use can lead to loss of Na, K from the burn wound.
- Some organisms can reduce nitrate to nitrite and this can rarely lead to methaemoglobinuria.
- It stains everything brown or black, and this is the principle reason it is not used routinely.

Silver sulphadiazine

- Used in *Burns dressings*.
- This is the most frequently used topical agent.
- It has a water-soluble base at a concentration of 1%.
- This will inhibit the growth of most sensitive organisms.
- It is applied every 12–24 hours and is active against Gram −ve and +ve organisms, *Candida* and herpes. It is not painful and is non-staining. It makes burn depth more difficult to assess as causes a pseudo-eschar to form.
- Toxicity is rare though leucopenia often occurs after 2–3 days of treatment.

- Clinical trials suggest that silver sulphadiazine reduces bacterial density and delays colonization with Gram −ve bacteria.

Simian crease

Seen in 1% of the normal population. 50% of Down's syndrome and trisomy 21 have a simian crease. They also have brachymesophalangia and syndactyly.

Simon's classification

Grading for *Gynaecomastia*.

- *1:* small enlargement with no skin redundancy.
- *2A:* moderate enlargement with no skin redundancy.
- *2B:* moderate enlargement with skin redundancy.
- *3:* marked enlargement with marked skin redundancy.

Simonart's band

- A soft tissue bridge in the setting of an otherwise complete cleft of the lip and alveolus.
- The definition supplied by Millard is probably the most accepted: 'soft tissue bridge located at the threshold of the nostril, or more internally, between segmented alveolar ridges.'
- Controversial and potentially confusing regarding the classification of complete versus incomplete cleft lip.
- Losee suggested abandonment of the term 'Simonart's Band'. Advocated instead distinguishing between soft tissue that bridges the nasal sill (therefore remains a complete cleft lip) between soft tissue that bridges the lip tissue inferiorly to the columella/philtral and alar/facial groove (therefore renders an incomplete cleft lip).

Sjögren's syndrome

Triad of dry eyes (keratoconjunctivitis sicca), dry mouth (xerostomia) and *Rheumatoid arthritis*.

Skew flap below knee amputation

- A technique of below knee amputation with well-vascularized flaps and a well-contoured stump.
- Stump length should be 10–15 cm below tibial plateau. Too short gives insufficient lever, too long requires a wide unsightly prosthesis. Skin blood flow at this level is predominantly from saphenous vein and sural artery.
- Mark level of amputation and measure circumference with tape. Mark point 2.5 cm lateral to tibial crest and mark half circumference from this. Divide tape into

quarters to mark midline of each flap and also the inferior point.

- A 2-cm proximal extension anteriorly allows access for bone section.
- Elevate flaps with fascia. Divide saphenous and sural nerves. Preserve arteries as long as possible.
- Divide anterior compartment muscles transversely. Divide interosseous membrane. Raise periosteum. Divide fibula high. Divide tibia in curved fashion. Hold lower leg to expose tibialis posterior which is cut transversely to reveal posterior and peroneal NVBs.
- Separate gastrocnemius/soleus from tibia. Divide vessels and divide gastrocnemius/soleus 15 cm distal to bone section. Ligate vessels and divide nerves under tension. Thin muscle tapering to aponeurosis. Remove muscle medially and laterally. Under-run soleal sinuses.
- Suction drain. Smooth bone ends. Secure posterior muscle flap to anterior tibial fascia with continuous suture. Suture skin under no tension.

Skier's thumb
See ULNAR COLLATERAL LIGAMENT.

Skin
Anatomy:
Epidermis:

- Stratified squamous epithelium 0.05–1.5 mm thick. Goal of skin is to maintain the waterproof *stratum corneum*. Cells migrate from the basal layer to the environment in 40 days.
- Comprised of basal cells, keratinocytes, melanocytes, _Merkel cells_ and _Langerhans cells_.
- *Stratum germinativum:* comprised of _Basal cells_ are the innermost layer. Columnar. BCCs arise from basal cells. These divide to form *keratinocytes*, which provide a barrier. These are attached by *desmosomes*. They are attached to basal lamina. They make keratin and cytokines. Also contains melanocytes.
- *Stratum spinosum:* 5–12 cells thick. Also called prickle layer. They are joined to each other by tonofibrils (prickles). SCC arises from these cells. They are polygonal and they flatten to become stratum granulosum.
- *Stratum granulosum:* with granules of keratohyalin in them. These dehydrate and flatten further to form stratum lucidum.
- *Stratum lucidum:* only present in the thick skin of palms and feet.

- *Stratum corneum:* keratinocytes die leaving keratin as a barrier. As the cells move through stratum corneum they become disorganized.

Dermis:

- Represents 90% of skin thickness. Provides a collagen matrix, holds dermal appendages and provides nutrients. The boundary is undulating. Basal cells are attached to basal lamina which attaches to dermis—this is the basement membrane. Acts as a barrier.
- *Papillary dermis:* is superficial and contains more cells and finer collagen.
- *Reticular dermis:* is deeper and contains fewer cells and coarser collagen.

Extracellular matrix:

- *Collagen:* thin outer layer of dermis is called the papillary layer. Collagen is randomly arranged and thin. Under this is the reticular layer with elastic fibres and thick aligned collagen. Type I:III ratio 5:1.
- *Elastin:* also produced by fibroblasts. They can reversibly stretch to twice the resting length.
- *Ground substance:* fills the remaining dermal space. Provide aqueous environment for cell migration. Mucopolysaccharide can hold 1,000 times its own volume of water. Produced by fibroblasts. Consists of glycosaminoglycans (GAGs), hyaluronic acid, dermatan sulphate and chondroitin sulphate.
- *Histiocytes and mast cells:* also in the dermis. Histiocytes are mobile macrophages, mast cells release histamine and heparin.

Sensory nerves: tactile sensation is detected by Meissner's (palm and sole only) and pressure by Pacinian corpuscles (mainly in palms and soles). Pain, itch and temperature is detected by unmyelinated nerve endings.

Hair follicles: develop from epithelial germ cells. Type of melanin gives hair its colour. Arrector pili smooth muscle is attached at the base of the hair. Innervated by adrenergic sympathetic supply. Action is to raise the hair and secrete sebum.

Sweat and sebaceous glands:

- *Apocrine:* sweat glands are stimulated by adrenergic sympathetic fibres. Found in axillae and anogenital region and become active after puberty. They are responsible for body odour which is from bacterial decomposition. The glands open into a pilosebaceous follicle.
- *Eccrine:* sweat glands are supplied by cholinergic sympathetic fibres. Found in palms, soles, axillae, forehead mainly, but

over most of the skin. Secrete odourless fluid by exocytosis. Control body temperature.

- *Sebaceous:* glands are appendages of hair follicles. They are under endocrine control. Found everywhere except palms and soles. They produce sebum, a mixture of fatty acids. Also lubricate hair.

Blood vessels: adrenergic sympathetic fibres innervate blood vessels. Flow is also mediated by histamine. Get plexus at dermal-subcutaneous junction and at papillary dermis. Glomus bodies are AV shunts which can greatly increase blood flow and control body temperature.

Function: protect from trauma. Resident bacterial count is reduced by sebum. It is flexible, elastic and tough. It regulates fluid and temperature. Normal daily loss of 500–800 ml.

Physical properties: collagen is convoluted, allowing stretching up to a certain point, after which there is sudden resistance. Return is by elastin fibres. If a load is prolonged, get irreversible extension. This viscoelasticity gives rise to *Creep.* During creep get a change in collagen fibre bonding. May be due to displacement of water from the ground substance.

Clinical implications:

- Resting tension is high over shoulders and sternum and may partly explain hypertrophy.
- *Wrinkles:* due to repetitive mechanical forces and reduced mass of collagen, and changing elastin. Muscle contraction and gravity pull collagen, which remodels.
- *Chronic ageing skin:* fibroblasts have reduced function, collagen cross-links increase. Skin is stiffer and thinner. Collagen is less convoluted. Dermis and epidermis thins. Ground substance which is responsible for skin turgidity is reduced.
- *Photo-ageing skin:* divided into 6 types. *See* ULTRAVIOLET RADIATION. Most DNA damage is repaired except in *Xeroderma pigmentosa.* Long-term changes are irreversible. In epidermis get thickened heterogeneous basal layer. In the dermis get tangled masses of elastin and collagen. Get reduced total collagen.
- *Racial differences:* darker skin has more layers of stratum corneum though it is the same thickness. Darker skin is photoprotective. Numbers of melanosomes per unit area is the same, but in darker skin they are more dispersed.

Histological terms: Acanthosis, *Papillomatosis, Hyperkeratosis*, parakeratosis.

Blister formation: pathological extracellular fluid in the skin. They can be intraepidermal or dermal-epidermal and further subdivided.

Skin creases: hand

- In the finger: at the DIP joint there is one crease just proximal to the DIPJ. There are 2 creases at the PIP joint and another at the distal palmar digital junction mid-proximal phalanx. The crease ends at mid-axial level. There is no fat at the level of crease and minor injury can easily penetrate the tendon sheath.
- The distal and proximal palmar creases run obliquely over the palm. A1 pulley lies under them.
- The crease at the base of the thenar eminence merges with the proximal palmar crease. The radial digital nerve to index follows this line.
- The second longitudinal crease runs from the base of the long finger to the radial edge of the hypothenar eminence.

Skin grafts

History:

- First described in Hindu texts 2500 years ago.
- Astley Cooper performed a skin graft in 1817, taking the skin of an amputated thumb to cover the stump.
- Reverdin, 1869 used pinch grafts to improve healing.
- Ollier, 1872 used skin grafts to treat ectropion.
- Wolfe used grafts for a fresh surgical wound.
- Blair and Barrett Brown, 1929 used split skin grafts.

Type:

- *Split-thickness skin grafts (STSG):* consist of epidermis and a portion of dermis, average thickness 0.3–0.4 mm. A method for harvesting them was developed by Thiersch in 1886.
- *Full-thickness grafts (FTSG):* include the entire thickness of skin, epidermis and dermis.

Properties:

- *SSG:* take well, but shrink, thinner, more fragile and abnormal pigmentation.
- *FTSG:* thicker and more robust, but require well-vascularized bed and limited by size.

Healing: in Fitzpatrick type I, II and III skin is initially white, then pink after a few days with capillary refill. By 2–3 weeks the graft surface thickens. Collagen replacement is complete by 6th week. Remodelling takes many months. Lymphatics are established by 5–6th day.

Graft take: 4 phases.

- *Adherence:* fibrin bonds form immediately. There are two phases of graft adherence. The first begins with placement of the graft on the recipient bed, to which the graft adheres because of fibrin deposition. This lasts approximately 72 hours. The second phase involves ingrowth of fibrous tissue and vessels into the graft.

- *Plasmatic imbibition:* during the first 48 hours allows the graft to survive. Diffusion of exudates allows access to nutrition and disposal of waste.
- *Revascularization:* by inosculation occurs next with anastomotic connections between graft and host.
- *Capillary ingrowth:* occurs at the same time with new vessels. Four theories have been proposed for graft revascularization:
  - ○ Neovascularization of the graft in which new vessels from the recipient bed invade the graft to form the definitive vascular structure of the graft;
  - ○ Communication occurs between existing graft vessels and those in the recipient site;
  - ○ There is a combination of ingrowth of new vessels and re-establishment of flow into existing vessels;
  - ○ The vasculature of the skin graft is made up, primarily, from its original vessels before transfer.
- *Remodelling:* architecture returns to normal.

Graft failure: due to haematoma, infection, seroma, shear and poor bed vascularity.

Pigmentation: varies with graft site. Grafts from thighs tend to darken and palms lighten with time. SSGs tend to become darker than FTSGs from the same site. Sunshine may affect pigmentation and should be avoided for 6 months. Pigmentation may be treated with dermabrasion.

Donor sites: the epidermis regenerates from adnexal structures, but dermis never regenerates. Therefore, donor sites can be recropped, but how many times is dependent on the thickness of the dermis and the thickness of the SSG.

Skin tag
See ACROCHORDON.

Skull base surgery
Tumours:
- *Malignant extracranial,* such as squamous cell carcinoma, adenoid cystic carcinoma.
- *Malignant intracranial,* such as malignant Schwannoma.
- *Malignant primary basicranial,* such as chondrosarcoma and osteogenic sarcoma.
- *Benign extracranial,* e.g. pleomorphic adenoma.
- *Benign intracranial,* e.g. primary adenoma.
- *Benign primary basicranial,* e.g. fibrous dysplasia.

Clinical findings: symptoms may be vague. Benign tumours present with signs of compression. Malignant tumours present with headaches, fits and cranial nerve paralysis.

Imaging:
- *CT scan with contrast:* provide information of bone involvement.
- *MRI with T1- and T2-weighted images:* for soft tissue information.
- *Angiography and naso-endoscopy.*

Surgical exposures:
- The transfacial approach allows safe access to a difficult area. Facial units are separated. Wide exposure is actually safer with clearer visualization of tumour and vital structures. 6 levels. The first 3 are intracranial and the latter 3 extracranial providing exposure to the midline skull base.
- *Level I Transfrontal approach:* to access tumours of the anterior cranial fossa. Performed through bicoronal scalp incisions. A bicoronal craniotomy is performed. A supra-orbital bar is removed.
- *Level II Transfrontal nasal approach:* to access anterior cranial fossa and tumours growing anteriorly. A bicoronal incision is performed and the supra-orbital bar including the nasal complex is removed.
- *Level III Transfrontal naso-orbital approach:* the approach is the same as level II but includes the lateral orbital wall, so that the superior orbital roof can be included to enable lateral globe retraction.
- *Level IV Transnasomaxillary approach:* for wide exposure of midline skull base. Through Weber–Ferguson incision. Le Fort II osteotomy performed.
- *Level V Transpalatal approach:* for small clival lesions. Through an intra-oral approach, a Le Fort I osteotomy is performed.
- *Level VI Transpalatal approach:* for lower clival and upper cervical. The palate is incised, mucoperiosteal flaps are raised and an osteotomy is performed in the hard palate.

SLAC: scapholunate advanced collapse
Also SNAC—scaphoid non-union with collapse.

Pathology:
- Rotary subluxation of the scaphoid following either acute rupture or chronic attenuation of the scapholunate ligament. The scaphoid palmar flexes with decreased surface area, but increase in joint contact forces between radius and scaphoid. Get carpal collapse with destruction of the capitolunate and lunohamate joints. In SLAC the radiolunate joint is preserved.

- Four stages:
  - *I:* stylocarpal arthritis;
  - *II:* scaphoid fossa involvement;
  - *III:* capitolunate arthrosis;
  - *IV:* diffuse wrist arthritis.

Surgery:
- Depends on the state of the proximal capitate and radiolunate articular surfaces. Two most common procedures are:
  - *Scaphoidectomy* with 4-corner arthrodesis (capitate-lunate-hamate-triquetrum);
  - *Proximal row carpectomy (PRC):* if the lunate fossa and proximal capitate are well preserved, PRC is better than arthrodesis.
- *Arthrodesis:* perform wrist arthrodesis if both articular surfaces are damaged.

SMAS: superficial musculo-aponeurotic system
- Layer of facial fascia. Contiguous with frontalis muscle, galea, temporoparietal fascia (superficial temporal fascia), platysma. It is tightly adherent to the zygomatic arch.
- In the parotid-masseteric area it is thick and attached to the parotid sheath. It becomes thin in the cheek region. The SMAS invests and extends into the external part of the superficial facial muscles, involving fibres of risorius, frontalis, platysma and peripheral part of orbicularis oculi.
- In the mandibular area the SMAS is in close contact with the superficial plane of platysma. The mandibular branch runs deep to platysma.
- Over the mastoid, SMAS is attached to dermis and fibrous tissue around the insertion of the sternoclavicular muscles.
- *Nasolabial fold:* SMAS is deep and thin here. Here it ends as a distinct layer.
- Sensory nerves are superficial and motor branches are deep to SMAS. The facial artery and vein lie deep to SMAS. Their perforating branches go through it.
- SMAS acts as a distributor of facial muscle contractions to the skin through its attachments to the dermis.

See FACE LIFT.

Smoking
- Get a thrombogenic state due to effects on dermal microvasculature and blood constituents.
- Nicotine increases vasoconstricting prostaglandins such as thromboxane A2. Carbon monoxide leads to tissue hypoxia and increased platelet adhesiveness.

- Smoking adversely affects procedures with extensive undermining, such as facelifts. There has been no proven adverse effect in free tissue transfer.
- Smoking one cigarette leads to a 42% reduction in blood flow velocity to the hand, which may adversely affect replants.

Snap test
For assessment of lower *Eyelid*. Pull the lower eyelid downward and assess how long it takes to return to the normal position. A return of less than 1 second is normal.

Snodgras repair: tubularized incised plate (TIP)
- Operative technique described in 1994 for the correction of distal shaft and mid-shaft *Hypospadias*.
- Use when urethral groove is wide and deep. Tubularize urethral plate *in situ*.
- Steps:

1. Midline central incision down urethral plate;
2. Vertical incisions down lateral edges of urethral plate to tubularize—need approximately 12 mm plate for this to work;
3. Close in layers using Dartos waterproofing layer over urethral suture line;
4. Glans is reconstructed over the Dartos layer.

Snuffbox: anatomic
Hollow on radial side of wrist. Contents of first dorsal compartment border the palmar side, EPL is dorsal, radial styloid proximal, and the base of thumb metacarpal distal. The radial artery traverses snuff box. Scaphoid in floor of snuffbox.

Snuffbox: ulnar
Depression immediately beyond ulnar styloid. Bordered by ECU and FCU tendons. Floor formed by triquetrum in radial deviation, and joint of triquetrum and hamate in ulnar deviation.

Sodium bicarbonate
- Sometimes added to local anaesthetics.
- Local anaesthetics are in a balanced solution between ionized and non-ionized forms. The non-ionized form goes into the nerve more rapidly.
- Alkalization of the solution changes the concentration of the non-ionized form and increases the rapidity of onset.
- Dose to give are 1 mEq/10 ml lignocaine and 0.1 mEq/20 ml bupivicaine.

Soft tissue tumours: upper limb
Most are benign. Foreign body granulomas and inclusion cysts are frequent. Most common benign lesion is a lipoma.

Location: often most useful sign. Ganglia—dorsal or volar wrist. DIPJ-mucous cyst. Retinacular cyst over volar aspect of finger at MCPJ. Palmar fibromas are found in the palm.

See EPIDERMOID INCLUSION CYST. *See* FIBROMA. *See* GANGLION. *See* GIANT CELL TUMOUR. *See* GRANULAR CELL TUMOUR. *See* MASON'S HAEMANGIOMA. *See* VASCULAR LEIOMYOMA. *See* SARCOMA.

Solar keratosis
See ACTINIC KERATOSIS.

Soleus flap
- A bipennate type 2 muscle flap.
- Major pedicle proximally from peroneal artery and variable minor pedicles distally from the posterior tibial artery.
- May be considered as a reconstructive option for mid-third lower limb defects.

Sonic hedgehog
Implicated in limb development in the AP plane. Sonic hedgehog (*SHH*) is a segment polarity gene. It is expressed in the posterior mesenchyme of limb buds. It patterns the AP limb axis. It may maintain the progress zone of the AER while acting as a positional signal along the AP axis.

See EMBRYOLOGY.

Speech and language
- Speech refers to the way in which sounds and words are said. Elements of speech include articulation, voice, resonance, fluency.
- Language refers to the words and signs and how we use them to communicate in society. Language can be spoken, signed or written. Language processing can be thought of in terms of receptive language (input) and expressive language (output).
- It is possible to have disorders of speech or language or both.
- Speech is a complex interaction between anatomy, physiology and cognitive processing. Thinking specifically about anatomy and physiology in the production of speech from diaphragm to lips:

  ○ *Respiration:* by the diaphragm to produce air flow;
  ○ *Phonation:* air passing through vocal cords to make sound;
  ○ *Resonance:* the shaping of the sound energy in the oral, nasal and pharyngeal cavities—velopharyngeal valve important here in regulating sounds energy. In the English language most sounds need velopharyngeal competence. The only sounds that don't need that are m/n/ng;

  ○ *Articulation:* tongue, teeth and lips shape the sounds into different pressure consonant types:
    ▪ Plosives;
    ▪ Fricatives;
    ▪ Affricatives.
  See CLEFT PALATE.

Speech restoration
See VOICE RESTORATION.

Spilled tea-cup sign
- Seen in volar lunate dislocation.
- Lunate displaced out of the fossa and into the carpal tunnel region.

Spina bifida
Failure of fusion of the neural groove.

Incidence: commonest CNS defect. 1:200–1,000. Related to folate deficiency. Inheritance is multifactorial.

Classification: 4 types:
- *Meningocoele:* meninges in herniation with no neurological defect.
- *Myelomeningocoele:* most common. Meninges and neural elements with neurological deficits.
- *Syringomyelocoele:* rare. Similar to meningomyelocoele, but with dilatation of the central canal of the cord.
- *Myelocoele:* rare. Exposed neural elements with no covering.

Clinical presentation:
- Spina bifida occulta presents with anomaly over the skin, such as a dimple, hair tuft, naevus or lipoma. XR shows a defect in the spinous processes and vertebra. A tethered cord may cause progressive neurological defect with growth.
- *Meningocoele:* usually lumbosacral bulge with poor or ulcerated skin. Bulge increases with crying.

Natural history: 90% survive, 25% have learning difficulties mostly due to infections, 85% walk with aids, 80% can become continent.

Treatment:
- Aim to close with 24–72 hours if cord exposed.
- 75% will close with wide relaxing incisions. Otherwise use bipedicled flaps, rhomboid flaps, latissimus dorsi or gluteus maximus. V-Y flaps based on paravertebral perforators.

See TRUNK RECONSTRUCTION.

Spitz naevus
- Also spindle cell naevus or benign juvenile melanoma.
- Mainly in children.

- Were thought to be melanoma, but is a compound naevus variant.
- Colour ranges from pink to purplish-red and a few are pigmented. Surface may be warty. Elevated firm nodules up to 2 cm in size. Vascular and may bleed.
- Often rapid initial growth over 3-6 months.
- Close histopathological resemblance to melanoma.
- Occur before puberty and may be present at birth.
- Most frequently found on the face.
- The incidence of melanoma transformation is no different than any other compound *Naevus*.
- Excise with narrow margins. If not excised completely they may recur.

Sporothrix schenkii

Occurs in nurserymen. Infection with subcutaneous erythematous nodules with centripetal pattern along the course of lymphatic drainage. Isolate on Sabouraud agar at 30°. *See* INFECTION.

Spurling's test

- Clinical test for cervical disc involvement. Tends to affect upper plexus.
- Seat patient, extend neck and apply pressure to vertex of scalp down cervical spine then flex head to affected side to narrow intervertebral foramen. Positive if elicits dermatomal paraesthesia.

  See THORACIC OUTLET SYNDROME.

Squamous cell carcinoma
Incidence:

- 25% of that of BCCs.
- Related to sun exposure, radiation, chemicals, chronic ulcers.

Sites: occur in areas of abnormal skin with sun damage, keratin horns, leucoplakia, chronic scar, *Solar keratosis*, *Bowen's disease*, *Pseudoepitheliomatous hyperplasia*.

Histology:

- SCCs arise from the keratinizing spindle cell layer (stratum spinosum) of the epithelium. Dysplastic epidermal keratinocytes extend through the basement membrane into the dermis. The presence of keratin pearls is characteristic.
- They may be well, moderate or poorly differentiated.
- Bad prognostic indicators are increased depth of invasion, vascular invasion, peri-neural invasion and lymphocytic infiltration.
- Initially smooth, verrucous or ulcerative then becomes inflamed and ulcerated. Verrucous may be deeply locally invasive, but less likely

to metastasize, whereas nodular have rapid growth and early ulceration. They are locally invasive and more likely to metastasize.
- *Dermoscopy:* central keratin plug with hairpin or arborizing vessels.
- SCCs >4 mm thick gives 35% metastatic rate.

Categorize:

Tumour risk can be more accurately stratified into low, high and very high risk.

- Tumour factors:

  o Low—tumour less than 2 cm, tumour thickness less than 4 mm, no perineural or lymphovascular invasion and well or moderately differentiated;

  o High—diameter 2-4 cm, thickness 4-6 mm, can have perineural invasion but only nerve diameter <0.1 mm, tumour site on ear or lip;

  o Very high—diameter >4 cm, thickness >6 mm, any bone invasion, peripheral nerve invasion >1 mm, any metastases.

- Margin status:

  o Low—clear margins >1 mm;

  o High—one or more close margins.

- Patient factors:

  o Immunosuppressed.

Staging AJCC 8:

- T1 <2 cm.
- T2 2-4 cm.
- T3 >4 cm or >6 mm depth of invasion beyond subcutaneous fat.
- T4a—gross cortical bone erosion.
- T4b—skull base invasion.

Management:

- Manage within an MDT for higher risk lesions.
- Surgery is the primary intervention. Non-surgical treatments only for carefully selected low-risk tumours and/or if primary surgery is not possible:

  o To be marked under bright lighting with magnification or dermoscopy:

    ▪ Low risk—4 mm;
    ▪ High risk—6 mm;
    ▪ Very high risk—at least 10 mm.

  o Histological margin should be at least 1 mm. For mobile lesions the deep margin should be in the next clear surgical plane. On the scalp always include the galea.

- Radiotherapy could be a primary treatment if all other options not available (e.g. patient not willing/too frail to undergo surgery). Consider adjuvant radiotherapy if clear but close margins or if involved margins and patient does not want/cannot undergo re-excision.

- Adjuvant immunotherapy—only 1 licensed drug for cSCC = *cemiplimab*—consider in metastatic or unresectable disease. Patient needs to be a fair performance status—needs a discussion with oncology team.
- Curettage and cautery—consider in immunocompetent patient with small (<1 cm) well-defined low-risk tumours.
- Only consider SLNB for specific high-risk primary SCC in the context of clinical trial or MDT discussion. For clinically suspicious nodes—do FNA. Do MTI for people with in-transit metastases or regional epineural invasion of named nerves. Offer therapeutic regional lymph node clearance for SCC with regional node metastases and adjuvant radiotherapy.

See BASAL CELL CARCINOMA.

Stahl classification
For XR changes in *Kienböck's disease*.
- *I:* compression fracture.
- *II:* sclerosis.
- *III:* sclerosis and mild collapse, IIIa without fixed scaphoid rotation, IIIb with fixed scaphoid rotation.
- *IV:* sclerosis, collapse, fragmentation.
- *V:* sclerosis, radiocarpal and midcarpal degeneration.

Stahl's ear
Congenital anomaly of the ear, which has a third crus.

Stainless steel
- A large group of iron–chromium–nickel alloys.
- They have a high degree of corrosion and implant failure.
- Galvanic current occurring between the screws and plates can result in corrosion. Vitallium and titanium corrode less due to protective oxide layer on their surface.

See ALLOPLASTS.

Staphylococci
- Gram positive organism which forms characteristic clusters on microscopy.
- *Staphylococcus aureus* and epidermis are the most common skin commensals.
- Resistance to beta-lactam antibiotics occurs though acquisition of *mecA* gene.
- *Scalded skin syndrome* is caused by *Staphylococcus aureus* and the release of *exotoxins*.

Steatoblepharon
Peri-orbital fat which is either excessive or pro-truding through a lax septum.
See BLEPHAROPLASTY.

Steele's classification
For base of phalanges intra-articular fractures.
- *Type 1:* non-displaced marginal fracture.
- *Type 2:* comminuted impaction fracture.
- *Type 3:* displaced intra-articular fracture.

Stelling classification
Classification of *Polydactyly*.
- *Type 1:* extra digit attached by skin bridge only.
- *Type 2:* extra digit articulating with metacarpal or phalanx.
- *Type 3:* extra digit articulating with extra metacarpal.

Stener lesion
Ulnar collateral ligament attaches deep to adductor aponeurosis. With complete disruption the adductor is interposed between UCL and proximal phalanx giving a Stener lesion.
See ULNAR COLLATERAL LIGAMENT

Stensen's duct
Excretory duct of the parotid gland. 7 cm long, runs over the masseter muscle and buccal fat pad then bends medially to pierce buccinator muscle ending intra-orally at the level of the second maxillary molar.
See PAROTIC DUCT.

Stepladder technique
- Used in *Lip reconstruction*.
- Use for defects up to 2/3s of the lower lip. It retains relatively good sensation and muscle continuity.
- The horizontal component measures one half the width of the defect, so 2–4 steps required. The vertical dimension of each step is 8–10 mm.

Stereognosis
The ability to recognize objects based on touch.
See MOBERG PICK-UP TEST.

Sternal cleft
- Rare and often dramatic presentation of central chest defect.
- Fusion from mesodermal plates occurs from above, so defects usually involve the lower or entire sternum.
- Deformities range from sternal clefts only, *Ectopia cordis* and Cantrell's pentalogy with multiple deformities of chest, heart, diaphragm and abdomen.
- Most sternal defects can be reapproximated and secured with wires.

See CHEST WALL RECONSTRUCTION.

Sternocleidomastoid

Origin: sternum and medial half of clavicle.

Insertion: lateral surface of mastoid process.

Blood supply:
- *Superior:* branches of occipital artery.
- *Middle:* branches of the superior thyroid artery.
- *Inferiorly:* branches of the thyrocervical trunk.

Innervation: spinal accessory nerve.

Sternocleidomastoid flap
- Can be raised on inferior or superior pedicle.
- The skin island is outlined over the inframastoid area. The skin paddle is not very reliable. The 11th cranial nerve is usually sacrificed.
- It can be used in a functional neck dissection for intra-oral reconstruction proximally based on superior thyroid and occipital vessels.

See ORAL CAVITY RECONSTRUCTION.

Sternotomy wounds
See CHEST WALL RECONSTRUCTION.

- 0.4–5% of median sternotomies get infected with a mortality of 5–50%.
- Related to internal mammary artery (IMA) use—Cosgrove reported no infection with saphenous vein, 0.3% with unilateral IMA and 2.4% with bilateral. Other associated factors are diabetes, smoking, hypertension.

Classification: by *Pairolero*.

- Can also be classified by anatomical site which can help in deciding the reconstruction into type A—upper half requiring pectoralis major reconstruction and Type B (lower half) and type C (whole sternum) requiring a combined pectoralis major and rectus abdominus bipedicled flap ('pec-rec' flap).

Reconstruction:
- Single stage debridement with muscle flap successful in 95% of cases.
- *Pectoralis major:* harvest through sternotomy wound. Detach muscle from ribs and sternum. Find pedicle and divide humeral attachment. Dissect from clavicle and advance medially. Bilateral flaps can be used for large defects. If the IMA is intact a turnover flap can be used. Ligate thoracoacromial pedicle and elevate from lateral to medial, preserving medial 2–3 cm of muscle.
- *Rectus abdominus:* use with pectoralis or if pectoralis not available. Based on the deep superior epigastric artery, a terminal branch of the IMA. Type III muscle (dual dominant supply). Midline incision, incise anterior

rectus sheath, divide muscle inferiorly, separate from posterior sheath and transpose. It can be used if the IMA has been harvested based on the 8th intercostal vessel, but vascularity is more tenuous.
- Combined pectoralis major and rectus abdominus bipedicled flap ('pec-rec' flap). Blood supply from the thoracoacromial artery superiorly and the deep inferior epigastric artery inferiorly. First a skin flap is raised then the plane deep to pectoralis major is developed. Rectus abdominus is elevated from the posterior rectus sheath. Lateral rectus abdominis and pectoralis major are divided.
- *Omentum:* used alone or with other flaps.
- Latissimus dorsi and external oblique (based on intercostals perforators) are used as back-up flaps.

See CHEST WALL RECONSTRUCTION.

Steroid
Hypertrophic scar: blunts the inflammatory response by stabilization of lysosomal membranes thus preventing the secretion of enzymes and cytokines. This leads to impaired capillary budding, inhibition of fibroblast proliferation, decreased protein synthesis and diminished epithelialization. Vitamin A counteracts the effects of steroids. Response rate of 30–100% with intralesional steroids but side-effects include atrophy, depigmentation, and telangiectasia.

Haemangiomas:
- *Action:* augments the sensitivity of the terminal vascular bed to catecholamines and inhibit fibroplasia.
- Dose is 2–3 mg/kg/day of prednisolone given systemically or orally over a 2–3-week period.
- Haemangiomas will respond within 7–10 days. After getting a response, lower the dose to 0.75 mg/kg/day. If they respond slowly, treat with a 4–6-week course then rest for 3–4 weeks, then another course. May see a rebound phenomenom. If so, treat with 2–3-week cycles with reducing doses. 1/3 respond quickly, 1/3 equivocal, 1/3 no response.
- Triamcinolone at a dose of 3–5 mg/kg can be used intralesionally. Usually require 3–5 injections at 6–8-week intervals.

See WOUND HEALING.

Stewart–Treves syndrome
See LYMPHANGIOSARCOMA.

Striae Caused by disruption of dermis with loss of continuity of elastic fibres.

Stickler syndrome
- One of the most commonly reported syndromes associated with cleft palate.
- Get myopia, retinal detachment, clefts and arthropathy.
- At least one form is due to a defect of collagen type II gene.
- It is autosomal dominant.
- Patients should be screened for vision.

See CRANIOFACIAL GENETICS.

Stork bite
See NAEVUS SIMPLEX.

Stranc and Robertson classification
Classification of nasal fractures: 3 groups.
- *Plane 1:* disruption of the cartilagenous septum. The nasal bones are unaffected.
- *Plane 2:* disruption of the bony septum and nasal bones.
- *Plane 3:* these injuries extend beyond the nasal skeleton into the piriform aperture and medial orbital rim. They represent mild naso-ethmoidal fractures.

Strawberry naevus
See HAEMANGIOMA.

Streptococcus
- Gram positive bacteria that microscopically form characteristics chains.
- Classified based on their haemolytic properties:
  - Alpha-haemolytic species cause oxidation of iron in haemoglobin. These include *S. pneumoniae* and *S. viridans*;
  - Beta-haemolytic species cause rupture of red blood cells. These include Group A and B haemolytic streptococci, which can be detrimental to wound healing and skin graft take.

Streptokinase
- It is the least expensive fibrinolytic agent, but highly antigenic with a high incidence of untoward reactions. It is produced by beta-haemolytic streptococci.
- It binds with free-circulating plasminogen or plasmin, which forms a complex that can convert additional plasminogen to plasmin. The active half-life is about 20 minutes. It can cause febrile reactions.
- It cannot be used safely a second time within 6 months.
- It is useful for breaking up clots in failing free tissue transfers.
- Use 5,000 units/ml and infuse 25,000–50,000 units, which will be effective locally, but not problematic systemically.

Struthers: arcade of
- One of the sites of potential *Ulnar nerve compression*.

- Formed from the medial intermuscular septum between biceps and triceps muscles in the arm.

Struthers: ligament of
- One of four sites of potential compression of the *Median nerve* in the forearm along with lacertus fibrosis, pronator teres and arch of FDS.
- The ligament may originate from a supracondylar process.
- It forms an accessory origin for pronator teres.

Sturge–Weber syndrome
- *Port-wine stain* with congenital glaucoma or ipsilateral leptomeningeal angiomatosis.
- Occurs in the distribution of the trigeminal nerve V1, V2 and V3 involvement (not V2 alone).
- There is a low risk of brain involvement.
- It can be associated with seizures, contralateral hemiplegia, and variable developmental delay of motor and cognitive skills.

Submucous cleft palate
- Cleft of the soft palate musculature with intact mucosa
- Cardinal triad of signs described by Calnan in 1954: bifid uvula, visible 'zona pellucida' and a palpable hard palatal notch in the midline at the hard/soft palate junction.
- Speech may be unaffected or can be associated with velopharyngeal dysfunction. Assess with a speech and language therapist and consider instrumental speech evaluation.
- An occult submucous cleft palate is a situation where velopharyngeal insufficiency exists in the absence of the classic triad of signs.
- Surgical management of submucous cleft palate if required is similar to an overt cleft palate. Common options include an intravelar veloplasty or a Furlow palatoplasty.

Succinylcholine in burns
- Succinylcholine is an acetylcholine agonist, which may cause a massive sometimes fatal release of potassium in burn patients.
- It has been documented as long as 18 months after a burn so its use is not recommended up to 2 years after a burn.
- Burn victims have an increased number of muscle receptor sites for acetylcholine.
- Non-depolarizing relaxants such as D-tubocurarine, pancuronium, atracurium and vencuronium are recommended, although burn patients have variable resistance with these.

Sudeck's osteoporosis
Seen in association with *Complex regional pain syndrome (CRPS)*. Diagnosed because of the apparent skeletal involvement. It frequently responds to intramuscular calcitonin treatment. Apart from the radiographic pattern it is indistinguishable from other forms of CRPS. The demineralization is similar to disuse, but more rapid than can be explained by disuse.

Sulphuric acid
• A strong acid and oxidizing agent.
• It is used in car batteries and electroplating.
• Strong thermal reaction occurs on contact with water.
• The skin is leathery and becomes red-brown, then grey. No systemic toxicity occurs. Upper and lower airway injury may occur.

See CHEMICAL INJURIES.

Supercharging
A method of augmenting the blood supply to a large pedicled flap by performing a micro-vascular anastomosis to a secondary pedicle of the flap. It is most often used for unipedicled TRAM flaps.

Superficial palmar arch
• Lies distal to the transverse carpal ligament (TCL) in a line from the base of the extended thumb to the hook of the hamate.
• Formed by the anastomosis of ulnar artery to superficial branch of radial artery.
• It gives off the common digital arteries, which divide at the base of the fingers to give off the digital arteries.

Superficial temporal artery
• Terminal branch of external carotid artery. Supplies the lateral aspect of the scalp and is the longest and largest of the scalp vessels.
• It arises from beneath the parotid anterior to the tragus. It travels along the temporoparietal fascia and bifurcates into an anterior and posterior branch 2 cm above the zygomatic arch. The main continuation is the posterior branch.

See SCALP RECONSTRUCTION.

Superior pedicle breast reduction
Operative technique: mark as for inferior pedicle with 90–100° angle. Limbs 8 cm and horizontal lines a little shorter. De-epithelialize around nipple/areolar complex. Cut nipple on pedicle 0.5 cm thick. Score inferior line and cut through dermis obliquely to the chest wall. Mobilize whole breast off pectoralis. Stabilize the breast and cut medial limb then vertical and lateral limb. Suture breast in two layers. Suture vertical limb to horizontal limb, which will rotate the breast tissue upward under the nipple to create projection. De-epithelialize the new areolar position and suture in the nipple.

Supraorbital nerve
• A sensory nerve from the ophthalmic branch of the trigeminal, supplying upper lid, conjunctiva, forehead and scalp up to the lambdoid suture.
• Exits orbit through the supra-orbital foramen, lateral to the supratrochlear nerve and courses deep to the corrugator supercilii and frontalis muscles.
• Block by inserting the needle under the midportion of the eyebrow while palpating the foramen.

Supratrochlear nerve
• A sensory nerve from the ophthalmic branch of the trigeminal supplying the medial aspect of the forehead, upper eyelid, skin of upper nose and conjunctiva.
• Exits orbit through the supratrochlear notch, medial to the supraorbital nerve and courses through the corrugator supercilii.
• Block by injecting medial portion of supraorbital rim lateral to the root of the nose.

Sural nerve
• *S1–2:* supplies skin of the lateral arch and lateral aspect of the heel.
• For nerve grafting, harvest through longitudinal or through stab incisions on the posterolateral aspect of the leg posterior to the lateral malleolus.

Sushruta
*c.*700 BC. Wrote in the *Samhita* (encyclopaedia). First to describe a facial (forehead) flap for the reconstruction of a nose.

Sutures
Absorbable:
• *Catgut:* from submucosal layer of sheep intestine. Hydrolysed by proteolytic enzymes within 60 days. Tensile strength lost within 10 days. Prolonged by chromatization.
• *Vicryl/Dexon:* synthetic. Minimal tissue reaction. Tensile strength lost in 1 month completely absorbed in 3 months. Both are braided sutures which can potentiate infection.
• *Polydiaxone (PDS):* synthetic absorbable monofilament. Minimally reactive. Retains tensile strength at 3 months, absorption complete by 6 months. Can spit out.
• *Maxon/monocryl:* absorbable monofilaments, similar to PDS, but retain tensile strength for only 3–4 weeks. Absorption complete by 3 and 4 months.

• So vicryl, dexon, monocryl, maxon, lose strength by 3 weeks, absorbed by 3 months. PDS loses strength by 3 months absorbed by 6 months.

Non-absorbable:
• Monofilament sutures (ethilon, prolene) have minimal inflammatory reaction, slide well, can easily be removed and retain tensile strength. Prolene keeps tensile strength better than ethilon.
• Braided sutures (ethibond, ticron, silk) give an inflammatory reaction.

See ALLOPLASTS.

Swan neck deformity
Hyperextension of the PIP joint with flexion of the DIP joint.

Causes of swan neck:
• *PIP:* volar plate deficiency.
• *Flexor:* rupture of FDS.
• *Intrinsics:* intrinsic muscle contractures.
• *Extrinsics:* chronic mallet finger, extensor tension, e.g. wrist deformity.

In RA: functional loss relates to loss of motion of PIP joint. 4 types determined by motion and joint space.

Classification:
• *I*—PIPJ flexible.
• *II*—flexion limited on MCP joint extension (intrinsic tightness).
• *III*—limited in all positions.
• *IV*—stiff with XR charges.

Type I—PIP flexible in all positions:
• Full passive motion of PIP joint.
• Deformity may originate in DIP or PIP joint.
• May start with stretching or rupture of terminal extensor tendon attachment giving a mallet deformity. This can be presumed when the DIP deformity is greater than the PIP deformity.
• In others the PIP joint is the cause of the problem when synovitis stretches the volar capsule or flexor rupture. Then DIP flexion is secondary.
• Treat by preventing PIP joint hyperextension and restoring DIP extension:
  ○ *Splint* around PIP joint;
  ○ DIP joint can be surgically fused;
  ○ Dermodesis (take ellipse of skin from volar aspect of PIP 5 mm wide);
  ○ Flexor tendon tenodesis (section one insertion of FDS proximally, pass through slit in A2 pulley and re-attach to itself);
  ○ Retinacular ligament reconstruction (ulnar lateral band free from extensor mechanism proximally, but left attached distally; passed volar to Cleland's fibres and suture to fibrous tendon sheath). *See* ORL.

Type II—PIPJ flexion limited in certain positions:
• PIP joint flexion is influenced by position of MCP joint. When the MCP joint is extended, passive PIP joint movement is limited. Though initially the limitation is only on MCP joint extension, eventually the PIP joint will become stiff.
• Need to relieve intrinsic tightness and correct any MCP joint problem such as subluxation.
• *Intrinsic release:* perform through dorso-ulnar longitudinal incision over proximal phalanx. Can be combined with DIP joint fusion or volar dermodesis.

Type III—limited PIPJ flexion in all positions:
• Significant loss of hand function. Often well-preserved joint spaces. Structures restricting movement are extensor mechanisms, collateral ligaments, and skin.
• Need to first restore passive motion.
• *PIP joint manipulation:* may be possible with an MUA, usually with intrinsic release or Swanson arthroplasty. Splint in flexion. May need K-wire fixation initially.
• *Skin release:* oblique incision which is left open—graft not needed. Perform just distal to joint.
• *Lateral band mobilization:* in established deformity lateral bands are displaced dorsally. Freeing them from the extensor tendon using two parallel incisions allows movement.
• *Flexor tenosynovitis:* tendon adherence and tenosynovitis can lead to stiff PIP joints.

Type IV—stiff PIPJ and poor XR appearance:
• Require fusion or arthroplasty. Tend to fuse index for stability.

Swanson classification
See CONGENITAL HAND ANOMALIES.

Swanson MCP joint arthroplasty: operative technique
• Transverse incision over dorsum over MCP joints. Expose extensor tendons, preserving all structures in between.
• Release intrinsics on ulnar side and reflect extensor tendon radially—usually requiring sagittal band division. Crossed intrinsic transfer—preserve intrinsic divided distally. Identify intrinsic on radial side and suture ulnar intrinsic to radial side of adjacent finger. Can be performed on middle, index and little finger.
• Try to preserve capsule, incise and reflect. Perform synovectomy. Put Mitchell trimmer and Howarth around metacarpal head and excise head with oscillating saw just around

the metacarpal flare. Hold head with towel clip and excise preserving collateral ligaments. Perform thorough synovectomy with rongeurs cleaning off volar plate and under metacarpal, but being careful not to injure NVBs. Put traction on finger to increase space.

- Now prepare bones for prosthesis. Start with broach then move to reamers. Ream metacarpal square, but angle proximal phalanx slightly to recreate normal arc of hand. When reaming phalanx hold finger to enable accurate gauging of position of reamer. Use sizers to determine prosthesis. Drill hole in distal radial side of metacarpal and stitch radial collateral with ticron, pass through hole and clip. Retract all soft tissue out of the way and using a no touch technique insert the prosthesis—long end proximally. Ensure a snug fit and tie collateral.
- Suture capsule with PDS and reef extensor if necessary. Place Swanson drain transversely and suture skin. Put in volar backslab in slight MCPJ flexion. After 1/52 put in outrigger.

Sweat glands
Two types.

- *Apocrine:* in axilla and groin. Start to function in puberty and give an odour due to bacterial decomposition. Sympathetic adrenergic.
- *Eccrine* glands are found throughout the body except lips and external genitalia. They are found more frequently in the eyelids, palms, feet and axilla. The eccrine glands on the sole of the foot and palm of hand differ from the rest of the body. Sympathetic cholinergic. The sweating of a graft follows that of the recipient site. Transplanted skin lacks lubrication until it is reinnervated.

Sweat gland tumours
- *Eccrine hidrocystomas.*
- *Syringomas.*
- *Cylindroma.*
- *Eccrine spiradenoma.*
- *Eccrine poroma.*

Symblepharon
Fusion of the eyelids to the globe. It is some-times caused by chemical burns. Localized areas may be corrected with Z-plasty, but the best method for correction is wide release of adhesions and conjunctival grafting. Larger areas will require mucosal grafts.

Symbrachydactyly
- Means short coalesced digits. Deficient bony framework leaves soft tissues unsupported. Get finger buds with nail appendages.
- Arises sporadically with mesodermal deficit in skeletal framework of fingers.

- There is a failure of formation and failure of differentiation in a longitudinal and transverse direction. Longitudinal deficiency centres around the middle phalanx, transverse affects index, middle, ring, little then thumb.
- Usually unilateral with no other abnormalities. 25–39% associated with ipsilateral pectoral or thoracic deficits.
- Short finger type is the most common. Usually the thumb is spared, but may get adduction of 1st web space. Categorize according to number of remaining phalanges (absence progresses from middle phalanx). All fingers affected but radial more severe. Some similarities in Apert's and constriction ring. It is the most common of the 4 types: 33–59%.

Classification: *Blauth and Gekeler.*

Treatment:
- If skin envelope is present, composite grafts can be inserted.
- May perform a reverse pollicization—transferring the index ray to the 3rd MC.
- Thumb reconstruction can be performed in a number of ways. Can use skin from cleft to widen 1st web space. Rotation osteotomy of border digits.

See CONGENITAL HAND ANOMALIES.

Sympathetic function testing
- The sympathetic nervous system controls vasomotor response, sweating and pilomotor activity. These 3 can be assessed along with trophic changes.
- *Trophic changes:* get atrophy and tapering of the fingers—'pencil-pointing effect'. Skin is smooth and finger prints disappear.
- *Vasomotor:* change in skin colour and temperature. May be blue or pink as heat regulatory capacity is lost. *Ninhydrin printing test* is the most accurate assessment. Wrinkle test assesses wrinkling after placing hand in water.

See SENSATION TESTING.

Symphalangism
- Originally described absent PIPJ with normal length of phalanges. Also used to describe stiffness of MCPJ and DIPJ and also includes shortened digits.
- Rare autosomal dominant inherited condition due to failure of differentiation. Can be seen in drug-induced anomalies and other non-inheritable anomalies such as Poland's and

Apert's. Most common in Caucasians, rare in those of African descent.

- Clinically no discernible finer creases, get square articular surfaces.

Classification:

- *3 types:* true (single or multiple) symbrachydactyly and symphalangism associated with other anomalies.
- *Cushing:* fusion of PIPJs most common.
- *Drey:* involvement of DIPJs of all fingers with hypoplastic nails.
- *Kermisson:* index to little finger severely malformed, absent nails and distal phalanges, short middle phalanges, fused PIPJs.
- *Fuhrman:* radiohumeral synostosis, carpal and tarsal fusion.
- *WL symphalangism:* brachydactyly syndrome. Autosomal dominant with conductive hearing loss, broad nose, pes excavatum.

Treatment:

- Arthroplasties have been tried, but none are successful in producing a mobile joint.
- Vascularized 2nd toe transfer. Operate at age 10 as exercise is very important.
- Alternatively perform osteotomies when the epiphyses are fused. Do it at 20°, 30°, 40°, 50° for D2, 3, 4 and 5, respectively.

Syndactyly

Two or more partially or completely fused digits. Arise because of failure of apoptosis (pro-grammed cell death).

Epidemiology:

- 1:2,000 births. 20% have a positive family history. M:F 2:1. Autosomal dominant with incomplete penetrance. Common in Caucasians.
- It may be associated with syndromes such as Apert's and Poland's. Linked to FGF receptor deficiency.
- Middle-ring web in 54% of cases, ring-little in 30%, middle-index in 15%, thumb-index 1%.

Classification:

- Complete (up to the tips of the fingers) or incomplete.
- Simple (only soft tissue), complex (soft tissue and bony connections), complicated (associated accessory digits or phalanges), acrosyndactyly (fingers fused distally with fenestrations between digits proximally—thought to be caused by constriction ring syndrome).

Treatment:

- Surgical release not usually before 1 year old, though earlier if 1st or 4th web involved due

to the length discrepancy. Also complex and acrosyndactyly are released earlier as the bony connections will affect growth.

- Only operate on one side of a finger at a time to avoid devascularizing digit.
- Do border digits first.
- Straight line scars may cause more contractures. Use a large proximally-based dorsal flap to create the web space and prevent web creep—many different designs have been described including rectangular, hourglass and gullwing flaps. Use interdigitating flaps volar and dorsal. Grafts may be required for the defects. Use interdigitating (Buck-Gramko) flaps from the hyponychium to reconstruct the lateral nail fold.

Synostosis

- Abnormal fusion of two bones which may be partial, permitting reduced motion or complete, with no motion.
- It can occur at any site in the upper limb where two bones are adjacent.
- Synostosis in the phalanges occur in complex *Syndactyly.*
- Forearm synostosis may require rotational osteotomy.

Synovectomy

See RHEUMATOID ARTHRITIS.

Syringocystadenoma papilliferum

- Usually a verrucous lesion that occurs most commonly on or near the scalp.
- A hamartomatous growth often in association with naevus sebaceous type.
- It begins to develop during childhood and may be bulbous.
- Basal cell epithelioma occur in about 10% of the lesions.
- Treat with excision of the lesion and any surrounding sebaceous nevus.

Syringomas

- Occur in adult women on the lower eyelids and upper cheeks, and also the trunk, neck, and extremities.
- Pink or yellow papules, usually 2–3 mm in diameter.
- They are often confused with trichoepitheliomas, xanthelasma or basal cell epithelioma.
- Removal for diagnosis and cosmesis with excision, cautery or laser.

Systemic lupus erythematosus (SLE)

- Usually young women (15–25 year). F:M 9:1.
- Varies from a mild to a fatal disease.

- When active get leucopoenia, anaemia, raised ESR, positive anti-nuclear factor and low serum complement with vasculitis.
- Hand deformities can resemble RA with volar subluxation and ulnar drift. XR show deformity with no erosive changes or joint space narrowing. Hand deformities are passively correctable as the ligaments are lax. Therefore, position can usually be maintained by splints though arthroplasty or arthrodesis maybe required.
- Skin grafts and flaps are not contraindicated in SLE patients and the benefits of steroid therapy in suppressing vasculitis outweigh the drawbacks.

Tagliacozzi to Two-point discrimination

Tagliacozzi
- *Gaspar Tagliacozzi:* sixteenth-century Italian surgeon from Bologna who defined the ideals of plastic surgery.
- 'We restore, repair and make whole those parts of the face which Nature has given but which fortune has taken away, not so much that they may delight the eye but that they may buoy up the spirit and help the mind of the afflicted.'
- He learnt and further developed the pedicled flap from arm for nasal reconstruction.

Tagliacozzi flap
- A random pattern flap of upper arm skin used for *Nasal reconstruction*. The original Tagliacozzi flap was based distally and required *Delay* with a cotton lint being placed under the flap to prevent reattachment.
- A more recent modification uses a proximally based flap that encompasses the axial vessel to the medial arm skin. A delay procedure is not necessary.
- After transfer, the upper extremity is immobilized for approximately 3 weeks until the pedicle is divided.
- Good quality skin is supplied but there is often a significant difference in quality from normal nasal skin and better options are usually available.

Tanzer classification
For congenital ear anomalies.
- *Type I:* anotia.
- *Type II:* microtia.
  - *A:* microtia with atresia of external auditory meatus;
  - *B:* microtia without atresia.
- *Type III:* hypoplasia of the middle third of the ear.
- *Type IV:*
  - *A:* constricted ear;
  - *B:* cryptotia;
  - *C:* hypoplasia of the upper third.

- *Type V:* prominent ear.
  See EAR.

Tanzini 1906:
performed a latissimus dorsi flap for breast reconstruction.

TAR syndrome
Thrombocytopenia Absent Radius. Autosomal recessive. The thumb is usually present. Usually get correction of the thrombocytopenia after 1 year with good prognosis.
See RADIAL CLUB HAND.

Targeted muscle reinnervation
- Technique by which the distal end of nerves divided at the time of limb amputation are coapted to smaller motor nerve branches of remaining muscles. Initially developed to motor myoelectric prostheses, but incidentally found to reduce phantom limb and neuroma pain following limb amputation. It is thought this is because you are 'giving the nerve somewhere to go and something to do.' Can be done primarily at time of amputation or as a delayed procedure.
- Indications are still contentious, but likely most effective for young trauma patients suffering chronic pain in a limb prior to amputation.
- For above knee amputations, address sciatic nerve. For below knee amputations, address tibial and peroneal nerves.
  - Divide sciatic nerve into common peroneal and tibial divisions. Coapt tibial division to motor branch to semimembranous and peroneal division to motor branch to biceps femoris;
  - Coapt tibial nerve to a motor branch to soleus;
  - Coapt superficial peroneal nerve to a motor branch to FDL or FHL.

Tarsal tunnel syndrome
- Results from compression of the posterior tibial nerve within the fibrous tunnel. Usually get a burning pain in the medial part of the

foot. Worsened by activity and at night. Tinel's sign positive along course of posterior tibial nerve. Sensation is decreased.

- May be confirmed by nerve conduction studies with prolonged latency and abnormal potentials.
- Treat by releasing the tunnel.

See LOWER LIMB RECONSTRUCTION.

Tarsorrhaphy

- Surgical closure of the eyelids indicated when any part of the cornea remains exposed when the eye is closed.
- A medial or lateral tarsorrhaphy can be performed. Pinch the eyelid to determine which side is best. A medial tarsorrhaphy keeps the puncta in touch with the globe. It is better cosmetically, but more difficult as the puncta and canaliculi need to be avoided.
- *Margaret Brand procedure:* pinch the lids together. Mark the correct length. Add amethocaine and LA. Incise along the grey line (behind the lash follicles). Make another incision parallel to the first 1-2 mm thick. Dissect this strip of tissue. Repeat on the upper lid. Suture together over bolsters. Ensure no lashes project inwards. Remove sutures after 2/52. Give chloramphenicol drops.
- *McLaughlin procedure:* incise lower lid margin along intermarginal line (the line where the lids touch anteriorly) medially from the lateral canthus for 5-6 mm. Remove a piece of anterior lamella of lower lid. Split the intermarginal line of the upper lid and remove a similar section of tarsus and conjunctiva. Evert upper lid and suture with a bolster.

Tattoo

- A foreign material entered into the dermis leaving an indelible mark. Depth varies. Professional tattoos are superficial and uniform and therefore more readily removable but have more ink than home-made tattoos. Tattoos were present in ancient Egypt. Polynesians had tattoos and this started the naval tradition.
- Medical tattoos are useful for vitiligo, nipple reconstruction, grafts. Also eyebrows and eyelids. Retattooing can cover up an offensive portion of a tattoo.

Safety:

- Dyes are generally safe. Patients can become sensitized to the pigment in a tattoo particularly the red from cinnabar. Usually it is a delayed hypersensitivity with itchy

glaucomatous lesions. Some are photoallergic.

- Using Q-switched laser with an allergy may worsen the allergy as the dye is broken up. There is a risk of transmission of infectious diseases.

Treatment:

- *Excision:* may be the best option, particularly if there is an allergy to the dye. May require serial excision, tissue expansion or a flap.
- *Laser:* short pulses disrupt tattoo material. Use Q-switched laser. Because the energy is high and the duration short, the pigment can be eliminated without injuring adjacent dermis. May develop scarring and hypopigmentation, response may be extremely variable. The most difficult to treat are the newer brightly coloured tattoos. Homemade tattoos are easier to treat as the load of ink is less. Match wavelength to colour:
  - Black ink: Nd:YAG (1064nm);
  - Blue/black/green ink: ruby (694nm) or alexandrite (755nm);
  - Red/orange/yellow ink: Nd:YAG (532nm)
- *Salabrasion:* skin is abraded and salt left on the wound allowing some pigment to leach out.
- *Tanic/oxalic acid:* use after abrasion to induce inflammation.
- *Dermabrasion:* the epidermis and superficial dermis is abraded. A dressing is changed daily allowing dye to leach onto the dressing. The problems are scarring and partial response. Also chemical peel and dermaplaning has been used.

Taylor classification

Nerve supply to muscles.

- *Type 1:* single unbranched nerve.
- *Type 2:* single nerve which branches.
- *Type 3:* multiple branches from same nerve.
- *Type 4:* multiple branches from different trunks.

See MUSCULOCUTANEOUS/MUSCLE FLAPS.

Teeth

Classification:

- *Universal system:* of notation of teeth. Adult/permanent maxillary teeth 1-16 from upper right third molar and mandibular teeth numbered 17-32 from lower left third molar. Baby/deciduous teeth are similarly counted using A-J for upper and T-K for lower.
- *Teeth names:* the 32 permanent teeth are divided into 4 quadrants. Each has a central incisor, lateral incisor, canine (cuspid), first

premolar (bicuspid), second premolar (bicuspid) and first second and third molars. The 20 deciduous teeth are also divided into four each having a central and lateral incisor, canine, and first and second molar.

Anatomy:

- The crown is visible and the root is attached to the bony walls by periodontal membrane fibres. The crown is covered with enamel and the root with cementum. The junction is the cervical line. Under enamel and cementum is the dentin. In the centre is the pulp chamber. The pulp tissue supplies nerve and blood vessels to the tooth through apical foramen.
- *Nerve supply:* lower teeth supplied by the inferior alveolar branch of the mandibular division of the trigeminal nerve. The upper teeth are supplied by the maxillary division of the trigeminal nerve which divides into the posterior superior alveolar branch from the pterygopalatine portion and the middle and anterior superior alveolar branches from the infra-orbital nerves.

Development:

- Get primary (deciduous, 'baby') and secondary (permanent, 'adult') dentition. At birth the maxilla and mandible contain the partially formed crowns of 20 deciduous teeth. All erupt in the first 2 years, starting with central incisors, then first molars, then second molars and canines. The first permanent teeth erupt at age 6 and take 6 years to complete (mixed dentition phase).
- All will be replaced by teeth of the same type except the primary molars which are replaced by bicuspids and the permanent 1-3 molars, which are posterior to the second primary molar. The third molars (wisdom teeth) erupt at cessation of jaw growth (17–21 years).
- *Missing teeth:* the most common congenitally missing tooth is the third molar. Several missing teeth (oligodontia) or anodontia is often associated with ectodermal dysplasia and oral–facial–digital syndrome.

Trauma: the most common tooth injury is fracture. A root fracture is most favourable if in the apical 1/3. Subluxed teeth can be intruded or extruded. If intruded they need repositioning. If extruded it should be replaced and splinted.

Occlusion: *see* ANGLE CLASSIFICATION.

Terminology:

- *Mesial:* toward the midline.
- *Distal:* away from the midline.
- *Lingual:* toward the tongue.
- *Buccal:* toward the cheek.

- *Crossbite:* an abnormal buccolingual relation of the teeth. Anterior crossbite is lingual crossbite of the upper incisors. Posterior crossbite is buccal crossbite of the maxillary premolars and molars.
- *Overbite:* vertical overlap of the incisors, where the upper incisors are in a lower than normal position. *Angle class* II: the buccal groove of the mandibular first molar is distal to the mesiobuccal cusp of the maxillary first molar.
- *Underbite: Angle* class III: the mandibular first molar is mesial to the mesiobuccal cusp of the maxillary first molar.
- *Overjet:* horizontal overlap of the incisors, where the upper incisors are positioned anterior to their normal position.
- *Open bite:* lack of contact between teeth in the mouth-shut position.
- *Tooth vitality:* sensate tooth with an intact pulpal nerve supply. (A tooth may have an adequate blood supply, but is non-vital if a nerve supply is not present.)
- *Curve of Spee:* curvature of the occlusal plane.
- *Centric occlusion:* position of the mandible where there is maximal intercuspation of the maxillary and mandibular teeth.
- *Centric relation:* the most retruded position of the mandible, where the condyles are comfortably seated in the glenoid fossae.
- *Centric occlusion and centric relation:* may be the same in a normal patient but may differ in cases of malocclusion. (Centric relation can exist in the absence of teeth.)
- *Ankylosis of a tooth:* solid fixation of a tooth resulting from fusion of the cementum and alveolar bone with obliteration of the periodontal ligament. (The tooth is 'locked' in bone and cannot be moved orthodontically.)
- *Retrogenia:* the chin is not necessarily small, but is positioned posterior to its desired location.
- *Retrognathia:* posterior positioning of the mandible.
- *Microgenia:* a small chin is present with an overall deficiency of bone, generally in all three planes.
- *Micrognathia:* the entire jaw is small.
- *Macrogenia:* the chin is large.
- *Mandibular prognathism:* anterior positioning of the mandible.
  See ORTHOGNATHIC SURGERY.

Telangiectasia

Dilation of the capillaries causing a red spider-like appearance on the skin.

- *Generalized essential telangiectasia:* onset varies widely, but is most common in adults. F:M 2:1. Get groups of pin-sized, vascular puncta in the lower extremities. The lesions extend proximally to form sheets of telangiectasias. Flashlamp pulsed dye laser therapy is relatively effective.

- *Cutis marmorata telangiectatica congenita* (Van Lohuizen syndrome).
- *Hereditary haemorrhagic telangiectasia* (HHT; Rendu–Osler–Weber syndrome).
- *Ataxia-telangiectasia (Louis–Bar syndrome).*

See VASCULAR MALFORMATIONS.

Telecanthus

- An increased distance between the medial canthi (a soft tissue structure).
- The outer canthal distance and inter-pupillary distance remain within normal limits.
- Associated with *Down's syndrome*, fetal alcohol syndrome, *Klinefelter's syndrome*, *Elhers-Danlos syndrome*
- Also known as pseudo-hypertelorism. Important to differentiate from *hypertelorism*, which is an increase in the interorbital distance at the dacryon.

Temporalis muscle

Origin:

- *Deep:* temporal fossa calvarium.
- *Superficial:* deep temporalis fascia.

Insertion: coronoid process and anterior ramus of mandible.

Innervation: mandibular division of trigeminal nerve (V3) anterior and deep temporal branches.

Blood supply: deep temporal fascia. Middle temporal branch of superficial temporal artery.

Action: anterior fibres are elevators and posterior fibres are retractors of the mandible.

Temporalis muscle flap

Based on the deep temporal vessels. First described by Golovine in 1898. It can be used to reconstruct the maxillofacial region and as a motor in facial nerve palsy when it can be detached from the origin as a turnover flap with a fascial extension or detached from the insertion on the coronoid process.

See ORAL CAVITY RECONSTRUCTION.

Temporomandibular joint (TMJ)

- Called a ginglymoarthrodial joint as it has both a hinged and a gliding motion. There is a meniscus separating superior and inferior joint compartments. The articular surface is lined with fibrocartilage.
- Both TMJs function as a single unit—the craniomandibular articulation. The end point is the position of dental occlusion.
- The articular disc separates the joint into two spaces. Hinge occurs in the inferior space and

sliding in the superior space. The joint surfaces consist of the mandibular condyle and temporal articular surface. The condyles are elliptical. They are surrounded by the fibrous joint capsule. The disc is a biconcave structure composed of dense fibrous connective tissue. It is anchored anteriorly to the superior head of the lateral pterygoid muscle and the eminentia articularis, inferiorly to the medial and lateral aspect of the mandibular condyle, and posteriorly in two zones.

- The main function of the disc is to distribute load evenly along the joint surfaces, as well as aiding in their lubrication and protection during translatory movements.

Temporomandibular joint dysfunction

- 30% of the Western population may have symptoms. F:M 3:1.
- Patients complain of pain, noise and limitation of movement. Look for asymmetry, dentition, malocclusion, joint movement.
- *Imaging:* XR, arthrography, CT and MRI.

Myofascial pain dysfunction syndrome (MPD): usually no anatomic abnormalities are seen in the TMJ. The cause is multifactorial and includes bruxism and anxiety and occlusal prematurity, which lead to spasm of the jaw muscles and pain. The aim of management is to break the spasm cycle. Treat occlusion problems with a splint. A splint at night will prevent bruxism. Also use NSAIDs, heat, diathermy and ultrasound.

Trauma: usually get anterior displacement of the disc trapping retrodisc tissues causing pain. Get premature wear of the articular surface. The management is stage-dependent but in the early stages treat as for MPD.

Ankylosis:

- Classified as true (intra-articular) or false (extra-articular) and bony or fibrous. Most commonly due to trauma, infection and juvenile arthritis.
- Get fibrous then bony fusion. Patients have oral hygiene problems. If the patient is young, mandibular growth will be retarded.
- Treatment with condylectomy or gap and interpositional arthroplasty. In severe cases replacement with costochondral graft harvested from contralateral 5th or 6th rib, and split longitudinally. Temporalis fascia is used between the graft and glenoid fossa.

TMJ dislocations:

- Acute dislocations of the TMJ occur as the condyle extends anteriorly beyond the eminence as a result of hypermobility

secondary to trauma or exaggerated mouth opening as in yawning. Spontaneous reduction usually follows, but in some cases the dislocation persists and requires manual reduction.
- With thumb inside and finger outside, push the mandible down and posteriorly. Muscle relaxants may be required.

Infective arthritis:
- Local spread or haematogenous spread with development of osteomyelitis and ankylosis of the TMJ.
- Treat with open drainage, intravenous antibiotics, and sequestrectomy if indicated.

Avascular necrosis:
- After trauma or devascularization at the time of TMJ surgery. The patient will present with the typical symptoms of TMJ syndrome including pain and limited jaw motion.
- Treat by debridement of the necrotic condyle and possible condylar replacement in severe cases.

Surgery treatment of TMJ problems:
- *TMJ arthroscopy:* lavage and debridement may improve symptoms. Long-term benefit has not been demonstrated.
- *TMJ arthrotomy:* through a preauricular incision the inferior border of the disc is incised. Disc displacement requires repositioning by resecting a wedge posteriorly. If there is significant degeneration then a total meniscectomy is performed. Osteophytes are shaved.
- *TMJ implants:* implants in young patients have caused significant problems. Implants are only indicated in severe ankylosis and degenerative disease.

Temporoparietal fascial flap
- Superficial temporal artery runs beneath subcutaneous tissues and within temporoparietal fascia. The vein is more superficial lying on the surface of the fascia.
- Temporoparietal fascia (TPF) is a thin fascial sheet which is an extension of SMAS layer that covers temporal, occipital and parietal scalp. Deep to TPF is the deep temporal fascia and temporalis muscle.
- A deep branch of the superficial temporal artery at the level of the zygoma separates to supply the deep temporal fascia.
- The deep temporal fascia can be dissected as a separate component to increase the size of the flap.

- There is an inconspicuous donor site scar, and the size of the flap can reach 14×17 cm though usually 8×10 cm.
- Dissection may cause alopecia.

Application:
- The tissue may be transferred on an ipsilateral pedicle or as a free flap. It may carry hair-bearing scalp and calvarial bone.
- It can be used to cover auricular cartilage and for a gliding surface in tendon reconstruction in the hand. It is good for facial soft tissue augmentation.

Technique:
- *Position:* supine.
- *Landmarks:* palpate the pulse anterior to the ear and mark the likely course of the pedicle. Mark *Pitanguy's line* to estimate course of frontal branch.
- *Markings:* Y incision with vertical limb in pre-auricular crease.
- Raise:
  - Subdermal skin flaps—careful not to injure the vein which lies superficially on the surface of the fascia;
  - Start the raise of the flap distally (superiorly)—a loose areolar plane between the superficial fascia and deep fascia allows the raise;
  - Narrow the flap as it nears the frontal branch of the facial nerve and isolate on the vascular pedicle.

Tendon
Anatomy: inelastic fibrils of type I collagen in a ground substance of dermatan sulphate. Fibrils are bundled into fibres. The main cell is the fibroblast. Tendon is covered with paratenon. Endotenon covers the central portions. Blood vessels run in paratenon from muscle and from bone. Also vincula system. Blood flow is low. Tendons within sheaths are covered with synovial fluid which is nutritive. Tendons contain few cells and those present include teno-cytes, synovial cells and fibroblasts.

Healing:
- Normally tendons are not very metabolically active. Healing occurs by adhesion from surrounding tissue and intrinsic healing driven by fibroblasts within the tendon. Both normally contribute to healing.
- *Extrinsic healing:* adhesion formation is maximized by immobilization and is similar to healing in other tissues. *See* WOUND HEALING.
- *Intrinsic healing:* depends much less on the inflammatory response. Early motion generates more intrinsic healing. Fibroblasts

migrate from epitenon into the damaged area facilitated by fibronectin. Neovascularization occurs. Collagen is synthesized by fibroblasts. Early motion gets quicker gains in tensile strength. Extensive injuries are more likely to heal with adhesion. Lunborg showed that tendons heal when wrapped in a semipermeable membrane and placed in the knee joint of a rabbit.

Surgical repair: careful apposition of ends is important. Reconstructing sheath has not been shown to improve healing.

Tendon harvest
- *Palmaris longus*.
- *Plantaris*.
- Long toe extensors. Make a transverse incision at the level of metatarsophalangeal joints. Long extensors are isolated proximal to the hood. Pass a stripper but when it gets stuck make further transverse incision and free the tendon then use the stripper again. Can take long extensor of 2nd, 3rd, 4th toes.

  See TENDON RECONSTRUCTION.

Tendon rupture in rheumatoid arthritis
In *Rheumatoid arthritis* due to attrition over bone, infiltration by synovium, ischaemia due to pressure from synovium. Ulnar subluxation of extensor tendons and PIN compression may cause confusion.

Extensor tendons:
- Get sudden loss of finger extension. Usually painless after trivial injury or activity. May go unrecognized. The factors causing an isolated rupture often lead to subsequent rupture often in order from little to index (*Vaughn-Jackson syndrome*). Often the tendons are abraded on the distal ulna.
- Tendon rupture can be mimicked by:
  - MCP joint dislocation (but patient cannot passively extend);
  - Ulnar subluxation of the extensor tendons between the metacarpal heads (patient can hold finger in extension if examiner extends passively);
  - Posterior interosseous nerve compression by elbow synovitis or subluxation of the radial head causing paralysis of the common extensor tendon. Tenodesis is preserved.

Management:
- *Single:* usually little finger. Amount of extensor lag depends on whether both tendons ruptured. If EDQM is ruptured may get 30° lag. Test EDC by holding other fingers flexed. if the extensor lag increases then EDC is still active. End to end repair may be

feasible. If not possible suture to adjacent (ring finger) tendon. Perform dorsal synovectomy. Remove bony spicules or ulna head. Transfer dorsal retinaculum deep to tendons if bone exposed.
- *Double:* if little and ring finger extensors are ruptured, can suture both to middle finger extensor. If the little finger extensor stump does not reach, can transfer ring to middle and use EIP or ECU transfer to little finger. If more than 2 tendons are ruptured, use FDS—can be brought through interosseus membrane (FDS middle to index and middle finger extensors, FDS ring for ring and little finger extensors). Palmaris longus, or, if the wrist is fused, a wrist extensor can be used as a bridge graft. Put the weave in tight as the muscle will stretch post-operatively.
- *Tendon ruptures with MCPJ disease:* first tackle the joints as unless the joints can be extended passively they won't benefit from tendon reconstruction.

Tendon transfers
- Used to restore balance to a hand with impaired function of extrinsic or intrinsic tendons. The transferred donor tendon remains attached to its parent muscle and the neurovascular pedicle remains intact.

General principles:
- Can remember principles to be considered with the mnemonic 'APOSTLES':
- **A**mplitude: *of tendon excursion:* should be adequate to restore function;
- **P**ower: donors lose one MRC power grade after transfer;
- **O**ne tendon, one function;
- **S**ynergy: the donor should ideally be synergistic to that which it is replacing. Finger flexion/wrist extension and finger extension/wrist flexion are synergistic;
- **T**issue equilibrium: accepting wound bed should be stable in terms of infection, scarring and healing;
- **L**ine of pull: aim for a straight line of pull as using a pulley weakens the donor;
- **E**xpendable: the donor muscle-tendon unit should be expendable;
- **S**table skeleton: fractures should be fixed first. Flaps may be required. Silicone rods may be required. Passive movement should be maintained.
- *Timing:* can be early, conventional or late. Conventional is performed when there is no reinnervation 3 months after the expected time. Early can be performed at the same time as nerve repair as a temporary substitute which may augment a suboptimal recovery.

- *Surgery:* mobilize the muscle carefully. The tendon should glide through a tunnel. Repair with a *Pulvertaft weave,* carefully tension. Immobilize for 3 weeks then gentle active ROM exercises.

Smith and Hastings algorithm:
- List all muscles that are functioning.
- List all muscles available for transfer, eliminating all that would leave an unacceptable deficit.
- Decide which functions need to be restored.
- Match available muscles with the needed functions.
- Consider other options such as arthrodesis and/or tenodesis.
- Divide the reconstruction into stages according to whether post-operative immobilization will be in flexion or extension.

Radial nerve palsy:
- Inability to extend wrist and fingers and abduct thumb. Biggest problem is the wrist instability. Sensory loss not a problem. Timing is controversial, some advocating early repair with the nerve repair. The more proximal the injury, the less likely is it that innervation will occur. Studies conflict as to the successfulness of repair. Results are less predictable with extensive injury, significant gap and older patients. In this group early transfer is indicated.
- Need to retain a wrist flexor. Preserve FCU as flexion and ulnar deviation is important for power grip, especially in PIN palsy as the ECU activity is lost.
- 3 options. All have PT → ECRB/L. Two have PL → EPL. Boyes uses FDS for wrist and thumb.

  ○ *Brand:* FCR to EDC, PL to EPL. Good for PIN palsy as keeps FCU and prevent wrist from radially deviating (ECRL remains intact in PIN palsy);
  ○ *Jones:* FCU to EDC, PL to EPL;
  ○ *Boyes:* FDSIII to EDC. FDS IV to EIP/EPL. FCR to APL/EPB.

Operative techniques:
- *FCU transfer:* inverted J incision over volar ulnar aspect of forearm. Transect at wrist crease. Mobilize PL, transecting distally. S incision on volar radial aspect of forearm. PT tendon divided from its insertion. ECRB transected at the musculotendinous junction. PT is rerouted to insert onto ECRB. A tunnel is made around the forearm and FCU is passed dorsally to lie across EDC. Perform end to side repair if some function might return. EPL is divided at the musculocutaneous junction

and passed to PL. Each EDC tendon is sutured to FCU.
- *FCR transfer:* can be exchanged for FCU.
- *Boyes sublimis transfer:* advocated as the excursion of FCU or FCR is not enough for EDC without using the tenodesis effect. The advantages are simultaneous wrist and finger extension, independent thumb and index extension and no reduced wrist strength. However, may get reduced grip and swan neck. Use FDS to ring and middle and pass through a window in the interosseous membrane. This window should be at least 4 cm long to allow gliding. EPL and EIP are woven to ring FDS, EDC to middle FDS.

Low median nerve palsy:
- If distal to the extrinsics, main problem is loss of thumb *Opposition* and sensory loss.
- FPB has dual innervation in 70% of patients so loss may be more difficult to detect.
- Prior to tendon transfers, need to ensure that no contractures develop. Release of the web space may be required.
- The direction of pull should come from the pisiform and insert into the dorso-ulnar base to produce pronation, so can pulley through a hole in the TCL or around the FCU tendon.
- The more distal the transfer in the palm, the greater the power of flexion.
- Perform early transfer in older patients with a poor prognosis for reinnervation. Early transfer will probably not be required if FPB is dual innervated. If not, patients may be able to achieve some abduction with APL if the arm is pronated. These patients would benefit from transfer.
- The benefits of opponensplasty are limited by sensory deficit which means fine motor movements remain difficult.

Opponensplasty techniques:
- *EIP transfer (Burkhalter—supplied by radial nerve):* transect. Repair stump to EDC to prevent extensor lag. Mobilize through two incisions proximal and distal to extensor retinaculum. Further incision in forearm to mobilize muscle. Make incision proximal to pisiform and pass EIP around the ulnar border then obliquely across the palm and woven into APB. By tenodesis, palmar flexion should give adduction.
- *FDS transfer (Royle-Thompson—supplied by median nerve more proximally):* isolate ring finger FDS and transect between A1 and A2 pulley. Bring out through distal forearm. Split FCU to create a pulley. Pass through this, across palm and into the radial aspect of MCPJ.

This is stronger with a greater length. May not be available. May get flexion contracture or swan neck. (Royles–Thompson) FDS ring is passed up the sheath of FPL to attach to superficial head of FPB and opponens pollicis.
- *PL (Camitz):* simple. Provides abduction but little pronation. Good for elderly patients with carpal tunnel syndrome. Dissect a strip of fascia with distal PL and extend into forearm. Fascia can be tubed. Develop tunnel to a mid-axial incision on the radial aspect of the MCP joint of the thumb. Suture to APB tendon.
- *ADM (Huber—supplied by ulnar nerve):* in children. Provides little abduction. Transect insertion and raise muscle, preserving NVB. Rotate and suture to APB.

High median nerve palsy:
Indications: loss of thumb opposition and also flexion to thumb and index. Often the middle finger can flex due to connection with the ring FDP. Functions which need restoring are thumb IPJ flexion and index PIP and DIPJ flexion.

Operations:
- *Thumb IPJ:* brachioradialis to FPL. Divide FPL at the musculotendinous junction and weave to BR. If there may be some recovery, weave end to side. FDP can be sutured to FDP of ring and little. If more power is required, transfer ECRL. ECU can be used as a thumb flexor or wrist pronator, wrist flexor and thumb abductor. Timing can be difficult. If seen late then perform transfers at the same time as nerve repairs.
- *Opposition:* EIP (Burkhalter) opponensplasty.
- *Index finger FDP:* ECRL transfer.

Low ulnar nerve palsy:
Indications: distal paralysis results in imbalance between flexors and extensors. Extension at the MCP joint is unopposed and the volar plate is weak. Flexion at the IPJs is unopposed. Grip is weak and flexion asynchronous. Function is improved by static or dynamic means on the MCP joint preventing hyperextension. Also get weak pinch due to adductor pollicis paralysis. Timing of transfers is based on probability of recovery. Consider early transfer if clawing is debilitating.

Operations to prevent clawing:
- *Static tendon transfers:* to prevent hyperextension of the proximal phalanx.
- Zancolli lasso *Volar plate* can be advanced to give 20° of flexion. Tendon graft can be attached to TCL, volar to deep transverse ligament then dorsally to radial lateral band.

Dynamic tendon transfers:
- Differ as to whether they provide MCP joint flexion or also IPJ extension. If the extrinsic extensors can fully extend IPJ then only MCP joint flexion is needed. So transfer can attach to A1 pulley (Zancolli), A2 pulley or drill hole in proximal phalanx. If central slip is attenuated, put transfer into lateral band. Using FDS does not increase grip whereas using a wrist flexor will.
- *MCPJ flexion only:* FDS to ring and little is divided distal to A1. Each is looped around A1 and sutured to itself. For a high palsy, motor the FDS lassos with ECRL or FCR.
- *MCPJ flexion and IPJ extension:*
  - *Modified Stiles-Bunnell transfer:* FDS to middle finger divided and split into two slips. Each is passed down the lumbrical canal of ring and little and sutured to the radial lateral band. If there is a total intrinsic palsy then FDS to middle and ring is used. The disadvantage is that the FDS is not expendable and may result in swan neck deformity:
    - Divide middle finger FDS proximal to PIPJ through radial mid-axial incision. Withdraw tendon through transverse distal palmar crease incision and split into 2;
    - Find radial lateral bands to ring and little finger through radial mid-axial incision and pass each slip down the lumbrical canal of the ring and little finger;
    - Suture to radial lateral band with MCPJ in 45° flexion and IPJ fully extended;
    - Should get intrinsic plus position with dorsiflexion;
    - Immobilize for one month with dorsal blocking splint—slight wrist flexion, and MCPJ 70° flexion. May need to split into 3 or for 4 fingers use FDS to middle and ring;
    - May get swan necking and, therefore, only use with mild PIPJ contractures.
  - *FDS expansion:* split FDS to middle into 4 and through a lateral incision to 3rd, 4th and 5th and medial incision to 2nd suture to lateral bands. Place hand on board with 70° MCPJ flexion to get tension right. Start with 5th then tension index until 5th just moves;
  - *ECRL/B transfers:* Paul Brand used ECRL with plantaris through lumbrical canals to the radial lateral bands of middle ring and little and the ulnar lateral band of the index finger. The tendon is rerouted around the radial border of the forearm. Plantaris is divided in half and split to give 4 tendon

grafts. Each is sutured to ECRL, passed through lumbrical canals, the slack is taken up and they are sutured to the lateral bands just proximal to the PIP joints. Brand also described a 4-tailed transfer with ECRB passing from dorsal to volar through the intermetacarpal spaces.

- *Correction of ulnar deviation of little finger:* detach ulnar half of EDM, pass volar to deep transverse intermetacarpal ligament, suture to radial collateral ligament of the MCP joint or loop under A2.
- *Thumb adduction:* ring finger FDS deep to flexor tendons of index and middle into a drill hole distal to adductor insertion. ECRB with tendon graft through 2nd intermetacarpal space, tunnelled beneath AP to its insertion.

High ulnar nerve palsy:
Grip strength can be improved by suturing FDP to adjacent tendons or by transferring FDS to middle. If ulnar deviation of the wrist is required, FCR should be transferred to FCU.

Tennison–Randall repair
- *Cleft lip* reconstruction with a *Z-plasty* of the cleft lip edges which reconstructs the Cupid's bow, but puts a scar across the philtral column. The middle limb of the Z is shared by the incised cleft margins.
- The length on noncleft side is measured from nostril sill to peak of Cupid's bow.
- *Advantages:* nostril sill closure is achieved by simple side-to-side approximation of medial and lateral nostril sill elements with minimal scar. Lip length can be accomplished even when medial element is very short. When the lateral lip element is short (often the case in complete clefts)—lateral lip height can be achieved without compromising Noordhof's point.
- *Disadvantages:* non-anatomical zigzag scar. Revisions may be challenging—z-plasty is in the middle of the lip.

Tenosynovitis
- Ligaments, pulleys and septa separate and restrain the tendons. Tendons are covered in tenosynovium. Any condition which changes the volume of the tenosynovium, tendon or canal will lead to stress and friction forces resulting in tenosynovitis with pain and disability. Most commonly occur in APL, flexors, FPL, FCR.
- Treatment is rest, splinting, NSAIDs, steroid injection and release.

Suppurative tenosynovitis:
see FLEXOR SHEATH INFECTION.

Rheumatoid tenosynovitis:
- The incidence is 50% with chronic *Rheumatoid arthritis*. Tendon attrition is caused by irregular bony prominences. 50% of patients undergoing prophylactic tenosynovectomy have been found to have tendon invasion.
- Because of the risk of tendon rupture and the difficulty of predicting it, tenosynovectomy is recommended if the tenosynovitis persists after 4 months of medical treatment. It will also treat the carpal tunnel syndrome which is as high as 65%. It also treats restricted movement and triggering.

Specific tenosynovitis:
- *Trigger thumb and finger.*
- *De Quervain's disease.*
- *Intersection syndrome.*
- *Extensor pollicis longus tenosynovitis.*
- *Flexor carpi radialis tendonitis.*
- *Flexor carpi ulnaris tenosynovitis.*

Tensor fascia lata
Origin: outer surface of anterior iliac crest between tubercle of the iliac crest and anterior superior iliac spine.

Insertion: iliotibial tract (anterior surface of lateral condyle of tibia).

Nerve: superior gluteal nerve (L4–5, S1).

Blood supply: lateral circumflex femoral artery.

Action: maintains knee extension and abducts the hip.

Tensor fascia lata flap
One of the earliest described free flaps, now mainly used pedicled.

Indications: good option for abdominal wall and pressure sores of the trochanteric area.

Blood supply: type I muscle supplied by lateral circumflex femoral vessels, which pierces the medial aspect of the flap 8–10 cm below ASIS. Can be sensate. Skin paddle reliable up to 5–8 cm above the knee. Fascia and skin can be transferred with minimal donor defect.

Procedure:
- Position—supine.
- Landmarks:
  - ASIS;
  - Lateral condyle of tibia (lies posterior to lateral border of patella).
- Pedicle—enters muscle 8–10 cm inferior to ASIS on a line from ASIS to lateral condyle.
- Markings:
  - Axis of the flap is where the pedicle enters—so skin paddle can be designed around this.

- Flap harvest:
  - Anterior incision first—through the fascia lata to identify anterior border of muscle;
  - Raise distal to proximal—pedicle on underside and visible middle third.
- Close in layers.

See ABDOMINAL WALL RECONSTRUCTION.

Tenzel flap

- Rotation flap extending high above outer canthus based superiorly for upper eyelid reconstruction and inferiorly for lower eyelid reconstruction.
- Cut semicircular flap of skin and orbicularis muscle which is high arched. Keep incision within the peri-orbital skin. Incision should not extend beyond the lateral part of the eyebrow. The orbital septum is freed, the conjunctiva mobilized and the lid pulled medially. Resuspend new lateral canthus to intact limb of lateral canthal tendon.

See EYELID RECONSTRUCTION.

Terry-Thomas sign

Widening of the scapholunate interval >3 mm. So named as it has the appearance of famous actor and comedian Terry-Thomas' gapped front teeth. Also *Cortical ring sign*.

See CARPAL INSTABILITY.

Tessier classification of craniofacial clefts

Classification of *Craniofacial clefts* by Paul Tessier.

- The orbit, nose and mouth are key landmarks.
- Clefts are numbered 0–14. 0–7 represent facial clefts and 8–14 the cranial extensions. Can have multiple and bilateral clefts.
- Broadly can be grouped into:
  - *Oral-nasal clefts:* those that disrupt the nose and lip, Tessier 0, 1, 2, 3;
  - *Oral ocular clefts:* those that disrupt the lip and orbit, Tessier 4, 5, 6;
  - *Lateral facial clefts:* lateral to mouth and orbit, Tessier 7, 8, 9;
  - *Cranial clefts:* affect the cranium, Tessier 10, 11, 12, 13, 14.
- If a cleft traverses both hemispheres then they generally follow the same pattern which adds up to 14: 0–14, 1–13, 2–12, 3–11 and 4–10. This is because 8 is the most lateral and subsequent clefts move medially.

Oral nasal clefts:
Cleft 0:

- Also called median craniofacial dysraphia. Midline cleft before nasal halves have fused. Severity depends on how much has developed. May have midline lack of fusion or midline

agenesis. May have bifid columella, nasal tip, septum etc. There may be a median cleft of the lip. Get diastasis between the central incisors. Orbital hypertelorism may occur or there may be absence of the nose and hypotelorism with associated brain malformation.
- The median cleft can extend cephalad as a 14 cleft or caudad as a cleft mandible, referred to as Tessier cleft 30. May be associated with encephalocoeles: Beware of midline cysts with intracranial extension.

Cleft 1:

- Nasoschisis or cleft of the lateral nose— paramedian craniofacial dysraphia.
- Extension cephalad is a Tessier 13.
- Originates at the lateral Cupid's bow and progresses into the nose. May be dysgenesis or a true cleft. If dysgenesis may get absent half of nose. Milder cases may have hypoplastic nose.

Cleft 2:

- Very rare. Paranasal cleft.
- The cleft originates at the lateral margin of Cupid's bow and extends to the middle third of the nostril as a deficiency and flattening of the soft tissue of the nose. There is absence of a true cleft.
- It may extend cephalad as a Tessier 12. It doesn't enter the orbit.

Cleft 3:

- Relatively common. Nasal ocular cleft or oblique facial cleft. Unilateral or bilateral.
- It can continue above the orbit as Tessier 10 or 11.
- The lip portion begins at the lateral margin of Cupid's bow. It then extends across the base of the nasal ala into the region of the normal union between the medial nasal process and the maxillary process.
- The nasolacrimal duct is blocked. Also have *Colobomas*. The cleft passes through the alveolus between lateral incisor and canine tooth. The frontal process of the maxilla may be absent.

Operations:

- Treatment of Tessier 0 is usually staged. The central lip defect is closed in a straight line or with a rotation. The nose cleft is opposed. If there is aplasia reconstruction is more difficult. Severe defects may require total nasal reconstruction.
- Repair of Tessier cleft 1 and 2 involve a hemirhinoplasty.
- Need to preserve vision in managing Tessier 3. The upper eyelid is usually not severely

involved. Local flaps can be used to close defects. Perform osseous reconstruction later with split calvarial grafts. Requires wide mobilization of lateral tissue. Lacrimal reconstruction usually fails. Multiple secondary surgeries are required.

Oral ocular clefts: the integrity of the nose is not disrupted. Also called oblique facial clefts.

Cleft 4:

- Always medial to the infra-orbital nerve. It may be bilateral and associated with other clefts.
- Treatment principles are similar to a Tessier 3. Discard the labial tissue between the ipsilateral philtral ridge and the cleft otherwise the lip is excessively wide. Use interdigitating flaps to increase the separation between the medial canthus and the nose.

Cleft 5:

- The rarest of the ocular clefts. The lip cleft is medial to the commissure and extends to the lateral third of the lower eyelid. There are varying degrees of ocular involvement. The skeletal deformities are lateral to the canine and extend lateral to the infra-orbital foramen. It enters the orbit in the lateral half. Much bone may be missing.
- Correct the soft tissue defect by increasing the distance between the mouth and the lower eyelid. Use local transposition flaps. The osseous restoration consists mainly of building an orbital floor and an anterior wall of the maxilla and filling the alveolar cleft with bone.

Cleft 6:

- Includes the incomplete form of *Treacher Collins*. Patients with *Nager's syndrome* possess the same cleft features.
- It is a transition form between the oral ocular and lateral facial clefts. The soft tissue deformity is more subtle than in Treacher Collins. It extends from lateral to the oral commissure to terminate in a coloboma of the lower lid in the lateral third. The ear is normal. There is usually a hypoplastic malar area. The palpebral fissures have an anti-mongoloid slant.

Operations: difficult and multistage. Emphasis is on preservation of the globe. Correction becomes urgent to save vision. The coloboma requires correction and the inferiorly dislocated lateral canthus requires repositioning. Extensive soft tissue mobilization is required. Tissue expansion can help. Multiple Z-plasties. Perform bone grafting at the age of 8.

Lateral facial clefts:

Cleft 7:

- Involves a lateral opening of the oral commissure. The most common craniofacial cleft. *See* MACROSTOMIA.

Cleft 8:

- Rare and usually exists with another rare cleft. Isolated to the orbital area. The cleft extends from the lateral canthus to the temporal region. The bony component is centred at the frontozygomatic suture. The soft tissue may just show a lateral canthal irregularity and a dermoid.
- Usually associated with *Goldenhar syndrome*. Reconstruction of the lateral commissure is achieved with local flaps.

Cleft 9:

- A transition from lateral clefts to orbital cranial clefts. Very rare. It involves the superolateral orbit dividing the eyelid into the lateral third and frequently the brow. Osseous defects occur in the superior orbital rim and temporal bone. It may be accompanied by encephalocoeles.
- Treatment consists of constructing a superior orbital rim, orbital roof and forehead. Local flaps are used for the soft tissue.

Treacher Collins syndrome clefts 6–8:
See TREACHER COLLINS.

Operations: a wide variety of operations. The lateral oral cleft of 7 is best repaired early by reapproximation of oral structures (*see* MACROSTOMIA) Lateral orbital clefts usually require proper positioning of the lateral canthus at the lateral orbital rim. Bone grafts may be required. The coloboma requires flaps from upper lid or rotation flaps. Most surgeons operate at age 6–8. Multidimensional distraction osteotomies should help correct these defects.

Cranial clefts: These extend superiorly from the lateral orbit to midline and traverse the frontal bone, and into the vault. May be isolated or with lower clefts. The larger the defect the greater the cerebral herniation and the more pronounced is the hypertelorism.

Cleft 10:

- Corresponds to no. 4. It is positioned in the centre of the upper lid, brow and orbit. The upper lid has a coloboma. The osseous component divides the superior orbital rim, cranial base and frontal bone. Associated encephalocoele will cause hypertelorism.
- An intracranial approach will be required to correct the asymmetric hypertelorbitism.

Cleft 11:

- Usually if not always with no. 3. Get a cleft of the medial eyebrow and lid with soft tissue irregularity of the forehead. The osseous deformity extends through the cranial base and into the ethmoid sinuses. Get orbital hypertelorism.
- Local flaps are used for the soft tissues and peri-orbital osteotomies for the hypertelorbitism.

Cleft 12:

- Extension of no. 2. Get an encephalocoele and disruption of the eyebrow medially. The bony cleft is severe and accompanied by hypertelorism.

Cleft 13:

- Cranial extension of no. 1. It extends through the olfactory groove giving a widened cribriform plate. Large defects may lead to massive encephalocoeles especially when bilateral. Get an irregular medial eyebrow with displacement into the orbit.

Cleft 14:

- Midline facial clefts with CNS abnormalities. The cranial extension of the Tessier 0 cleft but can occur alone. Produced by dysgenesis or agenesis. The holoprosencephalic malformations fall into this group. When a true cleft exists, herniation of the intracranial contents results in morphokinetic arrest of normal migration of the orbit. They remain in the embryonic position giving hypertelorism and cranium bifida. The nose may be widely separated. In severe cases, may get cyclopia or cebocephaly. Life expectancy is limited.

Operations: preserve brain function, re-establish the cranial vault and reposition facial structures. Correct the cleft early before rupture of meninges occurs.

Tessier classification of hypertelorism

Classifies *Hypertelorism* based on the inter-orbital distance:

- *Type I:* 30–34 mm.
- *Type II:* 35–39 mm.
- *Type III:* >39 mm.

Tetanus

- Caused by *Clostridium tetani*—anaerobic gram-positive bacillus.
- The neurotoxin tetanospasmin is produced which causes the clinical manifestations of hypertonia and painful muscle contractions.
- Wounds prone to tetanus include wounds older than 6 hours, contaminated, burn and crush injuries.
- Prophylaxis includes the tetanus toxoid vaccine (commonly administered as Rivaxis™)

which only protects for future exposures, and/or tetanus immunoglobulin which protects immediately and is used in high risk injuries.

TGF-β

See CYTOKINES AND GROWTH FACTORS.

Thalidomide

Used in 1950s and 1960s in early trimester nausea. One cause of limb malformations. Stopped in 1961. Cause intercalated *Transverse arrest*.

Thatte and Thatte classification

Classification of *Venous flaps*.

- *Type 1:* supplied by a single venous pedicle.
- *Type 2:* venous flow-through flaps supplied by a vein, which enters one side of the flap and exits from the other.
- *Type 3:* arterialized venous flaps.

Thenar flap

Vascularized pedicle flap from thenar skin which can be used in the reconstruction of *Fingertip injuries*. Base is perpendicular to thumb MP flexion crease. Divide after 2 weeks. Keep as high as possible on thenar eminence, as radial as possible. Minimize PIPJ flexion, release pedicle as soon as possible. More useful in children as the position of the finger leads to significant stiffness in the adult hand.

Thigh lift

Excision of lax thigh skin usually due to weight loss. If there is still a lot of fat patients benefit less as it is difficult to fix the skin into position. Medial thigh lift usually only benefits the upper inner thigh. Lateral thigh lift will benefit the buttock and thighs. Abdominoplasty can benefit anterior and medial thighs. Most patients will benefit from inner and outer thigh lift.

Markings: mark normal underwear. Make a transverse line just below the upper border which will be the planned eventual scar. Mark width of excision, laterally usually around 10–12 cm, 75% below the reference line. Medially 4–6 cm. Correct any mons descent.

Operation: place patient in the lateral position and infiltrate. The depth of incision is more superficial over the femoral triangle to leave some lymphatics intact. Suture superficial fascial system to Colles' fascia.

Thoracic outlet

- A space in the lower neck between the thorax and axilla.
- *Contents:* subclavian vein, subclavian artery and brachial plexus.
- Boundaries:
  - *Anterior:* clavicle;
  - *Posterior:* first thoracic rib;

- *Laterally:* insertion of pectoralis minor muscle onto coracoid process of humerus;
  - *Medially:* sternum.
- Subdivided into three areas:
  - Scalene triangle above the clavicle;
  - Costoclavicular space between the clavicle and first rib;
  - Subcoracoid space below the clavicle.

Thoracic outlet syndrome
Compression of the neurovascular bundle (subclavian artery and brachial plexus) passing between the thoracic outlet. T1 and lower plexus usually affected (so can look like an ulnar nerve lesion).

Symptoms:
- *Pain:* dull ache in shoulder but may radiate to hand.
- *Sensory disturbance: Dysaesthesia* and numbness C8 and T1.
- *Weakness:* T1 innervation in hand.
- *Vascular:* claudication, *Cold intolerance* and *Raynaud's.*

Examination:
- *General:* look at posture—kyphosis, slumping of shoulders, angle of root of neck, colour and temperature of upper limbs, examine brachial plexus.
- Vascular tests:
  - *Adson's test (adduction):* arm is adducted and neck extended and chin turned to affected side;
  - *Wright's hyperabduction test (right answer):* arm maximally abducted;
  - *Falconer's test (falcon diving):* military brace position;
  - *Roos test (I surrender):* abduct shoulder and flex elbow to 90 degrees.
- Neurological tests:
  - *Morley's compression test:* pressure over the plexus;
  - *Tinel's test:* percussion over the nerve.
- Other tests:
  - *Cervical rotation lateral flexion test:* test for first rib costotransverse joint dysfunction; the head is turned away from the side being examined and the neck is flexed; if the neck is not able to flex due to a bony block, this is positive; the block may be costotransverse joint subluxation;
  - *Spurling's test:* tests for cervical disc involvement.

Investigation:
- *XR:* chest and cervical spine.
- CT and MRI if mass suspected.

- *Nerve conduction studies:* may show slowed nerve conduction across supraclavicular fossa and can rule out distal nerve compression.

Treatment:
- Non-operative 50-100% improve:
  - First line therapy is conservative with exercises to strengthen the shoulder girdle, weight loss and occasionally breast reduction in women;
  - Analgesia.
- Operative—if conservative has not helped and for vascular or progressive neurological dysfunction:
  - Approach:
    - Supraclavicular (Adson);
    - Transaxillary approach (Roos);
    - Posterior parascapular (Claggett);
    - Transthoracic.
  - Resect first rib and excise anterior and middle scalene;
  - Neurolysis of supraclavicular plexus.

Thoracoepigastric flap
- A transposition flap option for reconstruction of lower chest wall defects.
- Medially based flaps vascularized by epigastric cascade whereas laterally based flaps vascularized by lumbar and intercostal arteries. An oblique design allows for the incorporation of multiple perforators.

Thrombus
- Exposure of collagen fibres is a trigger for platelet aggregation and degranulation. Releases ADP and thromboxane.
- These stimulate further platelet aggregation.

See COAGULATION CASCADE. See HEPARIN. See DEXTRAN. See ASPIRIN. See MICROSURGERY.

Thumb duplication
6% of congenital upper limb abnormalities. Aetiology is unknown, but rarely syndromic (Carpenter's).

Classification: *Wassel classification.* The most common level is duplication of the proximal phalanx (type IV). It occurs sporadically and unilaterally, though type VII (triphalangial thumb) may be hereditary and associated with big toe polydactyly.

Treatment principles: neither thumb is normal, all tissues are involved. The remaining thumb will be thinner and stiffer. The operation is not ablation of one of the thumbs but attempts to create the best possible thumb from the 2 abnormal digits.

Treatment options:
- Remove one duplicate and reconstruct the other. Use for Wassel type IV (most common).

Thumb hypoplasia

The ulnar digit is usually more developed and tends to be the one preserved. Need to reconstruct the radial collateral ligament. Usually perform with a periosteal flap from the amputated digit.
- Remove equal parts of both and combine the remaining to form a single finger. Usually for more distal duplications. An example is the *Bilhaut–Cloquet operation*.
- Remove unequal parts and combine.

See CONGENITAL HAND ANOMALIES. *See* POLYDACTYLY.

Thumb hypoplasia
- This is a radial longitudinal failure of formation. Thumb hypoplasia is on the spectrum of radial hypoplasia.
- Associated with ring D chromosome abnormalities, Holt–Oram syndrome, trisomy-18 syndrome, Rothmund–Thompson syndrome, thalidomide, VACTERL, TAR and Fanconi anaemia.
- A completely absent thumb is almost always associated with an absent radius except in Fanconi's syndrome when the thumb is present even though the radius is absent.

Examination of hand: compare with contralateral thumb:
- Look:
  - Size of thumb;
  - 1st webspace;
  - Lack of bulk in thenar eminence;
  - Joint creases for type 2 versus 3.
- Feel:
  - UCL laxity;
  - Also test RCL for type 2b as treatment is different;
  - CMCJ stability.
- Move:
  - APB—opposition.
- Donor sites:
  - Index finger flexibility.

Investigation:
- Bloods test for sign of anaemia.
- Xray to assess stability of CMCJ.
- Heart examination.
- Genetics—chromosome screening for Fanconi anaemia.

Classification: *Blauth*. Key is to decide whether the CMC joint is stable:
- *I:* minor hypoplasia, normally functioning.
- *II:* thumb small and less stable. Get adduction contracture of web space, thenar muscle hypoplasia and laxity of UCL (Type A =

uniaxial instability, Type B = multiaxial instability of both UCL and RCL).
- *III:* type II elements with skeletal hypoplasia, CMC vestigial, absent intrinsics, rudimentary extrinsics:
  - III-A has intact CMC;
  - III-B has basal metacarpal aplasia.
- *IV:* floating thumb without skeletal articulation — pouce flottant.
- *V:* total absence.

Treatment principles:
- Type I do not require treatment.
- Type II and IIIA (with stable CMC joints) are candidates for reconstruction. Web space needs deepening (commonly with 4-flap Z-plasty), extrinsic tendon rebalancing and *Opponensplasty* (Huber op FDS). Uniaxial UCL instability amenable to collateral ligament reconstruction whereas multiaxial instability requires chondrodesis.
- Type IIIB, IV and V require pollicization.

See CONGENITAL HAND ANOMALIES.

Thumb-printing/copper beaten sign
XR appearance of skull with raised intracranial pressure seen in *Craniosynostosis*.

Thumb reconstruction
Classification of thumb amputations by Lister and reconstruction options:
- Acceptable length with poor soft tissue cover—i.e. distal to IPJ:
  - Heal by secondary intention;
  - Moberg flap if <2 cm;
  - Free toe pulp if >2cm;
  - Foucher if not up to a free flap;
  - Revision amputation.
- Subtotal amputation with questionable remaining length:
  - Deepen first web to relatively lengthen stump.
- Amputation proximal to IPJ with preserved CMCJ:
  - Free toe—gold standard. If MCPJ involved, you have to use 2nd toe to preserve 1st MTPJ;
  - Metacarpal distraction lengthening;
  - Osteoplastic recon—bone graft covered with soft tissue flap.
- Total amputation with loss of CMCJ:
  - Pollicization.

Thyroglossal duct cysts
- A remnant from the descent of the thyroid from the base of the tongue. It usually reaches

the final position by 8 weeks of gestation and the duct disappears. It may remain at any point on the path.

- Commonly present in the 20s and in the midline at the level of the thyrohyoid membrane.
- Excision of the tract is required which may involve resection of hyoid bone. Thyroid scans should be performed to confirm the presence of other thyroid tissue. Usually present as a slow-growing mass in the midline. Often present when they are infected. They move up and down on swallowing. Image the neck and assess thyroid preoperatively.

Operation: horizontal skin incision. Retract strap muscles. Transect infrahyoid strap muscles to clear the junction of greater cornu and body of hyoid to enable the tract to be excised from the pharyngeal wall in continuity with the midpoint of the hyoid. As the tongue is approached, a finger is placed in the foramen caecum at the base of the tongue to find the tissue to be removed with the tract.

See HEAD AND NECK.

Thyroid nodule

- To diagnose, first determine TSH and thyroxine levels. If the patient is hyperthyroid, a scan will distinguish a hot from a cold nodule. A hot (hyperfunctioning) nodule does not require further investigation. If TSH is normal, do FNA. Around 5% of FNAs are suggestive of malignancy. Solitary benign nodules are treated with thyroid suppression therapy. In patients over 50 with atypia of follicular epithelium, thyroidectomy is recommended as the risk of malignant change is high.
- Prognostic factors predicting outcome are age, size, histology, spread, nodes and metastasis.

Tibia

- Blood supply is from metaphyseal vessels, periosteal vessels and nutrient artery, which is from the posterior tibial artery.
- The nutrient artery penetrates the tibialis posterior then follows the nutrient channel on the posterior surface of the tibia. It traverses intracortically. Once in the medulla it divides into proximal and distal branches, which supply the inner 2/3 of the cortex.
- Metaphyseal arteries anastomose with proximal branches.
- Periosteal vessels branch from major limb vessels and course perpendicular to the axis of the tibia thus both sides of a fracture may

derive the majority of their blood supply via these vessels as the other sources may be compromised by the fracture.

TILT: triquetral impingement ligament tear

- Ulnar wrist pain involving triquetrum.
- Triad of localized triquetral pain, hyperflexion injury and normal radiographs.
- Cuff of fibrous tissue becomes detached from ulnar sling mechanism and chronically impinges on triquetrum.
- Get synovitis, bony eburnation and pain. Find point tenderness on triquetrum just distal to ulnar styloid.

Tinel-Hoffman sign

- Percussion over a site of nerve regeneration elicits a tingling sensation in the nerve distribution.
- Commonly elicited at sites of suspected nerve compression or in the assessment of nerve repair where tingling represents the leading edge of regeneration.
- Can get a Tinel's sign in motor nerves such as the facial nerve, probably due to proprioceptor fibres.
- Birch listed values of the Tinel-Hoffman sign:

  1. A positive sign over a nerve lesion soon after an injury indicates rupture of axons;
  2. A migrating positive sign that is stronger than a sign at the point of injury suggests favourable prognosis for nerve regeneration;
  3. A positive sign which does not advance may represent misdirected extra epineurial growth cones;
  4. A positive sign is not seen in the setting of conduction block (neurapraxia).

Tissue-cultured skin

Human epidermal cells grown *in vivo*, stable enough for grafting.

- Whole skin is enzymatically digested with trypsin to produce a single cell suspension of keratinocytes which are grown as a monolayer on irradiated mouse fibroblasts. From a section of skin 2 cm^2, a 1 m^2 sheet can be made in 3-6 weeks.
- Used for areas of large skin loss such as burns or non-healing areas such as leg ulcers.
- A disadvantage is hyperkeratosis for long periods. It may be that the epidermis is hyperproliferative without the checks of the dermis. There may be a potential risk of malignancy as they are cultured in mitogens. They are also expensive and fragile.

Tissue expansion
- First performed by Charles Neumann who expanded preauricular skin in 1956. Then popularized by Chedomir Radovan in 1984.
- An expander is inserted subcutaneously and filled gradually over weeks until the desired degree of skin expansion has occurred.

Mechanism of expansion:
- 70% stretch (mechanical creep), 30% growth (biological creep).
- Mechanical creep refers to viscoelastic deformation, i.e. the elongation of skin under constant load over time. Collagen fibres stretch and realign, elastin fragments, water and insterstitial fluid is displaced. All occurs during intra-operative expansion. In addition, adjacent mobile soft tissue is recruited.
- Biological creep refers to the generation of new tissue due to a chronic stretching force and it is associated with increased collagen and ground substance.
- Stretch-relaxation describes reduction in the resistance of skin to stretching force with time.

Histology:
- *Epidermis:* thickens due to hyperplasia with increased mitoses.
- *Dermis:* thins, collagen realigns to become more parallel, elastin fibres rupture.
- *Adipose tissue:* cells atrophy with some permanent loss.
- Vascular supply is increased with increased VEGF.
- *Capsule:* Paysk described 4 zones within the capsule surrounding an expander:
  - Inner zone is a fibrin layer within the capsule surrounding the expander;
  - Central zone contains elongated fibroblasts and myofibroblasts;
  - Transitional zone of loose collagen fibres;
  - Outer zone contains blood vessels and collagen.

Principles:
- Expansion provides tissue that is most like the lost tissue and is sensate. Can expand hair-bearing scalp but follicles will be sparser in expanded skin. The donor defect is minimal, there is good contour and it is not a major procedure.
- May be a remote incision, or an incision orientated radially to the edge of the expander. Place incisions in stable tissue which will heal. Start injections one week after insertion if the wound is stable.

- To gauge the degree of expansion needed, measure the arc circumference and subtract the base diameter to give the amount of advancement. 20% of measured expansion is lost so over expand. Capsular scoring may improve advancement.
- It is limited by the amount of relaxation and growth of tissues. Irradiation and scar make it more difficult or impossible.

Complications:
- Migrations, extrusion, infection, rupture, wound dehiscence.
- It is contraindicated near malignancy, under skin graft, under tight tissue, near an open wound and in an irradiated field.

Rapid intra-operative tissue expansion:
- Uses cyclical loading or temporary expanders for 3–5 min of stretch and 2 min of relaxation.
- This takes advantage of the viscoelastic skin properties of mechanical creep and stretch-relaxation to cause incremental increase in length of the loaded skin. This is partly due to extrusion of fluid from between collagen fibres. Also due to recruitment of adjacent skin. May get 40% increase in surface area and flap length. At each expansion the end point is tautness of skin, not blanching. With larger expanders each inflation can last 20 minutes with 10 minutes rest.

Tissue plasminogen activator (t-PA)
- Second generation plasminogen activator with activity specific for fibrin. Fibrin possesses t-PA binding sites close to the plasminogen binding sites and therefore t-PA promotes plasminogen activation and lysis of clot.
- It has no antigenicity and no febrile or allergic reactions. It is more effective than streptokinase in acute limb ischaemia.

Titanium
Unalloyed it is very malleable. Titanium alloy (titanium-aluminium-vanadium has a tensile strength like vitallium and has a high biocompatibility). It is the least corrosive with the least artefact on CT/MRI.
See ALLOPLASTS.

Toe to hand transfer
- The first toe to hand transplant was performed by Nicoladoni in 1898 by attaching a pedicled toe to the hand for 3 weeks in a 5-year-old boy.
- Note the level of amputation and the dominance. Length, strength of grasp and sensation is more important for

the non-dominant hand as it grasps objects for the dominant side.
- Reconstruction is more difficult when there is agenesis as other structures will be abnormal. They are easier with constriction rings.
- The 2nd toe can be used for congenital absence as it hypertrophies. It is a preferable donor loss. Great toe atrophies to some degree. Attempts to improve size mismatch have been made and in particular the wrap-around though there is a functional loss.
- Great toe is the best option unless metacarpal is also required in which case 2nd toe can be used or big toe with 2nd metatarsal.
- Homotransplantation is possible, but problematic as skin provokes the strongest immune response.

Anatomy: many variations to the blood supply. The most common main supply is from the dorsalis pedis to the superficial first metatarsal artery. Next is the plantar first metatarsal artery either from plantar system or dorsal via a per-forating branch. The ideal system is the domin-ant dorsal system. A long vascular pedicle can be mobilized, which can reach mid forearm if needed.

Intra-operative drugs: heparin in saline 100 units/ml is used to irrigate the operative field. Dextran can be used. Papaverine 60 units/ml is used after anastomosis. For spasm, papaverine 6 units/ml can be used. Streptokinase can be used to flush out clots. Dilute to 5,000 units/ml and infuse 25,000–50,000 into the flap.

Technique: mark the pedicle on the upper sur-face to prevent a twist. Rotation can easily hap-pen and is disastrous. First fix the bone. Vasospasm is more severe in children and women.
See THUMB RECONSTRUCTION.

Tongue carcinoma
- Mainly in 60s, but also young and even adolescent.
- It is the most common site for intra-oral malignancy and most tongue cancers are in the anterior two-thirds on the lateral borders or the ventral surface.
- It usually presents as a lateral chronic non-healing ulcer and spreads locally to the floor of the mouth.
- It usually presents as a T2 lesion.
- It contains a rich lymphatic supply so that 40% have nodal involvement and 20% have bilateral nodes.

Treatment:
- T1: surgery or RT. Wedge resection under LA or *Brachytherapy*.

- T2 lesions will require partial glossectomy and possibly mandible if involved.
- ELND for T2 and T3 N0 necks. Give RT as well.

Results: 5-year survival rate is 50%.
See HEAD AND NECK CANCER. *See* GLOSSECTOMY.

Tonsil carcinoma
- Can be exophytic or deeply invasive.
- Tend to present late with 76% of patients having nodal involvement at presentation.
- Anterior tonsillar pillar lesions tend to have a better prognosis. Tonsillar fossa tumours tend to be more common and all are more radiosensitive than other sites.

Treatment:
- Most T1–T3 tumours can be cured with RT.
- Stage I and II are resected, and neck dissection performed. Stage III and IV have resection, neck dissection and radiotherapy.
See HEAD AND NECK CANCER.

Torre's syndrome
See SEBACEOUS ADENOMA. *See* MUIR–TORRE SYNDROME.

Torticollis
- 'Twisted neck'. Secondary to fixed shortening of sternocleidomastoid (SCM). The head tilts towards the affected side with the chin towards the opposite side.
- The incidence is 0.3%, rarely bilateral. M = F, left = right. Higher incidence in breech.
- The aetiology is unknown. Theories include muscle injury and haematoma at birth, venous occlusion and intrauterine malposition causing ischaemic fibrosis.
- *Pathology:* fibrous tissue, no muscle degeneration, no evidence of haematoma.

Classification:
- *Congenital:* muscular, vertebral.
- *Acquired:* 2° to muscle (trauma, infection), ocular, spasmodic (usually >40 years), psychogenic.

Clinical presentation:
- Usually a small tumour is felt in the first few weeks of birth, and the SCM feels short, stiff and cord-like.
- The head is tilted and rotated to the affected side with chin up and away to the opposite side. The shoulder may be higher on the affected side.
- The tumour may increase for some weeks then remain static then slowly resolve by 8 months.
- If it does not resolve, scoliosis capitis results. The mastoid, ear, jaw, maxilla and orbit can be growth restricted and pulled down giving facial asymmetry.

Treatment:
- *Non-operative:* reassurance, physiotherapy, stretching, botox.
- *Operative:* if it persists after 1 year. Options:
  - Perform total excision of the SCM (may leave a hollow);
  - Tenotomy;
  - Lengthening by dividing clavicular head in middle 1/3 and transposing to cranial end of sternal head;
  - Lengthening by vertical split and slide.

Outcome: from surgery excellent results. Best if <4 years. Beware spinal accessory nerve, recurrence, diplopia and instability.
See CRANIOSYNOSTOSIS.

Tourniquet time
- Tourniquet nerve damage will result in lower motor neuron damage with reduced pin prick, reduced vibration sense and reduced movement.
- MDU recommends:
  - Apply in healthy limbs;
  - TQ size 10 cm arm and 15 cm leg;
  - *Pressure:* arm 50–100 mmHg above systolic and leg double systolic or arm 200–250 mmHg, leg 250–350 mmHg;
  - Time absolute maximum 3 hours (recovers in 5–7 days), generally do not exceed 2 hours. Document duration and pressure.

Toxic shock syndrome (TSS)
- A systemic illness, which can occur following *Burns* due to colonization of the burn with toxin producing strains of *S. aureus.*
- TSST-1 is the most common toxin and is produced by *S. aureus.* It works by over-stimulating the immune system.
- It usually starts 3 days after a burn and can occur even in minor burns.
- Get fever, macular papular rash, myalgia, pain, nausea and gastrointestinal upset followed by hypotension and neurological symptoms (disorientation, altered consciousness). Blood results show lymphopaenia and hyponatraemia.
- Mortality of up to 50% if left untreated.
- Management is multidisciplinary with paediatrics, anaesthetics and microbiology:
  - Resuscitation and monitoring in high-care setting;
  - Inspect and clean burn wound;
  - Intravenous fluids (10–20 ml/kg);
  - Intravenous antibiotics to cover gram positive and negative bacteria;
  - Consider provision of passive immunity to help fight toxins: fresh frozen plasma (FFP)

(10 ml/kg over 1 hour) and/or immunoglobulin (IVIG) (e.g., Privigen™ liquid 10% 2g/kg).

Tracheostomy
Emergency: perform cricothyroidotomy. Make an incision through the cricothyroid membrane which lies superficially. The superficial tissue is relatively avascular apart from the anterior jugular veins. Emergency low tracheotomy is performed through a tracheal incision below the 2nd tracheal ring.

Elective: incise below the thyroid isthmus in the 2nd-3rd or 3rd–4th tracheal ring. Place sheet under patient to extend head and push back the shoulders. Incise transversely 4 cm, 2–3 cm above the suprasternal notch directly over the sternal opening. Incise vertically in the midline between the strap muscles. The isthmus may need to be ligated and divided. Place hooks in the trachea and incise once the balloon is deflated. Incise trachea vertically between the 3rd and 4th tracheal ring. Remove the ETT and insert the tracheostomy tube.

TRAM flap
Transverse rectus abdominus myocutaneous flap. Most frequently used for *Breast reconstruction.* Rectus is taken with overlying fat and skin. It may be pedicled on one or both superior epigastric arteries or free on the inferior epigastric artery.

Vascular anatomy:
Hartrampf initially described 4 vascular zones and these were later modified by Holm:
1. Ipsilateral central—supplied by the pedicle, i.e. musculocutaneous perforators from the deep inferior epigastric artery (DIEA) and superficial inferior epigastric artery (SIEA).
2. Ipsilateral peripheral—supplied by ipsilateral superficial circumflex iliac artery (SCIA). Choke vessels must open for it to be perfused by adjacent DIEA territory.
3. Contralateral central—supplied by the contralateral DIEA and SIEA.
4. Contralateral peripheral—supplied by contralateral SCIA and is commonly discarded.

Risk factors: obesity, smokers, abdominal scars, RT. Systemic diseases such as diabetes, heart disease.

Pedicled:
- Design the flap higher in the abdomen than a free flap because of the reduced vascularity.
- The flap can be made more reliable by:
  - *Delay:* ligate inferior epigastric artery 2 weeks prior to raising the flap;

○ *Supercharging:* anastomose the inferior epigastric vessels to the thoracodorsal vessels.

Free: dissect from side opposite to where the vessels are planned to be used first so that the position of the perforators can be assessed, then when doing the contralateral side they can be divided. Anastomose to thoracodorsal vessels or internal thoracic vessels. Better vascularity and less muscle taken than with a pedicled TRAM.

Complications: fat necrosis, partial loss and skin necrosis, abdominal hernias, wound dehiscence, size mismatch.

Contraindications: previous abdominoplasty, abdominal scars suggesting division of the superior epigastric artery would be a contraindication to a pedicled TRAM flap.

Alternatives: gluteal flap, latissimus dorsi flap, lateral thigh flap, Ruben's flap.

Tranquili–Leali flap
See ATASOY VOLAR V-Y FLAP.

TransCyte™
Human fibroblast-derived temporary skin substitute.

• TransCyte provides a temporary protective barrier.
• It consists of a polymer membrane and newborn human fibroblast cells. This nylon mesh is coated with porcine dermal collagen and bonded to silicone. As fibroblasts proliferate within the nylon mesh during the manufacturing process, they secrete human dermal collagen, matrix proteins and growth factors. Following freezing, no cellular metabolic activity remains; however, the tissue matrix and bound growth factors are left intact.

See BIOLOGICAL SKIN SUBSTITUTES.

Transplant immunology
Antigens:
• ABO blood group antigens.
• Major histocompatibility complex (MHC) antigens:
  ○ *Class 1:* including HLA-A and HLA-B found on nucleated cells and platelets;
  ○ *Class 2:* includes HLA-DR found on macrophages and dendritic cells.

Cells of immune response:
• *Antigen presenting cells:* of lymphoid origin. Bind antigen and process it. As well as presenting antigens to other cells, some, particularly macrophages, secrete <u>Cytokines</u>.
• *B cells:* produce antibodies.
• *T cells:* central in coordinating immune response. Divided into 2 subsets determined

by the presence of CD4 or CD8. CD4 cells are T-helper cells and secrete cytokines, whereas CD8 are T-cytotoxic and bind cells of particular antigen type and kill them. Natural killer cells respond without requiring presensitization. They have a role in tumour surveillance and they can detect cells not expressing self-antigens.

Graft rejection:
• *Hyperacute rejection:* minutes to hours after transplantation. Due to preformed antibodies to ABO or MHC molecules in the transplanted allograft. Complement is activated. This is a major obstacle to xenotransplantation.
• *Acute rejection:* days to weeks after transplantation. T cell-mediated.
• *Chronic rejection:* months to years after transplantation. Multifactorial and may be slowed by immunosuppression.

Immunological testing: as well as blood type, HLA-A, -B and -DR should be matched. A heterozygous individual with all matching would have six-antigen match. *See* MHC.

Clinical immunosuppression:
• Unless the immune system is partially suppressed, all tissue except in identical twins will eventually be rejected. Combinations are given.
• *Steroids:* downregulates all T-cell functions. Complications include hypertension, hyperglycaemia, osteoporosis and peptic ulcer.
• *Azathioprine:* interferes with nucleic acid synthesis. Inhibits differentiation and proliferation of lymphocytes. Can result in severe leukopenia. Also hepatic toxicity.
• *Methotrexate:* folic acid antagonist. Inhibits DNA and RNA synthesis.
• *Cyclosporine:* provides immunosuppression without marrow depression. Inhibits IL-2 and therefore T-cell differentiation. Nephrotoxic.
• *Biological agents:* monoclonal antibodies can suppress specific antigens.

Allotransplantation of tissues:
• *Bone:* frozen bone allograft is now common practice for reconstructing long bone defects. Either to bridge a gap or provide articular surface. They are devoid of living cells and become replaced by host bone. Immunosuppressants are not required though replacement is slow, starting at a year. Bone is removed in a theatre, soft tissue and marrow is removed and bone is frozen in a glycerol solution. Can also be freeze-dried. Also gamma-irradiated. They have been used for craniofacial procedures. Hand surgery

patients treated for enchondromas with allograft compared favourably to autograft from iliac crest. Good results have been obtained in children with congenital hand problems. Avascular necrosis of scaphoid has been treated successfully with allograft, which is used to replace the proximal fragment and achieve union.

- *Cartilage:* used for facial skeleton but high rate of resorption. It may be useful to resurface joints.
- *Skin:* primarily for burn victims. Risk of disease transmission. Rejection in around 14 days. Immunosuppression has been tried for children. Attempts to reduce the antigenicity of skin by exposing to UVB, stripping epidermis, and preserving in glycerol. Dermal scaffolds with all cellular elements removed have been produced. Alloderm™ is acellular dermis. Dermagraft™ is human neonatal dermal fibroblasts seeded onto a synthetic mesh.
- *Nerve:* has not been used much and immunosuppression is required for a short period.
- Vascularized composite allotransplantation.

Transposition flap
Rectangular flap, which rotates about a pivot point laterally into an adjacent area. Because it becomes shorter in length as it rotates, it is made longer than the defect. The pivot point is at the base distal to the defect. A backcut will reduce tension but will narrow the pedicle.
See ROTATION FLAP.

Transverse arrest: congenital hand
Complete: at any level, but most commonly at the junction of the proximal third and the middle third of the forearm. Treatment is usually non-surgical and involves the fitting of a suitable prosthesis.

Intercalated:
- Phocomelia is an intercalated deficiency of the upper limb. It was linked to thalidomide use in early pregnancy. Thalidomide is still used for treatment of leprosy.
- Phocomelia is divided into:
  ○ *Complete phocomelia:* the hand on the torso;
  ○ *Proximal phocomelia:* normal forearm and hand on torso;
  ○ *Distal phocomelia:* hand attached to upper arm and elbow.

Treatment:
- *Upper 1/3 forearm:* fit prosthesis by 6 months. Surgery to lengthen is not indicated. The Krukenberg procedure may help.

- *Carpus, metacarpus, phalanges.* Absence of digits may be transverse absence, cleft hand, constriction ring or *Symbrachydactyly.* Range of treatment is the same for all. Most have a normal wrist joint so palpate for skeletal parts. If the thumb metacarpal is present check the basal joint. Treat with distraction manoplasty—to lengthen skin envelope and toe phalangeal transfer. They survive well if performed before 15 months. Take periosteum and repair collateral ligaments. Bony distraction is performed for 4th or 5th metacarpal remnant. Toe transfer—function difficult to achieve as tendons and nerves are rudimentary.

Transverse carpal ligament
- The flexor retinaculum is a fibrous band arching over the carpus. Forming the roof of the carpal tunnel. *See* CARPAL TUNNEL SYNDROME.
- Medially it is attached to the pisiform and hook of the hamate and laterally to the tubercle of the scaphoid and ridge of trapezium.
- Palmaris longus and flexor carpi radialis are partly inserted into it, and the short muscles of the thumb and little finger take their origin from it.

Trapeziectomy: operative
- Incision from base of metacarpal curved towards FCR. Preserve radial artery and superficial branches of radial nerve.
- Establish position of CMC joint with needle and incise capsule to expose trapezium and base of metacarpal.
- Remove trapezium with combination of osteotome and rongeur. Preserve FCR in base.
- Expose area of metacarpal base and drill with a 2.3 mm rosehead burr.
- If desired, may perform a ligament reconstruction tendon interposition (LRTI) procedure, e.g. FCR sling. Through short transverse incisions expose FCR and place slings around. Pass prolene™ suture through one-third of the tendon proximally. Strip down distally. Divide proximally. Pass through the line of FCR into the CMC space.
- Pass wire through hole in metacarpal base and hook suture tied to tendon. Bring tendon through, then back around intact FCR. Suture tendon to metacarpal and onto intact FCR. Wrap twice and leave any remaining tendon as spacer.
- Close capsule, skin. K wire MCP joint and apply a POP backslab. Change in 4 days for a full plaster, leave for a further 5 weeks then apply a thermoplastic splint for a further 3 weeks.

Trapezium: fracture

- 5% of carpal bone injuries. Either through the body or the ridge. Fractures of the ridge are typically caused by a fall on the outstretched hand.
- Mechanism is either a direct blow or avulsion of TCL. Get volar point tenderness.

Classification: ridge fractures classified by Palmer:

- *Type I:* through base, heal well with immobilization.
- *Type II:* through tip. High incidence of non-union.

Treatment:

- Ridge fractures are treated conservatively.
- Body fractures are treated by open reduction if displaced.

Trapezius

Origin: external occipital protuberance, ligamentum nuchae, spinous processes of C7–T12.

Insertion: into clavicle, spine of scapula and acromion.

Blood supply: based on the superficial transverse cervical artery. Type II muscle with minor pedicles from the dorsal scapular artery, posterior intercostals and a branch of occipital artery.

Nerve supply: spinal root of accessory nerve (motor) and cervical nerves (C3 and C4) (pain and proprioception).

Action: elevates, retracts, depresses and rotates scapula.

See MUSCLES.

Trapezius flap

- Can be a lateral or lower musculocutaneous flap.
- Useful for midline defects of the upper spine and occiput. It may be used for Intra-oral reconstruction. Only the muscle under the skin and around the pedicle is raised.
- Shoulder strength can be preserved as long as the upper portion of muscle and the spinal accessory nerve are preserved. The lower region is functionally and aesthetically dispensable.

Technique:

- The flap pivots on the descending branch of the transverse cervical artery which runs along the deep aspect of the muscle and enters 5–7 cm lateral to the midline at the level of C7 spinous process.
- Mark C7 to T12 and the acromion. This triangle contains the trapezius.
- An extended flap can be used, but should be delayed.

- The skin island should be 8 cm wide. The larger the segment the more likely it is to contain perforators and to survive.
- Skin is incised down to muscle and lateral border is identified. Muscle is separated from paraspinous muscle. The vascular pedicle is found and the flap raised.

See TRUNK RECONSTRUCTION.

Trapeziometacarpal joint

- A biconcave saddle joint.
- The proximal surface is concave radioulnar and convex dorsopalmar.
- Base of metacarpal is saddle-shaped centrally with volar and dorsal peaks. The volar beak has no ligament.

Ligaments: intra- and extra-capsular.

- *Anterior oblique ligament:* the most important. Also called the beak ligament. From the palmar tubercle of trapezium to palmar tubercle of 1st metacarpal base (beak). Gets weak in OA leading to subluxation.
- *Posterior oblique ligament:* strong dorsal ligament running from dorsoulnar tubercle of trapezium to palmar tubercle of metacarpal. Tight in opposition and abduction.
- *Dorsoradial ligament:* intracapsular from dorsoradial tubercle of trapezium to metacarpal. Tight in adduction. Gets attenuated in OA.
- *First intermetacarpal ligament:* strong extracapsular ligament attached to the base of first and second metacarpal. Stretched in CMC OA allowing radial subluxation of the base of metacarpal.
- *Ulnar collateral ligament:* extracapsular from TCL to ulnar tubercle of base of 1st MC. Tight in extension, abduction and pronation.

Movement:

- Simple movements such as abduction, extension and complex movements, such as opposition and retroposition.
- Simple movement occurs in the saddle joint but complex movements also involve the articulation between the convex spheroidal surface of the trapezium and the radial slope of the base of first metacarpal. With adduction get internal rotation which helps pulp-to-pulp pinch of the thumb.

Trauma

Tissue damage due to the energy exchange between the patient and the environment.

Aetiology:

- *Mechanical:* blunt, penetrating, blast.
- *Thermal.*

- *Chemical.*
- *Electrical.*
- *Electromagnetic.*

Degree of energy exchange: low, medium or high.

Setting:
- Iatrogenic.
- Civilian trauma (RTA, industrial, etc.).
- Armed conflict (GSW, mine, chemical weapons, etc.).

Treacher Collins

Autosomal dominant condition involving first and second branchial arches. Described by Edward Treacher Collins in 1900. Also called Franceschetti syndrome and mandibulofacial dysostosis.

- TCOF Treacle gene on chromosome 5. *See* CRANIOFACIAL GENETICS.
- Incidence 1:25,000, M = F.
- *Tessier* cleft 6, 7 and 8 with malformation of structures derived from the first and second pharyngeal arches and pouch.
- Facial abnormalities are symmetric and bilateral.
- Get *Coloboma* of the lower eyelid with no. 6, absence of zygomatic arch with no. 7, absence of the orbital rim with no. 8.
- Hypoplasia of the supra-orbital area and zygoma.
- The face is narrow with depressed cheekbones, receding chin and large downturned mouth.
- 35% have a cleft palate. Also micrognathia.
- The external ears are absent, malformed, or malposed.
- Hearing is impaired due to variable degrees of aural atresia.
- The airway may be compromised with constricted nasal passages secondary to maxillary hypoplasia resulting in choanal stenosis or atresia. It may be worsened by cleft palate repair. Feeding and swallowing may also be affected.

Management at different timepoints:
- Neonatal—may require urgent intervention for airway and eye protection:
  - Airway due to narrow pharyngeal size and mandibular hypoplasia:
    - Nurse prone but must be monitored due to SIDS risk;
    - Nasopharyngeal airway;
    - Consider tracheostomy.
  - *Feeding:* may need NG tube if failing to thrive;
  - *Eyes:* protect with taping and if proptosis more severe may require tarsorrhaphy.

- Infancy:
  - *Hearing:* early banded hearing aids then bone anchored hearing aids (BAHA) at approximately 4 years;
  - *Speech: Cleft palate* repair at 9–12 months— may be wider than normal and also increased risk of post-op airway issues.
- Childhood:
  - Distraction of mandibular angle can be considered. Need to do before ear recon so that the new ear can be sited correctly;
  - Ear reconstruction if microtia or anotia.
- Adolescence—definitive correction of facial tissue at skeletal maturity:
  - Calvarial bone graft to augment orbital floor and zygoma;
  - *Orthognathic surgery:* bimaxillary osteotomies (bilateral sagittal split osteotomy (BSSO) for mandible and Le Fort 1 maxillary advancement for maxilla);
  - Lateral canthopexy, midface lifts and rhinoplasty.

Triangular fibrocartilage

Anatomy:
- *TFCC:* articular disc that is 1–2 mm thick originating from the base of the ulnar styloid and inserting into the sigmoid notch of the radius, the ulnocarpal ligament, the UCL and dorsal and palmar radioulnar joint. It is the major stabilizer of the *DRUJ*. It is a load-bearing structure between the carpus and ulna. 20% of load is transmitted across it, and the rest is across the radiocarpal joint.

Clinical: with a TFCC tear, the patient gets ulnar-sided wrist pain following a twisting injury. May get popping or catching. Assess stability of radioulnar joint. Traumatic peripheral tears can heal, central tears cannot.

Investigations:
- *XR:* look for ulna minus variance, ulnar styloid fracture which may disrupt the attachment of the TFCC. In *Pseudogout* get calcification of TFCC.
- Triple injection arthrogram, MRI.
- *Arthroscopy:* trampoline test—during arthroscopy the centre is balloted. It should feel firm. If not, a peripheral tear is suspected.

Classification: by Palmer, two types—traumatic and degenerative.

- *Class 1:* traumatic TFCC tears:
  - *Type A:* central perforation (most common);
  - *Type B:* avulsion from ulnar attachment;

○ *Type C:* avulsion from ulnocarpal ligaments;
○ *Type D:* avulsion from sigmoid notch.

• *Class 2:* degenerative tears:

○ *Stage 1:* TFCC wear;
○ *Stage 2:* wear with lunate/ulnar chondromalacia;
○ *Stage 3:* TFCC perforation, chondromalacia;
○ *Stage 4:* TFCC perforation, chondromalacia, lunotriquetral ligament perforation;
○ *Stage 5:* all above with ulnocarpal arthritis.

Treatment:
• For traumatic based on type of tear and length of ulna:

○ A: debride;
○ B: open or arthroscopic reattachment;
○ C: debridement or open repair;
○ D: as B.

• If positive ulnar variance, perform shortening ulnar osteotomy, *see* ULNOCARPAL IMPACTION SYNDROME.
• As long as the dorsal and palmar radio-ulnar ligaments are preserved, debridement of the central portion of the horizontal disc does not compromise stability of the radioulnar joint.

Triangular interval
• Teres major superiorly, long head of triceps medially, lateral head of triceps or humerus laterally.
• Through this interval emerges the radial nerve and profunda brachii artery.

See TRIANGULAR SPACE. *See* QUADRILATERAL SPACE.

Triangular ligament
• Formed by the transverse fibres, which connect the lateral bands of the *Extensor tendons* at the level of the proximal part of the middle phalanx, which may limit volar and lateral shifting of the lateral bands during flexion.
• It is attenuated in *Boutonnière deformity* contributing to volar subluxation of the lateral bands.

Triangular space
• Teres minor superiorly, teres major inferiorly, long head of triceps laterally.
• Through this space emerges the circumflex scapular artery and lymph nodes.

See SCAPULAR FLAP. *See* QUADRILATERAL SPACE. *See* TRIANGULAR INTERVAL.

Trichiasis
Eyelashes turned into the globe. Often associated with entropion.

Trichloro-acetic acid peels (TCA)
• A type of *Chemical peel*. Unlike phenol which is all or none response, the concentration of TCA can be varied. Light peel 10–25%, intermediate 30–35%, deep 50–60%. There is less toxicity than phenol. The desired degree of peel can be chosen.
• TCA has less effect on melanin metabolism so it may be better in darker patients and for regional peels. But the degree of penetration and neocollagen formation is less. It is, therefore, not so effective for coarse wrinkles.
• Skin is pretreated with tretinoin and hydroquinone. Retinoic acid affects the epidermis by decreasing the stratum corneum and increasing permeability. Hydroquinone suppresses melanocytic activity.
• Depth is judged by the appearance of the skin, the turgor and the time taken to return to normal colour after TCA application. A deeper peel is associated with frosting. If it is too deep the frosting becomes grey/white. Apply TCA with a gauze, leave for 30 seconds to 2 minutes after which it is neutralized.

Tricho-epithelioma
• Solitary or multiple lesions, generally benign and do not metastasize. Can be confused with BCC.
• Best described pathologically as a highly differentiated keratotic basal cell epithelioma.
• The multiple form is inherited as an autosomal dominant disorder.
• 2–5 mm diameter firm flesh-coloured papules developing early in life especially on the nose, nasolabial folds, forehead, upper lip and eyelids.
• Treatment is excision.

Trichofolliculoma
• Hair follicle naevus on the face or scalp.
• Skin-coloured papule with central pore containing white hairs.
• Resemble BCCs, but contain keratin-filled macrocysts.
• Treatment is excision.

Tricholemmal cyst
Also called Pilar cyst.
• 90% in the scalp. Derived from the outer hair sheath.
• They are true cysts consisting of a cell wall. The cyst content often has focal calcification.

See EPITHELIAL CYSTS.

Tricholemmoma
- Solitary facial papule. Rarely multiple papules occur as part of *Cowden disease*.
- Get buds of follicular sheath-type epithelial cells which show pallisading.
- It is benign, usually occurs on the scalp and is treated by excision.

Trigger thumb and finger
- Stenosing tenosynovitis of thumb or finger at the level of the A1 pulley resulting in hand pain with triggering or locking. Difficulty flexing or extending the finger depends on whether the tendon is caught distally or proximally to the A1 pulley.
- Most common in middle-aged women. Also secondary to RA, DM, gout when multiple digits may be affected. The ring and middle fingers are most commonly involved.
- Get fibrocartilaginous metaplasia of the inner layer of the pulley or synovial proliferative changes in the tendon. Rucking at the site of constriction leads to development of a nodule, which is aggravated by further movement. The primary lesion is in the sheath and Notta's node is a secondary phenomenon.

Treatment:
- *Conservative:* steroid injection and NSAIDS.
- *Operative:* percutaneous or open release of the A1 pulley. If the flexor tendon is enlarged then it may need to be reduced by excising a central portion of the tendon. Cut A1 pulley of thumb on the radial border as oblique pulley inserts into A1 on ulnar border and may also get cut if pulley is cut on ulnar border. Beware the radial digital nerve which crosses it obliquely. In the rheumatoid patient try to avoid cutting the A1 pulley to prevent ulnar drift or cut finger pulley on the radial side. In the rheumatoid patient, it may also be necessary to perform synovectomy, flexor tenoplasty, or decompress the sheath by excising one or two slips of FDS.

Congenital trigger thumb:
- Clinically similar to adults. 25% present at birth, 25% bilateral. 30% of congenital trigger thumbs seen at birth resolve spontaneously by one month but only 12% of those seen at 6 months resolve. The only known association is with trisomy-13—Patau's syndrome.
- Clicking is difficult to elicit in a child. A nodule (Notta's node) may be palpable over tendon of FPL proximal to A1 pulley.
- Surgical treatment involves release of A1 pulley.

Complications: digital nerve injury.

Triphalangeal thumb
- *Wassel Type 7:* duplication or isolated.
- Maybe autosomal dominant. M = F, most bilateral. Related to thalidomide.
- Associated with:
  - *Holt-Oram syndrome*;
  - *Fanconi's anaemia* is always associated with triphalangeal thumb;
  - Trisomy 13–15;
  - Juberg-Hayward syndrome.
- *3 types:* delta phalanx, short rectangular phalanx, normal length rectangular phalanx.
- The thumb is long and may be supinated with hypoplastic thenar muscles—may be extra finger, rather than a thumb.

Surgery:
- Often indicated for 5 problems:
  - Associated malformations;
  - Narrow web—*Four-flap Z-plasty*;
  - Abnormal shape extra phalanx—if small remove, in older child fuse to either distal or proximal phalanx;
  - Digits in same plane requires pollicization;
  - Thenar muscle deficiency—perform Huber opponensplasty.
- Complete operations by 6–24/12.

Tripier flap
Pedicled flap take from upper lid which can be uni- or bipedicled to reconstruct the lower lid.
See EYELID RECONSTRUCTION.

Triquetrum fracture
- Second most common carpal bone fracture (15%) usually due to a fall on the dorsal or palmar flexed wrist or avulsion of the radiotriquetral ligament. Isolated fracture more uncommon. Most fractures are associated with other carpal injuries, such as lunate injuries.
- Get dorsal cortical fracture due to avulsion of dorsal extrinsic ligaments and the body fracture caused by shear force on the ulnar styloid. Get point tenderness dorsally over the triquetrum. Check of VISI deformity or a break in *Gilula's lines*.
- Treat by splinting for 6 weeks.
See CARPAL INSTABILITY.

Triscaphe OA
Also known as scapho-trapezium-trapezoid (STT) OA.

Surgery: arthrodesis of the triscaphe articulation. If there is pantrapezial arthritis then resect trapezium and reconstruct beak ligament along with arthrodesis of the scapho-trapezoid articulation.

Trunk reconstruction
Indications:
- *Pressure sores.*
- Irradiation.
- Tumour.
- *Spina bifida.*

Management: divide into thirds.
- *Skeletal stabilization:* no consensus for indication for sternal fixation in setting of mediastinitis:
  - Can get sternal stabilization with wires or plates in setting of adequate bone stock and clean wound—may be preferable for younger patients or obese patients. Alternatively leave without fixation to be stabilised through scarring—tolerated better in older patients;
  - Can use mesh for rib stability: Prolene™, Gortex™, Permacol™;
  - If open and infected—avoid synthetic mesh—use TFL or anterior rectus sheath.
- *Soft tissue reconstruction:* traditionally with musculocutaneous flaps:
  - *Pectoralis major:* workhorse for median sternotomy wounds:
    - Advancement (based laterally on thoracodorsal trunk—may still need to divide at the humoral attachment to assist with medialization). May need bilateral for large defects;
    - Turnover (based medially on internal mammary).
  - *Rectus abdominis:* based superiorly on superior epigastric artery (termination of IMA—so has to be intact—can theoretically be harvested on 8th intercostal vessel if IMA previously harvested but tenuous vascularity)—good for inferior midline defects;
  - *'Pec-rec':* bipedicle muscle flap consisting of a superolaterally based (thoracoacromial) pectoralis major muscle flap and inferiorly based rectus abdominis muscle flap raised in continuity;
  - Latissimus dorsi (LD);
  - *Omentum:* either alone or in combination with other flaps. Can be accessed via the sternotomy wound via a diaphragm incision or a laparotomy incision;
  - *Serratus:* can be used on its own or with LD to help close dead space.
- Soft tissue reconstruction with perforator flaps preserves the muscles for secondary respiration (probably most needed by this patient group—an evolution from muscle flaps to FC flaps):
  - i. Regional: TDAP, LICAP, IMAP;
  - ii. Free: DIEP, ALT.

Tubed pedicle flaps
- Method of transporting tissue from distant sites in multiple stages often with the wrist as carrier, but seldom used now.
- First delay a flap, turning it into a tube. Once it has matured it is sutured to an intermediate carrier. After a delay, the base is detached and brought to final destination still attached at the wrist. Once healed it is separated.

Tuberous breast
See MASTOPEXY. Also called a constricted breast. Characterized by a deficient breast-base dimension, a tight and elevated inframammary fold, an elongated thin breast, herniation of the NAC and stretching of the areola.

Classification: by Heimburg.
- *Type 1:* hypoplasia of the inferior medial quadrant.
- *Type 2:* hypoplasia of both inferior quadrants with sufficient skin.
- *Type 3:* hypoplasia of both lower quadrants and subareolar skin shortage.
- *Type 4:* severely constricted breast base.

Surgery: a difficult problem. The principles include reducing the size of the areola, dividing constrictions in the breast parenchyma by radial scoring, lowering the inframammary fold, inserting implant or expander. A circumareolar mastopexy may also be required. Skin may need to be imported via a medially based thoraco-epigastric flap.
- *Type 1:* augment with submammary implant.
- *Type 2:* augment with internal flap—unfurling of breast tissue on chest wall. Perform through inferior areolar incision.
- *Types 3 and 4:* augment, internal flap, skin importation with Z-plasty, thoracoepigastric flap or tissue expansion.

Tuberous sclerosis
- Autosomal dominant condition with triad of cognitive impairment, epilepsy and facial skin rashes. Also get cardiac and renal tumours.
- Skin signs:
  - Angiofibromas in butterfly distribution;
  - Hypomelanotic macules;
  - Forehead fibrous patches;
  - Shagreen patches—thickened discoloured skin in lumbar region;
  - Fibromas from nails of hands and feet;
  - Profuse skin tags.

Tufted angioma

Or angioblastoma of Nakagawa.

- A rare vascular tumour that can be mistaken for a *Haemangioma*.
- An ill-defined, tender, purple indurated patch, several centimetres in size.
- More common in the upper trunk.
- Microscopically see cellular lobules ('tufts') throughout the dermis.
- The tumour may grow slowly and should be excised.

Tumescent anaesthesia

- Used in liposuction.
- Large volumes of dilute LA with adrenaline are injected to give good anaesthesia with reduced blood loss.
- Use 0.05% lignocaine with adrenaline 1:1 million NS. Add sodium bicarbonate. Inject twice as much as the amount of fat aspirated.
- High concentrations of lignocaine from 33 to 55 mg/kg have been reported. Lignocaine lasts longer in the tumescent technique than normal.

See LOCAL ANAESTHETICS.

Tumour necrosis factor

See CYTOKINES.

Turner syndrome

- *Sex differentiation defect* with 45,X karyotype.
- Short stature, high arched palate, webbed neck, shield-like chest, cardiac and renal anomalies, inverted nipples.

Turricephaly

Towering of the skull seen in severe *Craniosynostosis*.

Two-point discrimination (2PD)

- Method of *Sensation testing*. Over 6 mm is abnormal.
- Value varies with most patients having a normal static value at the pulp of 2–3 mm, reduced to 5–6 mm with heavy labour and 1–2 mm with blindness.
- A discrimination wheel is an easy way of testing this. Move prongs from distal to proximal. 7/10 consistent results are required to give a 2PD value.
- Dynamic 2PD has normal value of 2 mm. This returns before static 2PD.
- 2PD is the last sensory modality to return.

Ulna, distal: arthritis to Urbaniak classification

Ulna, distal: arthritis
Painful rotation. Treat by:
- Excision distal end ulna (*Darrach*).
- Hemiresection interposition arthroplasty.
- Resection and replacement (Swanson).
- Arthrodesis and pseudoarthrosis (*Sauvé-Kapandji*).

Ulna variance
- The length difference between the radius and the ulna is measured with the wrist in neutral (90° shoulder and 90° elbow flexion).
- Positive variance may be associated with wrist pain.
- It becomes more positive with forearm pronation or power grip.

Ulnar artery
Lies radial to FCU, passes superficial to TCL in Guyon's canal. A deep branch joins deep branch of nerve under FDM. It passes between transverse and oblique part of adductor pollicis to lie dorsal to adductor pollicis. A deep branch joins the radial artery to form the deep palmar arch, it then becomes the superficial palmar arch.

Ulnar artery flap
- Although the main blood supply to the hand, it can be safely raised as a flap and is less hair-bearing than the radial side. Perform an Allen's test first.
- The pedicle lies within the fascial septum of FCU and FDS. It can be made sensate by including the medial anti-brachial cutaneous nerve. It can also include PL and FCU.

Operation: incise border of flap through fascia. Elevate medial and lateral edges of flap to the septum. Artery is ligated proximally. A distally-based flap may occasionally get venous congestion and require anastomosing of a vein to a recipient vein in the hand.

Ulnar club hand
- 1/10th as common as *Radial club hand*.

- Can get a spectrum of abnormalities ranging from slight hypoplasia of the ulnar digits to total absence of the ulna.

It differs from radial club hand as the hand is stable at the wrist, but unstable at the elbow and partial absence is the most common finding.

Classification:
- *Type 1:* hypoplasia.
- *Type 2:* partial absence.
- *Type 3:* total absence.
- *Type 4:* fusion of radius to humerus—radiohumeral synostoses.

Treatment: depends of severity of deformity. Surgical treatment involves release of the fibrous anlage and realignment of the carpus and forearm.
  See CONGENITAL HANDS.

Ulnar collateral ligament
Anatomy: *see* THUMB MPJ.
- Range of motion of thumb MCP joint variable. Spherical heads have greater ROM. Little intrinsic stability.
- Strong proper collaterals run from metacarpal lateral condyles to volar third of proximal phalanx. Accessory collaterals (ACL) run more volar and insert into volar plate and sesamoids. Proper collaterals are tight in flexion and loose in extension and ACLs are the opposite. 3-sided ligament box differs from PIP joints as there is no flexor sheath and, therefore, no check rein ligament. Intrinsics insert into sesamoid bones embedded in distal volar plate.

Injury:
- *Acute UCL injury:* distal tears 5 times more common than proximal.
- *Stener lesion:* adductor aponeurosis interposes between distally avulsed ligament and its insertion, which prevents UCL healing. Not possible to reliably exclude a Stener lesion in the context of a complete tear,

therefore all clinically complete tears should be managed operatively.

- Important to distinguish between partial and complete tears. Assess clinically by comparing injured side to non-injured side. The injured joint must be examined under local anaesthetic to avoid patient actively resisting abduction. If the joint can be opened with no clear end point, this suggests a complete tear. Can be assessed by USS if not clear clinically.

Treatment:
- *Partial tear:* treat with splint for 4 weeks and protect for 3 months.
- *Complete tear:* treat by repair.
- *Chronic UCL injury:* use tendon graft to reconstruct.

Operative technique:
- Lazy S incision on ulnar border of thumb overlying MCP joint at junction of glabrous and non-glabrous skin and onto dorsum of hand to avoid crossing 1st webspace. Beware of dorsal sensory branch of radial nerve. Incise adductor aponeurosis 3 mm volar to ulnar border of EPL. Examine joint.
- Suture ligament or use bone anchor or pull-out suture. If primary repair is not possible, can use a PL graft to reconstruct. Secure distal end first. Ensure to recreate obliquity of the UCL.
- If there is a bony fragment it can be fixed with a small screw or a pull-out wire.
- After ligament repair:
  ○ Suture distal ligament to volar plate;
  ○ Repair dorsal ulnar capsule;
  ○ Test stability with radial stress;
  ○ K-wire in flexion and ulnar deviation, suture extensor expansion to adductor aponeurosis.

Ulnar dimelia
- Also called mirror hand.
- Very rare (only exceeded by multiple hands).
- 7 digits occur, but only the medial two are obviously little and ring.
- The forearm contains two ulnae, but no radial bones. The thumb is missing and there is an excess of fingers.
- The elbow is stiff and the forearm rotation reduced. The contralateral hand is usually not affected.

Treatment:
- Excise olecranon to increase elbow mobility.
- Excise excess fingers and pollicize. The finger to be pollicized will depend on observation.
- All fingers have their complement of tendons and these can be used in the pollicization and to rebalance the wrist.

Ulnar nerve
- In the forearm, ulnar nerve travels between FDS and FDP supplying FDP to ring and little finger.
- The ulnar nerve gives off a dorsal cutaneous branch 5-7 cm proximal to styloid process of ulna. It winds around the ulnar aspect of the forearm to supply the dorsum of the hand.
- The ulnar nerve divides into deep and superficial branches at the level of *Guyon's canal*.
- Superficial branch supplies palmaris brevis then splits into two branches to little and half of ring finger.
- The deep branch passes under the fibrous arch of the origin of FDM. It accompanies the *Deep palmar arch* passing between ADM and FDM, giving branches to the hypothenar muscles. It runs radially deep to palmar interosseous fascia and ends by passing between the two heads of AP. It supplies the *Interosseous muscles* and the 2 ulnar lumbricals. The interosseous branches enter the muscles on the palmar side and the lumbricals on the dorsal side.

Ulnar nerve compression
See CUBITAL TUNNEL SYNDROME. See GUYON'S CANAL.

Ulnar nerve palsy
Motor loss: by muscle.
- *Lumbrical: Duchenne's sign*—ring and little finger clawing, also *Bouvier's manoeuvre, Andre-Thomas sign*. Loss of normal flexion, which starts at MCP joint, instead curl from distal to proximal.
- *Interosseus: Pitres-Testut sign*—inability to abduct and adduct middle finger as well as cross the fingers, digital Froment's.
- *Hypothenar muscles: Masse's sign* of hypothenar wasting and *Wartenberg's sign* of the abducted little finger.
- *Adductor pollicis: Jeanne's* sign—loss of lateral pinch and *Froment's* sign with IPJ flexion.
- FDP 4th and 5th finger: Pollock's sign.
- *FCU:* partial loss of wrist flexion.
Sensory loss: to ulnar 1 1/2 digits.

Management:
- In hand MDT setting.
- Tendon transfers: aim of tendon transfers is not to restore the complex and intricate function of the ulnar nerve and intrinsic muscles but it is to improve function. Main priority to address the claw deformity using FDS to ring and little in either a static (Zancolli lasso with FDS to A1 pulley) or dynamic (Stiles-Bunnell with FDS to lateral bands) procedure to address MCPJ hyperextension. In addition, tendon transfers to address thumb adduction and index finger

abduction can be considered and if a high lesion transfers for ring and little DIPJ flexion.
- Nerve transfers such as AIN to ulnar nerve.

See TENDON TRANSFERS.

Ulnar translocation of the carpus

Carpal instability, which occurs after radiocarpal dislocation and commonly in rheumatoid arthritis.

Classification: by Taleisnik.

- *Type I:* entire carpus displaced ulnarly with widened radioscaphoid articulation.
- *Type II:* scapholunate interval is widened so scaphoid stays in place.

Ulnocarpal impaction syndrome

- Ulnar-sided wrist pain with ulnar positive *Variance*. Get erosion of carpus, synovitis, thinning of TFCC, and disruption of ulnocarpal ligaments.
- Caused by congenital or acquired positive variance—usually due to a malunion of a distal radius fracture or radioulnar instability (*Essex-Lopresti injury*).
- Treat by decompressing the ulnar side with *Darrach*, shortening osteotomy, or arthroscopic excision.

See TRIANGULAR FIBROCARTILAGE.

Ultraviolet radiation (UV)

- Harmful effects are due to electron excitation in the absorbing atoms and molecules, which induces damage in DNA and may be responsible for cell death and neoplastic transformation. Also get production of oxygen-free radicals, which damage cell membranes and nuclear DNA.
- Also may have an immunosuppressive effect with depletion of Langerhans cells.
- Adverse effects are reduced by hair, thick stratum corneum and melanin.
- Though most of the radiation reaching the human skin is UVA, UVB causes most of the problem with sunburn and neoplasia.

UVA: 320–400 nm.

- Contributes to erythema, carcinogenesis and photo-ageing.
- This is emitted by most sunbeds.
- Exposure is thought but not proved to increase the risk of developing *Melanoma*.

UVB: 290–320 nm. Causes sunburn, tan, pre-cancer and cancer.

UVC: 200–290 nm. Mostly filtered out by the ozone layer.

Umbilical sculpting

Technique: defat umbilicus and the reduce length of the pedicle by resecting upper portion of umbilicus. Suture edge of umbilicus to fascia. Mark position of new umbilicus on abdomen with some tacking sutures to skin edges. Excise a horizontal ellipse. Resect a core of fat. Lift skin flaps and cut an ellipse of fat away particularly from inferior margin. Put stay suture into edge of umbilicus to enable it to pull through opening. Once the abdomen is sutured pass stitch through and stitch with non-absorbable suture.

Unicameral bone cyst

- A cavity filled with yellow serous fluid.
- Occurs in long bones, 90% in proximal femur and proximal humerus.
- Presents in 10s–20s after a pathological fracture.
- Early lesions occur in the metaphysis abutting the physeal plate. Older lesions have moved away. They become multiloculated but don't undergo malignant degeneration.
- *XR:* an eccentric radiolucent cyst of variable size in the metaphysis of tubular bone.
- Treat by intralesional aspiration and injection with methylprednisolone.
- Larger lesions can be curetted and bone grafted. The natural history is spontaneous healing in adulthood.

See BONE TUMOURS.

Upper limb embryology

- Upper limb bud appears by the 26th day and consists of a core of mesoderm covered in a layer of ectoderm.
- Proximal/distal axis governed by the apical ectodermal ridge at the thickened ectodermal tip of the limb bud which secretes FGF.
- Radial/ulnar axis is governed by the zone of polarizing activity on the ulnar aspect of the limb bud which secretes sonic hedgehog (SHH).
- Dorsal/ventral axis is governed by the dorsal ectoderm, which secretes Wnt7a (wingless-type mouse mammary tumour).

Upton classification

See APERT'S HANDS.

Urbaniak classification   Classification of

Ring avulsion injuries. relates to microsurgical management.

- *I:* circulation adequate.
- *II:* circulation inadequate and microvascular reconstruction will restore circulation and function:
  - *IIA:* requires repair of digital arteries alone;
  - *IIB:* arteries, bone and tendon;
  - *IIC:* only the veins.
- *III:* complete degloving of skin. Microvascular reconstruction will restore circulation, but with poor function. Amputation is recommended.

VAC therapy to V–Y advancement

VAC therapy
Vm acuum-assisted closure. Also known as negative pressure wound therapy (NPWT). Developed by Louis Argenta in 1997.

- Uses intermittent or continuous vacuum through a sealed foam dressing to stimulate granulation tissue and speed healing.
- The principles are to remove exudates, provide a moist environment, remove oedema, increase blood flow, increase granulation, encourage epithelialization.
- It can be used over SSG at a lower pressure (50–100 mmHg) or on open wounds at 125 mmHg.

Action:
- Fluid removal improves O_2 delivery. Wound fluid also inhibits fibroblasts and keratinocyte activity and matrix metalloproteins break down collagen.
- Increases blood flow. This encourages granulation tissue formation.
- Micro-deformation—promotes mitotic activity and cell proliferation
- Macro-deformation—wound edges physically brought together. This encourages wound contraction.
- Decreases risk of infection.

Contraindications:
- Exposed vasculature or nerves.
- Exposed anastomotic structures.
- Exposed organs.
- Malignancy.
- Unexplored fistulae.

VACTERL association
- **V**ertebral anomalies.
- **A**nal atresia.
- **C**ardiac anomalies.
- **T**racheo-oesophageal fistula.
- **E**sophageal atresia.
- **R**enal disorders.
- **L**imb anomalies.

  See RADIAL CLUB HAND.

Vaginal agenesis
- Known as Mayer–Rokitansky–Küster–Hauser syndrome.

- 1:4,000 live female births.
- Results from failure of development of the paramesonephric duct (*see* EMBRYOLOGY).
- 50% associated with abnormalities of the urinary tract. Ovaries are usually normal. A vestigial vaginal dimple may be present. If no uterus, present with amenorrhoea. If uterus present, present with haematocolpos.

Investigation: examination may reveal a vaginal dimple. USS and IVP to assess upper urinary tract. EUA, chromosomal abnormality.

Vaginal reconstruction
For:
- Females born without a vagina (Mayer-Rokitansky–Küster–Hauser syndrome). Most have no uterus, but normal ovaries.
- After excision for neoplasm.
- Male to female gender reassignment.

Surgery:
- *McIndoe procedure:* cavity developed between rectum and bladder and lined with SSG. A stent is required. Complications are stenosis and fistulae. A mould is sutured in and left for 6 months.
- *FTSG:* similar to McIndoe procedure. Graft from either groin sutured together. Stent made with foam and condom. Post-operatively a candle is used covered in condom to stent the neovagina. Graft doesn't constrict.
- *Bowel:* vascularized ileum or colon. Disadvantage is the mucus and trauma during intercourse.
- *Dilatation:* if a dimple is present it can be dilated progressively.
- Also use flaps of labia minora and gracilis.

Van der Meulen hypospadias repair
- *Hypospadias* repair, a modification of the Duplay technique.
- It involves transposition of a flap based on the adjacent penile skin to form a neo-urethra followed by wraparound of the preputial skin. This moves the meatus distally, but does not sink it into the glans.

Van der Woude's syndrome

Associated with cleft lip and/or palate.

- Autosomal dominant.
- Lower lip pits that are accessory salivary glands are present in 80% of patients. Embryologically derived sinuses at the location of the lateral grooves in the lower lip. Classically located symmetrically bilateral paramedian. May have clear secretions but largely asymptomatic. Can be treated with surgical excision aiming to completely remove the sinus.
- Association with hypodontia: Missing central and lateral incisors, canines and bicuspids.
- There is a gene alteration in IRF6.

   See CRANIOFACIAL GENETICS.

Van Lohuizen syndrome

See TELANGIECTASES.

Vascular anomalies

- An umbrella term to describe a broad spectrum of vascular pathology.
- Originally classified by Mulliken and Glowacki. Updated classification by the International Society of the Study of Vascular Anomalies (ISSVA):

   - *Vascular tumours:*
     - Benign;
     - Locally aggressive or borderline;
     - Malignant.
   - *Vascular malformations:*
     - Simple;
     - Combined;
     - Of major named vessels;
     - Associated with other anomalies.

Vascular injuries: upper limb

Anatomy: *Ulnar artery, Radial artery.*

- *Aneurysms.* Pseudo aneurysms.
- *Arteriovenous fistulae.*
- *Buerger's disease.*
- Emboli.
- Thrombosis:

   - *Hypothenar hammer syndrome;*
   - It can also occur in the radial artery—particularly following cannulation. atherosclerosis is rare, digital ischaemia secondary to thrombosis of a persistent median artery has been described.

- *Vasospastic disorders:*

   - *Raynaud's.*

Vascular leiomyoma

Or dermal angiomyoma.

- A small tumour that arises from the tunica muscularis of small vessels and presents as a painless enlarging mass.

- Well encapsulated white lesions located in the dermis or subcutaneous layer.
- Histologically appear as bundles of smooth muscle surrounding vascular channels.

Vascular malformations

Pathology:

- *Malformation* describes a vascular anomaly with a normal endothelial turnover cycle. These are inborn errors of vascular channel morphogenesis formed by a combination of abnormal capillary, arterial, venous or lymphatic channels. It is present at birth and neither proliferates or involutes, but grows with the child. Some grow after a triggering factor.

Classification:

- Simple:

   - Capillary malformations;
   - Lymphatic malformations;
   - Venous malformations;
   - Arteriovenous malformations (high flow);
   - Arteriovenous fistula (high flow).

- Combined defined as two or more vascular malformations found in one lesion.
- Of major named vessels.
- Associated with other anomalies.

Associated syndromes:

- *Bonnet–Dechaume–Blanc.*
- *Sturge–Weber.*
- *Parkes–Weber syndrome.*
- *Klippel–Trenaunay syndrome.*
- *Rendu–Osler–Weber disease.*
- *Maffucci syndrome.*

Investigation:

- Clinical photographs.
- Do XR in venous malformations to look for phleboliths that can cause pain.
- (Duplex) USS—good initial screen.
- MRI with gadolinium enhancement is investigation of choice to assess flow characteristics and extent of lesion.
- Angiography if planning embolization.

Treatment:

- Non-operative:

   - Do nothing—conservative watch and wait;
   - Cosmetic camouflage;
   - Compression garments for venous malformations—simple and effective.

- Laser:

   - *Capillary malformations:* 585–595 Pulse dye laser (it is the most specific and safest laser)—target oxyhaemoglobin chromophore but can be blotchy. Small

V

lesions do better than large. Location matters—neck and upper torso do best. Treatment intervals: 2–3 months. 4-6 sessions required;
- *Venous:* has some role for superficial:
  - Long pulsed ND YAg—1064 nm—in reality only targets the small superficial vessels.
- Medical:
  - *Aspirin:* can help pheboliths in venous malformations;
  - *Oral sirilimus:* an immunosuppressant—inhibits vascular proliferation: can be used in VM and LMs.
- *Sclerotherapy:* causes inflammation and vessel sclerosis—most commonly alcohol, sodium tetradecyl sulphate (foam) and bleomycin. May need to be repeated. Can reduce pain and size of vessels:
  - Usually done under GA due to pain;
  - Day case;
  - *Imaging:* USS to find big channels and fluoroscopy—inject with radio-opaque dye to prevent you going into important vessels. This is the method to use in the face to reduce the risk of damage;
  - *Risks:* skin necrosis, nerve damage, DVT/PE, blindness in the face;
  - *Risk of bleomycin:* pulmonary fibrosis.
- Operative:
  - Small lesions can be excised;
  - Larger and intramuscular lesions can be debulked to improve pain, function (main indication) and appearance;
  - *Popescu sutures:* mattress sutures through skin to compress lesion.

Vascular tumours
Pathology:
- *Tumour:* describes an endothelial neoplasm characterized by increased cellular proliferation.
  - Haemangioma is the most common.

ISSVA classification:
- Benign:
  - Infantile haemangioma;
  - Congenital haemangioma;
  - Tufted angioma;
  - Pyogenic granuloma.
- Locally aggressive:
  - Kaposiform haemangioendothelioma;
  - Kaposi sarcoma.

- Malignant:
  - Angiosarcoma;
  - Epithelioid haemangioendothelioma.

Associated syndromes:
- *Kassabach-Merritt syndrome.*
- *PHACES.*

Investigation:
- Clinical photographs.
- Coagulation studies if any evidence of Kasabach-Merritt or venous malformation.
- *USS:* in haemangioma can show a soft tissue mass with fast-flow, decreased arterial resistance and increased venous drainage.
- *MRI with gadolinium enhancement:* in haemangioma can show isotense tumour on T1 and hypertense on T2—can also detect PHACES (posterior fossa malformations, facial haemangioma, arterial anomalies, cardiac defects, eye abnormalities, sternal cleft and supraumbilical raphe).
- Biopsy if any suggestion of malignancy:
  - Look for GLUT1 if sending any operative samples.

Treatment:
- Non-operative:
  - Most haemangiomas can be appropriately managed by a conservative watch and wait approach;
  - Medical treatment has become the standard of care for lesions that have complicating factors (intrinsic or extrinsic) or are present on cosmetically sensitive areas:
    - Propranolol (current first line treatment) blocks beta adrenergic receptors. 2mg/kg/day in three divided doses. Discovered inadvertently in 2008 in NEJM. Can be titrated up. Consider baseline ECG and glucose. Now a low threshold for using it;
    - Corticosteroids—lesser efficacy than betablockers in head-to-head studies;
    - 5FU and bleomycin.
  - Lasers—for residual sequelae.
- Operative:
  - Rarely indicated in the proliferative phase only if complications arise (bleeding, ulceration) or risk of damaging adjacent structures not adequately addressed by non-operative means;
  - May be indicated in the involuting or involuted phase to improve residual scars or fatty deposits:

- Tip of nose fibrofatty pad is difficult to manage (Cyrano de Bergerac deformity)—may have to do a rhinoplasty but technically challenging.

Vascularized composite allotransplantation (VCA)

- Transfer of a functional unit of multiple tissue types (skin, nerve, muscle, bone etc.). This differentiates VCA from solid organ transplant.
- VCA examples include _Hand transplant, Face transplant_ and _Abdominal wall transplant._
- Can provide like for like reconstruction in complex defects.
- Technically demanding and patients require lifelong immunosuppression due to the multiple tissues with different immunogenic and functional properties. A rapidly advancing field in reconstructive surgery requiring a highly specialized multidisciplinary approach working in a comprehensive institutional infrastructure.

Vasculitis

- Symptoms and signs include general malaise, high ESR, CRP, low complement, ischaemic lesions that are slow to heal due to increased coagulability of the blood.
- Need immunosuppression with steroids and cyclophosphamide.
- Classify according the size of vessels and the organs involved:
  ○ Large vessels are involved in periarteritis nodosa and temporal arteritis;
  ○ Small vessel involvement occurs in Henoch–Schönlein purpura, Waterhouse–Friderichsen syndrome and Wegener's syndrome.

Vasospastic disorders

- Get cold intolerance (occurs in 20% of premenopausal women) due to vasospasm or occlusion with inadequate microvascular perfusion.
- Primary vasospasm is _Raynaud's disease._
- Normally less than 10% blood flow goes through nutritional capillaries. Blood flow is dependent on vascular integrity and appropriate control mechanisms.
- Cutaneous circulation is controlled by alpha-adrenergic receptors via the sympathetic system.
- Primary Raynaud's has abnormal responsiveness of catecholamine receptors.
- Secondary Raynaud's has abnormal vessels.

Clinical:

- Repetitive trauma, drugs, smoking.
- Perform Allen's test, vascular studies. Stress test especially in collagen disease with

vascular occlusion. The difference between thermoregulatory flow and nutritional flow is difficult to distinguish. Vital capillaroscopy is one way of doing this by looking at finger with microscope.

Vastus lateralis flap

Anatomy: origin is the lateral surface of greater trochanter and inserts into the rectus femoris and upper lateral patella.

Blood supply: descending branch of the lateral circumflex femoral artery from the profunda femoris. Runs from medial to lateral coming from under rectus femoris. Enters the anterior belly 10 cm inferior to the ASIS. The distal third is supplied by perforating branches of the superficial femoral artery. Only the proximal two-thirds can be reliably elevated.

Reconstruction: perform through a lateral incision. Get significant weakness with knee instability.

See PRESSURE SORES.

Vaughn–Jackson syndrome

Ulnar prominence can lead to progressive rupture of EDC tendons. Primary repair is difficult due to frayed tendon ends. Usually treated with tendon transfers.

See CAPUT ULNA SYNDROME. _See_ TENDON RUPTURE IN RHEUMATOID ARTHRITIS.

Veau–Wardill–Kilner repair

For _Cleft palate_ reconstruction. V–Y advancement of the mucoperiosteum of the hard palate with the intention of lengthening the palate. Bone is left exposed to re-epithelialize, but this scar may contribute to maxillary growth disturbance.

VEGF—vascular endothelial growth factor

- An endogenous stimulator of angiogenesis and vascular permeability. It is expressed in developing blood vessels.
- It includes VEGF A, B, C, D, E and placental growth factor.
- VEGF-A is the most predominant protein. Experimentally it is found to be upregulated in flap ischaemia and administration may improve flap survival.

See GROWTH FACTORS.

Velocardiofacial syndrome

Also known as 22Q11.2 deletion syndrome, DiGeorge syndrome and CATCH 22.

- Most are sporadic, some are inherited.
- 83% of individuals have a deletion of long arm of chromosome 22q11.2.
- Associated with velopharyngeal insufficiency, cleft palate, cardiac anomalies, hypoplastic

thymus, unusual facies and learning difficulties.

- The facial feature includes a long face both physically and in expression, epicanthic folds, pinched nasal tip.
- Diagnosis—hemizygous deletion of chromosomes 22q11.2 using FISH method.
- Management is best led by a specialized and dedicated MDT and depends on age and phenotype. Speech difficulties are complex and multifactorial and may involve structural velopharyngeal insufficiency in combination with poor neuromuscular control and language problems (receptive and expressive).
- Speech surgery is complex and associated with poorer outcomes than non-syndromic overt cleft palate or submucous cleft palate. Velar musculature tends to be hypoplastic. In non-cleft VPD in the setting of 22Q11.2 deletion, a pharyngoplasty may be considered as a primary procedure. Medialized internal carotid arteries are seen in 25% of patients with velocardiofacial syndrome and MRA should be considered prior to speech surgery intervention.

Velopharyngeal dysfunction (VPD)
- Umbrella term for failure of velopharyngeal closure.
- Velopharyngeal valve is an anatomical sphincter which closes to separate the oral and nasal cavities during speech and mastication and opens to allow nasal breathing.
- VPD is associated with speech characteristics and regurgitation.

Anatomy:
- The velopharyngeal sphincter is a circular structure formed from the velum anteriorly, the palatopharyngeus within the posterior tonsillar columns of the lateral pharyngeal walls laterally and the superior pharyngeal constrictor within the posterior pharyngeal wall.
- Closure of the sphincter is mainly by the contraction of levator veli palatini and the superior pharyngeal constrictor.
- Opening of the sphincter is mainly by the palatopharyngeus and assisted by palatoglossus.

Causes of VPD:
- Velopharyngeal insufficiency implies a structural reason for VPD. Reasons for this include a cleft palate or submucous cleft palate.

- *Post-palate repair:* there may be a shortened soft palate, or inadequate lateral wall movement or central defect. Tonsils may cause VPD either by being too big and impeding velar movement or after resection due to increased pharyngeal volume (most commonly self-limiting).
- Velopharyngeal incompetence implies a neuromuscular reason for VPD in the presence of normal muscular anatomy.

Assessment:
Patients should be assessed in a specialized speech investigation clinic with a speech surgeon, speech therapist and psychologist. Investigation is multimodal:

- Patient reported outcome measure of speech function such as SPAR QL or CLEFT Q.
- Perceptual speech analysis such as GOS.SP. PASS score to identify speech characteristics in resonance, nasal emission, articulation and intelligibility.
- *Nasometry:* measures differential airflow between nose and mouth—get a percentage nasalance score. Normal <20%. Not definitive but useful for sequential measurement.
- Instrumental speech analysis:
  ○ Lateral video fluoroscopy to assess integrity of velopharyngeal valve during phonation. Can assess length of palate, point of lift, closure to the posterior pharyngeal wall and characteristics of the pharynx. Downside is exposure to XR. Most children will tolerate from 3 years old;
  ○ Nasendoscopy can help with analysis of closure pattern but may not be tolerated in a 3-year-old.
- Dynamic MRI is an evolving option to assess the position of the velar musculature and three-dimensional closure pattern of the velopharyngeal sphincter.

Management options:
In the setting of a structural velopharyngeal dysfunction, speech therapy will not be effective.

- *Surgical intervention:* aims to improve velopharyngeal closure but can be complicated by hyponasality and obstructive sleep apnoea. Surgery approaches can be categorized:
  ○ *Palatal optimization:* augment velar function in sphincter closure:
    ■ Re-repair may be indicated in the setting of anteriorly positioned velar musculature. Re-repair with an intravelar veloplasty aims to retro-position the muscles whereas re-repair with a Furlow double-opposing

Z-plasty may theoretically also lengthen the palate;
- Palatal lengthening with buccal flaps.
○ *Pharyngoplasty:* augment pharyngeal wall function in sphincter closure:
  - Sphincter-type pharyngoplasties involve the construction of myomucosal flaps from the lateral pharyngeal wall which are then sutured to the posterior pharyngeal wall. Includes the Hynes pharyngoplasty (set high above the soft palate and incorporates the salpingopharyngeus) and the Orticochea pharyngoplasty (set lower and incorporates the palatopharyngeus in the posterior tonsillar pillar);
  - Posterior pharyngeal flap involves a superiorly based flap from the posterior pharyngeal wall attached to the soft palate to create a midline obstruction with two lateral openings which remain open for respiration and close for oral consonants. Remains the most commonly used pharyngoplasty globally.
- *Prosthetics:* a palatal prosthesis, velar lift or velopharyngeal obturator may be used, particularly when there is adequate tissue but poor control of coordination and timing.

Venkataswami flap
- A homodigital neurovascular island flap. Sensate advancement digital flap based on the neurovascular bundle.
- Utilized for fingertip reconstruction.
- Oblique scars can cause problematic contractures. Evans step advancement flap may provide a better donor site.

Venous flaps
- Based on venous rather than arterial pedicles (but may be a misnomer as many venous pedicles have small arteries running alongside them).
- Mechanism of perfusion poorly understood—may be plasmatic imbibition, perfusion pressure, AV anastomosis, perivenous arterial networks, vein-to-vein interconnections and circumvention of venous valves.
- Have a tendency to become congested post-operatively and survival is inconsistent.
- Classified by the *Thatte and Thatte classification*.

See FLAPS.

Venous hypertension
Causes 80% of *Leg ulcers*. Occurs with long standing elevation of venous blood pressure.

Caused by incompetent valves, most commonly due to previous thrombophlebitis.

Anatomy:
- Deep veins are paired and run with the artery with crossing branches. Superficial veins do not travel with arteries and are not paired. Both systems have valves and connect via perforating veins.
- Perforating veins are principally found between the long saphenous and posterior tibial system. Perforators contribute to ulceration when the valves do not work.

Investigations:
- *Venogram:* invasive assessment now rarely performed.
- *Duplex scanning:* assesses anatomy and function.
- *Photoplethysmography and air plethysmography:* used to assess backward flow of blood.

Venous malformations
See VASCULAR MALFORMATIONS. Present at birth, but not always evident. They are slow flow and appear as a faint blue patch or a soft bluish mass. They can occur internally. They are usually solitary but multiple hereditary forms occur.

Treatment: for functional problems.
- Elastic support stockings.
- Low-dose aspirin (75 mg od) seems to minimize the occurrence of episodic, painful phlebothrombosis.
- *Sclerotherapy:* small cutaneous VM in any location can be injected with a sclerosant. A large VM, cutaneous or intramuscular, requires general anaesthesia and 'real-time' fluoroscopic monitoring during sclerotherapy. Sclerosis of a large VM is potentially dangerous. Compression and other manoeuvres prevent passage of the sclerosing agent into the systemic circulation. Local complications include blistering, full-thickness cutaneous necrosis, or neural damage. Systemic complications include renal toxicity and cardiac arrest. Multiple sclerotherapeutic sessions may be necessary, often at several-month intervals.
- *Surgical resection:* is considered to reduce tissue mass for functional or cosmetic indications. May be beneficial for intramuscular VMs or VMs of the hand/foot, particularly in the digits.

Familial glomangiomatosis:
- Rather common autosomal dominant syndrome of high penetrance.

- Multiple, often tender, blue nodular dermal venous lesions that can occur anywhere on the skin.
- Histologically, these differ from typical VM by the presence of numerous glomus cells lining the ecstatic venous channels.

Familial cutaneous-mucosal VM: inherited in an autosomal dominant mode.

Blue rubber bleb naevus (Bean syndrome):
- Sporadic combination of cutaneous and visceral VMs.
- The skin lesions are soft, blue and nodular; they can occur anywhere.
- Typically located on the hands and feet.
- The gastrointestinal lesions are sessile (submucosal–subserosal) or polypoid, located in the oesophagus, stomach, small and large bowel and mesentery.
- Recurrent intestinal bleeding can be severe, requiring repeated transfusions.

VMs are easily compressible and swell if dependent. They are often painful. Thrombosis and phleboliths occur. Limb VM rarely causes growth discrepancy. MRI is helpful. A coagulation profile can be performed as with extensive VM there is a risk of localized intravascular coagulopathy which is different to *Kasabach-Merritt phenomenon* as platelets are only minimally decreased, but fibrinogen is low.

Venous ulcers

Pathogenesis: not completely clear. Loss of valvular competence, raised venous blood pressure, extravasation of protein and blood cells into subcutaneous tissues, pericapillary fibrin cuff acts as a diffusion barrier, inflammation leads to scarring and lipodermatosclerosis (brawny oedema). This tissue is poorly vascularized and easily traumatized, and slow to heal.

Position: Gaiter region between malleoli and gastrocnemius. Possibly due to excessively high pressures in the perforating veins on contraction of gastrocnemius.

Investigation:
- ABPI.
- Wound swabs.
- Latest bloods.
- Biopsy any long-standing lesions for Marjolin's ulcer.
- Clinical photography.
- X-rays to exclude osteomyelitis.
- Consider vascular studies.

Conservative treatment:
Venous ulcers are usually treated conservatively with elevation, compression and dressings:
- Clean ulcer and debride necrotic tissue.

- Dress with simple non-adherent dressing.
- Avoid topical antibiotics (often become sensitizers)—only use systemic antibiotics for cellulitis.
- Graduated, multilayer compression bandages (from toe to knee) reduces capillary transudate—mean time to healing 5 months. Recurrence in 5 years 30%.
  - Orthopaedic wool;
  - Crepe bandage;
  - Elastic bandage;
  - Cohesive retaining layer.
- Compressive stockings are easier to use than multilayer bandaging.
- Vacuum dressings may be useful in some circumstances.

If ulcer fails to heal in 12 weeks—assess to rule out other causes, i.e. vasculitis, infection, autoimmune disease, sickle cell or tumour.

Surgery:
Required only when conservative management has failed or if pain is a prominent symptom. Involves debridement and soft tissue cover with grafts or flaps. Simple excision with grafts or flaps without addressing the underlying problem is prone to recurrence.

See LEG ULCERS.

Verruca vulgaris
- Caused by papovavirus, transmitted by direct contact or auto-inoculation.
- Get hyperkeratosis, acanthosis and parakeratosis.
- Treat with topical irritants, cryotherapy, excision or laser ablation.
- The basal epidermal layer is not invaded so re-epithelialization occurs rapidly.

Vicryl
- Braided synthetic suture composed of polyglactin 910 (90% glycoside, 10% L-lactide).
- It loses its strength in 3 weeks; it is absorbed in 3 months.
- It may be more prone to bacterial colonization due to its braided nature.
- It may provoke an inflammatory reaction.

Vincula
- Folds of mesotendon which provide connective support to the FDS and FDP tendons.
- The blood supply passes through these vincula via transverse communicating branches of the common digital artery. Each tendon is supplied by a short and long vincula, which enter the dorsal portion of each tendon.

• The short vincula are located close to the insertion point. The vinculum longum of FDP pierces superficialis close to PIP joint. Vessels run on the dorsum of tendons.

See FLEXOR TENDONS.

Vitallium
Cobalt-chromium-molybdenum alloy. High tensile strength so can be low profile.

See ALLOPLASTS.

Vitamin A
• Deficiency affects all stages of *Wound healing*.
• Counteracts the impairment in wound healing due to steroid administration by the labialization of lysosomes within inflammatory cells.
• Clinical use has been variable and definite improvements in healing have not been demonstrated.

Vitamin C
A cofactor required for the hydroxylation of pro-line and lysine. Deficiency causes cross-linking deficiency of collagen and impairment of *Wound healing* (a condition known as scurvy). Treat vitamin C deficiency with 100–1,000 g/day.

Vitamin E
A membrane stabilizer. Deficiency may inhibit healing.

Voice restoration
A laryngeal voice may be produced by air flow-induced vibration of the pharyngo-oesophageal mucosa by ingested air (oesophageal speech) or shunted air (fistula or tracheo-oesophageal speech).

Oesophageal speech: only 25% of patients can manage this. Only small amounts of air can be ingested and only 4–5 words can be expressed. Air must be able to pass freely through the neo-pharynx. Get a low-pitched voice with a lot of jitter (cycle-to-cycle pitch perturbation) and shimmer (cycle-to-cycle amplitude perturb-ation). A radial forearm flap may give more suc-cessful oesophageal speech than a jejunal flap.

Artificial larynx:
• This is a crude vibrator, which produces a focused tone electronically or pneumatically that mimics the vocal cords.
• When applied firmly to the neck or along the cheek, a penetrating signal enters the mouth. It is this new signal or voice that is used for speech.
• The user must learn to articulate vowels clearly with considerable exaggeration of mouth and tongue position. Only indicated when surgical reconstructive results are poor. It may be used while waiting for tracheo-oesophageal puncture (TEP) reconstruction.

Tracheo-oesophageal puncture and voice prosthesis placement:
• The addition of pulmonary air supply brings acoustic quality closer to normal. This is achieved with a TEF. The addition of a voice prosthesis allows for fluent speech.
• Developed in 1980, a one-way valve allows air to enter the oesophagus when the patient exhales with the tracheostoma occluded, but stops liquid and food entering the trachea when the patient swallows. Skin reconstruction gives better speech results.
• First the reconstruction is performed, preferably with a radial forearm flap. The Blom–Singer prosthesis can be inserted at the same time or as a separate procedure. With the neck extended a TEP is created by inserting a needle through the posterior wall of the tracheostoma just superior to the lower anastomosis. This hole is dilated to allow a size 14 catheter to be inserted as a stent. A week later the Blom–Singer voice prosthesis is inserted. This acts as a one-way valve, directing air into the oesophagus when a finger occludes it. The neo-oesophagus acts as the new vibratory segment. The frequency of voice is low.

Volar plate
• A thick ligament on the volar surface of the joints of the finger which resembles a swallow's tail. The space between allows the passage of the vincula.
• Distally the volar plate blends with volar periosteum of the middle phalanx, the strongest attachments being laterally.
• There are 3 layers. The dorsal layer has a proximal membranous portion and a distal meniscoid portion. The middle layer contains fibres which form the check rein ligament. The volar layer contains transverse fibres, which anchor the flexor sheath to the volar plate.
• A small recess separating the meniscoid portion from the middle phalanx allows the plate to hinge open with joint flexion.

See PROXIMAL INTERPHALANGEAL JOINT.

Volkmann's ischaemic contracture
• Occurs after an untreated *Compartment syndrome* in the upper limb due to insufficient arterial perfusion and venous stasis, often following a supracondylar fracture.
• There is an insensate hand due to injuries to the median and ulnar nerves with contractures due to muscle necrosis, fibrosis and shortening. The forearm is fixed in pronation, wrist flexed, MCP joints are

hyperextended, PIP and DIP joints are flexed. Tendons with the longest excursion are most severely affected, i.e. FDP and FPL.
- If only one compartment has been injured then tendon transfers may be possible.
A flexor slide may be indicated or free muscle transfers for severe cases. A delayed amputation may be required.

Vomer flap
- A mucoperiosteal flap raised from the vomerine bone in the nasal septum and based superiorly.
- Commonly used for reconstruction of a cleft involving the hard palate. Can be used as a single-layer closure at the same time as cleft lip reconstruction (described in the Oslo protocol) or as part of a two-layer closure of the hard palate to reconstruct the nasal layer in combination with oral mucoperiosteal mobilization for the oral layer.
- Proponents for the use of the vomer flap at the time of cleft lip reconstruction include making the definitive soft palate reconstruction easier, reducing the need for lateral releasing incisions and providing a good foundation for secondary alveolar bone grafting. There have been concerns that early use of the vomer flap may restrict mid-facial growth but this remains contentious in the literature.

Von Gräfe
Karl Ferdinand von Gräfe introduced the term 'plastic' in his 1818 book on nasal reconstruction called *Rhinoplastik*, describing the Italian and Indian method and the new German method. He used a free skin graft. He also described blepharoplasty and palatoplasty.

Von Langenbeck repair
- A technique for *Cleft palate* reconstruction described in 1859.
- The cleft palate is repaired using large bi-pedicled mucoperiosteal flaps raised from the hard palate. Approximation in the midline is achieved by lateral releasing incisions.

Von Recklinghausen's disease
Multiple *Neurofibromatosis*.

V–Y advancement
- A type of *Advancement flap* with forward advancement of a V without rotation and closure as a Y.
- Useful for lengthening the nasal columella, correcting whistle tip deformity of the lip, fingertip tissue loss and closure of cheek defects.
- An extended V–Y flap adds a transposition element to the side.

W-plasty to *Wucheri bancrofti*

W-plasty
- Used for reorientating the direction of a linear scar. Triangles of equal size are outlined on either side of the scar with the tip of the triangle on one side placed at the midpoint of the base of the triangle on the other side. At the ends of the scar the excised triangles should be smaller with the limbs of the W tapered.
- The main disadvantage is that the scar is not lengthened. The tension on the tissue is increased as tissue is sacrificed. Mainly used for scar revision. Limbs should not exceed 6 mm.

Wallace rule of 9s
- Used for the assessment of surface area in *Burns*. In adults:
  - Head and neck, 9%;
  - Arm, 9%;
  - Trunk anterior, 18%;
  - Each leg, 18%;
  - Genitalia, 1%.
- For children:
  - Head and neck, 18%;
  - Each leg, 14%;
  - For each year over 10, take 1% off head and neck and add to combined leg measurement.

Wallerian degeneration
The process of degeneration of the distal axonal segment in nerve injury. Has a ground-glass appearance of degenerated myelin and axonal material. These are phagocytosed by macrophages and Schwann cells and the space becomes occupied by columns of Schwann cell nuclei and their basement membranes. The collapsed columns of Schwann cells have a band-like appearance—the bands of Büngner.

Wart
See VERRUCA VULGARIS.

Wartenberg's sign
- Clinical sign in *Ulnar nerve palsy*.
- Abduction of the little finger with inability to adduct.

- Due to paralysis of the palmar interosseus muscles and unopposed action of extensor digiti minimi (EDM).

Wartenberg's syndrome
- Mononeuropathy caused by entrapment of the superficial branch of the radial nerve.
- Radial nerve divides into posterior interosseous nerve and superficial radial nerve 4 cm distal to lateral epicondyle. Superficial branch travels under brachioradialis and becomes superficial in the distal forearm (6-8 cm proximal to the radial styloid).
- Superficial branch of radial nerve may be compressed between ECRL and brachioradialis in mid-forearm during pronation-supination or it may be compressed at the wrist by bracelets or watches.
- Get pain in distribution of radial nerve, radiating proximally. Numbness and tingling on pronation with Tinel's over nerve. Forceful pronation against resistance useful test.

Treatment: non-operative management including avoiding repetitive pronation-supination or compressive jewellery or steroid injections. If unsuccessful, surgical decompression of superficial branch of radial nerve throughout its length. It may be entrapped by tendinous margin of brachioradialis, ECRL or the intervening fascia.

Washio flap
Transfer of retroauricular tissue on a temporal pedicle. It provides thin skin and cartilage with a hidden donor site. It is an axial pattern flap. It can be used as a free flap for nasal reconstruction.

Wassel classification for thumb duplication
- *Type I:* Bifid distal phalanx.
- *Type II:* Duplicated distal phalanx.
- *Type III:* Bifid proximal phalanx.
- *Type IV:* Duplicated proximal phalanx.
- *Type V:* Bifid metacarpal.
- *Type VI:* Duplicated metacarpal.

- *Type VII:* Triphalangia.
  See THUMB DUPLICATION.

Waterlow score
- Used to assess patients according to their risk of developing *Pressure sores*.
- The categories are:
  - BMI;
  - Skin type and risk areas;
  - Sex and age;
  - Appetite and weight loss;
  - Continence;
  - Mobility;
  - Special risks—tissue condition, neurology, major surgery, medication.
- The score in each section is summated to give the overall score, which indicates the relative risk:
  - 0–9: low risk;
  - 10–14: at risk;
  - 15–19: high risk;
  - 20+: very high risk.

Watson test
Scaphoid shift test.
- Test for scapholunate ligament incompetence.
- Put wrist in ulnar deviation, stabilize the scaphoid in extension. Grip left hand of patient with left hand.
- Bring wrist to radial deviation and resist scaphoid flexion with the thumb on volar surface, which forces the scaphoid dorsally.
- If the ligament is lax the scaphoid shifts dorsally. An audible painful clunk may occur.
- Many patients have mobility (36%), but clear instability with pain is a positive result.
  See CARPAL INSTABILITY.

Weber–Ferguson incision
Paranasal incision for access to the oral cavity.
  See ORAL CAVITY RECONSTRUCTION.

Weber 2-point discrimination
Test with callipers. Normal pulp values are 2–3 mm, but can be 5–6 mm in manual labourers and less in congenital blindness.

Webster operation
- Used for *Lip reconstruction*, a modification of *Bernard operation*.
- In this modification skin only is excised in *Burow's triangles*.
- The triangular excisions are further lateral, placing the scar in the nasolabial fold.
- Paramental Burow's triangles are created to ease inferior advancement of cheek tissue.
- Vermilion is advanced.
- Get improved sensation.

Werner's syndrome
- Adult *Progeria*.
- Autosomal recessive.
- *Scleroderma*-like skin changes, baldness, ageing, hyper/hypopigmentation, cataracts, diabetes, muscle atrophy, neoplasms.
- Plastic surgery is contraindicated due to microangiopathy.

Wet leather sign
Crepitus with tendon movement suggestive of an inflammation-induced change in synovium or synovitis.

Whitlow
See HERPES.

Whitnall's ligament
- A condensation of the superior sheath of levator palpebrae superioris which is a check ligament.
- This attaches medially to the pulley of superior oblique muscle and laterally to the lacrimal gland.
- It functions as a pulley to facilitate the change in direction of the levator action from horizontal to vertical.

Windblown hand
- Flexion and ulnar deviation of fingers and fixed flexion of thumb.
- Associated with craniocarpotarsal dystrophy and arthrogryphosis.
- Typically bilateral and worsens as the child grows.
- Most patients have 1st web space contracture and flexion deformity of the MCP joint.
- Windblown hand is a manifestation of many processes. Different processes may be responsible for a similar appearance such as thumb abnormalities, PIP joint changes, tendon subluxation. It may represent a combination of persistent intrinsic muscles with a disturbance of normal limb rotation.

Treatment:
- Try splintage initially.
- Correct skin contractures and splint. This may be all that is required and is needed before tackling other structures.
- Release at base of PIP joint and also release abnormal fascial bands.
- Subluxed extensors may require centralizing.
- Also the 1st web space contractures may require release and flexor and intrinsic muscles.

Wound A wound is an interruption in the anatomical and/or the functional integrity of a tissue.

Wound closure

Primary intention: where the wound edges are approximated directly such as a surgical wound. Collagen metabolism provides strength and epithelialization produces a thin scar.

Delayed primary: in a contaminated wound, first allow a few days for the host defences to debride the wound. Healing is as for primary.

Secondary: where the wound is left open and spontaneous re-epithelialization occurs, such as in a burn wound either from remaining epithelial elements or from the epithelial margin. The key processes are contraction and epithelialization. Myofibroblasts appear at day 3 and are gone by the time contraction is completed.

Tertiary: a wound not closed primarily and closed with imported tissue, such as a flap or graft.

Partial thickness: mainly epithelialization with minimal collagen deposition.

Wound healing

- Wound healing is the restoration of anatomical integrity to a traumatized tissue.
- Wounds heal by a combination of epithelialization, connective tissue deposition and contraction.
- Also describe healing by the surgical process as either primary intention, secondary intention or delayed primary closure. *See* WOUND CLOSURE.

Phases of wound healing:

- *Haemostasis:* occurs immediately. Exposed collagen causes platelet aggregation. Get clot, thrombus and vasospasm. Platelets initiate healing by releasing growth factors (PDGF, TGF-β). Fibrin is produced.
- *Inflammatory:* occurs in the first 24–48 hours. Platelets release *Growth factors and cytokines*, which are chemo-attractant for macrophages and neutrophils. Monocytes are called macrophages once they pass through the vessel wall. These remove necrotic debris. Neutrophils are the first to enter the wound and establish acute inflammation. Pro-inflammatory cytokines amplify the response. Monocytes are attracted to the wound especially by TGF-β. These are converted to macrophages, which continue to destroy bacteria and debride the wound. They also produce a lot of cytokines. The matrix is initially composed of fibrin.
- *Proliferative:* occurs approximately from day 2 to day 14. Fibroblasts arrive, attracted by *TGF-β* released from macrophages. They are usually located in perivascular tissue and migrate along networks of fibrin fibres.

Collagen is produced. Also glycosaminoglycans (GAGs) and elastin. GAGs become ground substance when hydrated. Also new capillaries.

- *Remodelling:* starts 2–4 weeks after the injury and lasts up to a year. Randomly laid down *Collagen* is cross-linked and orientated to increase strength. A well-healed wound reaches 70–80% of unhealed strength. After 21 days there is ongoing synthesis and degradation, and ECM is remodelled. Fibronectins are matrix molecules that are involved in wound contraction, cell–cell cell–matrix interaction, cell migration, collagen matrix deposition and epithelialization. They act as a scaffold for collagen deposition. They bind a wide variety of molecules. Their main function during repair is to promote cell–cell and cell–matrix interaction.
- *Epithelialization:* after a wound is created, basal cells flatten and hemidesmosomal attachments are lost allowing them to migrate. The leading epithelial cells phagocytose clot. Migration stops once another front is reached. After 2 days get basal cell proliferation. If the basement membrane is intact can get complete healing in 4 days. The epithelium comes from the edge and from hair follicles. Several growth factors modulate epithelialization. Epidermal growth factor (EGF) is a potent stimulator of epithelial mitogenesis and chemotaxis. Other factors, including basic FGF and keratinocyte growth factor (KGF), also stimulate epithelial proliferation.
- *Angiogenesis:* new capillaries originate as outgrowths from venules. Get endothelial cell migration. Vascular connections with other capillaries. Neovascularization remodels after flow established. Lots of angiogenic factors. O_2 tension is a potent stimulus.
- *Open wound contraction:* contraction is due to movement at the wound edges. Caused by myofibroblasts. Contain actin.

Delayed wound healing:
Systemic and local factors.

Systemic:
- Congenital: *Pseudoxanthoma elasticum, Ehlers–Danlos syndrome, Cutis laxa, Progeria, Werner's syndrome, Epidermolysis bullosa,* sickle cell.
- Acquired—systemic factors:
  - *Nutrition:* deficiency of *Vitamin A, Vitamin C, Vitamin E, Iron, Zinc* and copper. Albumin is an indicator of malnutrition. Low levels are associated

with poor healing, but malnutrition only affects healing when severe;

- *Pharmacological: Steroids*, NSAIDs, (decrease collagen synthesis), chemotherapy;
- *Endocrine: Diabetes*;
- *Ageing:* wounds take longer to heal with age. Connective tissue deposition is reduced. More fibroblasts in younger people. Macrophage function is reduced.
- *Smoking:* no proven relationship between smoking and delayed healing. *Nicotine* is vasoconstrictive and increases platelet adhesion and thrombus. CO competes with O_2. Cessation of smoking for 2 weeks give normal rates of healing.

Acquired—local factors:

- *Infection:* contamination does not necessarily impair healing and *Staph. aureus* accelerates healing. Infection alters every stage of the healing process. They prolong the inflammatory phase and interfere with epithelialization, contraction and collagen deposition.
- *Radiation.*
- *Hypoxia:* stimulates angiogenesis, but reduced O_2 tension impairs healing. Below 4.6 pKa fibroblasts can not replicate. In arterial disease reduced O_2 is due to reduced inflow and in venous disease due to reduced diffusion.
- *Trauma:* neoepidermis is disrupted by trauma.
- *Neural supply:* denervated tissue heal slowly.
- *Pressure.*
- Foreign material.

See SKIN.

Wright's hyperabduction test

- Clinical test in *Thoracic outlet syndrome*.
- Palpate radial artery with arm maximally abducted. Change in pulse or neurological signs is a positive test.
- Remember as student in classroom knowing the **right** answer.

Wrist ligaments
Interosseous: join adjacent bones.

- Lunate to triquetrum and scaphoid. They are short as the bones move in unison.
- Joining 4 bones of distal row—palmar and dorsal.
- Joining forearm bone to proximal carpal row. On palmar surface radioscapholunate and ulnolunate ligament. Dorsally is the radiocarpal ligament.

Transosseous: cross bones. Mainly tie radius to carpus on palmar side and attach radius to ulnar side of the carpus.

- Radioscaphocapitate.
- Radiolunatotriquetral.
- Triquetrohamitocapitate.

Wrist osteoarthritis
90% involve the scaphoid in 3 patterns—*SLAC*, *Triscaphe* (scapho-trapezium-trapezoid) and a combination of the two.

Wucheria bancrofti
A parasite transmitted by mosquitos that causes filariasis, a common cause of secondary lymphoedema in endemic countries. The resulting massive swelling in legs and genitalia is known as elephantiasis. Treated with dimethylcarbazine, but the lymphoedema is usually irreversible.

w

Xanthelasma palpebarum to Xeroderma pigmentosa

Xanthelasma palpebarum
- The most common kind of xanthoma. Occurs on the eyelids, usually near the inner canthi.
- Soft, thin, yellowish, slightly raised, elongated plaques, often symmetrically distributed.
- 50% have associated hyperlipoproteinemia.
- Also seen in context of biliary cirrhosis and in histiocytic disorders such as reticulohistiocytoma cutis, chronic multifocal Langerhans histiocytosis (previously known as Hand–Schüller–Christian disease) and xanthoma disseminatum.
- Treatment for cosmesis is excision, diathermy or trichloro-acetic acid.
- Recurrence occurs in 40% of the patients who undergo excision.

Xanthogranuloma
- Juvenile xanthogranuloma are self-limiting benign papules which occur in early infancy into adulthood.
- The typical lesion is papular and red to yellow, <1 cm diameter.
- They occur as single or multiple lesions in the head and neck.
- They usually involute spontaneously.
- 10% have visceral involvement with occasional eye involvement.

- Histologically they show an accumulation of histiocytes with a granulomatous infiltrate, which may contain foam cells, foreign body giant cells and Touton giant cells.

Xanthoma planum
Resembles xanthelasma, but may involve extensive areas beyond the eyelids, especially the palmar creases, axillae, flexor areas of the extremities, neck, inner thighs, trunk and shoulders.

Xeroderma pigmentosa
- Autosomal recessive disorder.
- Deficiency of thiamine dimerase.
- Thiamine absorbs light and forms dimers, which cannot be broken down.
- The build-up of thiamine dimers induces defects in DNA structure.
- Acute sensitivity to sunlight secondary to defective DNA repair mechanism results in multiple epitheliomas with malignant degeneration in the first two decades.
- May get neurological manifestations in 30%, including cognitive impairment, deafness, spasticity or seizures.
- Treat aggressively with sun protection, topical 5FU, excision and grafts.

See BASAL CELL CARCINOMA. *See* SKIN.

Y–V advancement flap

Y-V advancement flap

A type of *Advancement flap*. Used in serial fashion for release of scar contractures. The Y limb cuts across the scar contracture and the V advances into it.

Z-plasty to Zygomatic fractures

Z-plasty
- Described by Fricke in 1829 and William Horner in 1837.
- Two triangular flaps are interdigitated to gain length in the direction of the common limb and a change in direction of the common limb.
- The central limb is usually placed along the direction of the scar or contracture. The limbs are equal length and the angle varies from 30° to 90°.
- If there is tension, get immediate flap transposition. The wider the angle of the flaps the greater the difference between the long and short diagonals and the greater the lengthening so:
  ○ 30° gives 25% lengthening;
  ○ 45° gives 50% lengthening;
  ○ 60° gives 75% lengthening;
  ○ 90° gives 125% lengthening.
- Actual gains may be more or less than theoretical gains and depend on the ability of the skin at the base to fit in the new position.
- Multiple Z-plasties can produce as much lengthening as a larger single Z-plasty. Multiple Z-plasties do, however, produce less transverse shortening. It can also give a better cosmetic result.
- When a Z-plasty is used to change the direction of scars:
  ○ Draw the present scar—this will be the central limb;
  ○ Draw the intended final position of the scar—the same length and crossing the scar;
  ○ Join up adjacent ends;
  ○ The limbs which are the same length as the scar will make up the Z-plasty.

See FOUR-FLAP Z-PLASTY. *See* FIVE-FLAP Z-PLASTY (also called jumping man or double-opposing Z-plasties). *See* SIX FLAP Z-PLASTY.

Zinc
Required for DNA and RNA polymerase. Deficiency may retard epithelialization and fibroblast proliferation. Deficiency is seen in large burns, alcoholism and GI fistulae. *See* WOUND HEALING.

Zygomatic fractures
Anatomy:
- The zygoma is a pyramidal bone in the midface, which gives prominence to the cheek and forms the inferolateral border of the orbit.
- It has frontal, maxillary, temporal and orbital processes.
- It articulates with the frontal, temporal (arch), maxillary (medial orbit) and sphenoid bones (lateral orbit).

Fractures:
- Fractures tend to displace the zygoma downward, medial and posterior.
- Fractures tend to occur in a tetrapod fashion at its junction with:
  ○ Zygomatic process of the frontal bone (ZF suture);
  ○ Greater wing of the sphenoid in the lateral orbit;
  ○ Maxilla in the orbital margin, orbital floor and anterior wall of the maxillary sinus;
  ○ Temporal bone in the zygomatic arch.

Symptoms and signs:
- Bruising and swelling over the zygoma and inside the mouth.
- Malar depression.
- Palpable bony step.
- *Subconjunctival haematoma:* with no posterior limit as the fracture line extends behind the orbital septum. It will be bright red due to transconjunctival oxygenation.
- *Trismus:* when the zygomatic arch abuts the coronoid process of the mandible.
- *Epistaxis:* due to a tear in the mucosal lining of the maxillary sinus.
- *Paraesthesia:* in distribution of *Infra-orbital nerve* (presents as cheek numbness).
- *Enophthalmos* (rare with pure tetrapod fractures).
- *Dystopia.*

- *Diplopia:* usually on upward gaze due to trapping of inferior rectus muscle. Tethering can be detected by the forced duction test. The eye is anaesthetized. Gentle traction is applied to the inferior conjunctiva. Limitation in globe movement indicates tethering.
- *Decrease visual acuity:* due to retinal detachment.

Radiology: use the following.

- *XR:* PA. Lateral, *Water's views* (demonstrate maxillary sinus) and *Caldwell's views* (demonstrate ZF suture).
- CT and 3D CT.

Classification: by Knight and North.

- *Type I:* Undisplaced fractures.
- *Type II:* Isolated displaced fractures.
- *Type III:* Displaced body fractures (unrotated).
- *Type IV:* Medially rotated:
  a. Outward at the malar buttress;
  b. Inward at the FZ suture.

- *Type V:* Laterally rotated:
  a. Upward at the infraorbital margin;
  b. Outward at the FZ suture.
- *Type VI:* Any additional fracture lines across the main fragment.

Management:

- *Conservative:* usually for stable undisplaced fractures.
- *Gillies' lift:* for displaced fractures of zygomatic arch.
- *ORIF:* preferred method for many fractures. Plates are placed over the fracture lines:
  ○ *Fractures over ZF suture:* lateral brow incision;
  ○ *Fractures in the infra-orbital rim:* lower eyelid incision;
  ○ *Fractures in the maxilla:* upper buccal sulcus incision;
  ○ *Complex fracture:* bicoronal incision.

See FACIAL FRACTURES.

z

Abbreviations

2PD	two-point discrimination	**CIND**	carpal instability non-dissociative syndrome
5FU	5-fluorouracil		
AA	androgenic alopecia	**CL**	cleft lip
abs	antibodies	**CL/P**	cleft lip and palate
ACL	accessory collateral ligament	**CLAVM**	capillary, lymphatic, arteriovenous malformation
ADM	adductor digiti minimi		
ADP	adductor pollicis brevis	**CLM**	capillary lymphatic malformation
AER	apical ectodermal ridge	**CM**	capillary malformation
AIIS	anterior inferior iliac spine	**CMC**	carpometacarpal
AO	Arbeitsgemeinschaft für Osteosynthesefragen (from Swiss classification system)	**CMCJ**	carpometacarpal joint
		CMF	cyclophosphamide, methotrexate and 5-fluorouracil
AP	adductor pollicis	**CMN**	congenital melanocytic naevus
APB	abductor pollicis brevis	**CN**	chemotherapy
APL	abductor pollicis longus	**CNS**	central nervous system
aPTT	activated partial thromboplastin time	**CO**	carbon monoxide
ASIS	anterior superior iliac spine	**COAD**	chronic obstructive airway disease
ATLS	advanced trauma life support	**COHb**	carboxyhaemoglobin
AV	arteriovenous	**CP**	cleft palate
AVA	arteriovenous anastomosis	**CRP**	C-reactive protein
AVFs	arteriovenous fistulas	**CRPS**	complex regional pain syndrome
AVM	arteriovenous malformation	**CSAG**	Clinical Standards Advisory Group
AVPU	alert, vocal stimulus, painful stimulus, unresponsive	**CT**	computerized tomography
		CTD	connective tissue disease
BAHA	bone-anchored hearing aid	**CTS**	carpal tunnel syndrome
BBR	bilateral breast reduction	**CVLM**	complex combined vascular malformations
BCC	basal cell carcinoma		
BCNU	carmustine	**CVM**	capillary venous malformation
BDD	body dysmorphic disorder	**CW**	continuous wave
BEAM	bulbar elongation and anastomotic meatoplasty	**CXR**	chest X-ray
		DAB	dorsal abductor
BEE	basal energy expenditure	**DandV**	diarrhoea and vomiting
bFGF	beta fibroblast growth factor	**DBD**	dermolytic bullous dermatitis
BMI	body mass index	**DCIA**	deep circumflex iliac artery
BMPs	bone morphogenic proteins	**DCIS**	ductal carcinoma *in situ*
BOP	bilateral occipitoparietal flaps	**DHT**	dihydrotestosterone
BP	blood pressure	**DIEA**	deep inferior epigastric artery
BXO	*Balanitis xerotica obliterans*	**DIEP**	deep inferior epigastric perforator flap
ca	carcinoma		
CandL	Cormack and Lamberty	**DIP**	distal interphalangeal
CAVF	capillary-arteriovenous fistula	**DIPJ**	distal interphalangeal joint
CAVM	capillary arterial venous malformation	**DISI**	dorsal intercalated segmental instability
CCF	congestive cardiac failure	**DLE**	discoid lupus erythematosus
CDNH	chondrodermatitis nodularis helicis	**DM**	diabetes mellitus
CFNG	contralateral facial nerve grafting	**DMTA**	dorsal metatarsal artery
CGRP	calcitonin gene-related peptide	**DP**	deltopectoral
CIC	carpal instability complex	**DPA**	dorsalis pedis artery
CIC	congenital, involutional, cicatricial	**DRUJ**	distal radioulnar joint
CID	carpal instability dissociative syndrome	**DVT**	deep vein thrombosis
		EB	epidermolysis bullosa

EB	Epstein–Barr	IGF	insulin-like growth factor
ECM	extracellular matrix	IgG	Immunoglobulin G
ECOG	Eastern Co-operative Oncology Group	IgM	Immunoglobulin M
		IJV	inferior jugular vein
ECRB	extensor carpi radialis brevis	ILP	isolated limb perfusion
ECRL	extensor carpi radialis longus	IMA	inferior mammary artery
ECU	extensor carpi ulnaris	IMA	internal mammary artery
EDC	extensor digitorum communis	IMF	intermaxillary fixation
EDM	extensor digiti minimi	IOD	interorbital distance
EDQ	extensor digiti quinti	IPJ	interphalangeal joint
EGF	epidermal growth factor	IVP	intravenous pyelogram
EIP	extensor indicis proprius	K	potassium
ELND	elective lymph node dissection	KGF	keratinocyte growth factor
EM	extracellular matrix	KS	Kaposi's sarcoma
EMG	electromyelogram	LA	local anaesthetic
EORTC	European Organization for Research and Treatment of Cancer	LCIS	lobal carcinoma *in situ*
		LDH	lactate dehydrogenase
EPB	extensor pollicis brevis	LFTs	liver function tests
EPL	extensor pollicis longus	LLS	levator labii superioris
ESR	erythroctye sedimentation rate	LM	lymphatic malformation
EUA	examination under anaesthesia	LN	lymph node
FCR	flexor carpi radialis	LND	lymph node dissection
FCU	flexor carpi ulnaris	LT	lunotriquetral
FD	fibrous dysplasia	LVM	lymphaticovenous malformation
FDM	flexor digiti minimi	M	metastasis
FDMA	first dorsal metatarsal artery	MABC	medial antebrachial cutaneous
FDP	flexor digitorum profundus	MAGPI	meatal advancement and glansplasty
FDS	flexor digitorum longus	MC	metacarpal
FGF	fibroblast growth factor	MCP	metacarpophalangeal
FGFR2	fibroblast growth factor receptor 2	MCPJ	metacarpophalangeal joint
FLPD	flash lamp-pumped pulsed dye	MCR	mid-carpal radial
FNA	fine needle aspiration	MCU	mid-carpal ulnar
FOM	floor of mouth	MDU	Medical Defence Union
FPB	flexor pollicis brevis	MESS	mangled extremity severity score
FPL	flexor pollicis longus	MHC	major histocompatibility complex
F–S	Fasanella-Servat	MPB	male pattern baldness
FTSG	full thickness skin graft	MPD	myofascial pain dysfunction syndrome
G	grade		
GA	general anaesthetic	MRI	magnetic resonance imaging
GAGS	glycosaminoglycans	MRSA	methicillin-resistant *Staphylococcus aureus*
GCMN	giant congenital melanocytic naevus		
GHN	giant hairy naevus	MSH	melanocyte-stimulating hormone
GI	gastrointestinal	MT	muscle–tendon
GIT	gastrointestinal tract	MTP	metatarsophalangeal
GSW	gunshot wound	MTPJ	metatarsophalangeal joint
HA	hydroxyapatite	MUA	manipulation under anaesthetic
Hb	haemoglobin	Na	sodium
HBO	hyperbaric oxygen	NAC	nipple-areolar complex
HCL	hydrochloric acid	NAI	non-accidental injury
HHT	hereditary haemorrhagic telangiectasia	NandM	Nahai–Mathes
		NCS	nerve conduction studies
HLA	human leucocyte antigen	NGF	nerve growth factor
HS	hydradenitis suppuritiva	NGT	nasogastric feeding
HTA	high-tension abdominoplasty	NS	normal saline
IandD	incision and drainage	NSAID	non-steroidal anti-inflammatory drug
IF	interferon	NV	neurovascular
IGAP	inferior gluteal artery flap	NVB	neurovascular bundle

OA	osteoarthritis
od	every day
OP	operation
OPG	orthopantomograph
ORIF	open reduction and internal fixation
ORL	oblique retinacular ligament
PA	palmar aponeurosis
PA	postero-anterior view
PAD	palmar adductor
PCA	patient-controlled analgesia
PCD	programmed cell death
PCL	proper collateral ligament and
PDGF	platelet-derived growth factor
PDMS	policlymethylsiloxane
PDS	polydiaxone
PEEP	positive end expiratory pressure
PET	positron emission tomography
PGA	polyglycolic acid
PIN	posterior interosseous nerve
PIP	proximal interphalangeal
PIPJ	proximal interphalangeal joint
pKa	acid dissociation constant
PL	palmaris longus
PL	palmaris longus
PLLA	poly-1-lactic acid
PMN	polymorphonucleocyte
PNS	parasympathetic nervous system
POC	presurgical orthopaedic correction
POP	plaster of paris
PPT	photodynamic therapy
PR	cardiac conduction time
PRC	proximal row carpectomy
PSJ	pisotriquetral joint
Pt	patient
PT	pronator teres
PT	prothrombin time
PTCH	Patched gene
PTFE	polytetrafluoroethylene (Teflon)
PVA	polyvinyl alcohol
PVNS	pigmented villonuclear tenovaginosynovitis
PZ	progress zone
RA	rheumatoid arthritis
RADS	radiation absorbed dose (unit of measurement of radiation)
RBC	red blood cells
RhF	rheumatoid factor
ROM	range of movement
ROOF	retro-orbicularis oculi fat
RSD	reflex sympathetic dystrophy
RSTL	relaxed skin tension line
rt > lt	right greater than left
RT	radiotherapy
RTA	road traffic accident
r-TPA	recombinant tissue plasminogen activator

SCC	squamous cell carcinoma
SCM	sternocleidomastoid
SGAP	superior gluteal artery flap
Shh	Sonic hedgehog (gene)
SIADH	syndrome of inappropriate ADH (antidiuretic hormone)
SIEA	superior inferior epigastric artery
SIMON	single, introverted male, overly narcissistic
SIPS	sympathetically independent pain syndrome
SLAC	scapholunate advanced collapse
SLE	systemic lupus erythematosus
SLL	scapholunate ligament
SLNB	sentinel lymph node biopsy
SMAS	superficial musculo-aponeurotic system
SMPS	sympathetically maintained pain syndrome
SNAC	schaphoid non-union with collapse
SNAP	sensory nerve action potential
SOOF	suborbicularis oculi fat
SP	substance P
SSG	split skin graft
STSG	split-thickness skin graft
STT	scapho-trapezium-trapezoid
T	tumour site
TAR	thrombocytopenia absent radius
TATA	total anterior tenoarthrolysis
TB	tuberculosis
TBSA	total body surface area
TCA	trichloro-acetic acid
TCL	transverse carpal ligament
TEF	tracheo-oesophageal fistula
TENS	transcutaneous electrical nerve stimulator
TEP	tracheo-oeseophageal puncture
TFCC	triangular fibrocartilage
TFL	tensor fascia lata
TGF-β	tumour growth factor-beta
TICAS	trauma-induced cold-associated symptoms
TILT	triquetral impingement ligament tear
TMJ	temporomandibular joint
TNF-α	tumour necrosis factor alpha
TNM	tumour, node metastasis
t-PA	tissue plasminogenic activator
TPF	temporoparietal fascia
TPN	total parenteral nutrition
Tq	tourniquet
TRAM	transverse rectus abdominis muscle
TSH	thyroid-stimulating hormone
TSS	toxic shock syndrome
U&E	urea & electrolytes
UCL	ulna collateral ligament
US	ultrasound

USS	ultrasound scan		**VM**	venous malformation
UV	ultraviolet		**VPI**	velopharyngeal incompetence
UVA	ultraviolet irradiation		**VRAM**	vertical rectus abdominis muscle
VAC	vacuum-assisted closure		**VVs**	varicose veins
VCF	velocardiofacial		**WDR**	wide-dynamic range (neurons)
VEGF	vasoendothelial growth factor		**WHO**	World Health Organization
VF	ventricular fibrillation		**wt**	weight
VISI	volar intercalated segmental instability		**XR**	X-ray
			ZF	zygomatico-frontal
VM	vascular malformation		**ZPA**	zone of polarizing activity